American Academy of Pediatrics

141 Northwest Point Blvd
PO Box 927
Elk Grove Village, IL 60009-0927
Phone 708/228-5005
Fax 708/228-5097

President
Betty A. Lowe, MD

Vice President
George D. Comerci, MD

Past President
Howard A. Pearson, MD

Executive Director
Joe M. Sanders, Jr, MD

Board of Directors

Gilbert L. Fuld, MD
Keene, New Hampshire

Louis Z. Cooper, MD
New York, New York

Anthony DeSpirito, MD
Interlaken, New Jersey

Joseph R. Zanga, MD
Richmond, Virginia

Robert E. Hannemann, MD
Lafayette, Indiana

Thomas F. Tonniges, MD
Hastings, Nebraska

Carden Johnston, MD
Birmingham, Alabama

Donald E. Cook, MD
Greeley, Colorado

Leonard A. Kutnik, MD
San Diego, California

May 1994

I am pleased to enclose one of the most valuable benefits of your membership in the American Academy of Pediatrics — your copy of the *1994 Red Book.*

The *1994 Red Book: Report of the Committee on Infectious Diseases,* 23rd edition, is the most comprehensive to date. It offers important new information on a number of topics, including

- Updated recommendations on immunizations, including schedules and the National Standards for Pediatric Immunization Practices

- Vaccination against hepatitis B, *Haemophilus influenzae* type b, and pertussis

- Guidelines for measles immunization of children who recently received immune globulin

- Management and control of varicella, including indications for acyclovir

- Guidelines for chemoprophylaxis of group B streptococcal infection in newborns

- Recommendations for screening and treatment of tuberculosis

- Treatment of and prevention of sexually transmitted diseases

- Control of infectious diseases in out-of-home child care

- Updated guidelines for ribavirin therapy of RSV infections

- Drug tables, including recommendations for viral and parasitic infections

- HIV Infection

- Prevention and management of influenza

- Group A streptococcal infections

For your convenience in obtaining additional copies of the *1994 Red Book* at a special discount price, use the order form on the reverse side of this letter.

In the tradition of the Academy, this manual is written to promote the health of children, and we anticipate this new edition will assist you in serving children well.

Sincerely,

Betty A. Lowe, MD
President
American Academy of Pediatrics

Use this form to order additional copies of the *1994 Red Book*

Name: _____

AAP Member ID# _____

Organization: _____

Address: _____

City: _____

State: _____ Zip: _____

Please send me:

_____ Copies of *1994 Red Book: Report of the Committee on Infectious Diseases* at $54.95 each ($5 off the member price.)

_____ Canadian orders add 7% GST

_____ Shipping and Handling

_____ Total enclosed

Shipping & Handling	United States (UPS Ground)	Canada (Parcel Post)	Outside the US & Canada (Parcel Post)
Under $ 25	$4.50	$ 6.50	$ 8.50
$25 to $ 49	$6.50	$ 8.50	$10.50
$50 to $ 75	$8.50	$10.50	$12.50
$76 to $100	$9.95	$11.95	$13.95
Over $100	10% of order	15% of order	20% of order

Offer expires June 30, 1994

Return order form and payment to:

American Academy of Pediatrics
Publications Department
PO Box 927
Elk Grove Village, IL 60009-0927

Or charge your order by calling toll free 800/433-9016
Please allow 2-3 weeks for delivery

1994 Red Book:

Report of the Committee

on Infectious Diseases

Twenty-third Edition

Author: Committee on Infectious Diseases
American Academy of Pediatrics

Georges Peter, MD, Editor
Neal A. Halsey, MD, Associate Editor
Edgar K. Marcuse, MD, Associate Editor
Larry K. Pickering, MD, Associate Editor

American Academy of Pediatrics
PO Box 927
141 Northwest Point Blvd
Elk Grove Village, IL 60009-0927

23rd Edition
1st Edition - 1938
2nd Edition - 1939
3rd Edition - 1940
4th Edition - 1942
5th Edition - 1943
6th Edition - 1944
7th Edition - 1945
8th Edition - 1947
9th Edition - 1951
10th Edition - 1952
11th Edition - 1955
12th Edition - 1957
13th Edition - 1961
14th Edition - 1964
15th Edition - 1966
16th Edition - 1970
16th Edition Revised - 1971
17th Edition - 1974
18th Edition - 1977
19th Edition - 1982
20th Edition - 1986
21st Edition - 1988
22nd Edition - 1991

Suggested Citation: American Academy of Pediatrics. [chapter title cited]. In: Peter G, ed. *1994 Red Book: Report of the Committee on Infectious Diseases.* 23rd ed. Elk Grove Village, IL: American Academy of Pediatrics; 1994: [page no. cited]

Library of Congress Catalog Card No.: 93-74350
ISBN No.: 0-910761-48-5
MA0001

Quantity prices on request. Address all inquiries to:
American Academy of Pediatrics
PO Box 927, 141 Northwest Point Blvd
Elk Grove Village, IL 60009-0927

The recommendations in this publication do not indicate an exclusive course of treatment or serve as a standard of medical care. Variations, taking into account individual circumstances, may be appropriate.

Committee on Infectious Diseases
1991-1994

Caroline Breese Hall, MD, Chairperson

P. Joan Chesney, MD
James G. Easton, MD
Dan M. Granoff, MD
Donald S. Gromisch, MD
Neal A. Halsey, MD
Steve Kohl, MD
Edgar K. Marcuse, MD
S. Michael Marcy, MD

Melvin I. Marks, MD
George A. Nankervis, MD
James C. Overall, MD
Larry K. Pickering, MD
Gwendolyn B. Scott, MD
Russell W. Steele, MD
Ram Yogev, MD
Georges Peter, MD, *Ex Officio*

Liaison Representatives

Kenneth J. Bart, MD, National Vaccine Program Office
Ruth Berkelman, MD, Centers for Disease Control and Prevention
Claire Broome, MD, Centers for Disease Control and Prevention
M. Carolyn Hardegree, MD, Food and Drug Administration
Richard F. Jacobs, MD, American Thoracic Society
John R. LaMontagne, MD, National Institute of Allergy and
    Infectious Diseases
Noni MacDonald, MD, Canadian Paediatric Society
Walter A. Orenstein, MD, Centers for Disease Control and Prevention
N. Regina Rabinovich, MD, National Institutes of Health
Anthony Robbins, MD, National Vaccine Program Office

Consultants to the Editors

Leigh Grossman Donowitz, MD
John S. Finlayson, PhD
Walter T. Hughes, MD

George H. McCracken, Jr, MD
Carol F. Phillips, MD

iii

COLLABORATORS

On behalf of the American Academy of Pediatrics, the Committee gratefully acknowledges the invaluable assistance provided by the following individuals who served as contributors and reviewers in the preparation of this edition of the *Red Book*. Their expertise, critical review, and cooperation are essential in the Committee's continuing review and revisions of its recommendations for the management, control, and prevention of infectious diseases in children.

David G. Addiss, MD, MPH, Centers for Disease Control and Prevention, Atlanta, GA

Mercedes Albuerne, MD, Food and Drug Administration, Bethesda, MD

James P. Alexander, Jr, MD, Centers for Disease Control and Prevention, Atlanta, GA

Susan Alpert, MD, Food and Drug Administration, Bethesda, MD

Miriam J. Alter, PhD, Centers for Disease Control and Prevention, Atlanta, GA

Burt Anderson, PhD, Centers for Disease Control and Prevention, Atlanta, GA

Larry J. Anderson, MD, Centers for Disease Control and Prevention, Atlanta, GA

Bacom Anthony, MD, Food and Drug Administration, Bethesda, MD

Nancy H. Arden, MN, Centers for Disease Control and Prevention, Atlanta, GA

William L. Atkinson, MD, MPH, Centers for Disease Control and Prevention, Atlanta, GA

Carol E. Mosier Bach, MD, University of Washington, Seattle, WA

Carol J. Baker, MD, Baylor College of Medicine, Houston, TX

Julia Barrett, MD, Food and Drug Administration, Bethesda, MD

Barbara L. Bavins, ARNP, Children's Hospital & Medical Center, Seattle, WA

Judy Beeler, MD, Food and Drug Administration, Bethesda, MD

Thomas A. Bell, MD, MPH, Lewis County Health District, Chehalis, WA

Stuart M. Berman, MD, Centers for Disease Control and Prevention, Atlanta, GA

Richard E. Besser, MD, Centers for Disease Control and Prevention, Atlanta, GA

Martin J. Blaser, MD, Vanderbilt University School of Medicine, Nashville, TN

Michael D. Blum, MD, Food and Drug Administration, Bethesda, MD

William E. Brady, PA-C, MPH, Centers for Disease Control and Prevention, Atlanta, GA

Philip A. Brunell, MD, Cedars-Sinai Medical Center, Los Angeles, CA

Ralph T. Bryan, MD, Centers for Disease Control and Prevention, Atlanta, GA

Jane L. Burns, MD, University of Washington School of Medicine, Seattle, WA

Jay Butler, MD, Centers for Disease Control and Prevention, Atlanta, GA

John R. Campbell, MD, Oregon Health Sciences University, Portland, OR

Daniel T. Casto, PharmD, The University of Texas at Austin, San Antonio, TX

Martin Cetron, MD, Centers for Disease Control and Prevention, Atlanta, GA

Robert T. Chen, MD, MA, Centers for Disease Control and Prevention, Atlanta, GA

Stephen L. Cochi, MD, Centers for Disease Control and Prevention, Atlanta, GA

Lawrence Corey, MD, University of Washington, Seattle, WA

Charles A. Cowan, MD, Pacific Medical Center, Bellevue, WA

Philip Coyne, MD, Food and Drug Administration, Bethesda, MD

Robert B. Craven, MD, Centers for Disease Control and Prevention, Atlanta, GA
Adnan S. Dajani, MD, Wayne State University School of Medicine, Detroit, MI
Robert S. Daum, MD, University of Chicago, Chicago, IL
Jacqueline E. Dawson, MS, Centers for Disease Control and Prevention,
    Altanta, GA
Rebecca Devine, PhD, Food and Drug Administration, Bethesda, MD
Vance Dietz, MD, MPH, Centers for Disease Control and Prevention,
    Atlanta, GA
Ronald F. DiGiacomo, VMD, MPH, University of Washington, Seattle, WA
Ruth Ann Dunn, MD, Centers for Disease Control and Prevention, Atlanta, GA
Elias Durry, MD, MPH, Centers for Disease Control and Prevention, Atlanta, GA
Terry L. Dwelle, MD, University of North Dakota School of Medicine,
    Bismarck, ND
Paul V. Effler, MD, MPH, Centers for Disease Control and Prevention,
    Atlanta, GA
William Erhardt, MD, Food and Drug Administration, Bethesda, MD
David T. Estroff, MD, University of Washington, Tacoma, WA
Gary L. Euler, DrPH, Centers for Disease Control and Prevention, Atlanta, GA
Stephen Feinstone, MD, Food and Drug Administration, Bethesda, MD
Makonen Fekad, DVM, PhD, Centers for Disease Control and Prevention,
    Atlanta, GA
Patricia E. Ferrieri, MD, University of Minnesota Medical School,
    Minneapolis, MN
John Finlayson, PhD, Food and Drug Administration, Bethesda, MD
Susan Fisher-Hoch, MD, Centers for Disease Control and Prevention,
    Atlanta, GA
Julie Francis, MD, Children's Hospital and Medical Center, Seattle, WA
Carl Frasch, PhD, Food and Drug Administration, Bethesda, MD
Julia S. Garner, RN, MN, Centers for Disease Control and Prevention,
    Atlanta, GA
Robert Gaynes, MD, Centers for Disease Control and Prevention, Atlanta, GA
A. Russell Gerber, MD, Centers for Disease Control and Prevention, Atlanta, GA
Michael A. Gerber, MD, University of Connecticut School of Medicine,
    Farmington, CT
Anne A. Gershon, MD, Columbia University, New York, NY
G. Scott Giebink, MD, University of Minnesota Medical School,
    Minneapolis, MN
Ann E. Giesel, MD, University of Washington, Seattle, WA
Roger Glass, MD, PhD, Centers for Disease Control and Prevention, Atlanta, GA
Mary P. Glode, MD, University of Colorado, Denver, CO
Patricia M. Griffin, MD, Centers for Disease Control and Prevention,
    Atlanta, GA
Duane J. Gubler, ScD, Centers for Disease Control and Prevention, Atlanta, GA
William Habig, PhD, Food and Drug Administration, Bethesda, MD
Stephen C. Hadler, MD, Centers for Disease Control and Prevention, Atlanta, GA
Laraine Henchal, Food and Drug Administration, Bethesda, MD
S. Paul Herndon, MD, University of Washington, Seattle, WA
Kenneth L. Herrmann, MD, Centers for Disease Control and Prevention,
    Atlanta, GA

Barbara L. Herwaldt, MD, MPH, Centers for Disease Control and Prevention, Atlanta, GA

John C. Hierholzer, PhD, Centers for Disease Control and Prevention, Atlanta, GA

King K. Holmes, MD, University of Washington, Seattle, WA

Sandra Holmes, PhD, Centers for Disease Control and Prevention, Atlanta, GA

Margaret K. Hostetter, MD, University of Minnesota Hospital and Clinic, Minneapolis, MN

Lisa A. Jackson, MD, Centers for Disease Control and Prevention, Atlanta, GA

Hamid S. Jafari, MD, Centers for Disease Control and Prevention, Atlanta, GA

William R. Jarvis, MD, Centers for Disease Control and Prevention, Atlanta GA

Stephen M. Jones, DVM, Seattle Veterinary Association, Seattle, WA

Elaine C. Jong, MD, University of Washington Medical Center, Seattle, WA

Dennis D. Juranek, DVM, Centers for Disease Control and Prevention, Atlanta, GA

Edward L. Kaplan, MD, University of Minnesota Medical School, Minneapolis, MN

Samuel L. Katz, MD, Duke University School of Medicine, Durham, NC

Arnold F. Kaufmann, DVM, Centers for Disease Control and Prevention, Atlanta, GA

Jerome O. Klein, MD, Boston University School of Medicine, Boston, MA

Mark W. Kline, MD, Baylor College of Medicine, Houston, TX

Dennis Klinman, MD, PhD, Food and Drug Administration, Bethesda, MD

Jane Koehler, DVM, Centers for Disease Control and Prevention, Atlanta, GA

Peter J. Krause, MD, The University of Connecticut School of Medicine, Hartford, CT

Philip Krause, MD, Food and Drug Administration, Bethesda, MD

Ruth A. Lawrence, MD, University of Rochester School of Medicine and Dentistry, Rochester, NY

Brad Leissa, MD, Food and Drug Administration, Bethesda, MD

Roland Levandowski, MD, Food and Drug Administration, Bethesda, MD

Dale Little, PhD, Tulane University School of Public Health and Tropical Medicine, New Orleans, LA

Richard Lizambri, MD, Food and Drug Administration, Bethesda, MD

Murray Lumpkin, MD, Food and Drug Administration, Bethesda, MD

Charles Manclark, PhD, Food and Drug Administration, Bethesda, MD

Carol Marcus-Sekura, PhD, Food and Drug Administration, Bethesda, MD

Harold S. Margolis, MD, Centers for Disease Control and Prevention, Atlanta, GA

Lewis Markoff, MD, Food and Drug Administration, Bethesda, MD

Lauri Markowitz, MD, Centers for Disease Control and Prevention, Atlanta, GA

Barbara J. Marston, MD, Centers for Disease Control and Prevention, Atlanta, GA

Eric E. Mast, MD, Centers for Disease Control and Prevention, Atlanta, GA

David O. Matson, MD, PhD, Eastern Virginia Medical School, Norfolk, VA

Celia Maxwell, MD, Food and Drug Administration, Bethesda, MD

Kenneth McIntosh, MD, Harvard Medical School, Boston, MA

Kelly McKee, Jr, MD, MPH, Preventive Medicine Service, Fort Bragg, NC

Julia A. McMillan, MD, Johns Hopkins University School of Medicine, Baltimore, MD

Michael M. McNeil, MD, Centers for Disease Control and Prevention, Atlanta, GA

Anne K. Mellinger, MD, MPH, Centers for Disease Control and Prevention, Atlanta, GA

Zachary Miller, MD, University of Washington, Seattle, WA

Eric D. Mintz, MD, MPH, Centers for Disease Control and Prevention, Atlanta, GA

Carl J. Mitchell, ScD, Centers for Disease Control and Prevention, Atlanta, GA

Charles D. Mitchell, MD, University of Miami School of Medicine, Miami, FL

John Modlin, MD, Dartmouth School of Medicine, Hanover, NH

Nasim Moledina, MD, Food and Drug Administration, Bethesda, MD

Anne Moore, MD, PhD, Centers for Disease Control and Prevention, Atlanta, GA

John S. Moran, MD, Centers for Disease Control and Prevention, Atlanta, GA

Ardythe L. Morrow, PhD, Eastern Virginia Medical School, Norfolk, VA

John R. Mullen, MA, Centers for Disease Control and Prevention, Atlanta, GA

Dianne Murphy, MD, Food and Drug Administration, Bethesda, MD

Kenrad Nelson, MD, Johns Hopkins University, Baltimore, MD

Charles M. Nolan, MD, Seattle-King County Department of Public Health, Seattle, WA

Hans D. Ochs, MD, University of Washington School of Medicine, Seattle, WA

James G. Olson, PhD, Centers for Disease Control and Prevention, Atlanta, GA

Michael T. Osterholm, PhD, MPH, Minnesota Department of Health, Minneapolis, MN

Margaret J. Oxtoby, MD, Centers for Disease Control and Prevention, Atlanta, GA

Mark A. Pallansch, PhD, Centers for Disease Control and Prevention, Atlanta, GA

Claire Panosian, MD, UCLA Medical Center, Los Angeles, CA

Lynn A. Paxton, MD, MPH, Centers for Disease Control and Prevention, Atlanta, GA

Howard A. Pearson, MD, Yale University School of Medicine, New Haven, CT

Bradley A. Perkins, MD, Centers for Disease Control and Prevention, Atlanta, GA

Clarence J. Peters, MD, Centers for Disease Control and Prevention, Atlanta, GA

Robert W. Pinner, MD, Centers for Disease Control and Prevention, Atlanta, GA

Philip A. Pizzo, MD, National Institutes of Health, Bethesda, MD

Stanley A. Plotkin, MD, Pasteur-Mérieux-Connaught Biologicals, Paris, France

Jacquelyn A. Polder, RN, Centers for Disease Control and Prevention, Atlanta, GA

Louis B. Polish, MD, Centers for Disease Control and Prevention, Atlanta, GA

Bob Pond, MD, Centers for Disease Control and Prevention, Atlanta, GA

Neil S. Prose, MD, Duke University Medical Center, Durham, NC

Semour Rand, MD, Food and Drug Administration, Bethesda, MD

William C. Reeves, Jr, MD, Centers for Disease Control and Prevention, Atlanta, GA

Frank O. Richards, Jr, MD, Centers for Disease Control and Prevention, Atlanta, GA

Paul Richman, PhD, Food and Drug Administration, Bethesda, MD

Allen A. Ries, MD, Centers for Disease Control and Prevention, Atlanta, GA

Russell Rignery, PhD, Centers for Disease Control and Prevention, Atlanta, GA

Desiree V. Rodgers, MD, MPH, Centers for Disease Control and Prevention, Atlanta, GA

Martha F. Rogers, MD, Centers for Disease Control and Prevention, Atlanta, GA

Robert T. Rolfs, MD, Centers for Disease Control and Prevention, Atlanta, GA

Craig E. Rubens, MD, PhD, University of Washington, Seattle, WA

Andrea J. Ruff, MD, Johns Hopkins University, Baltimore, MD

Leigh Sawyer, DVM, Food and Drug Administration, Bethesda, MD

Lawrence A. Schachner, MD, University of Miami School of Medicine, Miami, FL

Peter M. Schantz, VMD, PhD, Centers for Disease Control and Prevention, Atlanta, GA

Lawrence B. Schonberger, MD, Centers for Disease Control and Prevention, Atlanta, GA

Anne Schuchat, MD, Centers for Disease Control and Prevention, Atlanta, GA

Benjamin Schwartz, MD, Centers for Disease Control and Prevention, Atlanta, GA

James Seidel, MD, PhD, UCLA School of Medicine, Torrance CA

Richard Sembo, Johns Hopkins University, Baltimore, MD

Craig N. Shapiro, MD, Centers for Disease Control and Prevention, Atlanta, GA

Stanford T. Shulman, MD, Northwestern University Medical School, Chicago, IL

R. J. Simonds, MD, Centers for Disease Control and Prevention, Atlanta, GA

David H. Sniadack, MD, Centers for Disease Control and Prevention, Atlanta, GA

Dixie E. Snider, Jr, MD, MPH, Centers for Disease Control and Prevention, Atlanta, GA

Jeffrey R. Starke, MD, Baylor College of Medicine, Houston, TX

Barbara W. Stechenberg, MD, Baystate Medical Center, Springfield, MA

Kathryn Stein, PhD, Food and Drug Administration, Bethesda, MD

John A. Stewart, MD, Centers for Disease Control and Prevention, Atlanta, GA

Katherine M. Stone, MD, Centers for Disease Control and Prevention, Atlanta, GA

Walter L. Straus, MD, MPH, Centers for Disease Control and Prevention, Atlanta, GA

Peter M. Strebel, MD, MPH, Centers for Disease Control and Prevention, Atlanta, GA

Raymond A. Strikas, MD, MPH, Centers for Disease Control and Prevention, Atlanta, GA

Roland W. Sutter, MD, MPH, TM, Centers for Disease Control and Prevention, Atlanta, GA

Ana Szarfman, MD, Food and Drug Administration, Bethesda, MD

Ofelia C. Tablan, MD, Centers for Disease Control and Prevention, Atlanta, GA

Glen Tamura, MD, PhD, University of Washington, Seattle, WA

Donald Tankersley, PhD, Food and Drug Administration, Bethesda, MD

Phillip I. Tarr, MD, University of Washington, Seattle, WA
Robert V. Tauxe, MD, MPH, Centers for Disease Control and Prevention, Atlanta, GA
Linda Teague, MD, Food and Drug Administration, Bethesda, MD
Fred C. Tenover, PhD, Centers for Disease Control and Prevention, Atlanta, GA
Moe Moe Thint, MD, Food and Drug Administration, Bethesda, MD
Margaret A. Tipple, MD, Centers for Disease Control and Prevention, Atlanta, GA
James K. Todd, MD, University of Colorado, Denver, CO
Thomas J. Török, MD, Centers for Disease Control and Prevention, Atlanta, GA
Theodore F. Tsai, MD, MPH, National Health Institute, Bethesda, MD
Paul Turkletaub, MD, Food and Drug Administration, Bethesda, MD
Jessica Tuttle, MD, Centers for Disease Control and Prevention, Atlanta, GA
Frank S. Virant, MD, University of Washington, Seattle, WA
Govinda S. Visvesvara, PhD, Centers for Disease Control and Prevention, Atlanta, GA
Duc J. Vugia, MD, MPH, Centers for Disease Control and Prevention, Atlanta, GA
Steven G. Wassilak, MD, Centers for Disease Control and Prevention, Atlanta, GA
John C. Watson, MD, MPH, Centers for Disease Control and Prevention, Atlanta, GA
Jay D. Wenger, MD, Centers for Disease Control and Prevention, Atlanta, GA
Peter N. Wenger, MD, Centers for Disease Control and Prevention, Atlanta, GA
Cynthia Whitman, MD, Centers for Disease Control and Prevention, Atlanta, GA
William L. Whittington, PhD, Centers for Disease Control and Prevention, Atlanta, GA
Catherine M. Wilfert, MD, Duke University School of Medicine, Durham, NC
Michael Williams, Food and Drug Administration, Bethesda, MD
Walter W. Williams, MD, MPH, Centers for Disease Control and Prevention, Atlanta, GA
Joseph Winfield, MD, Food and Drug Administration, Bethesda, MD
Robert Yetter, PhD, Food and Drug Administration, Bethesda, MD
Robert Yolken, MD, Johns Hopkins University, Baltimore, MD
Edward J. Young, MD, Baylor College of Medicine, Houston, TX
Kenneth M. Zangwill, MD, Centers for Disease Control and Prevention, Atlanta, GA

Committee on Infectious Diseases

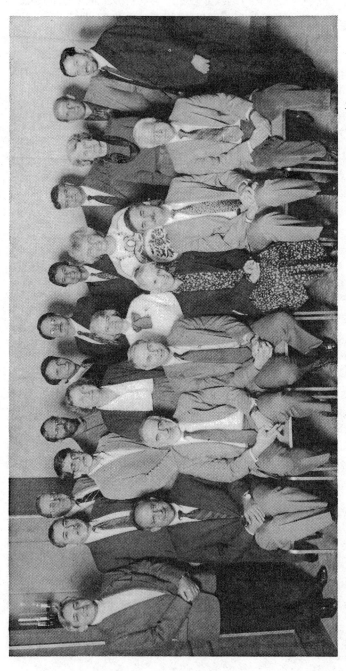

Front row: Edgar K. Marcuse; Neal A. Halsey; Georges Peter; Caroline B. Hall; Larry K. Pickering; Edgar O. Ledbetter *Second row:* Russell W. Steele; Kenneth J. Bart; Larry Anderson; Carol F. Phillips; Noni E. MacDonald; Gwendolyn B. Scott; Carolyn M. Hardegree; Walter A. Orenstein *Third row:* Donald S. Gromisch; Steve Kohl; Dan M. Granoff; Richard F. Jacobs; Melvin I. Marks; George A. Nankervis; Ram Yogev

PREFACE

To title the *1994 Red Book* a "Report of the Committee on Infectious Diseases" seems inappropriate, for it is a compendium of the cogitations and contributions of many consultants, though primarily the Committee. Special credit and commendation belong to the Associate Editors, Edgar Ledbetter, and most to Georges Peter. The perceptive wisdom, the painstaking diligence, the prescience, and the patience of "Saint Peter" have endowed him with omnipotence in our minds. "Report" also seems descriptively inadequate to indicate the perception in its conception, the interpretive and imaginative investment of it laborers. Often the color and tone of each word and phrase have been carefully chosen to complete a canvas that may convey correctly the subtleties of view . . .

This book is more than a "Report"
in the authors' close, chimeric view,
But a creative act combining
past experience with facts new.

The arduous, exacting process
gives just reverence to its birth;
But mortals are the parents
which should add to, not decrease, its worth.

Possessing no prognostic power
of a publisher on high,
Some parts may be antiquity
before the print of page is dry.

The words that now compose each line
were wrought, some fought, by mortal minds,
Their expertise defined, not divine,
by different training, views - and blinds.

Can any myriad of maestros
agree to speak, less write, as one?
Just as orchestral strings at times
may come to play in unison,

Their artistry comes from the varied tones
allowed in harmony
Thus, Astute Reader,
appreciate the passages in minor key

Which show the issues
over which "the experts" couldn't all agree.
For imperfect scales you'll sometimes hear
have tolerance, we plea. . .

To recommend that something
   "could" or "would" or "should" be done appears
To be a tune devoid of meter
   to discerning, scientific ears.

But guidelines most demanded
   are those for which there are no data yet;
If many data make the answer clear,
   no queries do we get.

We've also found each reader
   holds most dear his way - and Will of Rights,
Unfurled with might of voice and pen
   when impinged by what this Red Book cites. . .

And last, a dedication
   to our English teachers who warned us thus:
Unheeded dangling participles
   hang not themselves - but us.

Caroline Breese Hall

INTRODUCTION

The Committee on Infectious Diseases is responsible for formulating and revising guidelines of the American Academy of Pediatrics for the control of infectious diseases in children. At intervals of approximately 3 years, the Committee reviews and revises all of its recommendations and issues a composite summary, *Red Book: Report of the Committee on Infectious Diseases*. These recommendations represent consensuses developed by the members of the Committee in conjunction with liaison representatives from the Centers for Disease Control and Prevention, the Food and Drug Administration, the National Institutes of Health, the National Vaccine Program, and the Canadian Paediatric Society; the *Red Book* consultants; and the numerous collaborators whose expert advice the Committee solicits. This edition is based on information available as of December 1993.

Unanswered scientific questions, the complexity of medical practice, new information, and inevitable differences of opinion between experts result in inherent limitations of the *Red Book*. In the context of these limitations, the Committee endeavors to provide current, relevant, and defensible recommendations for the prevention and management of infectious diseases in children. In some cases, other committees and experts might differ in their interpretation of the data and resulting recommendations. In some instances, no single recommendation can be made, as several options for management are equally acceptable.

In making its recommendations, the Committee acknowledges these differences in viewpoints by judicious use of the phrases "most experts recommend. . ." and "some experts recommend. . .." Both phrases indicate valid recommendations, but the first signifies more support among experts, and the second, less support. Hence, "some experts recommend. . ." indicates a minority view that is based on data and/or experience and is sufficiently valid to warrant consideration.

Inevitably in clinical practice, questions arise that cannot be answered on the basis of currently available data. In such cases, the Committee attempts to provide guidelines and information that in conjunction with clinical judgment will facilitate well-reasoned decisions. We welcome questions, different perspectives, and alternative recommendations, as the resulting dialogue helps the Committee in its continuing review and periodic revisions of the *Red Book*. Through this process, the Committee seeks to provide a practical and authoritative guide for physicians in their care of children.

To aid the physician in assimilating current changes in the recommendations in the *Red Book*, a summary of major changes has been prepared. However, no list can be complete, and physicians are urged to consult individual chapters for other changes and additional guidelines. New information inevitably outdates some recommendations in the *Red Book* and necessitates that physicians remain informed of new developments and resulting changes in recommendations. Between editions, the Academy publishes new recommendations from the Committee in *AAP News* and *Pediatrics*.

Physicians, in using antimicrobials, should review the package inserts prepared by the manufacturers, particularly concerning contraindications and adverse reactions. No attempt has been made in the *Red Book* to provide this information, since it is readily available in the *Physicians' Desk Reference*. As in previous editions, recommended dosage schedules for antimicrobials are given (see Section 5, Antimicrobials and Related Therapy). Recommendations in the *Red Book* for drug dosages may differ from those of the manufacturer in the package inserts. Physicians should also be familiar with the information in the package inserts for vaccines and immune globulins, as well as the recommendations of other committees (see Sources of Vaccine Information, p 7).

This book could not have been prepared without the dedicated professional and administrative competence of Dr Edgar O. Ledbetter, Director of the Department of Maternal, Child, and Adolescent Health at the American Academy of Pediatrics. His wise counsel and support throughout the detailed 3-year process of preparation of a new edition of the *Red Book* has been invaluable. I am equally indebted to the Associate Editors, Drs Neal A. Halsey, Edgar K. Marcuse, and Larry K. Pickering for their expertise, tireless work, and immense contributions in their editorial and Committee work. The Associate Editors and I are also most appreciative of the guidance, dedication, and knowledge of the Committee Chairperson, Dr Caroline Breese Hall, whose suggestions and support are invaluable. She continues the exemplary leadership role in pediatric infectious diseases established by previous chairpersons of the Committee.

Special thanks are also given to Victoria K. Dahl of the American Academy of Pediatrics, and Charlotte A. Gauthier, secretary to the Editor, for their secretarial work, patience, and understanding, and to Felice Bassuk for editorial assistance. These individuals are only a few of the many major contributors whose long hours of work and sense of responsibility are integral and essential in the Committee's preparation of the *Red Book*.

Georges Peter, MD
Editor

TABLE OF CONTENTS

Section 2
Recommendations for Care of Children in Special Circumstances

Section 3
Summaries of Infectious Diseases

Section 4
Antimicrobial Prophylaxis

Section 5
Antimicrobials and Related Therapy

Appendices

SUMMARY OF MAJOR CHANGES IN THE *1994 RED BOOK*

Major changes in recommendations and related information in the *1994 Red Book* are summarized as follows:

1. *Immunization recommendations.* The schedules for routine immunization, including changes in recommendations for *Haemophilus influenzae* type b, hepatitis B, measles, and oral polio vaccines, have been revised (see Tables 1.3 and 1.4, pp 23 and 24). In view of the increasing complexity of the immunization recommendations for infants and children, particular attention should be given to the comments in the footnotes in these tables. In addition, since the licensure of new vaccines and revised recommendations after publication of the *Red Book* will result in continuing changes, the Committee anticipates publication of an updated immunization schedule each year in the interval before the next edition of the *Red Book* is published.

2. *Guidelines on active immunization.* New or revised recommendations have been made on vaccine handling and storage (see p 12 and Table 1.2, p 14), assessment of immunizations received in foreign countries in fulfilling vaccination requirements in the United States (see p 27), interchangeability of vaccine products (see p 22), vaccine injury compensation (see p 31), and reporting of vaccine-preventable diseases (see p 39).

3. *Standards for pediatric immunization practices* (see p 39 and Appendix II, p 602). These standards, as recommended by the National Vaccine Advisory Committee, approved by the United States Public Health Service, and endorsed by the AAP in 1993, are published in entirety in order to enhance timely and appropriate immunization of children.

4. *Immunization in special circumstances.* Recommendations for hepatitis B immunization of preterm infants have been revised (see pp 51 and 231). Guidelines for immunization of persons traveling to foreign countries have been updated (see p 67).

5. *Children in out-of-home child care.* The recommendations are similar to those in the previous edition of the *Red Book*, but the chapter has been revised to include the latest information concerning infectious diseases in child care (see p 83).

6. *Sexually transmitted diseases.* New guidelines on the prevention of these diseases in adolescents and young adults have been added (see p 105).

7. *Arboviruses*. The revised recommendations of the Centers for Disease Control and Prevention (CDC) for use of Japanese encephalitis vaccine, which was licensed in the United States in 1992, are summarized (see p 126).

8. *Chlamydia infections*. The recommendations for treatment of *Chlamydia trachomatis* infection have been revised, including guidelines for the management of infants born to mothers with previously untreated *C trachomatis* infection (see p 156).

9. *Cat scratch disease*. New information on the etiology (see p 150) and diagnostic tests (see p 151) for this disease.

10. *Escherichia coli diarrhea*. Recent information on *E coli* 0157:H7 (as well as that for other *E coli* pathogenic strains) and the complication from *E coli* 0157:H7 infection of hemolytic uremic syndrome are summarized (see p 187).

11. *Gonococcal infections and pelvic inflammatory disease*. Recommendations on treatment have been revised (see pp 197 and 353).

12. *Haemophilus influenzae infections*. The 1993 AAP recommendations on vaccination and related issues, including recently licensed conjugate vaccines, immunization schedules at different ages and in different circumstances, and rifampin chemoprophylaxis, are given (see p 205). In addition, an updated recommendation on the use of one of the conjugates (PRP-T) with DTP vaccine is given (see p 208).

13. *Hemorrhagic fevers caused by Bunyavirus, including Hantavirus*. Information on Hantavirus infection and the resulting epidemic in the southwestern United States in 1993 are provided in this chapter (see p 219).

14. *Hepatitis B*. In addition to the 1992 AAP recommendations on universal hepatitis B immunization, new recommendations on the immunization of preterm infants, clarification of the recommendations for immunization of preadolescents and adolescents, and guidelines on the immunization schedule in different circumstances (such as lapsed immunization and the flexibility in schedule) are given in detail (see p 227).

15. *Herpes simplex*. The recommendations on the management of infants exposed to herpes simplex virus (HSV) during delivery have been revised (see p 249). The changes, although not major, reflect recent epidemiologic findings and other information on HSV infection. Recommendations for antiviral therapy of HSV infection have been updated (see p 245). Guidelines on the prevention of transmission of HSV infection in athletic competition involving close contact, such as wrestling, are provided (see p 251).

16. *HIV infections and AIDS*. Changes include the revised surveillance definition for AIDS of the Centers for Disease Control and Prevention (CDC)

(see p 254), guidelines for the diagnosis of HIV infection in the first 6 to 18 months of life for infants born to HIV-infected mothers (see p 258), recommendations on antiviral therapy (see p 261), indications for intravenous immune globulin (IGIV) (see p 263), and recommendations of the AAP Task Force on Pediatric AIDS (now termed the Provisional Committee on Pediatric AIDS), as published in their statements on perinatal HIV serologic testing (see p 260), adolescent education (see p 265), school attendance and education (see p 266), and child care and foster care (see p 267). Related information on the prevention and management of *Pneumocystis carinii* pneumonia (see p 377) and *Mycobacterium avium* complex (MAC) infection (see p 503) in HIV-infected patients is given in the chapters on these infections. Since the guidelines on the management of children with suspected or proven HIV infection are complex and evolving, physicians should review these chapters for further information.

17. *Human herpesvirus-6 (roseola).* Because the etiology of roseola—human herpesvirus-6 (HHV-6)—has been identified, the title of this chapter has been changed and new information on HHV-6 infection is given (see p 272).

18. *Influenza.* Vaccine recommendations have been expanded to include possible indications for healthy children (see p 279) and timing of vaccination in steroid recipients, such as for children with asthma (see p 279). Recommendations for antiviral therapy and chemoprophylaxis have been revised to include rimantadine, which was approved by the Food and Drug Administration in 1993, and current dosage guidelines for this drug and its analogue, amantadine, are given (see pp 277 and 282).

19. *Kawasaki disease.* The recommendations on treatment, including guidelines on the use of intravenous immune globulin (IGIV), have been updated (see p 285).

20. *Measles.* Revisions include the recommended age of 12 to 15 months for the first dose of MMR vaccine (see p 314), timing of routine immunization of children who recently received immune globulin (see p 318), and indications for vitamin A in patients with measles (see p 310).

21. *Parainfluenza virus infection.* Treatment recommendations for children with croup have been expanded to include racemic epinephrine and dexamethasone (see p 342).

22. *Pediculosis.* The Committee's guidelines on treatment and prevention have been clarified (see p 350).

23. *Pertussis.* Major changes include the previously issued AAP statement giving recommendations for the use of acellular pertussis vaccine, ie, DTaP (see p 357), and delineation of the precautions and contraindications to pertussis vaccination (see p 364). A high-pitched cry after pertussis vaccination is no longer considered a precaution or contraindication to further pertussis immunization.

24. *Poliovirus infection.* The recommended age for the third dose of OPV in the routine childhood immunization schedule has been changed from 15-18 months to 6-18 months of age (see p 381).

25. *Group A streptococcal infections.* The indications for oral cephalosporins in the treatment of group A streptococcal pharyngitis have been revised (see p 435). The section *"Diagnostic Tests"* has been updated (see p 432). New information on the streptococcal toxic shock syndrome is given (see p 431).

26. *Group B streptococcal infections.* The 1992 AAP guidelines on the chemoprophylaxis of group B streptococcal infections are listed (see p 441).

27. *Syphilis.* Guidelines for the treatment of infants with possible congenital syphilis have been revised in an attempt to clarify the AAP recommendations (see p 450).

28. *Tuberculosis.* The recently published AAP recommendations on tuberculin skin testing, including indications, specific tests, and interpretation of the Mantoux test, are given (see p 482). New treatment recommendations, including the indications for four-drug therapy, are given (see p 487). In view of the complexities of management of patients with possible or proven tuberculosis, physicians caring for children with tuberculosis should review this chapter in detail.

29. *Varicella-zoster infections.* Changes include the 1993 AAP recommendations for oral acyclovir in children with varicella (see p 512), and guidelines on infection control in hospital exposures (see p 513). In addition, Varicella-Zoster Immune Globulin (VZIG) is no longer routinely recommended for healthy, susceptible adults exposed to a person with varicella (see p 514).

30. *Dexamethasone therapy for bacterial meningitis in infants and children.* The earlier AAP statement (see 1991 *Red Book*) has been revised (see p 558). Although the recommendations are similar to those in the previous statement, physicians should review this statement in order to make reasoned decisions about the use of dexamethasone in infants and children with bacterial meningitis.

31. *Ribavirin therapy of respiratory syncytial virus infection.* The 1993 AAP statement is included (see p 570).

32. *New chapters.* The following have been added:
    - Human Milk (see p 73). This chapter summarizes guidelines and recommendations on infectious disease issues in the management of infants who are receiving human milk. Many of the recommendations are also given in the disease-specific chapters in Section 3.
    - *Arcanobacterium haemolyticum* Infections (see p 127).
    - Astroviruses (see p 131).

- Bacterial Vaginosis (see p 135).
- *Microsporidia* Infections (see p 326).
- *Ureaplasma urealyticum* Infections (see p 509).

33. *Antimicrobial tables*. The tables on drug dosages and recommendations, including those for parasitic (see p 574), fungal (see p 560), and viral (see p 567) infections, have been updated. Drugs in each table are listed alphabetically.

Every effort has been made to identify major changes in order to aid physicians in adapting the new guidelines and recommendations of the *Red Book* in the care of their patients. However, since no list is complete, physicians are urged to review relevant chapters and sections of the *Red Book*. In addition, during the preparation of each edition, the entire book is reviewed and revised. Therefore, this edition has considerable new information to assist physicians in the diagnosis, management, and prevention of pediatric infectious diseases.

SECTION 1

ACTIVE AND PASSIVE IMMUNIZATION

Prologue

The ultimate goal of immunization is eradication of disease; the immediate goal is prevention of disease in individuals or groups. To accomplish these goals, physicians must maintain timely immunization, including both active and passive immunoprophylaxis, as a high priority in the care of infants, children, adolescents, and adults. The eradication of smallpox serves as a model for each disease that can be prevented by immunization. The global eradication of smallpox was achieved in 1980 by combining an effective immunization program with intense surveillance and adequate public health control measures worldwide.

Many infectious diseases can be prevented by immunoprophylaxis. With active immunization, a person is stimulated to develop immunologic defenses against future natural exposure. With passive immunization, a person already exposed, or about to be exposed, to certain infectious agents is given preformed human or animal antibody.

In the United States, immunization has sharply curtailed, or practically eliminated, diphtheria, measles, mumps, pertussis, poliomyelitis, rubella (congenital and acquired), tetanus, and *Haemophilus influenzae* type b disease. Yet, because these diseases persist in the United States as well as in other countries, immunizations need to be continued. Research on new vaccines involves molecular biologic techniques. Eventually, some of these experimental vaccines will be used routinely. Physicians must regularly update their knowledge about specific vaccines and their use because information about the safety and efficacy of vaccines and recommendations relative to their administration continue to develop after a vaccine is licensed.

Each edition of the *Report of the Committee on Infectious Diseases* (*Red Book*) presents recommendations for immunization of children and adolescents based on the knowledge, experience, and premises current at the time of publication. The recommendations represent a consensus with which reasonable physicians may at times disagree. No claim is made for infallibility, and the Committee acknowledges that individual circumstances may warrant decisions differing from the recommendations given here.

Sources of Vaccine Information

In addition to the *Red Book*, which is published at intervals of approximately 3 years, physicians should use the scientific literature and other sources for data or answers to specific questions encountered in practice. Among these sources are the following:

- *Pediatrics*. Statements developed by the Committee on Infectious Diseases (COID) and approved by the American Academy of Pediatrics (Academy), giving updated recommendations, are published in *Pediatrics* between editions of the *Red Book*. In addition, articles provide new information on infectious diseases and immunizations.
- *AAP News*. Policy statements from the COID are often initially published in *AAP News*, the Academy's monthly newspaper, to inform its membership promptly of new recommendations.
- *Morbidity and Mortality Weekly Report (MMWR)*. Published weekly by the Centers for Disease Control and Prevention (CDC), *MMWR* contains current vaccine recommendations, reports of specific disease activity, and changes in policy statements. Recommendations of the Advisory Committee on Immunization Practices (ACIP) of the United States Public Health Service are published periodically, usually as supplements. Subscriptions can be purchased from the following: Superintendent of Documents, US Government Printing Office, Washington, DC 20402-9235; Ochsner Clinic, 1514 Jefferson Highway, New Orleans, LA 70121; and *New England Journal of Medicine*, MMS Publications, CSPO, Box 9120, Waltham, MA 02254-9120. *Morbidity and Mortality Weekly Report* is now available by computer on DIALCOM.
- *Official package inserts*. Manufacturers provide product-specific information with each package of vaccine; the same information is also given in the *Physicians' Desk Reference (PDR)*. The package insert must be in full compliance with FDA regulations pertaining to labeling for prescription drugs, including indications and usage, dosages, routes of administration, clinical pharmacology, contraindications, and adverse reactions. The package insert lists preservatives, stabilizers, antibiotics, adjuvants, and suspending fluids, which may cause inflammation or elicit an allergic response. Health care providers should be familiar with the insert for each product they administer.
- *Health Information for International Travel*. This useful monograph is published annually by the CDC as a guide to requirements of the various countries for specific immunizations. It also provides information concerning vaccines that are not required but are recommended for travel for specific areas, and other information for travelers. It can be purchased from the Superintendent of Documents, US Government Printing Office, Washington, DC 20402-9235 (202/783-3238). For further sources of information on international travel, see Foreign Travel (p 67).
- *Control of Communicable Diseases in Man*. The American Public Health Association publishes this manual at intervals of approximately 5 years. It contains valuable information about most infectious diseases, their worldwide occurrence, diagnostic and therapeutic information, immunizations, and recommendations on isolation and other control measures for specific diseases.
- *Guide for Adult Immunization*. This publication by the American College of Physicians (Subscriber Services, Independence Mall, West Sixth Street at Race, Philadelphia, PA 19106-1572) provides useful information about infectious diseases and vaccine recommendations for adolescents and adults. The newest edition is scheduled for publication in 1994.

Physicians can consult members of the Committee by phone or letter. Specific questions may be addressed directly to the Academy at 141 Northwest Point Blvd, Elk Grove Village, IL 60009 (708/228-5005).

Consultation and printed material on immunizations can also be obtained from the Voice Information System (VIS) of the National Immunization Program, Centers for Disease Control and Prevention (404/332-4553). The VIS will provide the caller with the most up-to-date information by voice, mail, or FAX. Specific consultations with the National Immunization Program can be obtained by calling 404/639-8200. Other resources include the Food and Drug Administration (301/594-2000), infectious disease experts in medical schools, university-affiliated hospitals, and public health departments. Information can be obtained from local and state public health offices about current epidemiology of diseases, immunization recommendations, legal requirements, public health policies, foreign travel, and nursery school, child care, and school health concerns.

Informed Consent

Parents and patients should be informed about the benefits and risks of preventive and therapeutic procedures, including immunizations.

The patient, parent, and/or legal guardian should be informed about the benefits to be derived from vaccines in preventing disease in individuals and in the community, and about the risks of those vaccines. Benefit and risk information should be presented in lay terms. Questions should be encouraged so that the information is understood and coercion is avoided.

The National Childhood Vaccine Injury Act of 1986 included requirements for notifying patients and parents in both the private and public sectors about vaccine benefits and risks. This legislation requires development and distribution of standardized vaccine information pamphlets or comparable written information when administering vaccines for which vaccine injury compensation is available (see National Vaccine Injury Compensation Table, p 615). The requirements for information to be provided in these pamphlets were simplified by federal legislation in 1993, resulting in revised and shortened vaccine information materials scheduled to be issued in 1994. Providing the appropriate vaccine information became mandatory in 1992. Copies of the current vaccine information pamphlets can be obtained from the vaccine manufacturer, the Centers for Disease Control and Prevention (CDC), state and local health departments, and the Academy. For vaccines not now included in the National Childhood Vaccine Injury Act of 1986, such as *Haemophilus influenzae* type b conjugate vaccines and hepatitis B, no legally ratified vaccine information statements are available. The CDC has developed "Important Information" statements about these vaccines; these statements are revised periodically and are available from state health departments. The vaccine information pamphlets and "Important Information" statements may include space for the parents' or patients' signatures to indicate that they have read and understood the material. Such signatures are required whenever vaccines are administered that were purchased under the federal government contract. However, the Academy encourages physicians to obtain written informed consent for each immunization administered. Whether or not parents sign a form, those who administer vaccines should try to ensure that parents understand the information. If the parents' or patient's signature is not obtained, the fact that an informed request has been made should be recorded in the patient's record. (See also Vaccine Safety and Contraindications, p 29.)

Active Immunization

Active immunization involves administration of all or part of a microorganism or a modified product of that microorganism (eg, a toxoid, a purified antigen, or an antigen produced by genetic engineering) to evoke an immunologic response mimicking that of the natural infection but which presents little or no risk to the recipient. The immunization can result in antitoxic, anti-invasive, neutralizing activity, or other types of protective humoral or cellular response in the patient. Some immunizing agents provide complete protection against disease for life, some provide partial protection, and some must be readministered at intervals. The effectiveness of a vaccine is assessed by the evidence of protection against the natural disease. Induction of antibodies is frequently an indirect measure of protection, but in some circumstances (eg, in pertussis) the immunologic response correlated with protection is poorly understood, and serum antibody concentrations are not always predictive of protection.

Vaccines incorporating an intact infectious agent may be either live and attenuated or killed (inactivated). Currently licensed vaccines are listed in Table 1.1 (see p 11). Many viral vaccines contain live-attenuated virus. Although active infection (with replication) ensues after administration of these vaccines, little or no adverse host reaction usually occurs. The vaccines for some viruses and most bacteria are inactivated (killed) or subunit preparations. Inactive agents are incapable of replicating in the host; therefore, these vaccines must contain a sufficient antigenic mass to stimulate the desired response. Maintenance of long-lasting immunity with killed (inactivated) viral or bacterial vaccines often requires periodic administration of booster doses. Inactivated vaccines may not elicit the range of immunologic response provided by live attenuated agents. For example, an injected, inactivated viral vaccine may evoke sufficient serum antibody or cell-mediated immunity but fail to evoke local antibody in the form of secretory immunoglobulin A (IgA). Thus, mucosal protection after administration of inactivated vaccines is generally inferior to the mucosal immunity induced by live vaccines, and local infection or colonization with the agent can occur, although systemic infection is prevented or ameliorated by the presence of serum and cellular factors. However, inactivated vaccines cannot replicate or be excreted as infectious agents by the vaccinee and thereby adversely affect the immunosuppressed host.

The mechanics of immunization are critical to the success of immunization procedures. Recommendations for dose, route, technique of administration, and schedules should be followed for predictable, effective immunization.

The physician must be certain that vaccines are stored at the appropriate temperature and handled correctly (see Vaccine Handling and Storage, p 12, and Table 1.2, p 14). When multidose vials are used, scrupulous care must be taken to prevent bacterial contamination.

TABLE 1.1–Vaccines Licensed in the United States and Their Routes of Administration

Vaccine[a]	Type	Route[b]
Anthrax	Inactivated bacteria	SC
BCG	Live bacteria	ID (preferred) or SC
Cholera	Inactivated bacteria	SC, IM, or ID
DTP	Toxoids and inactivated bacteria	IM
DTaP	Toxoids and bacterial products or fractions	IM
Hepatitis B	Inactivated viral antigen: yeast-derived recombinant; plasma-derived	IM
Hib conjugates	Saccharide-protein conjugate[c]	IM
Hib conjugate and DTP combination (HbOC-DTP)	Saccharide-protein conjugate with toxoids and inactivated bacteria	IM
Influenza	Inactivated virus (whole-virus); viral components (split-virus)	IM IM
Japanese encephalitis	Inactivated virus	SC
Measles	Live virus	SC
Meningococcal	Polysaccharide	SC
MMR	Live viruses	SC
MR	Live viruses	SC
Mumps	Live virus	SC
Pertussis[d]	Inactivated bacteria	IM
Plague	Inactivated bacteria	IM
Pneumococcal	Polysaccharide	IM or SC
Poliovirus (trivalent)		
OPV	Live virus	Oral
IPV	Inactivated virus	SC
Rabies	Inactivated virus	IM or ID[e]
Rubella	Live virus	SC
Tetanus and Td, DT (adsorbed)	Toxoids	IM
Tetanus (fluid)	Toxoid	SC
Typhoid		
Parenteral	Inactivated bacteria	SC (boosters may be ID)
Oral	Live bacteria	Oral
Varicella[f]	Live virus	SC
Yellow fever	Live virus	SC

[a]Vaccine abbreviations: BCG = bacillus Calmette-Guerin (tuberculosis) vaccine; DTP = diphtheria and tetanus toxoids and pertussis vaccine; DTaP = diphtheria and tetanus toxoids and acellular pertussis vaccine; Hib = *Haemophilus influenzae* type b conjugate vaccine; MMR = live measles, mumps, and rubella viruses vaccine; MR = measles and rubella virus vaccine; OPV = oral poliovirus vaccine (containing attenuated poliovirus types 1, 2, and 3); IPV = inactivated poliovirus vaccine; Td = tetanus and diphtheria toxoid (for children ≥7 y and adults); DT = diphtheria and tetanus toxoids (for children <7 y).

[b]Route abbreviations: SC = subcutaneous; ID = intradermal; IM = intramuscular.

[c]See Table 3.7 (p 208).

[d]Distributed by the Division of Biologic Products, Michigan Department of Public Health, North Lansing, MI.

[e]The intradermal dose is different from the subcutaneous and intramuscular doses, and is used only for preexposure vaccination.

[f]Investigational vaccine, currently under consideration for licensure, as of December 1993.

Immunizing Antigens

Physicians should become familiar with the major constituents of the products they use. These are listed in the package inserts. If a vaccine is produced by different manufacturers, some differences may exist in the active and inert ingredients contained in the various products. The major constituents of vaccines include the following:

1. *Active immunizing antigen.* In some vaccines this antigen is a highly defined, single constituent (eg, pneumococcal polysaccharide, or tetanus or diphtheria toxoid); in others, it is complex and/or less well defined (eg, live viruses or killed pertussis bacteria).

2. *Suspending fluid.* The suspending fluid frequently is as simple as sterile water for infection or saline, but it may be a complex tissue-culture fluid. This fluid may contain proteins or other constituents derived from the medium and biologic system in which the vaccine is produced (eg, egg antigens or tissue-culture-derived antigens).

3. *Preservatives, stabilizers, and antibiotics.* Trace amounts of chemicals (eg, mercurials, such as thiomersal, and certain antibiotics such as neomycin or streptomycin) are frequently necessary to prevent bacterial growth or to stabilize the antigen. Allergic reactions may occur if the recipient is sensitive to one or more of these additives. Whenever feasible, these reactions should be anticipated by identifying known host hypersensitivity to specific vaccine components.

4. *Adjuvants.* An aluminum compound is frequently used to increase immunogenicity and to prolong the stimulatory effect, particularly for vaccines containing inactivated microorganisms or their products (eg, hepatitis B and diphtheria and tetanus toxoids). Newer adjuvants are being investigated and may be incorporated into vaccines in the future.

Because of possible hypersensitivity to vaccine components, vaccines should be administered only when emergency equipment and drugs, such as epinephrine, are readily available (see Hypersensitivity Reactions to Vaccine Constituents, page 36).

Vaccine Handling and Storage

Inattention to vaccine storage conditions can contribute to vaccine failure. Certain vaccines, such as oral poliovirus vaccine (OPV), measles, and yellow fever vaccine, are very sensitive to increased temperature. Others are sensitive to freezing. These include diphtheria and tetanus toxoids and pertussis vaccines (DTP, DTaP, DT, Td), inactivated poliovirus vaccine (IPV), and *Haemophilus influenzae* conjugate, hepatitis B, and influenza vaccines. Some products may show physical evidence of altered integrity (eg, DTP vials containing clumps of antigen that cannot be resuspended by vigorous shaking of the vial), but others may retain their normal appearance despite a loss of potency. Therefore, all personnel responsible for handling vaccines in an office or clinic setting should be familiar with standard procedures designed to minimize the risk of vaccine failure. Recommended storage conditions for commonly used vaccines are listed in Table 1.2 (p 14). New vaccines and new formulations of currently available products may have storage requirements different from those listed in the table. Recommendations for the handling and storage of selected biologicals are summarized in the package insert for each product and in the publication *Vaccine Management*, available from the CDC.* The most current information concerning recommended vaccine storage conditions and handling instructions can be obtained directly from manufacturers of immunobiologicals whose phone numbers can be found in the package insert and in the *Physicians' Desk Reference (PDR)*,† published yearly. The following guidelines are suggested as part of a quality control system for safe handling and storage of vaccines in an office or clinic setting:

Personnel
1. Designate one individual as the vaccine coordinator, and assign to this person responsibility for ensuring that vaccines and other biologic products are carefully handled in a safe, documentable manner.
2. Inform all individuals who will be handling vaccines about specific storage requirements and stability limitations of the products they will encounter (see Table 1.2, p 14). The details of proper storage conditions should be posted on or near each refrigerator or freezer used for vaccine storage or should be readily available.

Equipment
1. Ascertain that refrigerators and freezers in which vaccines are to be stored are working properly.
2. Equip each refrigerator with a thermometer located at the center of the storage compartment.
3. Keep a log book in which temperature readings are systematically recorded daily and the date and time of any mechanical malfunctions or power outages are noted.
4. Place in the refrigerator a tray in which all opened vials of vaccine are kept. To avoid mishaps, do not store other pharmaceuticals in the same tray.
5. Equip refrigerators with several bottles of chilled water and freezers with several ice trays or ice packs to fill empty space to minimize temperature fluctuations, should brief electrical or mechanical failure occur.
6. Consider purchasing and placing vaccine cold chain monitor cards‡ in refrigerators. These cards provide a means of establishing whether vaccines have been exposed to potentially harmful temperatures during intervals between manual measurement of the refrigerator's core temperature.

Procedures
1. Acceptance of vaccine
   Upon receiving a shipment of vaccine:
   - Check that the delivered product has not expired.
   - Examine the merchandise and its shipping container for any evidence of damage during transport.

---

*Centers for Disease Control. Vaccine Management: Recommendations for Handling and Storage of Selected Biologicals. Atlanta, GA: US Department of Health and Human Services, Public Health Service; March 1991.
†*Physicians' Desk Reference.* 48th ed. Montvale, NJ: Medical Economics Data; 1994.
‡Available from 3M Pharmaceuticals, St Paul, MN.

TABLE 1.2–Recommended Storage Conditions for Commonly Used Vaccines*

Vaccine	Recommended Temperature	Duration of Stability	Normal Appearance
Diphtheria and tetanus toxoids and acellular pertussis vaccine adsorbed (DTaP)	2°-8°C. Do not freeze. As little as 24 hours at <2°C or >25°C may cause antigens to fall from suspension and be very difficult to resuspend.	Not more than 18 mo from the time of issue from manufacturer's cold storage.	Markedly turbid and whitish suspension. If product contains clumps of material that cannot be resuspended with vigorous shaking, it should NOT be used.
Diphtheria and tetanus toxoids and whole-cell pertussis vaccine adsorbed (DTP)	2°-8°C. Do not freeze. As little as 24 hours at <2°C or >25°C may cause antigens to fall from suspension and be very difficult to resuspend.	Not more than 18 mo from the time of issue from manufacturer's cold storage.	Markedly turbid and whitish suspension. If product contains clumps of material that cannot be resuspended with vigorous shaking, it should NOT be used.
Diphtheria and tetanus toxoids, whole-cell pertussis vaccine adsorbed, and Haemophilus b conjugate vaccine (DTP-HbOC)	2°-8°C. Do not freeze. As little as 24 hours at <2°C or >25°C may cause antigens to fall from suspension and be very difficult to resuspend.	Not more than 18 mo from the time of issue from manufacturer's cold storage.	Markedly turbid, white suspension. If product contains clumps of material that cannot be resuspended with vigorous shaking, it should NOT be used.
Diphtheria toxoid adsorbed	2°-8°C. Do not freeze.	Not more than 2 y from the time of issue from manufacturer's cold storage.	Turbid and white, slightly gray, or slightly pink suspension.
Haemophilus b conjugate vaccine: HbOC (diphtheria CRM$_{197}$ protein conjugate)	2°-8°C. Do not freeze.	Not more than 2 y from date of issue from manufacturer's cold storage.	Clear, colorless liquid.

Vaccine	Storage	Dating	Appearance
Haemophilus b conjugate vaccine: PRP-D (diphtheria toxoid conjugate)	2°-8°C. Do not freeze.	Not more than 2 y from date of issue from manufacturer's cold storage.	Clear, colorless liquid.
Haemophilus b conjugate vaccine: PRP-OMP (meningococcal protein conjugate)	Lyophilized formulation: 2°-8°C. Do not freeze. Diluent should not be frozen. Reconstituted formulation: 2°-8°C. Do not freeze.	Not more than 2 y from date of issue from manufacturer's cold storage. Reconstituted vials should be used within 24 h.	Lyophilized: white to off-white powder. Reconstituted: after agitation, slightly opaque, white suspension.
Haemophilus b polysaccharide conjugate vaccine (tetanus toxoid conjugate; PRP-T)	Lyophilized formulation: 2°-8°C. Do not freeze. Diluent should not be frozen. Reconstituted formulation: 2°-8°C. Do not freeze.	Not more than 2 y from date of issue from manufacturer's cold storage.	Lyophilized: white to off-white powder. Reconstituted: clear and colorless.
Hepatitis B virus vaccine inactivated (recombinant)	2°-8°C. Storage outside this temperature range may reduce potency. Freezing substantially reduces potency.	Vaccine should be used immediately when reconstituted. 2 y from date of issue from manufacturer's cold storage.	After thorough agitation, a slightly opaque, white suspension.
Influenza virus vaccine (Subvirion)	2°-8°C. Freezing destroys potency.	Vaccine is good only the year for which it is manufactured; antigenic composition differs annually.	Clear, colorless liquid.

TABLE 1.2–Recommended Storage Conditions for Commonly Used Vaccines* (continued)

Vaccine	Recommended Temperature	Duration of Stability	Normal Appearance
Measles virus vaccine, live	Lyophilized formulation: 2°-8°C, but may be frozen. Protect from light, which may inactivate virus. Diluent: may be stored at room temperature or refrigerated. Reconstituted formulation: 2°-8°C. Protect from light, which can inactivate virus.	1 to 2 y (depends on manufacturer) from date of issue from manufacturer's cold storage. Discard reconstituted vaccine after 8 h.	Reconstituted: clear, yellow solution. Reconstituted vaccine that is cloudy should NOT be used.
Mumps virus vaccine, live	Lyophilized formulation: 2°-8°C, but may be frozen. Protect from light, which may inactivate virus. Diluent: may be stored at room temperature. Reconstituted formulation: 2°-8°C. Protect from light, which can inactivate virus.	1 to 2 y (depends on manufacturer) from date of issue from manufacturer's cold storage. Discard reconstituted vaccine after 8 h.	Reconstituted: clear, yellow solution. Reconstituted vaccine that is cloudy should NOT be used.
Pneumococcal vaccine, polyvalent	2°-8°C. Freezing destroys potency.	Not longer than indicated by expiration date on vial.	Clear, colorless, or slightly opalescent liquid.
Poliovirus vaccine, inactivated	2°-8°C. Do not freeze.	Not more than 1 y from date of issue from manufacturer's cold storage.	Clear, colorless suspension. Vaccine that contains particulate matter, develops turbidity, or changes in color should NOT be used.

Poliovirus vaccine, live, oral (OPV)	Must be stored at <0°C. Because of sorbitol in the vaccine, it will remain fluid at temperatures above minus (−)14°C. Refreezing the thawed product is acceptable (maximum of 10 thaw-freeze cycles), if the temperature never exceeded 8°C, and the cumulative thawing time is <24 h.	Not more than 1 y from date of issue from manufacturer's cold storage.	Clear solution, usually red or pink in color, from phenol red (pH indicator) it contains. May have a yellow color if shipment was packed with dry ice. Color changes that occur during storage or thawing are unimportant, provided the solution remains clear.
Rubella virus vaccine, live	Lyophilized formulation: 2–8°C, but may be frozen. Protect from light, which may inactivate virus.	1 to 2 y (depends on manufacturer) from date of issue from manufacturer's cold storage.	Reconstituted: clear, yellow solution. Reconstituted vaccine that is cloudy should NOT be used.
	Diluent: may be stored at room temperature.		
	Reconstituted formulation: 2°–8°C. Protect from light, which can inactivate virus.	Discard reconstituted vaccine after 8 h.	
Tetanus and diphtheria toxoids adsorbed (DT & Td)			
Tetanus toxoid adsorbed			

*Instructions for new vaccines may be different from those for products listed in the table. Also, any changes in the formulation of currently available immunizing agents may alter their appearance, stability, and storage requirements. **Questions regarding the stability of biologicals subjected to potentially harmful environmental conditions should be addressed to the manufacturer of the product in question.**

- Consider whether the interval between shipment from the supplier and arrival of the product at its destination is excessive (more than 48 hours), and whether the product has likely been exposed to excessive heat or cold that might alter its integrity. Check vaccine cold chain monitor cards if included in the vaccine shipment.
- Do not accept shipment if reasonable suspicion exists that the delivered product may have been damaged by environmental insult or improper handling during transport.
- Contact the vaccine supplier or manufacturer when unusual circumstances raise questions regarding the stability of a delivered vaccine. Store suspect vaccine under proper conditions until viability is determined.

2. Refrigerator inspection
- Measure the temperature of the central part of the storage compartment daily, and record this temperature in a log book.
- Inspect the unit for outdated vaccine at least monthly, and dispose of expired products appropriately.

3. Routine procedures
- Promptly remove expired vaccine from the refrigerator or freezer and dispose of it appropriately, at the earliest possible time, to avoid its accidental use.
- Keep opened vials of vaccine in a tray, so that they are readily identifiable.
- Indicate on the label of each vaccine vial the date and time it was reconstituted or first opened:
   - for multidose vials of vaccines that contain a bacteriostatic agent, discard opened vials promptly when outdated or if contaminated.
   - discard opened vials of vaccine that do not contain a bacteriostatic agent after 24 hours.
   - discard reconstituted measles-mumps-rubella (MMR) vaccine after 8 hours.
   - discard reconstituted PedvaxHIB (PRP-OMP)* after 24 hours.
- Store vaccines in the refrigerator throughout the office day.
- Do not open more than one vial of a particular vaccine at a time.
- Store vaccine only in the central storage area — not on the door shelf or in peripheral areas of the unit, where temperature fluctuations are greater.
- Do not keep food in refrigerators where vaccine is stored, as this practice will lead to more frequent opening of the unit and greater chance for thermal instability.
- Do not store radioactive materials in the same refrigerator in which vaccines are stored.
- Publicize among all clinic or office personnel any violation of handling protocol or any accidental storage problem (eg, electrical failure), and contact vaccine suppliers regarding the handling of the affected vaccine.

Haemophilus influenzae type b conjugate vaccine, available from Merck & Co, West Point, PA.

Vaccine Administration

General Instructions for Persons Administering Vaccines

Personnel administering vaccines should take appropriate precautions to minimize the risk of spread of disease to or from patients. Such personnel should be immunized against measles, mumps, rubella, hepatitis B, and influenza, as well as tetanus and diphtheria. Hands should be washed before and after each new patient contact. Gloves are not required when administering vaccines unless the health care worker has open hand lesions or will come into contact with potentially infectious body fluids. Syringes and needles must be sterile and preferably disposable. Disposable needles and syringes should be discarded promptly in puncture-proof, labeled containers to prevent accidental needlesticks or reuse. Different vaccines should not be mixed in the same syringe unless specifically licensed and labeled for such use.

Site and Route of Immunization

Oral vaccines. Breast-feeding does not interfere with successful immunization with oral poliovirus vaccine (OPV). If the patient immediately spits out, fails to swallow, or regurgitates OPV, the dose should be repeated. If the second dose is not retained, neither dose should be counted and the vaccine should be readministered at the next visit.

*Parenteral vaccines.** Injectable vaccines should be administered in a site as free as possible from the risk of local neural, vascular, or tissue injury. Data in the medical literature do not warrant recommendation of a single preferred site for all injections, and many manufacturers' product recommendations allow some flexibility in site of injection. Preferred sites include the anterolateral aspect of the upper thigh and the deltoid area of the upper arm for vaccines administered either subcutaneously or intramuscularly.

Recommended routes of administration are included in the package inserts of vaccines and are listed in Table 1.1 (p 11). The recommended route is based on the results of prior clinical use that demonstrated maximum safety and efficacy. To minimize untoward local or systemic effects and ensure optimal efficacy of the immunizing procedure, vaccines should be given according to the recommended route.

For intramuscular (IM) injections, the choice of site is based on the volume of the injected material and the size of the muscle. In children younger than 1 year (ie, infants), the anterolateral aspect of the thigh provides the largest muscle and is the preferred site. In older children, the deltoid muscle is usually large enough for IM injection. Some physicians prefer to use the anterolateral thigh muscles for toddlers. Parents and children, however, often prefer the deltoid muscle for children 18 months and older because of less discomfort in the affected extremity and in ambulating.

Ordinarily, the upper, outer aspect of the buttocks should not be used for immunizations in infants because the gluteal region consists mostly of fat until the child has been walking for some time and because of the possibility

---

*For an informative review on intramuscular injections, see Bergeson PS, Singer SA, Kaplan AM. Intramuscular injections in children. *Pediatrics.* 1982;70:944-948

of damaging the sciatic nerve. When the upper, outer quadrant of the buttocks is used for immunization, care must be exercised to avoid injury to the nerve. The site selected should be well into the upper, outer mass of the gluteus maximus, away from the central region of the buttocks, and the needle should be directed anteriorly—that is, if the patient is lying prone, perpendicular to the table's surface, not perpendicular to the skin plane. The ventrogluteal site may be less hazardous for IM injection because it is free of major nerves and vessels. This site is the center of a triangle whose boundaries are the anterior superior iliac spine, the tubercle of the iliac crest, and the upper border of the greater trochanter. However, clinical information on the use of this area is limited. Because of diminished immunogenicity, hepatitis B and rabies vaccine should not be given in the buttock at any age. Persons who were given hepatitis B vaccine in the buttock should be tested for immunity and revaccinated if antibody concentrations are inadequate.

Vaccines containing adjuvants (eg, aluminum-adsorbed DTP, DTaP, DT, Td, hepatitis B, and PedvaxHIB [PRP-OMP]*) must be injected deep in the muscle mass. They should not be administered subcutaneously or intracutaneously because they can cause local irritation, inflammation, granuloma formation, and necrosis. The needles used for IM injections should be long enough to reach the substance of the muscle. Ordinarily, a needle 7/8 in. or longer is required to ensure penetration of the muscle in a normal 4-month-old infant. A 22- or 23-gauge needle is appropriate for most IM vaccines.

Immunizing agents requiring IM injection include DTP, DTaP, DT, Td, hepatitis B, and rabies (human diploid cell) vaccine for postexposure prophylaxis (see Table 1.1, p 11). Immune Globulin (IG), Rabies Immune Globulin (Human), and other similar products for passive immunoprophylaxis are also injected intramuscularly. Serious complications of IM injections are rare. Reported events include broken needles, muscle contracture, nerve injury, bacterial (staphylococcal, streptococcal, and clostridial) abscesses, sterile abscesses, skin pigmentation, hemorrhage, cellulitis, tissue necrosis, gangrene, local atrophy, periostitis, cyst or scar formation, and inadvertent injection into a joint space. Sterile or bacterial abscesses at the injection site are estimated to occur approximately once per 100,000 to 166,000 doses of DTP. The incidence of other complications is unknown.

Subcutaneous (SC) injections can be given in the anterolateral aspect of the thigh or the upper arm by inserting the needle in a pinched-up fold of skin and subcutaneous tissue. Recent data demonstrate that immune responses after SC administration of hepatitis B and recombinant rabies vaccine have been reduced compared to those after IM administration. In patients with a bleeding diathesis, the risk of bleeding after IM injection can be minimized by administration immediately after the patient's receipt of replacement factor, use of a 23-gauge (or less) needle, and application of direct pressure to the vaccination site for at least 2 minutes. However, certain vaccines (eg, pneumococcal polyvalent polysaccharide, *Haemophilus influenzae* vaccines, and meningococcal quadrivalent polysaccharide) recommended for IM injection may be given subcutaneously to persons at risk for hemorrhage after IM injection, such as those with hemophilia. For

---

Haemophilus influenzae type b conjugate vaccine, available from Merck & Co, West Point, PA.

these vaccines, immune responses and clinical reactions after either IM or SC injection have generally been reported to be similar.

Intradermal (ID) injections are generally given on the volar surface of the forearm. Because of the decreased antigenic mass administered with ID injections, attention to technique is essential to ensure that the material is not injected subcutaneously.

For SC or ID injections, a 25-gauge needle 5/8 to 3/4 in. long is recommended.

Syringes and needles for vaccine injections must be sterile and preferably disposable to minimize the chances of contamination. Changing needles between drawing the vaccine into the syringe and injecting it into the child is not necessary. After use, needles and syringes should not be recapped and should be discarded in specially labeled impermeable containers to prevent accidental inoculation or theft.

The patient should be adequately restrained before any injection. When multiple vaccines are administered, separate sites should ordinarily be used if possible, especially for DTP-containing vaccines. When necessary, two vaccines can be given in the same limb at a single visit. The thigh is the preferred site for two simultaneous IM injections because of its greater muscle mass. The distance separating the two injections is arbitrary but should be spaced so that local reactions are unlikely to overlap. Multiple vaccines should not be mixed in a single syringe unless specifically licensed and labeled for administering in one syringe. A different needle and syringe should be used for each injection. Before the injection is given, the needle should be inserted in the site and the syringe plunger pulled back to see if blood appears; if so, the needle should be withdrawn and a new site selected. The procedure is repeated until no blood appears.

Scheduling Immunizations

A vaccine is intended to be administered to an individual who is capable of an appropriate immunologic response and who will likely benefit from the protection afforded. However, optimal immunologic response for the individual must be balanced against the need to achieve effective protection against disease. For example, DTP and poliovirus vaccines in early infancy are less immunogenic than later in infancy, but the benefit of conferring early protection in infants at high risk from these diseases dictates that immunization should proceed despite a lessened immunologic response. In some situations in the developing world, poliovirus vaccine is given at birth, in accordance with recommendations of the World Health Organization.

With parenterally administered live-virus vaccines, the inhibitory effect of residual specific maternal antibody determines the optimal age of administration. For example, live-virus measles vaccine in use in the United States has suboptimal rates of successful immunization during the first year of life because of transplacentally acquired maternal antibody.

An additional factor in selecting an immunization schedule is the need to achieve a uniform and regular response. With some products, a response is achieved after one dose; for others, it is achieved only after multiple doses. Live rubella vaccine is an example of a vaccine that evokes a regular, predictable response at highly acceptable rates after a single dose. In contrast, some individuals respond to only one or two types of poliovirus(es) after a single dose of

OPV. Hence, at least three doses are given to produce antibody against all three types, thereby ensuring complete protection for the individual and maximum response rates for the population. A single dose of some vaccines (mostly inactivated or killed antigens) confers less than optimal response in the individual. As a result, several doses are used to complete the primary immunization, and periodic booster doses (eg, with tetanus and diphtheria toxoids) are administered to maintain immunologic protection.

Most of the widely used vaccines are considered safe and effective when administered simultaneously, although limited data are available for many products at this time. This information is particularly important in scheduling immunization for children with lapsed or missed immunizations and for persons preparing for foreign travel (see Simultaneous Administration of Multiple Vaccines, p 25). Theoretical concerns exist about impaired immune responses to two live-virus vaccines given within 30 days of each other, but no evidence substantiates this concern with present vaccines. Hence, when feasible, live-virus vaccines not administered on the same day should be given at least 30 days apart. Recent receipt of OPV is **not** a contraindication to MMR, which should be given at the first available opportunity (according to age-specific recommendations).

Tables 1.3 (p 23) and 1.4 (p 24) give the recommended immunization schedules in the United States for infants and children, including those who were not appropriately immunized in the first year of life. Special attention should be given to the "Comments" and boldfaced footnotes in these tables, as they indicate the flexibility the physician has in scheduling immunizations, especially during the second year of life. The MMR vaccine may be given at 12 to 15 months of age except in communities experiencing measles, where it should be administered promptly at age 12 months (see also Measles, p 312). The third dose of OPV should be administered between 6 and 18 months. DTaP or DTP and OPV can be given concurrently with MMR, hepatitis B, and *Haemophilus influenzae* type b conjugate vaccines. The fourth dose of DTP should be given between 12 and 18 months of age; this dose may be given as DTaP between 15 and 18 months of age. Although administration of DTaP or DTP at 18 months of age is still appropriate, administration of this vaccine at 15 months is equally acceptable and has often been the practice in public health clinics in order to enhance immunization rates at the recommended ages. For those not immunized on schedule, simultaneous vaccination with multiple products allows more rapid protection. Physicians who choose to avoid multiple simultaneous injections and elect a multiple visit schedule should administer MMR vaccine between the ages of 12 and 15 months.

The immunization schedule used in the United States may not be appropriate for developing countries because of different disease risks, age-specific immune responses, and vaccine availability. The schedule recommended by the Expanded Programme on Immunization (EPI) of the World Health Organization should be consulted (see Table 1.5, p 25). Modifications may be made by the ministries of health in individual countries, based on local considerations.

Interchangeability of Vaccine Products

Comparable vaccines made by different manufacturers may differ in their components and formulation, and they may elicit different immune responses.

Table 1.3–Recommended Schedule for Immunization of Healthy Infants and Children[a]

Recommended Age[b]	Immunization(s)[c]	Comments
Birth	HBV[d]	
1-2 mo	HBV[d]	
2 mo	DTP, Hib,[e] OPV	DTP and OPV can be initiated as early as 4 wk after birth in areas of high endemicity or during outbreaks.
4 mo	DTP, Hib,[e] OPV	2-mo interval (minimum of 6 wk) recommended for OPV.
6 mo	DTP, (Hib[e,f])	
6-18 mo	HBV,[d] OPV	
12-15 mo	Hib,[e] MMR	MMR should be given at 12 mo of age in high-risk areas. If indicated, tuberculin testing may be done at the same visit.
15-18 mo	DTaP or DTP	The 4th dose of diphtheria-tetanus-pertussis vaccine should be given 6 to 12 mo after the third dose of DTP and may be given as early as 12 mo of age, provided that the interval between doses 3 and 4 is at least 6 mo and DTP is given. DTaP is not currently licensed for use in children younger than 15 mo.
4-6 y	DTaP or DTP, OPV	DTaP or DTP and OPV should be given at or before school entry. DTP or DTaP should not be given at or after the 7th birthday.
11-12 y	MMR	MMR should be given at entry to middle school or junior high school unless 2 doses were given after the 1st birthday.
14-16 y	Td	Repeat every 10 y throughout life.

[a]Table is not completely consistent with all package inserts. For products used, also consult manufacturer's package insert for instructions on storage, handling, dosage, and administration. Biologics prepared by different manufacturers may vary, and package inserts of the same manufacturer may change from time to time. Therefore, the physician should be aware of the contents of the current package insert.

[b]These recommended ages should not be construed as absolute. For example, 2 mo can be 6 to 10 wk. However, MMR usually should not be given to children younger than 12 mo. If measles vaccination is indicated, monovalent measles vaccine is recommended, and MMR should be given subsequently, at 12-15 mo.

[c]Vaccine abbreviations: HBV = Hepatitis B virus vaccine; DTP = diphtheria and tetanus toxoids and pertussis vaccine; DTaP = diphtheria and tetanus toxoids and acellular pertussis vaccine; Hib = *Haemophilus influenzae* type b conjugate vaccine; OPV = oral poliovirus vaccine (containing attenuated poliovirus types 1, 2, and 3); MMR = live measles, mumps, and rubella viruses vaccine; Td = adult tetanus toxoid (full dose) and diphtheria toxoid (reduced dose), for children ≥7 y and adults.

[d]See Table 3.13 (p 232). An acceptable alternative to minimize the number of visits for immunizing infants of HBsAg-negative mothers is to administer dose 1 at 0-2 mo, dose 2 at 4 mo, and dose 3 at 6 to 18 mo.

[e]See Table 3.8 (p 211).

[f](Hib: dose 3 of Hib is not indicated if the product for doses 1 and 2 was PedvaxHIB [PRP-OMP], available from Merck & Co, West Point, PA).

TABLE 1.4–Recommended Immunization Schedules for Children Not Immunized in the First Year of Life

Recommended Time/Age	Immunization(s)[a,b]	Comments
Younger Than 7 Years		
First visit	DTP, Hib[c], HBV, MMR, OPV	If indicated, tuberculin testing may be done at same visit. If child is 5 y of age or older, Hib is not indicated.
Interval after first visit:		
1 mo	DTP, HBV	OPV may be given if accelerated poliomyelitis vaccination is necessary, such as for travelers to areas where polio is endemic.
2 mo	DTP, Hib,[c] OPV	Second dose of Hib is indicated only in children whose first dose was received when younger than 15 mo.
≥8 mo	DTP or DTaP,[d] HBV, OPV	OPV is not given if the third dose was given earlier.
4-6 y (at or before school entry)	DTP or DTaP,[d] OPV	DTP or DTaP is not necessary if the fourth dose was given after the fourth birthday; OPV is not necessary if the third dose was given after the fourth birthday.
11-12 y	MMR	At entry to middle school or junior high school.
10 y later	Td	Repeat every 10 y throughout life.
7 Years and Older[e,f]		
First visit	HBV,[g] OPV, MMR, Td	
Interval after first visit:		
2 mo	HBV,[g] OPV, Td	OPV may also be given 1 mo after the first visit if accelerated poliomyelitis vaccination is necessary.
8-14 mo	HBV,[g] OPV, Td	OPV is not given if the third dose was given earlier.
11-12 y	MMR	At entry to middle school or junior high.
10 y later	Td	Repeat every 10 y throughout life.

[a]Abbreviations for vaccines are explained in the footnotes to Table 3. If all needed vaccines cannot be administered simultaneously, priority should be given to protecting the child against those diseases that pose the greatest immediate risk. In the US, these diseases for children younger than 2 y usually are measles and *Haemophilus influenzae* type b infection; for children older than 7 y, they are measles, mumps, and rubella (MMR).

[b]DTP or DTaP, HBV, Hib, MMR, and OPV can be given simultaneously at separate sites if failure of the patient to return for future immunizations is a concern.

[c]See *Haemophilus influenzae* Infections, p 210, including Table 3.9 (p 212).

[d]DTaP is not currently licensed for use in children younger than 15 mo of age and is not recommended for primary immunization (ie, first 3 doses) at any age.

[e]If person is 18 y or older, routine poliovirus vaccination is not indicated in the US.

[f]Minimal interval between doses of MMR is 1 mo.

[g]Priority should be given to hepatitis B immunization of adolescents (see Hepatitis B, p 232).

Table 1.5–Immunization Schedule Recommended by the Expanded
Programme on Immunization (EPI) of the World Health Organization

Age*	Immunization†
Birth	BCG, OPV, and HBV‡
6 wk	DTP, OPV, and HBV‡
10 wk	DTP and OPV
14 wk	DTP and OPV
9 mo	Measles and HBV‡
Women of childbearing age	Tetanus toxoid

*In many countries, OPV is administered to all children on the same day in national immunization campaigns. This strategy has been very effective in eliminating transmission of wild-type poliomyelitis virus.

†Vaccine abbreviations: BCG = bacillus Calmette-Guerin; OPV = oral poliovirus vaccine; DTP = diphtheria and tetanus toxoids and pertussis vaccine; HBV = hepatitis B vaccine.

‡HBV is recommended for all children in countries where hepatitis B surface antigenemia among adults has a prevalence of 2% or greater. Where perinatal transmission contributes a significant proportion of childhood infections, the first dose should be given at birth.

Comparable vaccines made by different manufacturers, when administered according to their licensed indications, have been considered interchangeable, although for some vaccines the data documenting interchangeability are limited. Vaccines that can be used interchangeably according to their licensed indication during a vaccine series include diphtheria and tetanus toxoids, whole-cell and acellular pertussis vaccines, live and inactivated polio vaccines, hepatitis B vaccines, and rabies vaccines. At this time, use of acellular pertussis vaccine is licensed only for use as the fourth and fifth doses. Human diploid cell rabies vaccine (HDCV) and rabies vaccine adsorbed (RVA) are interchangeable when given by IM injection for preexposure and postexposure prophylaxis, but RVA should not be used intradermally.

Currently licensed *Haemophilus influenzae* type b conjugate vaccines induce different immunologic responses in infants. Limited data suggest that infants given sequential doses of different vaccines produce a satisfactory antibody response after a complete primary series. Pending further data, the primary vaccine series for children younger than 15 months of age, if feasible, should be completed with the same conjugate vaccine. Any of the licensed conjugate vaccines can be used for the recommended booster dose at 12 to 15 months of age (see *Haemophilus influenzae* Infections, p 210).

Simultaneous Administration of Multiple Vaccines

Most vaccines can be safely and effectively administered simultaneously. No contraindications to the simultaneous administration of multiple vaccines routinely recommended for infants and children are known. Immune responses to one vaccine generally do not interfere with those to other vaccines; exceptions include interference among the three oral poliovirus serotypes in trivalent OPV and concurrent administration of cholera and yellow fever vaccines. Simultaneous administration of MMR, DTP, and OPV has resulted in rates of seroconversion and of side effects similar to those observed when the vaccines are administered at separate times. Because simultaneous administration of common vaccines is not known to affect the efficacy or safety of any of the routinely recommended childhood vaccines, if return of a vaccine recipient for further immunization is doubtful, simultaneous administration of all vaccines (including DTP or DTaP, OPV, MMR, hepatitis B, and *Haemophilus influenzae* type b vaccines) appropriate for the age and previous vaccination status of the recipient is recommended. Evidence suggests that the simultaneous administration of multiple needed vaccines can potentially raise immunization rates by 9% to 17%.

For persons preparing for foreign travel, multiple vaccines can generally be given concurrently. An exception is the simultaneous administration of yellow fever and cholera vaccines. Antibody responses to both cholera and yellow fever vaccines are decreased if given simultaneously or within a short time of each other. If possible, these vaccines should be separated by at least 3 weeks. If both vaccines are necessary and time constraints exist, these vaccines can be given simultaneously or within a 3-week period with the understanding that antibody responses may not be optimal. However, the currently used cholera vaccine provides only limited protection of brief duration, and few indications for its use exist.

When vaccines commonly associated with local or systemic reactions (eg, cholera, parenteral typhoid vaccines, and plague) are given simultaneously, the reactions can be accentuated. Thus, in most circumstances, if feasible, these vaccines should be given on separate occasions.

Lapsed Immunizations

A lapse in the immunization schedule does not require reinstitution of the entire series. If a dose of DTP, OPV, *Haemophilus influenzae* type b conjugate, or hepatitis B vaccine is missed, immunization should occur on the next visit as if the usual interval had elapsed. The charts of children in whom immunizations have been missed or postponed should be flagged to remind health care providers to complete immunization schedules at the next available opportunity.

Reimmunization

Epidemics of measles involving large numbers of high school and college-aged students led to the decision to recommend universal measles reimmunization. Some data suggest that control of mumps may require reimmunization. A second dose of MMR, therefore, should be given to all children entering middle school, enrolling in college, or traveling abroad. Some states follow the recommendations of the Advisory Committee on Immunization Practices (ACIP) of the US Public Health Service and require MMR reimmunization at entry to primary school. In states and localities where the law mandates revaccination at or before school entry, the pediatrician should revaccinate at a younger age, but where the law is mute the pediatrician should explain to the parents why revaccination at a later age (11 or 12 years) is preferred by the Academy. In any case, a child who has received two doses of MMR at least 1 month apart beginning at age 12 months or older should be considered adequately immunized. Reactions to reimmunization are no greater than those seen after primary immunization and are likely to be less common, since many recipients are already immune.

Unknown or Uncertain Immunization Status

The physician may encounter some children with an uncertain immunization status. Many young adults and some children have no adequate documentation of immunizations, and recollection by the parent or guardian may be of questionable validity. In general, these individuals should be considered susceptible and appropriate immunizations should be administered. No evidence indicates that administration of MMR, *Haemophilus influenzae*, hepatitis B, or poliovirus vaccine to already immune recipients is harmful. Td, rather than DTP, or DTaP should be given to those 7 years or older.

Immunizations Received Outside the United States

Persons vaccinated in other countries including international adoptees, refugees, and exchange students should be immunized according to recommended schedules in the United States for healthy infants, children, and adolescents (see Tables 1.3 and 1.4, pp 23 and 24). Only written documentation should be accepted as evidence of prior immunization. Although occasional vaccines of inadequate potency have been produced in other countries, the majority of vaccines used worldwide, including those in developing nations, are produced with adequate quality control standards and are reliable. In general, written immunization records may be considered valid if the vaccine, date of administration, interval between doses, and age of the patient at the time of vaccination would be appropriate for a comparable vaccine produced in the United States.

Vaccine Dose

The recommended doses of vaccines are derived from theoretical considerations, experimental trials, and experience. Reduction in the recommended doses can result in an inadequate response and leave the recipient susceptible. Exceeding the recommended dose may also be hazardous because excessive local concentrations of injectable, inactivated vaccines might result or because an excessive dose of a live vaccine might be given (a theoretical, but unproven, risk).

The Committee does not recommend reducing or dividing doses of DTP or any vaccine, including those given to premature or low-birth-weight infants. The efficacy of this practice in reducing the frequency of adverse events associated with DTP has not been demonstrated. Such a practice might also confer less protection against disease than that which is achieved with the recommended doses. A diminished antibody response in both term and premature infants to reduced doses of DTP has been reported (see Preterm Infants, p 51). A previous immunization with a dose that was less than the standard dose or one administered by a nonstandard route should not be counted and the patient should be revaccinated as appropriate for age.

Active Immunization of Persons Who Recently Received Immune Globulin

In general, live-virus vaccines given parenterally have diminished immunogenicity when given shortly before or during a period of several months after receipt of immune globulin (IG). Recent evidence demonstrates that high doses of IG inhibit the response to measles vaccine for a prolonged period. The duration of inhibition varies directly with the dose of IG administered. Inhibition of immune response to rubella vaccine, while of shorter duration, has also been demonstrated. The appropriate suggested interval between IG administration and measles vaccination will vary with the indication for IG (which determines the dose). Suggested intervals are given in Table 3.30 (p 319; see also Measles, p 318). If IG must be given within 14 days after the administration of measles or measles-containing vaccines, these live-virus vaccines should be administered again after the period specified in Table 3.30, unless serologic testing indicates immunity, ie, adequate serum antibodies were produced.

In contrast, concurrent administration of recommended doses of Hepatitis B Immune Globulin (HBIG), Tetanus Immune Globulin (TIG), or Rabies Immune Globulin (RIG), and the corresponding inactivated vaccine or toxoid in postexposure prophylaxis, does not impair the immune response to these vaccines and provides immediate protection and active or passive immunity. Standard doses of the corresponding vaccines should be used, and increases in the vaccine dose volume or number of immunizations are not indicated. Vaccines should be administered at sites different from that of IG. (See chapters on specific diseases in Section 3 for further discussion.)

Immune globulins have been reported not to interfere with the immune response to OPV and yellow fever vaccine. Hence, these live vaccines can be administered simultaneously with IG to individuals such as travelers whose departure is imminent. Similarly, data indicate that IGs do not significantly affect the responses of infants to DTP. However, maternally acquired passive antibodies may complicate the evaluation of responses in young infants.

Tuberculin Testing

Recommendations for tuberculin testing (see Tuberculosis, p 485) are independent of those for immunization. Tuberculin testing at any age is not a prerequisite before administration of live-virus vaccines, such as MMR. A tuberculin skin test can be applied in the same visit that MMR is administered. Because measles vaccine can temporarily suppress tuberculin reactivity, if tuberculin testing is indicated and cannot be done at the same time as measles vaccination, tuberculin testing should be postponed 4 to 6 weeks.

Record Keeping

Patient's personal immunization record: Each state health department has developed an official immunization record. This record should be given to the parents of every newborn infant and should be accorded the status of a birth certificate or passport and retained with vital documents for subsequent referral. The Committee urges physicians to cooperate with this endeavor by recording immunization data in this record and by encouraging patients not only to preserve the record but also to present it at each visit to a health care provider.

The immunization record is especially important for patients who move frequently. It will facilitate an accurate patient medical record, enable the physician to evaluate the child's immunization status, and fulfill the need for documentation of immunizations for child care and school attendance and admission to other institutions and organizations.

Until computer-based immunization registries are functioning reliably throughout the United States, parents and physicians must rely on the personal immunization record to document each child's immunization status.

Physicians' immunization records: Every physician should maintain the immunization history of each patient in a permanent office record that can be reviewed easily and updated when subsequent immunizations are administered. The format of the record should facilitate identification and recall of patients in need of immunization.

Records of children whose immunizations have been postponed should be flagged to indicate the need to complete immunizations. For all immunizations, the following data should be entered into the patient's permanent medical record and the patient's personal immunization record: (1) month, day, and year of administration; (2) vaccine or other biologic administered; (3) manufacturer; (4) lot number and its expiration date; (5) site and route of administration; and (6) name, address, and title of the health care provider administering the vaccine.

The National Childhood Vaccine Act of 1986 requires that the above information be recorded in the patient's personal medical record for childhood-mandated vaccines. As of December 1993, those vaccines included diphtheria, tetanus, pertussis, poliovirus, measles, mumps, and rubella vaccines. In addition, reporting of selected events that occur after vaccination is required (see Reporting of Adverse Reactions, p 30).

Vaccine Safety and Contraindications

Risks and Adverse Events

Although modern immunizing agents are generally considered safe and effective, they are neither completely safe nor completely effective. Some vaccinees may have an untoward reaction, and some will not be protected. The goal in vaccine development is to achieve the highest degree of protection with the lowest rate of untoward effects.

Risks associated with the use of vaccines vary from trivial and inconvenient to severe and life threatening. In developing recommendations for the use of a vaccine, vaccine benefits and safety, and the risks of the natural disease are weighed. The resulting recommendations attempt to minimize the risk by providing specific advice on dose, route, and timing of the vaccine and by delineating circumstances that warrant precaution in, or abstention from, administering the vaccine.

Vaccine side effects are usually mild to moderate in severity, with no permanent sequelae. Because such reactions are intrinsic to the immunizing antigen or some component of the vaccine, they may occur frequently and are unavoidable. Examples include fever or local irritation after administration of DTP vaccine and fever and rash after administration of live measles virus vaccine.

Sterile abscesses have occurred after injection of a number of killed vaccines. The abscesses presumably result from the irritating nature of the vaccine or its adjuvant vehicle; in some instances they may be caused by inadvertent SC inoculation of a vaccine intended for IM use.

On rare occasion, serious consequences of vaccination may also occur. These result in permanent sequelae or may even be life threatening. These individual events are usually not predictable (eg, paralytic poliomyelitis after administration of OPV to an otherwise healthy child).

The occurrence of a clinical event after the administration of vaccine does not prove that the vaccine caused the symptoms or signs. Vaccines are administered to infants and children during a period in their lives when certain clinical conditions most often become manifest (eg, seizure disorders). For most live-virus vaccines, definitive etiologic association between the vaccine and a subsequent clinical illness requires isolating the vaccine strain from the patient. However, even this generalization has exceptions. For example, vaccine-type poliovirus is commonly found in the stool of vaccinees for several weeks or more after immunization. The occurrence of a neurologic syndrome during this period (eg, encephalitis) does not prove that the poliovirus vaccine caused the illness. Better evidence can be obtained by isolating the agent from normally sterile body fluids or tissues, such as the brain or the cerebrospinal fluid. Association of an adverse clinical event with a specific vaccine is suggested if vaccinees experience the event at a rate significantly higher than that in nonvaccinated groups of similar age and residence. Unusual clustering of a condition in vaccinees in a limited interval after vaccination may also suggest a causal association.

Although a specific condition occurring in a single individual after immunization does not provide sufficient evidence to link that condition to the vaccine, reporting of each of these occurrences is important because, in conjunction with other reports, it may provide clues to a new or unanticipated adverse reaction.

Reporting of Adverse Reactions

Before administering a subsequent dose of any vaccine, parents and patients should be questioned concerning side effects and possible reactions after previous doses, and physicians should be alert to possible deviations from the expected outcome. No recommendations can anticipate all possible contingencies, particularly with newly developed vaccines. Unexpected events occurring soon after administration of any vaccine, particularly those severe enough to require medical attention, should be noted; a detailed description of the occurrence should be recorded; and a report should be made, as subsequently described.

The National Childhood Vaccine Injury Act of 1986 requires physicians and other health care providers who administer vaccines to maintain permanent vaccination records and to report occurrences of certain adverse events stipulated in the Act, as originally posed (see Table 1.6, p 32). The vaccines to which these requirements apply are measles, mumps, rubella, polio, pertussis, diphtheria, and tetanus (see Record Keeping, p 28).

Health-care providers are required to report selected events occurring after vaccination to the Vaccine Adverse Events Reporting System (VAERS).*

Adverse events other than those listed in Table 1.6 (p 32), or those occurring after administration of other vaccines, especially events that are serious or unusual, should also be reported to VAERS. Forms from VAERS (see Figure 1, p 34) and instructions are also available in the *FDA Drug Bulletin* and the *PDR*.

All reports of suspected adverse events after administration of any vaccine, irrespective of the age of the recipient, will be accepted. Submission of a report does not necessarily denote that the vaccine caused the adverse event.

All patient-identifying information will be kept confidential. Written notification that the report has been received is provided to the person submitting the form. Staff from VAERS will contact the person for follow-up of the patient's condition at 60 days and at 1 year after serious adverse events.

Vaccine Injury Compensation

The National Vaccine Injury Compensation Program is a system in which compensation is made on behalf of an individual who was injured or died after a vaccine-related event. The program is intended as an alternative to civil litigation in the traditional tort system in that negligence need not be proven. The program became effective in 1988.

The Act established a Vaccine Injury Compensation Table (see p 615) listing the vaccines covered by the program as well as the injuries, disabilities, illnesses, and conditions (including death) for which compensation may be made. As of December 1993, this table is subject to change for prospective cases. The table also defines the period of time during which the first symptom or significant aggravation of the injury must appear. This period often differs from that required for reporting. Additional information about the program is available from the following:

National Vaccine Injury Compensation Program
Health Resources and Services Administration
Parklawn Building, Room 8-05
5600 Fishers Lane
Rockville, MD 20857
Telephone: 800/338-2382

Persons wishing to file a claim for a vaccine injury should call or write to the following:

United States Court of Federal Claims
717 Madison Place, NW
Washington, DC 20005-1011
Telephone: 202/219-9657

---

*See Directory of Telephone Numbers, p 601.

TABLE 1.6–Reportable Events Following Immunization[a]

Vaccine/ Toxoid[b]	Adverse Event	Interval From Vaccination to Onset of Event	
		For Reporting[c]	For Compensation[d]
DTP, P, DTP/ Poliovirus combined	A. Anaphylaxis or anaphylactic shock	24 h	24 h
	B. Encephalopathy (or encephalitis)[e]	7 d	3 d
	C. Shock-collapse or hypotonic-hyporesponsive collapse[f]	7 d	3 d
	D. Residual seizure disorder[g]	(See footnote g)	3 d
	E. Any acute complication or sequela (including death) of above events	No limit	Not applicable
	F. Events described as con-traindications to additional doses of vaccine (see manufacturer's package insert[h])	(See package insert[h])	
Measles, Mumps, and Rubella; DT, Td, T	A. Anaphylaxis or anaphylactic shock	24 h	24 h
	B. Encephalopathy (or encephalitis)[e]	15 d for measles, mumps, and rubella vaccine; 7 d for DT, Td, and T	15 d for measles, mumps, and rubella vaccine; 3d for DT, Td, and T
	C. Residual seizure disorder[g]	(See footnote g)	15 d for measles, mumps, or rubella vaccine; 3 d for DT, Td, and T
	D. Any acute complication or sequela (including death) of above events	No limit	
	E. Events described as contra-indications to additional doses of vaccine (see manufacturer's package insert[h])	(See package insert[h])	
OPV	A. Paralytic poliomyelitis		
	• in a nonimmunodeficient recipient	30 d	30 d
	• in an immunodeficient recipient	6 mo	6 mo
	• in a vaccine-associated community case	No limit	Not applicable
	B. Any acute complication or sequela (including death) of above events	No limit	Not applicable
	C. Events described as contra-indications to additional doses of vaccine (see manufacturer's package insert[h])	(See package insert[h])	

| Vaccine/ Toxoid[b] | Adverse Event | Interval From Vaccination to Onset of Event | |
		For Reporting[c]	For Compensation[d]
Inactivated Polio Vaccine	A. Anaphylaxis or anaphylactic shock	24 h	24 h
	B. Any acute complication or sequela (including death) of above events	No limit	Not applicable
	C. Events described as contra-indications to additional doses of vaccine (see manufacturer's package insert[h])	(See package insert[h])	

[a]As of December 1993.

[b]The vaccine/toxoid abbreviations, in alphabetical order, are: DT = diphtheria and tetanus toxoids; DTP = diphtheria and tetanus toxoids and pertussis vaccine (pediatric); OPV = oral poliovirus vaccine, live, trivalent; P = pertussis vaccine; T = tetanus toxoid; and Td = tetanus and diphtheria toxoids (for adult use).

[c]Adverse events that are required by *National Childhood Vaccine Injury Act of 1986* (NCVIA) to be reported to Vaccine Adverse Events Reporting System (VAERS) if their onset is within the indicated interval after vaccination.

[d]Adverse events that may be compensable under NCVIA if the onset is within this interval after vaccination.

[e]Encephalopathy means any significant acquired abnormality of, injury to, or impairment of function of, the brain. Among the frequent manifestations of encephalopathy are focal and diffuse neurologic signs, increased intracranial pressure, or changes lasting at least 6 h in level of consciousness, with or without convulsions. The neurologic signs and symptoms of encephalopathy may be temporary with complete recovery or may result in various degrees of permanent impairment. Signs and symptoms such as high-pitched and unusual screaming, persistent inconsolable crying, and bulging fontanel are compatible with an encephalopathy, but in and of themselves are not conclusive evidence of encephalopathy. Encephalopathy can usually be documented by slow-wave activity on an electroencephalogram.

[f]Shock-collapse or hypotonic-hyporesponsive collapse may include signs or symptoms such as decrease or loss of muscle tone, paralysis (partial or complete), hemiplegia, hemiparesis, loss of color or turning pale white or blue, unresponsiveness to environmental stimuli, depression of or loss of consciousness, prolonged sleeping with difficulty being aroused, or cardiovascular or respiratory arrest.

[g]Residual seizure disorder may have occurred if no other seizure or convulsion unaccompanied by fever or accompanied by a fever of <102°F occurred before the first seizure or convulsion after the administration of the vaccine involved, and if, in the case of measles-, mumps-, or rubella-containing vaccines, the first seizure or convulsion occurred within 15 d after vaccination, or, in the case of any other vaccine, the first seizure or convulsion occurred within 3 d after vaccination, and, if 2 or more seizures or convulsions unaccompanied by fever or accompanied by a fever of <102°F occurred within 1 y after vaccination. The terms "seizure" and "convulsion" include grand mal, petit mal, absence, myoclonic, tonic-clonic, and focal motor seizures and signs.

[h]Refer to the CONTRAINDICATION section of the manufacturer's package insert for each vaccine/toxoid. Adapted from Update on adult immunization: recommendations of the Immunization Practices Advisory Committee (ACIP). *MMWR*. 1991;40(RR-12):53-54.

VAERS

VACCINE ADVERSE EVENT REPORTING SYSTEM
24 Hour Toll-free information line 1-800-822-7967
P.O. Box 1100, Rockville, MD 20849-1100
PATIENT IDENTITY KEPT CONFIDENTIAL

For CDC/FDA Use Only

VAERS Number _____

Date Received _____

Patient Name:	Vaccine administered by (Name):	Form completed by (Name):
Last First M.I.	Responsible Physician _____	Relation ☐ Vaccine Provider ☐ Patient/Parent to Patient ☐ Manufacturer ☐ Other
Address	Facility Name/Address	Address *(if different from patient or provider)*
City State Zip	City State Zip	City State Zip
Telephone no. (_____)_____	Telephone no. (_____)_____	Telephone no. (_____)_____

1. State	2. County where administered	3. Date of birth / / mm dd yy	4. Patient age	5. Sex ☐ M ☐ F	6. Date form completed / / mm dd yy

7. Describe adverse event(s) (symptoms, signs, time course) and treatment, if any	8. Check all appropriate: ☐ Patient died (date ___/___/___) mm dd yy ☐ Life threatening illness ☐ Required emergency room/doctor visit ☐ Required hospitalization (_____days) ☐ Resulted in prolongation of hospitalization ☐ Resulted in permanent disability ☐ None of the above

9. Patient recovered ☐ YES ☐ NO ☐ UNKNOWN	10. Date of vaccination	11. Adverse event onset
12. Relevant diagnostic tests/laboratory data	/ / mm dd yy Time_____ AM PM	/ / mm dd yy Time_____ AM PM

13. Enter all vaccines given on date listed in no. 10

	Vaccine (type)	Manufacturer	Lot number	Route/Site	No. Previous doses
a.					
b.					
c.					
d.					

14. Any other vaccinations within 4 weeks of date listed in no. 10

	Vaccine (type)	Manufacturer	Lot number	Route/Site	No. Previous doses	Date given
a.						
b.						

15. Vaccinated at: ☐ Private doctor's office/hospital ☐ Military clinic/hospital ☐ Public health clinic/hospital ☐ Other/unknown	16. Vaccine purchased with: ☐ Private funds ☐ Military funds ☐ Public funds ☐ Other /unknown	17. Other medications

18. Illness at time of vaccination (specify)	19. Pre-existing physician-diagnosed allergies, birth defects, medical conditions (specify)

20. Have you reported this adverse event previously?	☐ No ☐ To health department ☐ To doctor ☐ To manufacturer	*Only for children 5 and under*
		22. Birth weight _____ lb. _____ oz.	23. No. of brothers and sisters

21. Adverse event following prior vaccination (check all applicable, specify)

	Adverse Event	Onset Age	Type Vaccine	Dose no. in series	*Only for reports submitted by manufacturer/immunization project*
☐ In patient					24. Mfr. / imm. proj. report no.	25. Date received by mfr. / imm. proj.
☐ In brother					26. 15 day report?	27. Report type
or sister					☐ Yes ☐ No	☐ Initial ☐ Follow-Up

Health care providers and manufacturers are required by law (42 USC 300aa-25) to report reactions to vaccines listed in the Vaccine Injury Table. Reports for reactions to other vaccines are voluntary except when required as a condition of immunization grant awards.

Form VAERS -1

Precautions and Contraindications

Precautions and contraindications are described in specific *Red Book* chapters on vaccine-preventable diseases and in the manufacturers' package insert; they indicate circumstances in which the physician should be cautious in administering vaccines. In some of these situations, vaccine administration may still be indicated after the benefits and risks to the child have been carefully assessed.

Minor illness and fever. Most vaccines are intended for use in healthy individuals or in those whose diseases or conditions are not affected by immunization. For optimal safety, vaccines should not be used if an undesirable side effect or adverse reaction to the vaccine may be seriously accentuated by an underlying illness. A common situation is the child scheduled for immunizations who has an acute illness. Minor illnesses do not contraindicate the use of vaccines, particularly when a child frequently has a minor upper respiratory tract infection or allergic rhinitis. In this situation, no evidence indicates an increased risk from immunization. Deferring immunization in such situations frequently results in unimmunized children who will need to "catch up" with immunizations at a later age or who develop vaccine-preventable disease.

For the child with an acute, febrile illness, guidelines for immunization are based on the physician's assessment of the child's illness and the specific vaccines the child is scheduled to receive. Fever per se is not a contraindication to immunizations. However, if fever or other manifestations suggest a moderate or serious illness, the child should not be vaccinated until he or she has recovered. Vaccine-specific recommendations are as follows:

- *Live-virus vaccines.* Minor respiratory, gastrointestinal, or other illnesses with or without fever do not contraindicate the use of live-virus vaccines such as MMR. The preponderance of evidence demonstrates that children with febrile upper respiratory infections have serologic responses similar to those of well children after vaccination. No evidence indicates an increased risk of adverse events from vaccination of children with minor illnesses with or without fever. Deferring vaccination of children with minor illness frequently results in failure to immunize a large proportion of young children at the desired age. The potential benefit of immunization at the recommended age, irrespective of the presence of a minor illness, outweighs the possible increased risk of vaccine failure.

- *DTP and DTaP.* Mild illnesses (eg, upper respiratory illnesses) do not contraindicate administration of DTP or DTaP. However, a moderate or severe illness with or without fever is a contraindication, as the vaccine may be blamed for the signs and symptoms associated with the illness.

- *Child with frequent febrile illnesses.* In the circumstance of the child who repeatedly has moderate or severe febrile illnesses at the time of scheduled immunizations, the child should be asked to return as soon as the current febrile illness is terminated so that immunization can be completed.

- *Immunocompromised children.* Special consideration needs to be given to immunocompromised children, such as those with congenital immunodeficiencies, HIV infection, or malignancy, or recipients of immunosuppressive therapy. Immunization of children with these problems is discussed in detail in the section on Immunodeficient and Immunosuppressed Children (see p 53).

A concise summary of contraindications and precautions (as of May 1992) to immunizations is given in the *Standards for Pediatric Immunization Practices* (see p 602).

Hypersensitivity Reactions to Vaccine Constituents

Hypersensitivity reactions to constituents of vaccines are rare. In some instances, although symptoms appear soon after a vaccine is administered, differentiation between allergic reaction to the vaccine and reaction to an environmental allergen is impossible.

Four types of hypersensitivity reactions believed related to vaccine constituents are (1) allergic reactions to egg or egg-related antigens, (2) mercury sensitivity in some recipients of immune globulins or vaccines, (3) antibiotic-induced allergic reactions, and (4) hypersensitivity to some component of the infectious agent or other vaccine components.

Allergic reactions to egg-related antigens. Current measles, mumps, yellow fever, and influenza vaccines contain small amounts of egg proteins. Skin testing with the vaccine has been recommended before administration in individuals with a history of systemic anaphylactic symptoms (generalized urticaria, shock, or manifestations of upper or lower airway obstruction) after egg ingestion. The predictive value of such skin testing with MMR vaccine has recently been questioned because the data suggest that anaphylactic reactions to the vaccine may not be related to hypersensitivity to egg antigens but to some other, as yet undefined, component. At the present time, particularly in view of recommendations in the package inserts, continued skin testing of persons with a history of anaphylactic symptoms after egg ingestion seems advisable even though the value is uncertain.

Less severe or localized manifestations of allergy to egg or to feathers are not contraindications to vaccine administration and do not usually warrant vaccine skin testing.

An egg-sensitive individual can be tested with the vaccine before it is used in the following manner:

1. *Scratch, prick, or puncture test.* A drop of 1:10 dilution of the vaccine in physiologic saline is applied at the site of a superficial scratch, prick, or puncture on the volar surface of the forearm. Positive (histamine) and negative (physiologic saline) control tests should also be used. The test is read after 15 to 20 minutes. A positive test is a wheal 3 mm larger than that of the saline control, usually with surrounding erythema. The histamine control must be positive for valid interpretation. If the result of this test is negative, an intradermal (ID) test is performed.

2. *Intradermal test.* A dose of 0.02 mL of a 1:100 dilution of the vaccine in physiologic saline is injected; positive and negative control skin tests are performed concurrently. A wheal 5 mm or larger than the negative control with surrounding erythema is considered a positive reaction.

Some investigators have recommended the use of a puncture test using undiluted vaccine or an ID test using a 1:100 dilution as the only skin test necessary for MMR vaccine.

Note: Scratch, prick, or puncture tests with other allergens have resulted in fatalities in highly allergic individuals. Although such untoward effects have not been reported for vaccine testing, all skin tests and "desensitization" procedures should be performed by trained personnel who can treat acute anaphylaxis. Necessary medications and equipment should be readily available (see Treatment of Anaphylactic Reactions, p 49).

"Desensitization." If the child has a history of severe egg sensitivity and has a positive skin test to the vaccine, the child still may be given the vaccine using a "desensitization" procedure if immunization is imperative. A suggested protocol is subcutaneous (SC) administration of the following successive doses at 15- to 20-minute intervals:

1. 0.05 mL of 1:10 dilution
2. 0.05 mL of full strength
3. 0.10 mL of full strength
4. 0.15 mL of full strength
5. 0.20 mL of full strength

This type of skin testing and "desensitization" should be undertaken only if supervised by a physician experienced in the management of anaphylaxis and with necessary equipment immediately available.

Mercury sensitivity in some recipients of immune globulins or vaccines. Mercury from the organic mercurial preservatives used in the preparation of immune globulin (IG) for intramuscular use can accumulate in individuals given repeated injections. Only one case of proven mercury sensitivity (acrodynia) has been reported. Intravenous immune globulin (IGIV) does not contain preservatives. Exposure to vaccines containing mercury can elicit hypersensitivity, usually manifested as a local, delayed-type hypersensitivity reaction. Even when results of patch or local ID tests indicate hypersensitivity, most patients do not react to thiomersal administered as a vaccine component.

Antibiotic-induced allergic reactions. Antibiotic reactions have been suspected in individuals with known allergies who received vaccines containing trace amounts of antibiotics. Proof of a causal relationship is difficult and often impossible to confirm.

Inactivated poliovirus vaccine (IPV) contains trace amounts of streptomycin and neomycin. Live measles, mumps, and rubella vaccines, singly or in combination, contain an extremely small amount of neomycin (25 µg). Some persons allergic to neomycin may experience a delayed-type, local reaction 48 to 96 hours after administration of MMR or IPV. The reaction consists of an erythematous, pruritic papule. This minor reaction is of little importance when weighed against the benefit of immunization, and should not be considered a contraindication. However, if the person has a history of anaphylactic reaction to neomycin, neomycin-containing vaccines should not be used.

No currently recommended vaccine contains penicillin or its derivatives.

Hypersensitivity to some component of the infectious agent or other vaccine components. DTP vaccine (and, to a lesser extent, parenterally administered typhoid, plague, and cholera vaccines) is associated with local and occasionally systemic reactions, usually of a toxic rather than a hypersensitivity nature. Such reactions are less frequent with DTaP vaccines, in which the pertussis component is acellular. On occasion, urticarial or anaphylactic reactions have occurred in DTP, DT, Td, or tetanus toxoid vaccine recipients. Tetanus and diphtheria antigen-specific antibodies of the IgE type have been identified in some of these patients. Although attributing a specific sensitivity to vaccine components is very difficult, an immediate, severe, or anaphylactic allergic reaction to one of these vaccines is a contraindication to subsequent immunization of the patient with the specific product. A transient urticarial rash, however, unless it occurs immediately after immunization, is not a contraindication to further doses. (For more detailed discussion, see Pertussis, p 361.)

Persons who have high serum concentrations of tetanus IgG antibody, usually as the result of frequent booster immunizations, can have an increased incidence and severity of reactions to subsequent vaccine administration (see Tetanus, p 463).

Reactions resembling serum sickness have been reported in approximately 6% of patients after a booster dose of human diploid rabies vaccine, probably due to sensitization to human albumin that had been altered chemically by the virus-inactivating agent.

Japanese encephalitis virus vaccine has been associated with generalized urticaria and angioedema, sometimes with respiratory distress and hypotension occurring within minutes of vaccination to as long as 2 weeks after vaccination. The pathogenesis of such reactions is not understood. Persons with history of urticaria are at increased risk for an adverse reaction. Vaccinees should be observed for 30 minutes after vaccination and warned about the possibility of delayed urticaria and potentially life-threatening angioedema.

Significant hypersensitivity reactions occurring as a result of pneumococcal, *Haemophilus influenzae*, and hepatitis B vaccines appear to be extremely rare.

An unusual sensitivity to killed measles virus vaccine (KMV) has been documented. This vaccine has not been available for more than 25 years, but it was received by many patients between 1963 and 1967 in the United States. A moderate-to-severe local reaction, occasionally with systemic symptoms, was observed in KMV recipients when live measles virus vaccine was administered months or years later. In some KMV recipients, exposure to natural (wild) measles virus as many as 16 years later resulted in atypical measles (often a severe illness with fever, pulmonary infiltrates, polyserositis, and a vesicular and/or hemorrhagic rash resembling Rocky Mountain spotted fever). Immunologically, the local reaction and atypical illness represent either an Arthus reaction, a delayed hypersensitivity reaction (cell-mediated immune reaction), or both.

Misconceptions Concerning Vaccine Contraindications

Some health care providers inappropriately consider certain conditions or circumstances to be contraindications to vaccination. Conditions most often inappropriately regarded as routine contraindications include the following:

- **Mild acute illness with low-grade fever or mild diarrheal illness in an otherwise well child.**
- **Current antimicrobial therapy or the convalescent phase of illness.**
- **Reaction to a previous DTP dose that involved only soreness, redness, or swelling in the immediate vicinity of the vaccination site or temperature of less than 105°F (40.5°C).**
- **Prematurity.** The appropriate age for initiating most immunizations in the prematurely born infant is the usual recommended chronologic age. Vaccine doses should not be reduced for preterm infants. (See Preterm Infants, p 51, and Hepatitis B, p 231.)
- **Pregnancy of mother or other household contact.**

- **Recent exposure to an infectious disease**.
- **Breast-feeding**. The only vaccine virus that has been isolated from breast milk is rubella vaccine virus. No evidence indicates that breast milk from women immunized against rubella is harmful to infants.
- **A history of nonspecific allergies or relatives with allergies**.
- **Allergies to penicillin or any other antibiotic, except anaphylactic reactions to neomycin or streptomycin** (see Hypersensitivity Reactions to Vaccine Constituents, p 36). These reactions occur rarely, if ever. None of the vaccines licensed in the United States contains penicillin.
- **Allergies to duck meat or duck feathers**. No vaccine available in the United States is produced in substrates containing duck antigens.
- **Family history of convulsions in persons considered for pertussis or measles vaccination** (see Children With Personal or Family History of Seizures, p 59).
- **Family history of sudden infant death syndrome in children considered for DTP vaccination**.
- **Family history of an adverse event, unrelated to immunosuppression, after vaccination**.
- **Malnutrition**.

Reporting of Vaccine-Preventable Diseases

Nearly all vaccine-preventable diseases are reportable throughout the United States. Public health officials depend on health care providers to report promptly to state or local health departments suspected cases of vaccine-preventable disease. These reports are transmitted weekly to the CDC and are used to detect outbreaks, monitor disease, control strategies, and evaluate national immunization practices and policies.

Standards for Pediatric Immunization Practices

In 1992, national *Standards for Pediatric Immunization Practices*, recommended by the National Vaccine Advisory Committee, were approved by the United States Public Health Service and endorsed by the Academy. These standards are recommended for use by all health professionals providing care in public or private health care settings who are involved in the administration of vaccines or management of immunization services for children. Their use is intended to augment preschool immunization rates, control vaccine-preventable disease outbreaks, and, as a result, meet the national health objectives for immunization by the year 2000 or before. Although not all providers have the resources necessary to fully implement the *Standards* immediately, providers by adopting these standards can enhance their policies and practices for delivery of vaccines.

The *Standards* are given in Appendix II (p 602).

Passive Immunization

Passive immunization entails administration of preformed antibody to a recipient. It is indicated in the following general circumstances for the prevention or amelioration of infectious diseases:

- When persons are deficient in synthesis of antibody as a result of congenital or acquired B-lymphocyte cell defects, alone or in combination with other immunodeficiencies.
- When a person susceptible to a disease is exposed to that infection, especially when that person has a high risk of complications from the disease (eg, a child with leukemia exposed to varicella or measles), or when time does not permit adequate protection by active immunization alone (eg, some postexposure situations involving measles, rabies, or hepatitis B).
- Therapeutically, when a disease is already present, antibody may ameliorate or aid in suppressing the effects of a toxin (eg, food-borne or wound [not infant] botulism, diphtheria, or tetanus).

Passive immunization or serotherapy has been accomplished with several different types of products. The choice is dictated by the types of products available, the type of antibody desired, the route of administration, timing, and other considerations. These products include Immune Globulin (IG) (Human) and specific ("hyperimmune") immune globulins (Human), all of which are intended for intramuscular administration; Immune Globulin Intravenous (IGIV) (Human); human plasma; and antibodies of animal origin.

Indications for administration of IG other than those relevant to infectious diseases are not reviewed in the *Red Book*. Examples include idiopathic thrombocytopenia purpura and treatment of certain poisonous snake bites.

Blood components and whole blood for transfusion (including plasma) from registered blood banks in the United States are tested to prevent transmission by these products of blood-borne pathogens, including syphilis, hepatitis B, hepatitis C, HIV viruses, and human T-cell leukemia viruses (HTLV-1 and -2). A similar array of tests is performed by US-licensed establishments that collect plasma used only for manufacture into plasma derivatives such as IGIV, IG, and specific immune globulins. US-licensed IGIV, IG, and specific immune globulins have not transmitted any of these diseases.

Immune Globulin

Immune Globulin (Human) is derived from the pooled plasma of adults by an alcohol-fractionation procedure. It consists primarily of the immunoglobulin fraction (at least 95% IgG and trace amounts of IgA and IgM), is sterile, and is not known to transmit hepatitis, HIV, or any other infectious disease agent. It is a concentrated protein solution (approximately 16.5%; that is, 165 mg/mL).

Immune globulin contains specific antibodies in proportion to the infectious and immunization experience of the population from whose plasma it was prepared. Large numbers of donors (at least 1,000 donors per lot of final product) are used to ensure inclusion of a broad spectrum of antibodies.

Immune globulin is currently recommended for intramuscular administration. Since some recipients of intramuscular IG experience local pain and most feel some local discomfort, IG should be administered deep in a large muscle mass, usually in the gluteal region. Ordinarily, no more than 5 mL should be administered in one site in an adult or large child; lesser amounts (1 to 3 mL) should be given to small children and infants. Seldom should more than 20 mL be given at any one time, even to an adult.

Peak serum concentrations of antibodies are usually achieved 48 to 72 hours after IM inoculation. The serum half-life is generally 3 to 4 weeks. Some investigators have used slow SC administration in immunodeficient patients.

Intravenous use of IG is contraindicated. Intradermal use of IG is not recommended.

Indications for the Use of Immune Globulin

Replacement Therapy in Antibody-Deficiency Disorders. The usual dose is 100 mg/kg (equivalent to 0.66 mL/kg) per month. Customary practice is to administer two times this dose initially and to adjust the interval (2 to 4 weeks) between administration of the doses, based on the trough IgG concentrations and on the clinical response (absence of, or decrease in infections). In most cases, this form of therapy has been replaced by IGIV.

Hepatitis A Prophylaxis. Immune globulin can prevent clinical disease resulting from hepatitis A virus in exposed susceptible individuals when given within 14 days of exposure. The usual dose is 0.02 mL/kg (maximum dose 2 mL), given as soon as possible after exposure. For pre-exposure use for prolonged travel to countries where hepatitis A is prevalent, a higher dose is warranted (see Hepatitis A, p 224).

Measles Prophylaxis. Immune globulin administered to exposed, measles-susceptible individuals will prevent or modify infection if given within 6 days of exposure (see Measles, p 311). Immune globulin is especially indicated for susceptible household or hospital contacts younger than 6 months. A single dose of 0.25 mL/kg (maximum, 15 mL) is given as soon after exposure as possible. If IG is given for this purpose in the recommended dose, the individual should receive live-virus measles vaccine 5 months later, unless contraindications are present or the individual is not yet 15 months old. If the risk of severe morbidity from the disease is extremely high, as in the immunosuppressed patient, 0.5 mL/kg is given and live-virus measles vaccine is administered 6 months later. A child regularly receiving IGIV at a dose of 100 to 400 mg/kg ordinarily need not receive an additional dose of IG if exposure to measles occurs within 3 weeks of exposure. The usual dose should be more than sufficient for postexposure measles prophylaxis for at least 3 weeks and perhaps longer.

Nonproven Uses of Immune Globulin

- *Hepatitis B prophylaxis.* Immune globulin is prepared from normal adult plasma, whereas Hepatitis B Immune Globulin (HBIG) (Human) is prepared from plasma preselected for high antibody titer against hepatitis B surface antigen (HBsAg). Hence, HBIG should be used for hepatitis B prophylaxis, generally in conjunction with hepatitis B vaccine (see Hepatitis B, p 228).
- *Hepatitis C.* Results of studies evaluating the prophylactic value of IG have been equivocal. Now that screening of plasma donors for anti-HCV is recommended, with the resulting exclusion of anti-HCV-positive persons from

the donor pool in the United States, IG manufactured in this country does not contain antibodies to HCV and is unlikely to prevent hepatitis C (see Hepatitis C, p 239).

- *Hepatitis E (enterically transmitted non-A, non-B hepatitis).* No evidence indicates that US-manufactured IG will prevent this infection.
- *Asthma or severe allergic diatheses.* No evidence supports the use of IG in these conditions.
- *Burn patients.* Evidence for reduction of infection by IG is contradictory at best. Large doses (1 mL/kg daily for 3 days) of IG resulted in a 50% reduction of infections in one study, but one half that dose was nonbeneficial in another investigation.
- *Most acute infections.* Despite the frustration experienced by physicians confronted with severe, even life-threatening, acute bacterial or viral infections, little convincing evidence indicates benefit from IG administration. Of particular note is the lack of efficacy in reduction or modification of undifferentiated, repetitive upper respiratory tract infections.
- *Other clinical circumstances.* Immune globulin has not proved beneficial in infants who are septic, debilitated, or malnourished; who are ill because of chronic or persistent infection; who are failing to thrive, or are premature; or who have non-B-cell immunodeficiencies.

Precautions in the Use of Immune Globulin
- Immune globulin is recommended for clinical use only in situations where its efficacy has been established.
- Immune globulin should be given intramuscularly in a large muscle mass (see p 40).
- Caution should be used in giving IG to a patient with history of adverse reactions to IG.
- Although systemic reactions to IG are rare (see Adverse Reactions to Immune Globulin, below), epinephrine and other means of treating acute reactions should be immediately available.
- Immune globulin should not be given to patients with severe thrombocytopenia or any coagulation disorder that would preclude IM injection.
- Screening for IgA-deficiency is not routinely recommended for potential recipients of IG (see Adverse Reactions to Immune Globulin, below).

Adverse Reactions to Immune Globulin
- The most common problem encountered with the use of IG is discomfort and pain at the site of administration. Less common reactions include flushing, headache, chills, and nausea.
- Serious reactions are uncommon; these may involve chest pain or constriction, dyspnea, or anaphylaxis and systemic collapse. An increased risk of systemic reaction results from inadvertent or deliberate IV administration. Persons requiring repeated IM doses have been reported to experience systemic reactions such as fever, chills, sweating, uncomfortable sensations, and shock.
- Because IG contains trace amounts of IgA, persons who are selectively serum IgA-deficient in rare cases can develop anti-IgA antibodies and react to a subsequent dose of IG, whole-blood transfusion, or plasma infusion

with systemic symptoms, particularly chills, fever, and shock-like symptoms. In those rare cases in which reactions related to anti-IgA antibodies have occurred, use of IgA-depleted IGIV preparations may reduce the likelihood of further reactions. Because of the rarity of these reactions, routine screening for IgA deficiency is not recommended.

- Healthy persons given IG may manufacture antibodies against IgG allotypes that differ from their own. Usually, this phenomenon has no clinical significance; however, on rare occasion, a systemic reaction can result.
- One case of acrodynia caused by the mercury in thiomersal in IG has been reported in a young adult who had been receiving IG since early infancy for agammaglobulinemia.

Specific Immune Globulins

Specific immune globulins or "hyperimmune globulins" differ from IG in the selection of donors and the number of donors whose plasma is included in the pool from which the product is prepared. Donors known to have high titers of the desired antibody, either naturally acquired or stimulated by immunization, are selected. These globulins are prepared by the same procedure as IG, and they contain 10% to 18% protein (IG has approximately 16.5% protein). Specific immune globulins for use in infectious diseases include Hepatitis B Immune Globulin (HBIG) (Human), Rabies Immune Globulin (RIG) (Human), Tetanus Immune Globulin (TIG) (Human), Varicella-Zoster Immune Globulin (VZIG) (Human), and Cytomegalovirus Immune Globulin Intravenous (CMV IGIV). Recommendations for use of these globulins are given in the discussion of specific diseases in Section 3. The precautions and adverse reactions for IG and IGIV are also applicable to the specific immune globulins.

Immune Globulin Intravenous (IGIV)

Immune Globulin Intravenous (IGIV) (Human) is derived from the pooled plasma of adults by an alcohol-fractionation procedure; it is then modified to be suitable for IV use. The donor pool is like that of IG. All preparations must have adequate measles, tetanus, and polio antibody titers. Antibody concentrations against common pathogens, such as *Streptococcus pneumoniae*, vary widely between products and even among lots of the same product. Intravenous IG consists primarily of the immunoglobulin fraction (more than 95% IgG and trace amounts of IgA and IgM). The protein content varies, depending on the product; both liquid and dried products are available. Intravenous IG does not contain thiomersal and can be used in mercury-sensitive individuals.

Indications for the Use of Intravenous Immune Globulin

Approval by the Food and Drug Administration (FDA) of specific indications for a manufacturer's IGIV product is based on the availability of data from one or more clinical trials. Therapeutic differences between IGIV products of different manufacturers may exist but have not been demonstrated. A listing of FDA-approved indications by trade name and manufacturer is in *The Medical Letter.** Recommended and possible indications in children and adolescents include the following:

- *Replacement therapy in antibody deficiency disorders.* The usual dose of IGIV in immunodeficiency syndromes is 300 to 400 mg/kg body weight administered once a month by IV infusion. Dose or frequency of infusions, however, should be based on the effectiveness in the individual patient, and effective doses have ranged from 200 to 800 mg/kg monthly. Maintenance of a trough IgG concentration of 500 mg/dL has been demonstrated to correlate with clinical response.

- *Kawasaki disease.* Intravenous IG administered within the first 10 days of the illness shortens the duration of fever and decreases the frequency of coronary abnormalities (see Kawasaki Disease, p 285).

- *Pediatric AIDS.* The benefit of IGIV to HIV-infected children has been controversial. Some centers advocate treating all infected children with IGIV monthly or biweekly. Intravenous IG can delay the time to development of bacterial infections in infants with peripheral T-helper (CD4) lymphocyte counts of $200/mm^3$ or greater, but it does not affect survival. Intravenous IG therapy may be beneficial, especially in combination with an antiviral agent, for children with hypogammaglobulinemia (serum IgG less than 250 mg/dL), those with recurrent bacterial infections, or those who fail to form antibodies to common antigens, including measles vaccine (see HIV Infections and AIDS, p 265).

- *Hypogammaglobulinemia in chronic lymphocytic leukemia.* Intravenous IG in adults with this disease has been demonstrated to reduce the incidence of serious bacterial infections, although its cost-effectiveness has been questioned.

- *Bone marrow transplantation.* Results of limited trials in pediatric bone marrow recipients suggest that IGIV may reduce the incidence of infection and death but not acute graft-versus-host disease (GVHD). Studies in adult transplant recipients indicate that IGIV decreases the incidence of interstitial pneumonia (presumably caused by cytomegalovirus), may reduce the risk of bacterial infection, decreases the incidence of GVHD and death, and, in conjunction with ganciclovir, is effective in the treatment of some patients with cytomegalovirus pneumonia.

- *Low-birth-weight infants.* Results of some clinical trials have indicated that IGIV decreases the incidence of late-onset infections in infants less than 1,500 g in birth weight, but other studies have not confirmed these results. Trials have varied in IGIV dose, time of administration, and other aspects of study design. A National Institutes of Health Consensus Development Panel concluded in 1990 that although the use of IGIV in the prevention of late-onset infection in preterm neonates had a rational basis, the available data did not support the routine use of IGIV in low-birth-weight infants, including those less than 1,500 g. A recent large multicenter placebo-controlled

*Intravenous immune globulin. In: *The Medical Letter.* 1992;34:116-118

trial, however, did conclude that IGIV was beneficial in very-low-birth-weight infants. At present, IGIV is not recommended for routine use in preterm infants to prevent late-onset infection.

Precautions in the Use of Intravenous Immune Globulin
- Intravenous IG is recommended for clinical use only in situations where its efficacy has been established.
- Intravenous IG should be given only intravenously; other routes have not been evaluated.
- Caution should be used in giving IGIV to a patient with a history of adverse reactions to IG.
- Because systemic reactions to IGIV may occur (see Adverse Reactions to Intravenous Immune Globulin, below), epinephrine and other means of treating acute reactions should be available immediately.
- Adverse reactions can often be alleviated by reducing either the rate or the volume of infusion. For patients with repeated severe reactions unresponsive to these measures, hydrocortisone, 1 to 2 mg/kg, can be given intravenously 30 minutes before infusion.
- Seriously ill patients with compromised cardiac function, who are receiving large fluid volumes of IGIV, may be at increased risk of vasomotor or cardiac complications manifested by elevated blood pressure and/or cardiac failure.
- Screening for IgA-deficiency is not routinely recommended for potential recipients of IGIV (for further information, see Adverse Reactions to Intravenous Immune Globulin, below).
- As with any biologic or pharmacologic product, the potential for new or previously unrecognized adverse events should be anticipated.

Adverse Reactions to Intravenous Immune Globulin
The reported incidence of adverse events associated with the administration of IGIV ranges from 1% to 15%, but is usually less than 5%. Most of these reactions are mild and self-limited. Severe reactions occur very infrequently and usually do not contraindicate further IGIV therapy.

Adverse events include the following:
- Pyrogenic reactions marked by high fever and systemic symptoms.
- Minor systemic reactions with headache, myalgia, fever, chills, lightheadedness, nausea, or vomiting.
- Vasomotor or cardiovascular manifestations, marked by changes in blood pressure and tachycardia.
- Aseptic meningitis.
- Hypersensitivity reactions.

Anaphylactic reactions induced by anti-IgA can occur in patients with primary antibody deficiency who have a total absence of circulating IgA and antibodies to IgA. These reactions are extremely rare in panhypogammaglobulinemic individuals and potentially more common in patients with selective IgA deficiency and subclass IgG deficiencies. In those rare instances when reactions related to anti-IgA antibodies have occurred, use of IgA-depleted preparations will reduce the likelihood of further reactions. Avoidance of anaphylactic reactions, however, may require the use of material completely devoid of IgA. Because of the extreme rarity of these reactions, screening for IgA deficiency is not routinely recommended.

Human Plasma

The use of human plasma in the control of infectious diseases should be limited. Human plasma has been administered to burn patients in an attempt to control *Pseudomonas* infections, but the data are insufficient to substantiate this use. Plasma infusions have been useful in treating infants who have protein-losing enteropathy. Plasma infusions have also been substituted for IG in some patients with IgG antibody deficiency when these individuals develop adverse reactions to IG or fail to respond to treatment with IG; however, these immunodeficient patients can be managed with IGIV (or by slow subcutaneous administration of IG).

Antibodies of Animal Origin (Animal Antisera)

Products of animal origin available in the United States are derived from the serum of horses. Experimental products prepared in other species may also be available. These products are derived by concentrating the serum globulin fraction with ammonium sulfate. Some, but not all, products are also subjected to an enzyme digestion process in an attempt to decrease reactions to foreign proteins.

The use of the following products is discussed in the disease-specific chapters in Section 3:

• Botulism Antitoxin Types A, B, E
• Diphtheria Antitoxin
• Tetanus Antitoxin
• Antirabies Serum

Indications for Use of Animal Antisera

Antibody-containing products prepared from animal sera pose a special risk to the recipient, and the use of such products should be strictly limited to certain indications, in which specific IGs of human origin are not available (eg, diphtheria and botulism).

Reactions to Animal Sera

Before any animal serum is injected, the patient must be questioned about asthma, allergic rhinitis, urticaria, and previous injections of animal sera. Patients with history of asthma or allergic symptoms, especially on exposure to horses, can be dangerously sensitive to the animal sera and should be given serum only with the utmost caution.

Sensitivity Tests for Reactions to Animal Sera

Each patient who is to be given an animal serum should be tested before its administration, as follows:

1. *Scratch, prick, or puncture test.** Apply one drop of a 1:100 dilution of the serum in normal saline to the site of a superficial scratch, prick, or puncture on the volar aspect of the forearm. Positive (histamine) and neg-

---

*Antihistamines may inhibit reactions in the scratch, prick, or puncture test, and in the ID skin test. Hence, testing should not be done for at least 24 or, preferably, 48 hours after receipt of these drugs.

ative (physiologic saline) control tests should also be applied. A positive test is a wheal with surrounding erythema at least 3 mm larger than the negative control test, read at 15 to 20 minutes. The histamine control must be positive for valid interpretation. If the scratch test is negative, an ID test is performed.

2. *Intradermal test.* A dose of 0.02 mL of 1:1,000 saline-diluted serum (enough to raise a small ID wheal) is administered. If the test is negative, it should be repeated using a 1:100 dilution. In persons with negative history for animal allergy and for prior exposure to animal serum, only the 1:100 dilution may be used. Interpretation of the ID test is done as with the scratch test. Positive and negative control tests should be applied as described above.

Whereas ID skin tests have resulted in fatalities, the scratch test is usually safe. Therefore, scratch tests should always precede the ID tests. These skin tests should always be performed by trained personnel familiar with the treatment of acute anaphylaxis (see Treatment of Anaphylactic Reactions, p 49).

Positive tests indicate the probability of sensitivity, but a negative skin test is not an absolute guarantee of lack of sensitivity. Therefore, animal sera should be administered with caution, even in individuals whose tests are negative.

If the skin test is positive or if the history for systemic anaphylaxis after previous administration of serum is highly suggestive in a person for whom the need for the serum is unquestioned, "desensitization" can be undertaken (as described in "Desensitization" for Animal Sera, below).

If the history and sensitivity tests are negative, the indicated dose of serum can be given intramuscularly. An IV injection may be indicated if a high concentration of serum antibody is imperative, such as occurs in the treatment of diphtheria. In these instances, a preliminary dose of 0.5 mL of serum should be diluted in 10 mL of either physiologic saline or 5% glucose solution. This preparation should be given as slowly as possible, and the patient should be observed for 30 minutes for reactions. If no reaction occurs, the remainder of the serum, diluted 1:20, may be given at a rate not to exceed 1 mL/min.

"Desensitization" for Animal Sera

Tables 1.7 (p 48) and 1.8 (p 49) serve as guides for the "desensitization" procedure for administration of animal sera. Either the IV (Table 1.7) or the ID/SC/IM (Table 1.8) route may be chosen. The IV route is considered safest because it offers better control. The desensitization procedure should be performed by trained personnel familiar with the treatment of anaphylaxis and with appropriate drugs and equipment available (see Treatment of Anaphylactic Reactions, p 49). Some physicians advocate the concurrent use during the procedure of an oral or IM antihistamine (such as diphenhydramine), with or without intravenously administered hydrocortisone or methylprednisolone. If signs of anaphylaxis occur, aqueous epinephrine should be administered immediately (see Treatment of Anaphylactic Reactions, p 49). Administration of sera under the protection of a desensitization procedure must be continuous. Once administration is interrupted, protection from desensitization is lost.

TABLE 1.7–"Desensitization" to Serum – Intravenous Route

Dose Number*	Dilution of Serum in Normal Saline	Amount of Injection (mL)
1	1:1,000	0.1
2	1:1,000	0.3
3	1:1,000	0.6
4	1:100	0.1
5	1:100	0.3
6	1:100	0.6
7	1:10	0.1
8	1:10	0.3
9	1:10	0.6
10	undiluted	0.1
11	undiluted	0.2
12	undiluted	0.6
13	undiluted	1.0

*Administer at 15-min intervals.

Types of Reactions to Animal Serum

The following reactions can occur as the result of animal serum administration. The first two are not mediated by IgE antibodies and, therefore, are not predicted by previous skin testing.

- *Acute febrile reactions.* These reactions are usually mild and can be treated with antipyretics. Severe febrile reactions should be treated with antipyretics, tepid water sponge baths, or other available methods to reduce the temperature.
- *Serum sickness.* Manifestations consist of fever, urticaria, or maculopapular rash (90% of cases); arthritis or arthralgia; and lymphadenopathy, which usually begin 7 to 10 days (occasionally as late as 2 to 3 weeks) after the primary exposure to the foreign protein. Local edema can occur at the serum injection site a few days before the systemic signs and symptoms appear. Angioedema, glomerulonephritis, Guillain-Barré syndrome, peripheral neuritis, and myocarditis can also occur. However, serum sickness may be mild and resolve spontaneously within a few days to 2 weeks. Persons who have previously received serum injections are at an increased risk after readministration; manifestations in these patients occur shortly (from hours to 2 to 3 days) after administration of serum. Drugs that can be helpful in the management of serum sickness include antihistamines for alleviation of pruritus, edema, and urticaria. Fever, malaise, arthralgia, and arthritis can be controlled in most patients by aspirin (30 to 60 mg/kg/d, in four divided doses; maximum single dose, 650 mg) or other nonsteroidal anti-inflammatory agents. Corticosteroids may be helpful in controlling serious manifestations that are poorly alleviated by other treatment modalities. Prednisone in therapeutic doses for 7 days is an acceptable approach.
- *Anaphylaxis.* The rapidity of onset and the overall severity of anaphylaxis vary considerably. Anaphylaxis usually begins within minutes of exposure

TABLE 1.8–"Desensitization" to Serum – Intradermal (ID), Subcutaneous (SC), and Intramuscular (IM) Routes

Dose Number*	Route of Administration	Dilution of Serum in Normal Saline	Amount of Injection (mL)
1	ID	1:1,000	0.1
2	ID	1:1,000	0.3
3	SC	1:1,000	0.6
4	SC	1:100	0.1
5	SC	1:100	0.3
6	SC	1:100	0.6
7	SC	1:10	0.1
8	SC	1:10	0.3
9	SC	1:10	0.6
10	SC	undiluted	0.1
11	SC	undiluted	0.2
12	IM	undiluted	0.6
13	IM	undiluted	1.0

*Administer at 15-min intervals.

to the etiologic agent, and, in general, the more rapid the onset, the more severe the overall course. Major manifestations are the following: (1) cutaneous, including pruritus, flushing, urticaria, and angioedema; (2) respiratory, with hoarse voice and stridor, wheeze, dyspnea, and cyanosis; and (3) cardiovascular, with a rapid, weak pulse, hypotension, and arrhythmias. Anaphylaxis is a major medical emergency.

Treatment of Anaphylactic Reactions

Personnel administering biologic products or serum should be prepared to treat anaphylaxis. The necessary medications, equipment, and staff competent to maintain the patency of the airway and to manage cardiovascular collapse must be immediately available.

The emergency treatment of anaphylactic reactions is based on the type of reaction. In all instances, epinephrine is the primary drug. Mild symptoms of pruritus, erythema, urticaria, and angioedema should be treated with epinephrine injected subcutaneously, followed by diphenhydramine, hydroxyzine, or other antihistamine given orally or parenterally (see Tables 1.9 and 1.10, pp 50 and 51). Epinephrine administration may be repeated within 10 or 20 minutes. If the patient improves with this management and remains stable, a long-acting epinephrine injection may be given, and an oral antihistamine prescribed for the next 24 hours.

Treatment of more severe or potentially life-threatening systemic anaphylaxis involving severe bronchospasm, laryngeal edema, shock, and cardiovascular collapse necessitates additional therapy. Intravenous epinephrine may be indicated; for this use, it must be diluted from the 1:1,000 aqueous base using physiologic saline (see Table 1.9, p 50). A slow, continuous infusion is prefer-

TABLE 1.9–Epinephrine (Adrenalin) in the Treatment of Anaphylaxis*

Subcutaneous or Intramuscular Administration

- Epinephrine 1:1,000 (aqueous): 0.01 mL/kg per dose repeated every 10 to 20 min. Usual dose:
  Infants: 0.05 to 0.1 mL
  Children: 0.1 to 0.3 mL

- Long-acting epinephrine suspension (Sus-Phrine): 0.005 mL/kg per dose as a single dose. The usual dose in infants and children is one half that of epinephrine 1:1,000 (see above). This medication should be given for more prolonged effect only after initial management.

Intravenous Administration

- Epinephrine 1:1,000 (aqueous): 0.1 cc/kg diluted to 1:10,000 with physiologic saline. Dose may be repeated every 10 to 20 min. A continuous infusion should be started if repeated doses are required. One milligram (1 mL) of 1:1,000 dilution of epinephrine added to 250 mL of 5% dextrose in water, resulting in a concentration of 4 µg/mL, is infused initially at a rate of 0.1 µg/kg/min, and increased gradually to 1.5 µg/kg/min to maintain blood pressure.

Maintenance of an airway is critical, in addition to administering epinephrine.

---

able to repeated bolus administration. Nebulized albuterol or IV aminophylline is indicated for bronchospasm (see Table 1.10, p 51). Rapid IV infusion of physiologic saline, Ringer lactate, or other isotonic solution adequate to maintain blood pressure must be instituted to compensate for the loss of circulating blood volume that occurs.

In some cases, the use of an alpha-adrenergic pressor agent titrated to maintain blood pressure may be necessary (eg, dopamine 200 mg in 250 mL of saline, given at a rate of 5 to 50 µg/kg/min). The combination of H_1 and H_2 blocking agents (Table 1.10, p 51) can be synergistic in their effect and should be used. Airway maintenance measures and oxygen administration should be instituted promptly. Corticosteroids should probably be used in all cases of anaphylaxis except those that are mild and have responded promptly to therapy (Table 1.10). Corticosteroids do not exert an immediate effect, however, and should not be considered primary drugs.

All patients showing signs and symptoms of anaphylaxis, regardless of severity, should be observed for several hours. Biphasic and protracted anaphylaxis (5 to more than 24 hours) has occurred in spite of adequate initial management. Hence, even patients with apparent remissions of immediate symptoms need careful follow-up.

Anaphylaxis occurring in persons already taking beta-adrenergic blocking agents presents a unique situation. In such individuals, the manifestations are likely to be more profound and significantly less responsive to epinephrine and

TABLE 1.10–Dosages of Commonly Used Secondary Drugs in the Treatment of Anaphylaxis

Drug	Dose*
Antihistamines (H$_1$ blocking agents):	
Diphenhydramine	Oral, IM, IV: 1 mg/kg every 4-6 h (50 mg, maximum)
Hydroxyzine	Oral, IM: 10-25 mg every 4-6 h
H$_2$ blocking agents (also antihistamines):	
Cimetidine	IV: 5 mg/kg, slowly, every 8 h
Ranitidine	IV: 1 mg/kg, slowly, every 8 h
Corticosteroids:	
Hydrocortisone	IV: 100-200 mg every 4-6 h
Methylprednisolone	IV: 20-40 mg every 4-6 h
Prednisone	Oral daily ("burst") dose: 30, 25, 20, 15, 10, and 5 mg (ie, daily decrease); entire dose given in the morning
B$_2$ agonist:	
Albuterol	Nebulizer solution: 0.5% (5 mg/mL), 0.05-0.15 mg/kg per dose in 2-3 mL normal saline, maximum of 2.5 mg per dose every 20 min for 1-2 h or 0.5 mg/kg/h by continuous nebulization (maximum dose, 15 mg/h)
Aminophylline	IV: 4-6 mg/kg in 20 mL saline by rapid drip every 6 h

*IM = intramuscular; IV = intravenous

other beta-adrenergic agonist drugs. More aggressive therapy with epinephrine may be adequate to override the receptor blockade in some patients. The use of intravenous glucagon for cardiovascular manifestations and inhaled atropine for bronchospasm has also been recommended.

Immunization in Special Clinical Circumstances

Preterm Infants

Prematurely born infants, including those of low birth weight, should be immunized at the usual chronologic age, in most cases. Vaccine doses should not be reduced for preterm infants.

If an infant is still in the hospital at the time immunizations are scheduled, DTP and *Haemophilus influenzae* conjugate vaccines should be given. To avoid nosocomial transmission of poliovirus vaccine strains in the nursery, the oral poliovirus vaccine (OPV) series should be initiated on discharge. If the infant is discharged at 2 months of age, OPV should be given at that time with the other recommended vaccines.

Preterm infants exposed to a mother who is HBsAg-positive should receive HBIG within 12 hours of birth and the appropriate dose of hepatitis B vaccine should be given concurrently (at a different site), or as soon as possible thereafter, and always within the first month of life (see Hepatitis B, p 231).

The optimal time to initiate hepatitis B vaccination in preterm infants with birth weight less than 2 kg, whose mothers are HBsAg-negative, has not been determined. Seroconversion rates in very-low-birth-weight infants, in whom vaccination was initiated shortly after birth, have been reported in some studies to be lower than in those in preterm infants vaccinated later or in term infants vaccinated shortly after birth. Hence, initiation of vaccination in preterm infants with a birth weight of less than 2 kg, whose mothers are HBsAg-negative, should be delayed until just before hospital discharge if the infant weighs 2 kg or more, or until approximately 2 months of age when other immunizations are given (see Hepatitis B, p 231).

Preterm infants who develop chronic respiratory disease should be given influenza immunization at 6 months of age. To protect these infants and those with other chronic conditions before this age, the family and other caretakers, including hospital personnel, should be immunized against influenza (see Influenza, p 280).

Pregnancy

Vaccination during pregnancy poses special theoretical risks to the developing fetus. Although no evidence indicates that vaccines in use today have ill effects on the fetus, pregnant women should receive vaccines only when the vaccine is unlikely to cause harm, the risk for disease exposure is high, and the infection would pose a significant risk to the mother or fetus. The only vaccines routinely recommended for administration during pregnancy in the United States are those for tetanus and diphtheria, provided they are otherwise indicated (either for primary or booster immunization). Influenza and pneumococcal immunization can be given if the pregnant woman is at high risk for serious or complicated illness from these infections. Pregnancy is not a contraindication to hepatitis B vaccination if indicated. Although data on the safety of hepatitis B vaccines for the developing fetus are not available, no risk would be expected because the vaccines contain only noninfectious hepatitis B surface antigen (HBsAg). In contrast, hepatitis B infection in a pregnant woman can result in severe disease in the mother and chronic infection in the newborn.

Pregnancy is a contraindication to administration of all live-virus vaccines, except when susceptibility and exposure are highly probable and the disease to be prevented poses a greater threat to the woman or fetus than does the vaccine. Although no evidence for the theoretical risk to the fetus of a live-virus vaccine exists, the background rate of anomalies in uncomplicated pregnancies might result in a defect that could be attributed to a vaccine; therefore, live vaccines should be avoided. However, both yellow fever vaccine and live oral poliovirus vaccine (OPV) may be given to pregnant women who are at substantial risk of imminent exposure to infection, such as in some circumstances of international travel. Alternatively, inactivated poliovirus vaccine (IPV) may be considered if immunization can be completed before anticipated exposure. Some experts prefer to administer OPV to pregnant women because a single study reported an increased risk of malignancy in the offspring of pregnant women who received IPV.*

No evidence indicates that commonly used, inactivated bacterial or viral vaccines have adverse effects on the mother or fetus. Tetanus immunization is routinely administered in pregnancy in areas with high incidence of neonatal tetanus, without evidence of adverse effects and with striking reductions in the occurrence of neonatal tetanus. Pregnant women who are not fully immunized against tetanus should receive the needed Td doses.

Because measles, mumps, and rubella vaccines are contraindicated in pregnant women, efforts should be made to immunize susceptible women with MMR before they become pregnant. Although of theoretical concern, accumulated evidence demonstrates that inadvertent administration of rubella vaccine to susceptible pregnant women is very unlikely, if at all, to cause congenital defects.

Immunodeficient and Immunosuppressed Children†

Indications for active immunization of the altered host are an important consideration. Experience with vaccine administration in immunodeficient or immunosuppressed children is limited. For many persons and with most vaccines, theoretical considerations are the only guide because experience with the vaccine in patients with a specific disorder is lacking or because adverse consequences have not been reported. However, considerable data acquired in HIV-infected infants provide reassurance about the lack of adverse events in these patients when vaccinated. Although the contraindications and lack of efficacy of immunizations in immunodeficient and immunosuppressed patients are emphasized in these guidelines, certain immunosuppressed children benefit from immunization with vaccines, such as *Haemophilus influenzae*, pneumococcal, meningococcal, and influenza vaccines.

Live-bacterial and live-virus vaccines are contraindicated in patients with congenital disorders of immune function. Fatal poliomyelitis, vaccinia, and measles virus infections have occurred in children with these disorders after administration of live-virus vaccines. If an inactivated vaccine is available for a given disease (eg, IPV in poliomyelitis prophylaxis), it should be administered. Children with deficiency in antibody-synthesizing capacity may be incapable of responding to vaccines; these children receive regular doses of IG that provide passive protection against many infectious diseases. Specific immune globulins

---

*Heinonen OP, Shapiro S, Monson RR, Hartz SC, Rosenberg L, Slone D. Immunization during pregnancy against poliomyelitis and influenza in relation to childhood malignancy. *Int J Epidemiol.* 1973;2:229-235.

†For further information, see Centers for Disease Control and Prevention. Recommendations of the Advisory Committee on Immunization Practices (ACIP): Use of vaccines and immune globulins for persons with altered immunocompetence. *MMWR.* 1993;42(RR-4):1-18.

(eg, Varicella-Zoster Immune Globulin) are available for postexposure prophylaxis for other infections.

Immunologically normal siblings and other household contacts of persons with an immunologic deficiency should not receive oral poliovirus vaccine (OPV) because the vaccine strains are transmissible to the immunocompromised individual. However, these siblings and household contacts can receive live measles, rubella, and mumps (MMR) vaccines because transmission of these vaccine viruses does not occur.

Inactivated vaccines are not a risk to immunocompromised persons, although their efficacy in these individuals may be substantially reduced. The ability to develop a quantitatively normal immunologic response usually returns between 3 months and 1 year after discontinuing immunosuppressive therapy.

Because patients with congenital or acquired immunodeficiencies may not have an adequate response to immunizing agents, they may remain susceptible despite having received an appropriate vaccine. If feasible, specific serum antibody titers or other immunologic responses should be determined after immunization to assess immunity and guide management of future exposures and further immunization.

For the child receiving immunosuppressive therapy, several factors are considered in immunization, including the underlying disease, the specific immunosuppressive regimen (dose and schedule), and the infectious disease and immunization history of the patient. Live-virus vaccines are generally contraindicated because of the risk of serious adverse effects. An exception appears to be the judicious use of live varicella vaccine in children with acute lymphocytic leukemia in remission, in whom the risk of natural varicella outweighs the risk from the attenuated vaccine virus. This investigational vaccine may be obtained on a compassionate-use protocol for patients 12 months to 17 years of age who have acute lymphocytic leukemia in remission.*

Inactivated vaccines and IGs should be used when appropriate. The immune responses of immunosuppressed children to some inactivated vaccines (eg, DTP and influenza) can be inadequate. If possible, influenza vaccine should be given to children with malignancy 3 to 4 weeks after chemotherapy is discontinued and when they have peripheral granulocyte and lymphocyte counts greater than 1,000/mm^3.

After cessation of immunosuppressive therapy, live-virus vaccine is generally withheld for an interval of no less than 3 months after all immunosuppressive therapy has been discontinued. This interval is based on the assumption that immunologic responsiveness will have been restored in 3 months, and that the underlying disease for which the immunosuppressive therapy was given is in remission or under control. However, because the interval may vary with the intensity and type of immunosuppressive therapy, radiation therapy, underlying disease, and other factors, a definitive recommendation for an interval after cessation of immunosuppressive therapy when live-virus vaccines can be safely and effectively administered is often not possible.

Patients with leukemia in remission, whose chemotherapy has been terminated for at least 3 months, may receive live-virus vaccines for infections to which they

*Available from Varivax Coordinating Center, Bio-Pharm Clinical Services, Inc, 4 Valley Square, Bluebell, PA 19422 (215/283-0897).

are still susceptible (ie, those diseases that the child neither had nor was vaccinated against, before developing leukemia).

Corticosteroids. Children can become immunocompromised because of corticosteroid therapy. For the purpose of immunization guidelines, patients treated with corticosteroids are categorized as follows:

1. *Previously healthy children who are on a short-term (less than 2 weeks), low to moderate, daily maintenance dose of systemic corticosteroids; or on a low- or moderate-dose, long-term, alternate-day treatment with short-acting systemic corticosteroids for a condition which, in itself, is not associated with a compromised immune system.* These patients, who are receiving only maintenance physiologic doses of corticosteroids and who have no underlying immune defects, can receive live-virus vaccines. Also, the administration of topical corticosteroids, either on the skin or in the respiratory system or eyes, and intra-articular, bursal, or tendon injections of steroids usually does not result in immunosuppression that would contraindicate live-virus vaccines. However, live-virus vaccines should be avoided if systemic immunosuppression results from prolonged topical application.

2. *Healthy children treated with large amounts of systemic corticosteroids.* Children in this category should not be given live-virus vaccines. The exact amount of systemic corticosteroids and the duration of administration needed to suppress the immune response in an otherwise healthy child are not well defined, however. The immunosuppressive efforts of steroid treatment vary, but many clinicians consider a prednisone dose equivalent to or greater than either 2 mg/kg of body weight or a total of 20 mg/d to raise concern about the safety of immunization with live-virus vaccines at this time.

3. *Children with a disease which, in itself, is considered to suppress the immune response and who are receiving either systemic or locally administered corticosteroids.* These children are at risk and should not be given live-virus vaccines, except under special circumstances.

Hodgkin's Disease. Patients who are 24 months or older, including adults, should be immunized with pneumococcal vaccine; they should also receive *Haemophilus influenzae* type b conjugate vaccine, according to age-specific recommendations (see *Haemophilus influenzae* Infections, p 210). These patients are at increased risk for invasive pneumococcal infection; most experts believe that they are also at increased risk for invasive *Haemophilus influenzae* type b infection. The antibody response is likely to be best when patients are immunized at least 10 to 14 days before initiation of therapy for Hodgkin's disease. During active chemotherapy and shortly thereafter, the antibody responses to the pneumococcal and *Haemophilus influenzae* vaccines are impaired. However, the ability of these patients to respond improves rapidly, and immunization as early as 3 months after the cessation of chemotherapy is reasonable.

Transplant Recipients. A special situation is a child recovering from successful bone marrow transplantation. Many factors can affect the child's immunity to vaccine-preventable diseases, including the donor's immunity, type of transplant (ie, autologous or allogeneic), interval since the transplant, receipt of immunosuppressive medications, and graft-versus-host disease (GVHD). Although many children who are transplant recipients acquire the immunity of the donor, some will lose serologic evidence of immunity. Consequently, some experts base the decision to reimmunize against diphtheria and tetanus on serologic titers against tetanus and diphtheria toxoids obtained 1 year after transplantation. Other experts elect to reimmunize all children without serologic evaluation, and some obtain titers to determine the number of doses of diphtheria and tetanus toxoids that should be given. Based on one study, reimmunization with three doses of tetanus toxoid is necessary to achieve an adequate immune response. Data on which to base recommendations for reimmunization against *Haemophilus influenzae* type b are not available; until relevant information is available, considerations similar to other bacterial vaccines are applicable.

At 2 years after bone marrow transplant, MMR vaccine is often given, since recent data indicate that healthy survivors at that time can receive these live-virus vaccines without untoward effects. However, patients with chronic GVHD should not receive MMR vaccine because of concern about resulting chronic latent virus infection that could lead to chronic central nervous system sequelae.

A decision to immunize against polio should be based on the child's likelihood of exposure, as determined by reported cases of poliomyelitis in areas where the child resides or will be visiting. Serologic tests for antibody titers against polioviruses are not readily available in commercial or state laboratories. **Only inactivated polio vaccine (IPV) should be given to transplant recipients and their household contacts.**

Other vaccines that should be considered for the bone marrow recipient include pneumococcal and influenza vaccines. Data indicate that pneumococcal vaccine is not immunogenic in the first year after marrow transplantation or in patients with chronic GVHD, but two or more years after transplantation, patients without GVHD do respond to this polysaccharide vaccine. Similarly, influenza immunization is not effective when given within the initial months after marrow transplantation but does appear to be effective when given later. Thus, vaccination against pneumococcal and influenza infection should be initiated between 12 and 24 months after transplantation.

Children who are scheduled to have a solid-organ transplantation and who are older than 12 months, if previously vaccinated, should have serologic titers measured against measles, mumps, and rubella. Those who have negative titers should be given MMR vaccine before transplantation. The preferred time to give this vaccine is at least 1 month before transplantation. Measles antibody titers should be measured in all patients 1 and 2 years after transplantation. Information about the use of live-virus vaccines in patients after solid-organ transplantation is limited. The use of passive immunization with immune globulin (IG or IGIV) should be based on negative antibody titers and exposure to disease.

Because of the limited data on immunizations of transplant recipients, immunization schedules vary in different centers. Physicians managing these patients are encouraged to develop immunization protocols and schedules in conjunction with experts in infectious diseases and immunology.

HIV Infection (see also HIV Infection and AIDS, p 263). Data on the use of currently available live-virus and bacterial (oral polio, measles, mumps, rubella, and BCG) vaccines in children who are known to be HIV-infected are limited, but complications, to date, have been reported only after BCG vaccination. Because of reports of severe measles in symptomatic HIV-infected children, including fatalities in as many as 40% of cases, measles vaccination (given as

MMR) is recommended for these children regardless of clinical status. In accordance with the usual schedule of childhood immunizations, the recommended age of administration is 12 to 15 months (see Measles, p 311). If the risk of exposure is high, such as in a measles outbreak, the vaccine should be given at the earlier age. Children with symptomatic HIV infection should receive DTP, influenza, hepatitis B, and *Haemophilus influenzae* conjugate vaccines, and those 2 years of age or older should receive pneumococcal vaccine (see Table 3.21, p 264). **Inactivated polio vaccine should be given in place of oral polio vaccine.** In the United States, as of December 1993, BCG is currently contraindicated in HIV-infected patients. In areas with high incidence of tuberculosis, however, the World Health Organization recommends giving BCG to HIV-infected children who are asymptomatic.

Routine or widespread screening to detect asymptomatic HIV-infected children before routine immunization is not recommended. Children without clinical or epidemiologic manifestations of HIV infection should be immunized in accordance with the recommendations for routine childhood immunization.

Household contacts of an adult or child with proven or suspected HIV infection should not receive OPV, since the vaccine virus can spread from person to person, particularly in households. Although no cases of poliovirus-vaccine-associated poliomyelitis have been reported in HIV-infected persons, only IPV should be used in polio immunization of household contacts.

Asplenic Children

The asplenic state results from (1) the surgical removal of the spleen; (2) certain diseases, such as sickle-cell disease (functional asplenia); or (3) congenital asplenia. All asplenic infants, children, and adults, regardless of the reason for the asplenic state, have an increased risk for fulminant bacteremia, which is associated with a high mortality rate. Susceptibility to fulminant bacteremia is influenced considerably by the underlying disease. In comparison with healthy children who have not had splenectomy, the incidence of mortality from septicemia is increased 50-fold in children who have had splenectomy after trauma, approximately 350-fold in children with sickle-cell disease, and may it be higher in children who have had splenectomy for thalassemia. The risk of bacteremia is higher in younger than in older children, and it may be greater in the years right after splenectomy. Fulminant bacteremia has been reported in adults as many as 25 years after splenectomy.

Streptococcus pneumoniae, Haemophilus influenzae type b, and *Neisseria meningitidis* are the most important pathogens in asplenic children. Less common causes of bacteremia include other streptococci, *Escherichia coli, Staphylococcus aureus,* and Gram-negative bacilli, such as *Klebsiella* species, *Salmonella* species, and *Pseudomonas aeruginosa.* Persons who are functionally or anatomically asplenic are also at increased risk for fatal malaria and severe babesiosis. Polyvalent pneumococcal vaccine may be of value in reducing the risk of fulminant pneumococcal bacteremia in asplenic children, and it is recommended for all asplenic children 2 years and older (see Pneumococcal Infections, p 374). Immunization against *H influenzae* type b infections should be initiated in infancy, as recommended for otherwise healthy young children (see *Haemophilus influenzae* Infections, p 213). Quadrivalent meningococcal polysaccharide vaccine (see Meningococcal Infections, p 326) should also be administered to asplenic children 2 years and older. The efficacy of meningococcal vaccine in asplenic children is not certain, although this vaccine is probably as effective as pneumococcal polysaccharide vaccine. No known contraindication exists to giving these vaccines at the same time in separate syringes at different sites. Since the currently licensed pneumococcal and meningococcal vaccines are unconjugated polysaccharide vaccines, they may not be as effective in preventing disease in children younger than 5 years of age as they are in older persons.

Daily antimicrobial prophylaxis is recommended for many asplenic children, irrespective of vaccination status. For infants with sickle-cell disease, oral penicillin prophylaxis against invasive pneumococcal disease should be initiated before 4 months of age (see Pneumococcal Infections, p 375). This recommendation is based on a multicenter study demonstrating that oral penicillin V (125 mg twice daily) given to children with sickle-cell disease reduced the incidence of severe bacterial infection by 84% in comparison to placebo-treated children. In an earlier study, monthly intramuscular benzathine penicillin tended to lower the number of episodes of pneumococcal bacteremia in children with sickle-cell disease in comparison to children who did not receive penicillin. Although the efficacy of antimicrobial prophylaxis has been proven only in patients with sickle-cell disease, substantial agreement exists that asplenic children with malignancies, thalassemia, and other diseases with particularly high risk for fulminant bacteremia should receive daily chemoprophylaxis; less agreement exists about the need in children who have had splenectomy after trauma. In general, antimicrobial prophylaxis (in addition to vaccination) should be strongly considered for asplenic children younger than 5 years and considered for older children. Some experts continue prophylaxis throughout childhood and in adulthood in particularly high-risk patients with asplenia. The age at which prophylaxis is discontinued in individual patients remains an empirical decision, as studies of this question are in progress.

For antimicrobial prophylaxis, oral penicillin V (125 mg twice daily for children younger than 5 years and 250 mg twice daily for children 5 years and older) is usually recommended. Some experts have recommended amoxicillin (20 mg/kg/d) or trimethoprim-sulfamethoxazole (4 mg/kg/d [TMP] – 20 mg/kg/d [SMX]) for children younger than 5 years.

When antimicrobial prophylaxis is used, its limitations must be stressed to parents and patients; they should recognize that some bacteria that can cause fulminant bacteremia are not susceptible to the antimicrobials given for prophylaxis. In all situations, parents should be aware that all febrile illnesses are potentially serious, and that immediate medical attention should be sought because the initial signs and symptoms of fulminant bacteremia can be subtle. When bacteremia is a possibility, the physician should hospitalize the child, obtain samples of blood (and cerebrospinal fluid or other body fluids as indicated) for culture, and immediately treat with intravenous ceftriaxone, cefotaxime, or another antimicrobial regimen effective against *S pneumoniae*, *H influenzae*, and *N meningitidis*. In some clinical situations, other antibiotics such as aminoglycosides may be indicated. If an asplenic child travels or resides in an area where medical care is not accessible, an appropriate antibiotic should be made available and the child's caretaker instructed in its use.

Whenever possible, alternatives to splenectomy should be considered. These include postponement of splenectomy for as long as possible in congenital hemolytic anemias, preservation of accessory spleens, performance of partial splenectomy for benign tumors of the spleen, conservative (nonoperative) management of splenic trauma, or, when feasible, repair rather than removal, and, if possible, avoidance of splenectomy when immunodeficiency is present (eg, Wiskott-Aldrich syndrome).

Children With Personal or Family History of Seizures

Infants and children with personal and family history of convulsions are at increased risk for having a convulsion after receipt of either pertussis (as DTP) or measles (usually as MMR) vaccine. In most cases, these seizures are brief, self-limited, and generalized, and occur in conjunction with fever. These characteristics indicate that such vaccine-associated seizures are usually febrile convulsions. No evidence indicates that these seizures (1) cause permanent brain damage or epilepsy, (2) aggravate neurologic disorders, or (3) affect the prognosis in children with underlying disorders.

In the case of pertussis immunization during infancy, however, administration of DTP may coincide with or hasten the recognition of an inevitable disorder associated with seizures, such as infantile spasms or epilepsy, and cause confusion about the role of pertussis vaccination. Hence, pertussis immunization in infants with recent seizures should be deferred until a progressive neurologic disorder is excluded or the cause of the earlier seizure has been diagnosed. In contrast, measles immunization is given at an age when the cause and nature of the recent convulsion and the child's neurologic status are more likely to be established. This difference provides the basis for the recommendation that measles immunization should not be deferred in children with personal history of one or more convulsions.

A family history of convulsive disorders is not a contraindication to pertussis or measles vaccination, or a reason to defer immunization. Postvaccination seizures in these children are usually febrile in origin, have a generally benign outcome, and are not likely to be confused with manifestations of a previously unrecognized neurologic disorder. In addition, many children have a family history of convulsion and would remain susceptible to pertussis and measles if family history were a contraindication to immunization.

Parents whose children may be at increased risk of a seizure after pertussis or measles immunization, either from personal or family history of convulsions, should be informed of the risks and benefits of these immunizations in these circumstances. Advice should be provided about appropriate medical care in the unlikely event of a seizure. Infants and children with personal or family history of convulsive disorders may benefit from antipyretic prophylaxis, especially in the case of DTP immunization.

Additional discussion and recommendations for pertussis and measles immunization of children with personal or family history of convulsions is given in the chapters on measles (see p 317) and pertussis (see p 362). Detailed discussion and recommendations are also provided on pertussis immunization of children with neurologic disorders.

Children With Chronic Diseases

Some chronic diseases render children more susceptible to the severe manifestations and complications of common infections. In general, immunizations recommended for healthy children should be given to children with these disorders. However, for children with immunologic disorders, live vaccines are usually contraindicated; exceptions include children with HIV infection, and varicella vaccine for children with acute lymphocytic leukemia (see Immunodeficient and Immunosuppressed Children, p 53). Children with certain chronic diseases (eg, cardiorespiratory, allergic, hematologic, metabolic, and renal disorders, and cystic fibrosis) may be more susceptible to complications of influenza and pneumococcal infection and should receive influenza and/or pneumococcal vaccines (see Influenza, p 280, and Pneumococcal Infections, p 374).

The appropriateness of administering a live-virus vaccine to a specific child with a rare disorder (eg, galactosemia or renal tubular acidosis) is problematic. The experience in some of these disorders is minimal or nonexistent, and the physician should seek guidance from experts before administering the vaccine(s).

Active Immunization After Exposure to Disease

Since not all susceptible persons receive vaccines before exposure, active immunization in an individual who has been exposed to a specific disease may be considered. The following situations are most commonly encountered (see the chapters on the specific disease in Section 3 for details):

Measles. Live measles virus vaccine given within 72 hours of exposure will provide protection against measles in some cases because immunity induced by parenterally administered, live measles virus vaccine appears more rapidly than that induced by natural measles. Infected individuals can spread measles virus for 3 to 5 days before the appearance of a rash (and 1 to 2 days before the onset of symptoms). Thus, those in continuous contact with such individuals, as in households, child care, and school settings, would have been exposed before the appearance of clinical manifestations.

Immune globulin (IG) intramuscularly in a dose of 0.25 mL/kg (maximum dose, 15 mL), given within 6 days of exposure, can be given to prevent or modify measles in a susceptible person. Since measles morbidity is high in children younger than 1 year of age, IG is indicated for infants exposed to measles. Subsequently, after age 12 months and at least 5 months after receiving IG, they should receive live-virus measles vaccine. Immune globulin may also be given to older, susceptible children who have been exposed within 6 days (assuming that they were not given vaccine after exposure), and live-virus measles vaccine is then given at least 5 months later. Exposed immunodeficient or immunocompromised individuals should receive 0.5 mL/kg of IG (maximal dose, 15 mL). Live-virus measles vaccine should not be administered subsequently if the immunodeficiency persists, except in the case of HIV-infected children (see HIV Infection and AIDS, p 263). If vaccination is indicated, it should be given at least 6 months after the child received IG.

Hepatitis B. Postexposure vaccination is highly effective if combined with passive antibody. Administration of Hepatitis B Immune Globulin (HBIG) does not inhibit active immunization with the hepatitis B vaccine. For postexposure prophylaxis in a newborn whose mother is a hepatitis B surface antigen (HBsAg) carrier, hepatitis B vaccination in addition to HBIG is essential. For accidental percutaneous or mucosal exposure to HBsAg, combined active and passive immunization is recommended. Children with continuing household contact with an HBsAg carrier should also be vaccinated.

Tetanus. In wound management, the use of Tetanus Immune Globulin (TIG) depends on the nature of the wound and the immunization history of the individual (see Table 3.45, p 461). In addition, unimmunized or incompletely immunized individuals should be given tetanus toxoid immediately (Td, DT, or DTP); the type of vaccine will depend on the patient's age.

Rabies. Postexposure immunization is an essential feature of the immunoprophylaxis of rabies even for individuals who have received preexposure rabies immunization. Most rabies exposures occur because of unanticipated animal contact (bite, scratch, or mucosal contamination). In an unimmunized individual, both Rabies Immune Globulin (RIG) (Human) and rabies vaccine should be administered as appropriate for the circumstances of the exposure.

Mumps. Exposed susceptible persons are not necessarily protected by postexposure live-virus vaccine administration. However, a common practice in mumps exposure is to administer live mumps virus vaccine to presumed susceptible persons so that if mumps does not occur as a result of the current exposure, permanent immunity will be afforded by the immunization. Administration of live mumps virus vaccine is recommended for exposed adults born after 1956 who have not previously had mumps or mumps vaccination.

Rubella. Although rubella may be modified by IG, the benefits are so questionable that IG administration is not recommended for children. Pregnant women exposed to rubella who are presumed or proven to be susceptible and who choose not to undergo therapeutic abortion may be given IG, but congenital rubella can still occur and may be the result of maternal infection without discernible rash or other clinical manifestations. Postexposure rubella vaccination is not known to be effective.

Children in Residential Institutions

Children housed together in institutions pose special problems for control of certain infectious diseases. Ensuring appropriate immunization of these children is important because of the risk of transmission within the facility and because the conditions that led to institutionalization may increase the risk of complications from the disease. All children entering a residential institution should have received appropriate routine immunizations for their age (see Tables 1.3 and 1.4, pp 23 and 24). If they have not, arrangements should be made to complete these immunizations as rapidly as possible. Employees should be familiar with procedures for handling contaminated blood and body fluids and accidents involving these fluids, and they should be aware of children infected with hepatitis B virus in order to ensure prompt and appropriate management in this circumstance. Specific diseases of concern include the following (see chapters on specific diseases in Section 3 for details):

Measles. Epidemics can occur among susceptible children in institutional settings. Recommendations for managing children in an institutional setting when a case of measles is recognized are as follows: (1) administer live measles virus vaccine as MMR immediately to all susceptible children 1 year or older for whom vaccination is not contraindicated, and (2) administer IG (0.25 mL/kg, or 0.5 mL/kg for immunocompromised children, 15 mL maximum dose) as soon as possible to all exposed, susceptible children younger than 1 year. These IG recipients will still require live measles virus vaccine at 12 to 15 months of age or thereafter, depending on the age and dose of IG administration (see Table 3.30, p 319, for the appropriate interval between IG administration and vaccination).

Mumps. Epidemics may occur among susceptible, nonimmunized children in institutions. The major hazards are disruption of activities and the need for acute nursing care in difficult settings. The occasional serious complication is a hazard for the child and the susceptible adult attendant.

If mumps is introduced into a setting where susceptible persons reside, no prophylaxis is available to limit the spread or modify the disease in an individual. Immune globulin is not effective. Although mumps virus vaccine may not be effective after exposure, the vaccine should be administered to susceptible persons to protect against future exposures.

Influenza. This illness can be devastating in a residential or custodial institutional setting. Rapid spread, intensive exposure, and underlying disease can result in a high risk for severe disease that may affect many residents simultaneously or in close sequence. Current measures for control of influenza in institutions include (1) an immunization program with the current influenza vaccine timed to provide immunity well in advance of possible exposure, and (2) appropriate use of chemoprophylaxis during influenza A epidemics (see Influenza, p 282). Amantadine and rimantadine are not effective in preventing influenza B infection. In considering the use of chemoprophylaxis, the physician can often obtain information on which strains of influenza are prevalent in the community from local and state health departments.

Pertussis. Since progressive developmental delay is an indication for deferral of pertussis immunization, some children in an institutional setting may not be immunized against pertussis. If pertussis is recognized, patients should be treated with erythromycin, and close contacts of infected patients should receive chemoprophylaxis with erythromycin.

Hepatitis A. Infection may be a risk to residents and attendants if fecal-oral spread is likely. Although symptomatic infection in infants is infrequent, it can be severe in adults. In custodial institutions (eg, facilities for the developmentally disabled or jails), infection may be readily transmitted. If an outbreak occurs, residents and staff members in close personal contact with patients should receive IG (0.02 mL/kg, intramuscularly). Investigational hepatitis A vaccines appear effective and one or more products may be licensed in the United States in the near future. Indications for immunization may include outbreaks and residential institutions in which hepatitis A is endemic.

Hepatitis B. Children living in residential institutions and their caretakers are assumed to be at increased risk for acquiring hepatitis B infection. The high prevalence of hepatitis B virus (HBV) markers among children living in residential institutions for the mentally retarded indicates that HBV infections have the propensity for spread in an institutional setting, presumably by exposure to fluids containing HBV. Factors that can be associated with high prevalence of HBV markers include crowding, high staff-client ratios, and lack of in-service educational programs for the staff. In the presence of such factors, the prevalence of HBV increases with the duration of time spent at the institution. Thus, individuals entering or already residing in residential institutions for the developmentally disabled should be vaccinated against HBV; screening for HBV markers is probably not cost-effective since the prevalence of markers will be low.

After parenteral or sexual exposure to an institutionalized patient recognized to be a hepatitis B surface antigen (HBsAg) carrier, unimmunized, susceptible attendees and/or staff should receive active and passive immunoprophylaxis (see Hepatitis B, p 234).

Haemophilus influenzae type b infections. Because these infections can spread within institutions, in outbreaks involving two or more cases, rifampin chemoprophylaxis is indicated if residents include unvaccinated or incompletely vaccinated children, as is the case in child care centers (see *Haemophilus influenzae* Infections, p 206).

Varicella. This disease is very contagious and can occur in a high percentage of susceptible children in an institutional setting. No prophylactic measures are currently recommended unless susceptible children with an underlying disease are exposed, rendering them prone to serious complications or death. Administration of Varicella-Zoster Immune Globulin (VZIG) is warranted for such high-risk individuals. The availability of varicella vaccine in the future should decrease the need for VZIG.

Other infections that spread in institutions, for which no immunization is currently available, include *Shigella*, *Streptococcus pyogenes*, *Staphylococcus aureus*, respiratory viruses, rotaviruses, cytomegalovirus, *Giardia lamblia*, scabies, and lice.

Children in Military Populations

In general, children of active-duty military personnel require the same immunizations as their civilian counterparts. If delay in pertussis immunization is recommended for any reason, parents should be warned that the risk of contracting the disease in countries where pertussis immunization is not routinely given is significantly higher than that in countries where effective vaccine is used. For military dependents going overseas, the risk of exposure to hepatitis A and B, measles, pertussis, polio, rubella, yellow fever, Japanese encephalitis virus, and other infections may be increased and necessitate additional immunizations (see Foreign Travel, p 67). In these instances, the choice of immunizations will be dictated by the country of proposed residence, expected travel and residence, and the age and health of the child. Information on the risk of specific diseases in different countries and preventive measures is provided in the yearly publication *Health Information for International Travel* (see p 8) and by the Centers for Disease Control and Prevention Information

Service on International Travelers Hotline (see Directory of Telephone Numbers, p 601).

As of 1992, no active-duty United States military personnel were receiving smallpox vaccine.

Adolescents and College Populations

Teenagers and young adults may not be protected against vaccine-preventable diseases. This age group can include individuals who escaped natural infection and who (1) were not immunized with all recommended vaccines; (2) received appropriate vaccines but at too young an age (eg, live measles virus vaccine before 12 months); (3) received incomplete vaccination regimens (eg, only one or two doses of poliovirus vaccine or of DTP); or (4) failed to respond to vaccines administered at the appropriate ages.

School immunization laws encourage "catch-up" programs for older adolescents. Accordingly, school and college health services should establish a system to ensure that all students are protected against vaccine-preventable diseases. Many colleges are implementing the American College Health Association (ACHA) recommendations for prematriculation immunization requirements, mandating protection from measles, mumps, rubella, tetanus, diphtheria, and polio.

Measles. Many colleges and universities experienced measles outbreaks in recent years, impeding efforts to eliminate this disease from the United States. To prevent measles outbreaks and ensure high levels of immunity among young adults on college and university campuses, the ACHA has recommended that colleges and universities require two doses of measles vaccine as a condition for matriculation. In addition, the Academy recommends a two-dose measles vaccination schedule, preferably given as MMR vaccine, for persons born after 1956 in post-high-school educational settings.

Rubella. Adolescents and adults should be considered susceptible to rubella if documentation of immunity is lacking. Vaccinating adolescents or adults in college reduces the chance of outbreaks.

Hepatitis B. Hepatitis B vaccination is recommended for all adolescents whenever possible. Special efforts should be made to vaccinate adolescents who have one or more risk factors for hepatitis B, such as those with multiple sexual partners (defined as more than one within the previous 6 months), those who have had a sexually transmitted disease, sexually active homosexual or bisexual males, intravenous drug users and those whose occupation or training involves contact with blood or blood-contaminated body fluids (see Hepatitis B, p 232).

Tetanus/diphtheria. Td (adult-type tetanus and diphtheria toxoid) should be given if 10 or more years have elapsed since the last DT, Td, DTP, or DTaP administration.

Influenza. Epidemic influenza can affect any closed population. Physicians responsible for health care in schools and colleges should consider influenza vaccination of students, particularly those residing in dormitories or who are members of athletic teams, to minimize disruption of routine activities during epidemics (see Influenza, p 281).

The probable occurrence of diseases such as measles, mumps, rubella, hepatitis B, pertussis, and influenza in a school or college should be reported promptly to local health officials.

Because adolescents and young adults frequently undertake international travel, their immunization status and travel plans should be reviewed 2 or more months before departure to allow time to administer any needed vaccines (see Foreign Travel, p 67).

Some physicians are unaware of the risks of vaccine-preventable diseases to adolescents and young adults, and do not give priority to immunization. Pediatricians should assist in providing information on immunization and vaccine-preventable disease to others who care for adolescents in their communities and should work to heighten awareness of the importance of immunizing adolescents and young adults.

Health Care Personnel

Adults whose occupations place them in contact with patients with contagious diseases are at increased risk for contracting vaccine-preventable diseases and, if infected, for transmitting them to their patients. Health care personnel, including physicians, nurses, students, and auxiliary personnel, should protect themselves and susceptible patients by receiving appropriate immunizations, following the usual guidelines for each disease and vaccine. Physicians, hospitals, and schools for health professionals should play a major role in implementing these policies. Infections of special concern to those involved in the care of children follow (see the specific diseases in Section 3 for details).

Rubella. Outbreaks of rubella among health care workers have been reported. Although the disease is mild in adults, the risk to the fetus necessitates documentation of rubella immunity in hospital personnel of both sexes. Individuals for whom the risk of rubella infection is heightened include hospital workers in obstetrics and pediatrics, physicians and nurses working in pediatric and obstetric offices and clinics, and all those working in health care areas in which pregnant women are encountered. Persons should be considered immune only on the basis of serologic tests or documented proof of live rubella virus immunization; history of rubella is unreliable and should not be used in judging immune status. All susceptible individuals should be immunized with live rubella virus vaccine or MMR before initial or continuing contact with pregnant patients.

Measles. Because measles in health care workers has contributed to the spread of the disease during outbreaks, evidence of immunity to measles should be required for health care personnel born after 1956 who are beginning employment and will have direct patient contact. Proof is established by a physician-documented illness, a positive serologic test for antibody, or documented receipt of two doses of live-virus measles vaccine on or after the first birthday. Workers born before 1957 generally have been considered immune to measles. However, since measles cases have occurred in health care workers in this age group, health facilities should consider offering at least one dose of measles-containing vaccine to such workers who lack proof of immunity to measles, particularly in communities with ongoing measles transmission.

Mumps. Mumps transmission in health care facilities can be disruptive and costly. Adults born before 1957 have generally been considered immune to mumps; those born in 1957 or later may be considered immune if they have documentation of a single dose of mumps vaccine received after their first birthday, a record of physician-diagnosed mumps, or laboratory evidence of immunity.

Hepatitis B. Any health care worker who comes in contact with blood is at risk for acquiring hepatitis B. Hepatitis B vaccine is recommended for all health care personnel, including physicians, who are likely to be exposed to blood or body fluids. In 1991, the Occupational Safety and Health Administration of the US Department of Labor issued a regulation requiring employers of workers at risk for occupational exposure to hepatitis B to offer these employees hepatitis B vaccine at the employer's expense.

Among physicians in the United States caring for children, 10% to 20% have evidence of previous hepatitis B infection, indicating an appreciable occupational risk.

Influenza. Certain groups of patients, such as those with chronic cardiovascular or pulmonary disease, are at high risk for serious or complicated influenza infection. Because medical personnel can transmit influenza to their patients, and because nosocomial outbreaks can occur, influenza immunization programs for hospital workers and other health care professionals should be organized each fall. Since infants younger than 6 months cannot be protected by immunization, vaccination of personnel working in nurseries and infant wards is highly advised.

Varicella. The virus can spread readily in hospitals, and varicella can be a devastating disease in immunosuppressed children or in adults. To facilitate varicella infection control, some experts advise that immune status to varicella should be determined by serology on all patient-care hospital personnel who do not have a history of disease, particularly those working with or likely to be exposed to children. A minority (10% to 15%) of these persons will be seronegative. If a patient with varicella or zoster is admitted, previously identified susceptible personnel should be excluded from contact. When a licensed varicella vaccine becomes available, immunization of susceptible personnel may be advisable.

Refugees

Prevention of infectious diseases in refugee children presents special problems because of the diseases to which these children have been exposed and the immunization practices unique to their native countries. Whereas most of these children will be free of contagious diseases, certain infections are more common in refugees than in residents of the United States (see Table 2.10, p 112).

Children who come from refugee camps in southeast Asia will usually have received DTP, OPV, MMR, and hepatitis B vaccines as appropriate for their ages before entry into the United States. However, some children may not have been completely immunized before arrival. Refugee children from eastern Europe and countries of the former Soviet Union are less likely to be fully immunized than children from southeast Asian refugee camps. For these refugee children whose immunizations are not up-to-date for age, OPV, DTP (or DT, DTaP, or Td), MMR, *Haemophilus influenzae* conjugate, and hepatitis B vaccines should be administered simultaneously, as indicated for their ages, particularly when follow-up care is likely to be disrupted by relocation.

Tuberculosis is the most important public health problem of refugees. Approximately 1% to 2% of refugees have had active tuberculosis on entry into the United States, and about one half the refugees have positive tuberculin skin tests. The number who have received BCG vaccination is unknown. All refugee children should be skin tested with Mantoux tuberculin test at the time of the first visit and 3 months later to identify recently acquired infection. Previous BCG vaccination (which many of these children will have received) is not a contraindication to skin testing, although a vaccinated individual may have a positive tuberculin skin test. However, since tuberculin hypersensitivity resulting from BCG is neither great nor persistent, a positive skin test cannot be attributed to BCG (see Tuberculosis, p 484). A chest roentgenogram is usually indicated if the skin test is positive in BCG-vaccinated infants or children.

The physician should be aware that all refugees are screened for tuberculosis, and if found to have tuberculous disease they must receive treatment until they are no longer infectious before they may enter the United States. Some refugees will arrive before treatment is completed; those individuals will have been given enough medication to last until they are evaluated by the local health department. All refugees with active or suspected active tuberculosis are provided with copies of medical records that summarize roentgenographic findings, laboratory studies, and treatment, and the local health department is notified at the time of the refugee's arrival in the United States. Some refugees will develop active tuberculosis after arrival. Evaluation of these patients must include efforts to obtain the organism for culture and antibiotic susceptibility testing. Initial therapy should be with a regimen recommended for possible drug-resistant bacteria (see Tuberculosis, p 489).

The prevalence of hepatitis B surface antigen (HBsAg) carriers in eastern Asian refugees is estimated to be 10% to 15%. Most of these persons are asymptomatic, and transmission can be limited by universal infant hepatitis B immunization and administration of hepatitis B vaccine to susceptible household contacts. Serologic screening of pregnant refugee women for HBsAg is necessary to prevent perinatal transmission by active and passive immunoprophylaxis (see Hepatitis B, p 234).

Refugees from endemic areas, particularly eastern Asia and Africa, should be serologically screened for HBsAg. If a carrier is found, all susceptible household contacts should be vaccinated. Even if no carriers are found within a family, vaccination should be considered for susceptible children (see Hepatitis B, p 232). Person-to-person (horizontal) transmission of this infection has been documented in immigrant populations from endemic areas among preschool children without a known carrier in the family.

Foreign Travel

Foreign travel requires consideration of additional vaccines as well as the recommendations for routine childhood immunizations. Vaccines such as yellow fever may be required for entry into certain countries, and immunization against typhoid fever, meningococcal meningitis, rabies, or Japanese encephalitis may be recommended, depending on destination, planned activity, and length of stay. Immune globulin may be given to prevent hepatitis A in persons traveling to areas with unsanitary conditions. Hepatitis B is a particular risk in countries of Asia and Africa, where as many as 15% of the general population are asymptomatic, chronic carriers. Travelers to some tropical and subtropical areas risk exposure to chloroquine-resistant malaria, dengue fever, and other viral diseases for which vaccines are not available. For travelers at risk, malaria chemoprophylaxis and insect precautions are important preventive behaviors.

An excellent source of comprehensive information is the annually revised publication *Health Information for International Travel* (see p 8). The CDC also publishes the biweekly *Summary of Health Information* (known as the "Blue Sheet"), which lists areas infected with yellow fever and cholera and gives changes reported by the World Health Organization (WHO) in the official recommendations for entry to certain countries. Local and state health departments can be consulted for updated information before travel. Information is also available from the CDC Information Service or International Travelers Hotline, which is accessible from a touchtone telephone 24 hours a day, 7 days a week, and provides information by FAX as well (see Directory of Telephone Numbers, p 601).

Special attention should be given to ensure that infants and children embarking on international travel receive routine immunizations appropriate for their ages, including DTP, poliovirus, *Haemophilus influenzae* conjugate, MMR, and hepatitis B vaccines (see Tables 1.3 and 1.4, pp 23 and 24). To ensure immunity, some vaccines may have to be given at an accelerated rate before departure. Infants 6 to 15 months traveling to geographic areas where polio is endemic should receive their third dose of oral polio vaccine (OPV) before departure.

Since some cases of measles in the United States result from exposure in foreign countries, persons traveling abroad should be immune to measles (see Measles, p 315). Unless a contraindication exists, a single dose of a measles-containing vaccine should be given to all persons born after 1956 traveling abroad who have not already received two doses of measles vaccine or do not have other proof of immunity. For children traveling to areas in which measles is present, the age for initiation of measles vaccination should be lowered. Infants 6 to 11 months should receive a dose of monovalent measles vaccine (or MMR if monovalent vaccine is not available); those 12 to 14 months should receive MMR vaccine before departure. Those vaccinated before 12 months should be given MMR at 12 to 15 months, provided at least 1 month has elapsed since the preceding dose. Since immune globulin (IG) can interfere with the immunologic response to measles vaccine, the need for IG should be considered in scheduling measles immunization (see p 70).

Hepatitis B vaccine is recommended for travelers of all ages going to areas where the infection is highly endemic and who will have close contact with the local people, or are likely to have blood or sexual contact with residents of these areas. An accelerated dosing schedule is approved for one hepatitis B vaccine (Energix*); the first 3 doses are given at 0, 1, and 2 months, and a fourth dose is given at 12 months. It may benefit travelers who have insufficient time (ie, less than 6 months) before departure to complete the standard three-dose primary series.

Depending on destination and length of stay, additional required or recommended travel immunizations can include vaccines against yellow fever, typhoid fever, meningococcal disease, and rabies. Health authorities at the destination should be consulted if a prolonged stay is contemplated. Recommendations for vaccine-preventable diseases for international travelers are listed in Table 1.11, p 69 (see specific disease chapter in Section 3 for details).

---

*Available from SmithKline Beecham, Philadelphia, PA.

TABLE 1.11–Recommendations for Travelers to Developing Countries[a]

Preventive Measures	Length of Travel[b]		
	Brief (<2 wk)	Intermediate (2 wk to 3 mo)	Long-Term Residential (>3 mo)
Immunizations			
Review and complete age-appropriate childhood schedule[c]	+	+	+
– DTP may be given at 4-wk intervals	+	+	+
– OPV may be given at 4-6-wk intervals[d]	+	+	+
– OPV: 3rd dose given if 6-14 mo old	+	+	+
– Measles: extra dose given if 6-11 mo old at 1st dose	±	+	+
– Hepatitis B	±	±	+
Yellow fever[e]	+	+	+
Typhoid fever[f]	–	±	+
Meningococcal meningitis	±	±	±
Rabies[g]	–	±	+
Japanese encephalitis	–	±	+
Immune globulin for hepatitis A	±	0.02 mL/kg	0.06 mL/kg every 5 mo
Tuberculosis skin test (PPD)	±	+	+
Chemoprophylaxis for malaria[h]	+	+	+

[a]See specific disease chapters in Section 3 for details. For further information, see text.
[b] " + " = recommended; " ± " = consider; " – " = not recommended.
[c]See Table 1.3 (p 23) and Table 1.4 (p 24).
[d]If necessary to complete the primary series before departure.
[e]For endemic regions of Africa and South America (see *Health Information for International Travel*, p 8).
[f]Indicated for travelers who will consume food at nontourist facilities.
[g]May be indicated for individuals with high risk of wild animal exposure and for spelunkers.
[h]See Malaria (p 303) for recommendations for specific countries.

Yellow fever vaccine is required by some countries as a condition of entry from infected areas for travelers as young as 6 months of age. Whenever possible, immunization with this live-attenuated-virus vaccine should be delayed until age 9 months or older to avoid the risk of vaccine-associated encephalitis. Since infants younger than 4 months are more susceptible, yellow fever vaccine should not be given to infants of this age (see Arboviruses, p 125).

The currently available cholera vaccine has limited efficacy and is no longer required by any country. If cholera vaccine is given, it should be administered, if possible, at least 3 weeks apart from yellow fever vaccine. If this schedule is not possible, the yellow fever vaccine should be given first (see Simultaneous Administration of Multiple Vaccines, p 25).

Typhoid vaccine is recommended for those who expect to consume food and water at nontourist facilities and to children who will reside in endemic areas. An oral typhoid vaccine given in a four-dose schedule is now available (see *Salmonella* Infections, p 416). Since the antimalarial mefloquine can affect the immune response, for persons taking this drug, oral typhoid vaccine should probably be given at least 24 hours before or after a dose.

Meningococcal polysaccharide vaccine (quadrivalent groups A/C/Y/W-135) should be considered for travelers to endemic areas in central Africa and Brazil, and to countries with current meningococcal A or C epidemics. The duration of protection is not established but is likely to be less than 3 years for group A meningococcal infection in children immunized when younger than 4 years of age. Such children should be revaccinated after 2 or 3 years if they continue to be at risk of exposure.

Rabies immunization should be considered if children will be living in areas where they may encounter rabid animals. The three-dose series may be given as an intradermal or intramuscular injection, depending on the vaccine product given (see Rabies, p 394). Since administration of chloroquine for malaria chemoprophylaxis may decrease the efficacy of intradermal rabies immunization, rabies vaccine by this route is not indicated when the person is taking chloroquine or a related antimalarial, such as mefloquine.

Japanese encephalitis, spread by mosquitoes, is a problem in the eastern part of the Commonwealth of Independent States, Asia, and Southeast Asia. Travelers to rural farming areas are at most risk. An inactivated Japanese encephalitis vaccine (JEV) was recently licensed in the United States (see Arboviruses, p 126). Immunization requires three doses administered subcutaneously on days 0, 7, and 30. The last dose should be administered at least 10 days before travel to an endemic area. If time constraints necessitate an abbreviated schedule, vaccine can be given at 0, 7, and 14 days.

Influenza vaccination may be warranted for foreign travelers, depending on the destination, duration of travel, risk of acquisition (based, in part, on the season of the year), and possible consequences to the traveler (see Influenza, p 281).

Immune globulin may be given to prevent hepatitis A if food and water will be consumed in nontourist facilities or if extended periods of travel are planned. Since hepatitis A in children younger than 4 years of age is usually a benign illness providing long-lasting immunity, some experts do not advise IG for very young travelers. However, since young children are often sources of infection for parents and siblings, IG for all household members including young children is prudent (see Hepatitis A, p 224). Since IG can interfere with the response to MMR, vaccine should be given 2 weeks before or 3 months after IG is administered for hepatitis A prophylaxis for international travel. If a larger dose is given, a longer delay is necessary to ensure that the response to MMR is not inhibited (see Table 3.30, p 319). Investigational inactivated hepatitis A virus vaccines may be licensed in the United States in the near future for travelers at risk for hepatitis A. These vaccines are already licensed in at least eight other countries and are highly effective, beginning within 2 weeks after administration of the first dose of the recommended three-dose schedule.

Skin testing for tuberculosis before departure is recommended for intermediate and long-term travelers who will reside and work in Asia or Africa. Some countries may require bacillus Calmette-Guerin (BCG) vaccine for issuance of work and residency permits for expatriate workers and their families.

Of all the diseases faced by international travelers going to the tropics, malaria is probably the greatest threat. Prophylaxis requires daily or weekly doses of antimalarial drugs (see Malaria, p 303).

Prevention of mosquito bites is important in minimizing the risk of malaria, dengue fever, and other arboviruses. Wearing long-sleeved cotton clothing, using window screens and bednets, and judiciously using repellents containing DEET* and insect sprays containing permethrin are appropriate in high-risk areas.

Travelers' diarrhea is a significant problem that may be mitigated by attention to the foods and beverages ingested. Chemoprophylaxis is not recommended for general use, but provision of an antibiotic for the treatment of travelers' diarrhea is a useful precaution (see *Escherichia coli* Diarrhea, p 191). Giardiasis is commonly transmitted in some areas by contaminated water supplies.

---

*N, N-diethyl-m-toluamıde.

SECTION 2

RECOMMENDATIONS FOR CARE OF CHILDREN IN SPECIAL CIRCUMSTANCES

Human Milk

Breast-feeding provides numerous health benefits to young infants, including protection against morbidity and mortality from infectious diseases of bacterial, viral, and parasitic origin. While providing an ideal source of infant nutrition, largely uncontaminated by environmental pathogens, human milk contains protective factors, including cells, specific secretory antibodies, and nonimmune factors such as glycoconjugates, for infants. Evidence of protection by human milk is most clearly established for pathogens causing gastrointestinal tract infection. In addition, human milk appears to provide protection against otitis media, *Haemophilus influenzae* type b, respiratory syncytial virus, and other causes of lower respiratory tract infections.

The AAP Committee on Nutrition issues statements on infant feeding that provide further information about the benefits of breast-feeding and recommended feeding practices (see *Pediatric Nutrition Handbook*, 1993[*]). This handbook addresses questions about immunization of lactating mothers and nursing infants, transmission of infectious agents via human milk, and potential effects on nursing infants of antimicrobial agents administered to lactating mothers.

Immunization of Mothers and Infants

Effect of maternal immunization. Women who have not received the recommended immunizations before or during pregnancy may be immunized postpartum regardless of lactation status. No evidence exists for concern about the potential presence in maternal milk of live virus from vaccines if the mother is immunized during lactation. Lactating women may be immunized, as recommended for other adults, to protect against measles, mumps, rubella, tetanus, diphtheria, influenza, and hepatitis B. If previously unvaccinated or if traveling to a highly endemic area, a lactating mother may be given inactivated poliovirus vaccine (IPV). Although rubella vaccine virus has been detected in milk after maternal immunization, no evidence indicates that administration of rubella vaccine to the postpartum mother has any potential for harm to the term or preterm infant. Thus, rubella seronegative mothers who could not be immunized during pregnancy should be immunized postpartum.

---

[*]American Academy of Pediatrics, Committee on Nutrition. *Pediatric Nutrition Handbook*. 3rd ed. Elk Grove Village, IL: American Academy of Pediatrics; 1993

Efficacy of immunization in breast-fed infants. The efficacy of currently recommended vaccines is not affected by the mode of infant feeding. Although high concentrations of antipoliovirus antibody in milk of some mothers theoretically could interfere with the immunogenicity of oral polio vaccine (OPV), no such association has been demonstrated. Similarly, studies of vaccines against rubella and *H influenzae* type b have failed to establish any adverse effects of breast-feeding on vaccine efficacy. Thus, infants should be immunized according to the recommended schedule regardless of the infant's mode of feeding.

Transmission of Infectious Agents Via Human Milk

Bacteria.

Mastitis and breast abscesses have been associated with the presence of bacterial pathogens in human milk. In general, infectious mastitis resolves with continued lactation during antibiotic therapy, and it does not pose a significant risk for the healthy term infant. Breast abscesses occur rarely but have the potential to rupture into the ductal system, releasing large numbers of organisms, such as *Staphylococcus aureus*, into milk. Thus, in general, feeding an infant using a breast affected by an abscess is not recommended. However, some experts recommend that infant feeding using the affected breast may resume once the mother is adequately treated with an appropriate antimicrobial agent and the abscess is drained surgically.

Women with active tuberculosis who are suspected to be contagious should refrain from breast-feeding, based on the potential for transmission through respiratory droplets during close contact with their infants. Women who have been treated for 2 or more weeks or who are otherwise considered to be noncontagious may breast-feed. *Mycobacterium tuberculosis* rarely causes mastitis or a breast abscess, but if a breast abscess caused by *M tuberculosis* is present, breast-feeding should be discontinued.

Expressed human milk can become contaminated with a variety of bacterial pathogens including *Staphylococcus* spp and Gram-negative enteric bacilli. Outbreaks of Gram-negative bacterial infections in neonatal intensive care units occasionally have been traced to contaminated human milk specimens that have been collected or stored improperly. Freezing at −20°C limits growth but does not destroy viable bacteria, whereas pasteurization (62.5°C for 30 minutes) effectively eliminates most organisms. Guidelines regarding the collection, processing, and storage of milk specimens, as well as evaluation for bacterial contamination, have been established by the Human Milk Bank Association of North America.

Viruses.

Cytomegalovirus (CMV). Virus may be shed intermittently in human milk. Although transmission through human milk has occurred, disease in the neonate usually does not result, presumably because of passively transferred maternal antibody. Preterm infants, however, are at greater potential risk of symptomatic disease and sequelae than term infants. Infants born to seronegative women who seroconvert during lactation and premature infants with low concentrations of transplacentally acquired maternal antibodies can develop symptomatic disease with sequelae from CMV acquisition through breast-feeding. Decisions regarding breast-feeding of premature infants by CMV-positive mothers should consider both the potential benefits of human milk and the risk of CMV transmission. Possible means of diminishing the risk of transmission to breast-fed infants include pasteurization or freezing of milk at −20°C for 7 days before use. Some experts recommend freezing for only 3 days.

Hepatitis B. Hepatitis B surface antigen (HBsAg) has been detected in milk from HBsAg-positive women. However, studies from Taiwan and England have indicated that breast-feeding by HBsAg-positive women does not significantly increase the risk of infection among their infants. In the United States, infants born to known HBsAg-positive women should receive both hepatitis B immune globulin and hepatitis B vaccine, effectively eliminating any theoretical risk of transmission through breast-feeding. Immunoprophylaxis of infants with hepatitis B vaccine alone also provides some protection (see Hepatitis B, p 227).

HIV. Type 1 virus has been isolated from human milk, and breast-feeding has been implicated in the transmission of HIV, especially in the case of women who acquire HIV during lactation (ie, postpartum). In some studies, breast-feeding among women infected with HIV before delivery has been associated with an increase in the rate of mother-to-infant HIV transmission. The precise risk of transmission through breast-feeding has not been established. Therefore, in populations such as in the United States where infectious diseases and malnutrition are not the major causes of death, and where safe, alternative, and effective sources of feeding are readily available, HIV-infected women should be advised to refrain from breast-feeding their infants or from donating milk. Women of unknown serostatus who are at risk for infection (including postpartum acquisition) should be counseled and screened for HIV infection. In areas where infectious diseases and malnutrition are important causes of mortality early in life, however, the World Health Organization recommends that mothers should be advised to breast-feed their infants regardless of the mother's HIV status (see HIV Infection and AIDS, p 269).

Human T-cell leukemia virus type 1 (HTLV-1). This retrovirus, which is endemic in Japan, the Caribbean, and parts of South America, is associated with development of malignancies and neurologic disorders among adults. Epidemiologic and laboratory studies suggest that mother-to-infant transmission of HTLV-1 occurs primarily through breast-feeding. Women in the United States who are HTLV-1 seropositive should be advised not to breast-feed.

Herpes simplex virus type 1 (HSV-1). Virus has been isolated from human milk in the absence of vesicular lesions or drainage from the breast, or concurrent positive cultures from the maternal cervix, vagina, or throat. Several cases of HSV-1 transmission after breast-feeding in the presence of maternal breast lesions have been reported. Since development of extragenital lesions appears to occur more often with primary HSV infection, some experts have recommended that women with primary mucocutaneous disease should not breast-feed their infants until all lesions have resolved and viral shedding has ceased. However, because identification of primary HSV infection is often difficult, implementation of these recommendations is problematic. Women with herpetic lesions on their breasts should refrain from breast-feeding; active lesions elsewhere should be covered.

Rubella. Both wild and vaccine strains of rubella virus have been isolated from human milk. However, the presence of rubella in human milk has not been associated with significant disease in infants, and transmission is more likely to occur through other routes. Therefore, women with rubella or those who have just been immunized with live-attenuated rubella vaccine need not refrain from breast-feeding.

Human milk banks. Some conditions, such as premature delivery, may preclude breast-feeding. In these cases, milk collected from an infant's mother, from unrelated individual donors, or from pooled milk may be fed to the infant. The potential for transmission of infectious agents through human milk requires appropriate selection of donors and careful collection, processing, and storage of milk. Currently, seven human milk banks belonging to the Human Milk Banking Association of North America voluntarily follow guidelines drafted by the Centers for Disease Control and Prevention (CDC). These guidelines include screening of all donors for HIV, HTLV-1, and HBsAg, and pasteurization of all milk specimens. Holder pasteurization (62.5°C for 30 minutes) reliably inactivates HIV and CMV, and it will eliminate or significantly decrease titers of most other viruses and bacteria. Heat treatment at temperatures less than Holder pasteurization does not reliably eliminate CMV. Freezing at –20°C will eliminate HTLV-1 and will decrease the concentration of CMV, but it will not destroy most other viruses or bacteria. Although few data are available regarding appropriate microbiologic quality standards for expressed milk, the Human Milk Banking Association of North America recommends use of only specimens with less than 10^4 CFU/mL of nonpathogenic bacteria. The presence of Gram-negative bacteria, *S aureus* or alpha- or beta-hemolytic streptococci precludes use of milk specimens.

Antimicrobial Agents in Maternal Milk

Antimicrobial agents taken by a lactating mother can often appear in her milk. A general guideline is that an antimicrobial agent is safe to administer to a lactating woman if it is safe to administer to an infant. The AAP Committee on Drugs has reviewed the risks to infants of specific antimicrobial agents taken by lactating mothers.* Recommendations are included in Tables 2.1 (p 77) and 2.2 (p 78). Although important exceptions exist, the majority of antimicrobial agents that might be taken by lactating mothers are compatible with breast-feeding..

If chloramphenicol or metronidazole is administered, breast-feeding is precluded during the course of therapy. Maternal chloramphenicol use is not compatible with breast-feeding because of the theoretical risk of idiosyncratic bone marrow suppression in the nursing infant. When treatment with metronidazole is indicated for the lactating mother, the infant's exposure can be minimized by alteration of the dosing schedule and temporary interruption of breast-feeding. For example, for treatment of *Trichomonas vaginalis* infection, a single 2-g dose of metronidazole may be taken by the lactating mother; she should pump

---

*AAP Committee on Drugs. The transfer of drugs and other chemicals into human milk. *Pediatrics.* 1994;93:137-150.

TABLE 2.1–Antimicrobial Agents Taken by Mothers That Are Not Compatible With Breast-feeding or Are Cause for Concern

Maternal Antimicrobial Agent	Reported Sign or Symptom in Infant or Possible Cause for Concern	Committee on Drugs Evaluation
Ciprofloxacin	Theoretically may affect cartilage development of weight-bearing joints; case report of pseudo-membranous colitis in a 2-mo-old nursing infant.	Not evaluated
Norfloxacin	Theoretically may affect cartilage development of weight-bearing joints.	Not evaluated
Ofloxacin	Theoretically may affect cartilage development of weight-bearing joints.	Not evaluated
Chloramphenicol	Possible idiosyncratic bone marrow suppression.	Unknown effect on nursing infant but may be of concern.
Metronidazole	In vitro mutagen; may discontinue breast-feeding 12-24 h to allow excretion of dose when single-dose therapy is given to mother.	Unknown effect on nursing infant but may be of concern.
Isoniazid	None; acetyl metabolite also secreted; may be hepatotoxic.	Usually compatible with breast-feeding.
Nalidixic acid	Hemolysis in infant with G-6-PD* deficiency.	Usually compatible with breast-feeding.
Nitrofurantoin	Hemolysis in infant with G-6-PD* deficiency.	Usually compatible with breast-feeding.
Sulfapyridine	Caution in infant with jaundice or G-6-PD* deficiency, and in ill, stressed, or premature infant.	Usually compatible with breast-feeding.
Sulfisoxazole	Caution in infant with jaundice or G-6-PD* deficiency, and in ill, stressed, or premature infant.	Usually compatible with breast-feeding.

*Glucose-6-phosphate dehydrogenase.

and discard her milk for 24 hours, then resume nursing. The alternative is a 10-day course with a 10-day cessation in breast-feeding.

The AAP Committee on Drugs considers maternal use of isoniazid to be generally compatible with breast-feeding. However, potential hepatotoxicity in nursing infants necessitates concern (see Tuberculosis, p 491). Although not evaluated by the Committee on Drugs, maternal use of the fluoroquinolones, including ciprofloxacin, norfloxacin, and ofloxacin, is not recommended during

TABLE 2.2–Antimicrobial Agents Listed by Committee on Drugs as Usually Compatible With Breast-feeding

Acyclovir	Dapsone*,†
Amoxicillin	Erythromycin‡
Aztreonam	Kanamycin
Cefadroxil	Moxalactam
Cefazolin	Pyrimethamine
Cefotaxime	Quinine
Cefoxitin	Rifampin
Cefprozil	Streptomycin
Ceftazidime	Sulbactam
Ceftriaxone	Tetracycline†,§
Chloroquine	Ticarcillin
Clindamycin	Trimethoprim-sulfamethoxazole†

*Sulfonamide detected in infant's urine.
†Some experts recommend that drug should be avoided in lactating women.
‡Concentrated in human milk.
§Negligible absorption by infant.

breast-feeding by some experts because these compounds are excreted in human milk in high concentrations and, based on experimental data in immature animals, may affect cartilage development of weight-bearing joints of infants. In addition, a case has been reported of pseudomembranous colitis in a 2-month-old breast-fed infant associated with ciprofloxacin self-administered by the mother. However, in one study, norfloxacin has been found not to be excreted in detectable concentrations in human milk. Therefore, some experts consider the use of norfloxacin to be compatible with breast-feeding.

Maternal use of tetracycline is usually compatible with breast-feeding, since absorption of the drugs by the nursing infant is negligible. However, some experts recommend that use of tetracycline by a lactating mother should be avoided, if possible, because of the potential for dental staining in the infant's unerupted teeth.

The amount of drug an infant receives from a lactating mother depends on a number of factors, including maternal dose, frequency and duration of administration, absorption, and distribution characteristics of the drug. When a lactating woman receives appropriate doses of an antimicrobial agent, the concentration of the compound in her milk is usually less than the equivalent of a therapeutic dose for the infant. Therefore, a breast-fed infant who requires antimicrobial therapy should receive recommended doses directly, even if the same agent is administered to his or her mother. In theory, an infant could develop bacterial resistance to an antimicrobial agent by receiving subtherapeutic doses in maternal milk, but in practice no known cases of therapeutic failure caused by lactational exposure have occurred.

The characteristics of the recipient infant should be considered when assessing the potential effect of specific antimicrobial agents taken by the mother. The maturity of the infant at birth, the chronologic postpartum age, the infant's clinical problems, and the pattern of breast-feeding will alter the possible risk. If an infant has a glucose-6-phosphate dehydrogenase deficiency, maternal use of nalidixic acid, nitrofurantoin, or sulfonamides should be avoided (see Table 2.1, p 77). With premature, stressed, or ill infants, maternal use of sulfonamide compounds should be avoided. In addition, pharmacokinetic properties of the antimicrobial agent may be helpful in deciding about the safety of a new agent whose appearance in milk is not known. If the drug is not orally bioavailable (ie, it must be given parenterally), it will not be absorbed from milk by the infant.

Another consideration is the potential for interaction of the drug the mother is receiving and that which an infant is receiving. Hence, physicians caring for infants who are breast-feeding should be aware of the medications the mother is taking and their potential for adverse interaction with drugs that might be prescribed for the infant.

In making the decision about use of appropriate antimicrobial agents for a lactating woman, the physician should weigh the benefits of breast-feeding against the potential risk to the nursing infant of exposure to a drug. In most cases, the benefits exceed the risks. The circumstance would be rare in which the only effective medication for treatment of maternal infection would be contraindicated because of risks to the infant.

Children in Out-of-Home Child Care*

Infants and young children who are brought together in groups for care have a higher rate of infection, greater severity of illness, and increased risk for acquisition of resistant organisms. Prevention and control of infection in out-of-home child care (day care) settings is influenced by (1) the caregivers' practice of personal hygiene, (2) environmental sanitation, (3) food handling procedures, (4) the ages and immunization status of the children, (5) the ratio of children to caregiver, and (6) the physical space and quality of the facilities. Adequately addressing the problems of infection control in child care settings requires the collaborative efforts of public health officials, licensing agencies, child caregivers, physicians, nurses, parents, employers, and the community.

Child care programs should require that all children receive appropriate immunizations and routine health care. In addition, these programs have the opportunity to provide young, inexperienced parents with day-to-day instruction in child development, hygiene, appropriate nutrition, and management of minor illnesses.

Classification of Care Service

Child care services are commonly classified by the type of setting, the number of children in care, ages of the children, and their health status. **Small-family child**

---

*This section is modified from the recommendations originally formulated by a joint committee of the American Academy of Pediatrics (AAP) and the American Public Health Association and published in 1992 (*Caring for Our Children. National health and safety performance standards: guidelines for out-of-home child care programs.* Washington, DC: American Public Health Association; 1992.)

care is defined as out-of-home care provided in a private residence where a provider cares for fewer than six unrelated children. **Large-family child care** is also provided in a private residence and consists of seven to 12 children. These programs usually provide care only for well children, although some family child care settings accept mildly ill children. **Center child care** is provided in a nonresidential facility and usually serves 13 or more children in a part-day or full-day program. These programs may be structured to provide care for well and for mildly ill children. **Sick child care** describes specialized programs designed to provide care for mildly ill children who are excluded from regular child care programs. All 50 states license out-of-home child care; however, licensing is directed toward center-based child care; few states or municipalities license small- or large-family or sick child care programs.

Grouping of children by age varies in different programs but in child care centers often consists of **infants** (birth to 12 months), **toddlers** (13 to 35 months), **preschoolers** (36 to 59 months), and **school-aged** children (5 to 12 years).

Infants and toddlers require diapering or assistance in toileting, explore the environment with their mouths, are careless about their secretions, have immature immune systems, and require hands-on contact with care providers. In addition, toddlers have frequent direct contact with other toddlers. Therefore, child care programs that provide infant and toddler care need to give special attention to infection control measures.

Management and Prevention of Illness

The major pathogens that can be transmitted within child care settings are listed in Table 2.3 (p 81). In most instances, the risk of introducing an infectious agent into a child care group is directly related to its prevalence in the population and to the number of susceptible children in that group. Transmission of the agent within the group depends on (1) such characteristics as mode of spread, infective dose, and survival in the environment; (2) the frequency of asymptomatic infection or carrier state; and (3) immunity to the respective pathogen. Transmission can also be affected by characteristics of the child care center, particularly hygienic aspects of child handling, environmental practices, and ages of the children enrolled. Appropriate and thorough hand washing is the most important factor for reduction of transmission of disease in child care settings. Infected children in a child care group can subsequently transmit infection not only within the group but also within their households and the community.

The major options for management of ill or infected children in child care and for controlling spread of infection include (1) antimicrobial treatment or prophylaxis when appropriate, (2) exclusion of ill or infected children from the facility, (3) provision of alternative care at a separate site, (4) cohorting (ie, inclusion of infected children in a group with separate staff and facilities), and (5) closing the facility (an option exercised rarely). Specific recommendations for control of spread of specific infectious agents differ according to the epidemiology of the pathogen (see chapters on specific diseases in Section 3).

Certain general and disease-specific infection control procedures in child care programs reduce the acquisition and transmission of communicable diseases within and outside the programs. Among these procedures are the following: (1) acquisition and review of child and employee illness records and current immu-

TABLE 2.3–Pathogens and Infections That Can Be Transmitted in Child Care

Mode of Transmission	Bacteria	Viruses	Parasites and Fungi

Fecal-oral	Campylobacter
	Clostridium difficile
	Escherichia coli
	   0157:H7
	Salmonella
	Shigella
		Astrovirus
		Calicivirus
		Enteric adenovirus
		Enteroviruses
		Hepatitis A
		Rotaviruses
			Cryptosporidium
			Enterobius
			   vermicularis
			Giardia lamblia

Respiratory	Bordetella
	   pertussis
	Haemophilus
	   influenza type b
	Mycobacterium
	   tuberculosis
	Neisseria
	   meningitidis
		Adenovirus
		Influenza
		Measles
		Parainfluenza
		Parvovirus B19
		Respiratory
		   syncytial virus
		Rhinovirus
		Rubella
		Varicella	

Person-to-person via skin contact	Group A
	   streptococci
	Staphylococcus
	   aureus
		Herpes simplex	Pediculosis
			Scabies
			Tinea capitis
			Tinea corporis

Contact with blood, urine, or saliva		Cytomegalovirus Hepatitis B Herpes simplex	

nization records for children and staff; (2) hygienic and sanitary procedures for toileting and toilet training; (3) hand washing procedures (the single most important measure for preventing infection) and enforcement of these procedures; (4) environmental sanitation; (5) personal hygiene for children and staff; (6) sanitary handling of food; and (7) management of pets. Specific staff policies that include training procedures for full- and part-time employees, and staff illness exclusion policies, also aid in the control of infectious diseases. Health departments should have plans for responding to reportable and nonreportable communicable diseases in child care programs, and should provide training, written information, and technical consultation to child care programs. Evaluation of the health status of each child should be performed by a qualified staff member each day, both upon entry of the child at the site and during the day. Parents should be encouraged to share information with child care staff about their child's acute and chronic illnesses and current immunization status.

Recommendations for Inclusion or Exclusion

Mild illness is common among children, and many children will not need to be excluded from their usual source of care for respiratory illnesses of mild severity, since transmission is likely to have occurred before the child became symptomatic or from children with asymptomatic infection. Illness risk can be reduced by following common-sense hygienic practices.

Exclusion of sick children (and adults) from out-of-home child care settings has been recommended when it has the potential of reducing the likelihood of secondary cases. In many situations, the expertise of the program's medical consultant and the responsible local and state public health authorities are helpful in determining the benefits and risks of excluding children from their usual care program. Most states have laws regarding isolation of persons with communicable diseases. Local or state health departments should be contacted regarding these laws, and authorities in these areas should be notified about cases of communicable diseases involving children or adults in the child care environment.

Children need not be excluded for a minor illness unless any of the following exists:

- The illness prevents the child from participating comfortably in program activities.
- The illness results in a greater care need than the staff can provide without compromising the health and safety of the other children.
- The child has any of the following conditions: fever; lethargy, irritability, persistent crying, difficult breathing, or other signs of possible severe illness.
- Diarrhea that is not contained by diapers or toilet use or stools that contain blood and/or mucus.
- Vomiting two or more times in the previous 24 hours, unless the vomiting is determined to be caused by a noncommunicable condition and the child is not in danger of dehydration.
- Mouth sores associated with an inability of the child to control his or her saliva, unless the child's physician or local health department authority states that the child is noninfectious.
- Rash with fever or behavior change, until a physician has determined the illness not to be a communicable disease.
- Purulent conjunctivitis (defined as pink or red conjunctiva with white or yellow eye discharge, often with matted eyelids after sleep and eye pain or redness of the eyelids or skin surrounding the eye), until examined by a physician and approved for readmission, with or without treatment.
- Tuberculosis, until the child's physician or local health department authority states that the child is noninfectious.
- Impetigo, until 24 hours after treatment has been initiated.
- Streptococcal pharyngitis, until 24 hours after treatment has been initiated, and until the child has been afebrile for 24 hours.
- Head lice (pediculosis), until the morning after the first treatment.
- Scabies, until after treatment has been completed.
- Varicella, until the sixth day after onset of rash or sooner if all lesions have dried and crusted (see Varicella-Zoster Infections, p 513).
- Pertussis (for definition, see Pertussis, p 357), until 5 days of appropriate antibiotic therapy (currently, erythromycin) has been completed (total course of treatment is 14 days).
- Mumps, until 9 days after onset of parotid gland swelling.
- Hepatitis A virus infection, until 1 week after onset of illness or jaundice (if symptoms are mild) or until immune globulin has been administered to appropriate children and staff in the program, as directed by the responsible health department (see Hepatitis A, p 223).

Most infections do not constitute a reason for excluding a child from child care. Examples that do not necessitate exclusion include nonpurulent conjunctivitis (defined as pink conjunctiva with a clear, watery eye discharge and without fever, eye pain, or eyelid redness); rash without fever and without behavior change; cytomegalovirus infection; hepatitis B virus carrier; and HIV infection. Asymptomatic children who excrete an enteropathogen usually do not need to be excluded, except when *Escherichia coli* 0157:H7 or *Shigella* infection has occurred in the child care program. Since these infections are transmitted easily and can be severe, exclusion is warranted (see *Escherichia coli* Diarrhea, p 191, and *Shigella* Infections, p 423) until a stool culture is negative for the organism.

During the course of an identified outbreak of any communicable illness at the child care setting, a child may be excluded if she or he is determined to be contributing to the transmission of the illness at the program. The child may be readmitted when the risk of transmission is determined to be no longer present.

Infectious Diseases—Epidemiology and Control

(See also chapters on the specific diseases in Section 3.)

Enteric Diseases

The close, personal contact and poor hygiene of young children provide ready opportunities for spread of enteric bacteria, viruses, and parasites in child care groups. Although many enteropathogens can cause diarrhea among children in child care, rotavirus, *Giardia lamblia*, enteric adenoviruses, *Shigella*, *E coli* 0157:H7, and *Cryptosporidium* have been the principal organisms implicated in outbreaks; infrequently, *Salmonella*, *Clostridium difficile*, and *Campylobacter jejuni* have been problems in child care.

The most important aspect of child care that is associated with increased frequencies of enteric illness and hepatitis A is the presence of young children who are not toilet trained. Fecal contamination of the environment is frequent in child care programs and is highest in infant and toddler areas where enteric disease and hepatitis A are known to occur most often. Enteropathogens can be spread fecally or orally, either directly (by person-to-person transmission) or indirectly (by toys and other objects, environmental surfaces, and food). The risk of food contamination can be increased when staff caring for diapered children also prepare or serve food. Several enteric pathogens, including rotavirus, hepatitis A virus, *Giardia* cysts, and *Cryptosporidium* oocysts survive on environmental surfaces for periods ranging from hours to weeks.

Child care programs can be a major source of hepatitis A spread within the community. Hepatitis A differs from most other diseases in child care centers in that symptomatic illness occurs primarily among adult contacts of infected, asymptomatic children. To recognize outbreaks and take appropriate control measures (ie, administration of immune globulin), health care personnel and staff need to be aware of this epidemiologic characteristic (see Hepatitis A, p 222).

The single most important procedure to minimize fecal or oral transmission is frequent hand washing combined with staff training and monitoring of staff procedures. A child who develops acute diarrhea or jaundice while in child care should be moved to a separate area, away from contact with other children, until the child can be removed by a parent or guardian. Exclusion for acute diarrhea should continue until the diarrhea ceases; children with *Shigella* infections should also receive antimicrobial therapy before readmission. The child with symptomatic hepatitis A should be excluded until 1 week after the onset the illness. Specialized child care facilities, which care for mildly ill children, could be provided for children with enteric illness and hepatitis A. Asymptomatic children without diarrhea who excrete enteropathogens other than *E coli* 0157:H7 or *Shigella* do not require treatment or exclusion from child care in the absence of specific public health indications. Asymptomatic excretion illustrates the need for frequent hand washing and environmental cleaning in out-of-home child care facilities.

Respiratory Diseases

Diseases spread by the respiratory route include those causing acute upper respiratory tract infections or invasive diseases caused by pathogens, such as *Haemophilus influenzae* type b, *Streptococcus pneumoniae*, *Neisseria meningitidis*, *Bordetella pertussis*, and *Mycobacterium tuberculosis*. Possible modes of spread of respiratory tract viruses include aerosols, respiratory droplets, direct hand contact with contaminated secretions, toys, and other objects. The viral pathogens responsible for respiratory tract disease in child care settings are those causing disease in the community, including respiratory syncytial virus, parainfluenza virus, influenza virus, adenovirus, and rhinovirus. The incidence of respiratory tract virus infections is increased in child care settings, and outbreaks can occur.

Hand washing may decrease the incidence of acute respiratory tract disease among children in child care. However, exclusion from child care of children with respiratory tract symptoms associated with the common cold, croup, bronchitis, pneumonia, and otitis media will probably not decrease spread. Children with such conditions should be separated from other children in the program if their illness is characterized by one or more of the following conditions: (1) it has a specified etiology, which requires exclusion; (2) it limits the child's comfortable participation in child care activities; or (3) it results in a greater care need than can be provided by the staff without compromising the health and safety of other children.

Transmission of *H influenzae* type b is likely among unvaccinated young children in group child care, especially those younger than 24 months. Transmission can originate from an asymptomatic carrier or a carrier with a respiratory tract infection. Immunization of children with an *H influenzae* type b conjugate vaccine according to current recommendations prevents the occurrence of disease and decreases carriage rate, thereby decreasing the risk of transmission to others. In an outbreak of invasive *H influenzae* disease in attendees, defined as two or more cases within 60 days, rifampin prophylaxis is indicated for all children and personnel with unvaccinated or incompletely vaccinated children attending child care; after a single case of *H influenzae*, the need for rifampin is controversial (see *Haemophilus influenzae* Infections, p 206).

Infections caused by *N meningitidis* occur in all age groups. The highest attack rates occur in children younger than 1 year. Close contact, for an extended time, of children and staff exposed to an index case of meningococcal disease predisposes to secondary transmission, and outbreaks have occurred. Thus, rifampin chemoprophylaxis is indicated for child care contacts.

Group A streptococcal infection among children in child care has generally not been a common problem, but child care outbreaks of streptococcal pharyngitis have been reported. A child with proven group A streptococcal infection should be excluded from classroom contact until 24 hours after initiation of antibiotic therapy.

Infants and young children with tuberculosis are not as infectious to others as adults, since they are less likely to have cavitary pulmonary lesions and are unable to forcefully expel large numbers of organisms into the air. If approved by health officials, they may attend a child care group after chemotherapy is begun and when they are considered noninfectious to others. Infants and young children who have both HIV and *M tuberculosis* infection may need to be excluded from group child care. Because an adult with tuberculosis poses a hazard to children in a child care group, tuberculin screening with a Mantoux skin test of all adults who have contact with children in a child care setting is strongly recommended before contact with the children. The need for periodic, repeat tuberculin testing of persons without clinically important reactions should be based on their risk of acquiring new infection and local health department recommendations. If found to have active tuberculosis, care providers should not be allowed to care for children until chemotherapy has rendered them noninfectious to others (see Tuberculosis, p 480).

Parvovirus B19. The spectrum of illness produced by parvovirus B19 includes, but is not limited to, asymptomatic infection in 20% of infected persons and erythema infectiosum, which is the most common manifestation of illness and usually occurs in children. Results of studies to date indicate that isolation or exclusion of persons with parvovirus B19 infection in child care settings is unwarranted, since little or no virus is present in respiratory tract secretions at the time of occurrence of the rash of erythema infectiosum, and resulting diagnosis. In addition, since fewer than 1% of pregnant teachers during erythema infectiosum outbreaks would be expected to experience an adverse fetal outcome, exclusion of pregnant women from employment in child care or teaching for this reason is not recommended (for more information, see Parvovirus B19, p 345).

Vaccine-Preventable Diseases

Routine immunization at the appropriate age is particularly important for children in child care because preschool-aged children have the highest age-specific incidence of measles, rubella, *H influenzae* type b disease, and pertussis. Outbreaks of mumps in child care settings have not been reported, but any cluster of susceptible persons can sustain transmission.

All children enrolling in child care should provide written documentation of satisfactory immunizations appropriate for age. Unless contraindications exist, children should demonstrate the following:

- One dose of DTP vaccine by 3 months, two doses by 5 months, three doses by 7 months, and four doses by 19 months.
- One dose of trivalent poliomyelitis vaccine, either OPV or IPV, by 3 months, two doses by 5 months, and three doses by 19 months.
- One dose of MMR vaccine by 16 months.

- One or more doses of *Haemophilus influenzae* type b conjugate vaccine by 16 months; for younger children, see the age-appropriate recommendations (see *Haemophilus influenzae* Infections, p 207).
- Two doses of hepatitis B vaccine by 6 months and three doses by 18 months.

Children who have not been immunized in an age-appropriate manner before enrollment should have their immunization series initiated as soon as possible—no later than within 1 month of enrollment—and completed according to Tables 1.3 (p 23) and 1.4 (p 24). In the interim, unimmunized or inadequately immunized children should be allowed to attend child care unless a vaccine-preventable disease to which they are susceptible occurs in the child care program. In such a situation, all underimmunized children should be excluded for the duration of possible exposure or until after they have completed their immunizations.

Child care providers should be current for all immunizations routinely recommended for adults. All staff should have completed a primary series for tetanus and diphtheria, and should receive a booster every 10 years. All staff should have been immunized against measles, mumps, rubella, and poliomyelitis, according to guidelines for adult immunization of the Advisory Committee on Immunization Practices (ACIP) of the US Public Health Service and the American College of Physicians. Consideration should be given to annual immunization of child care providers against influenza. Hepatitis B vaccination should also be considered, especially for providers who may manage blood spills.

Because the highest age-specific incidence of rubella now occurs in preschoolers, children and staff members in child care programs are probably at higher risk of exposure than the general population. Of particular concern are susceptible women of childbearing age (staff members and mothers of young children) who might deliver an infant with congenital rubella if infected while pregnant. Child caregivers who have not been immunized against poliomyelitis and who will be caring for infants and children receiving oral polio vaccine (OPV) may become infected and have a small risk of vaccine-associated paralytic poliomyelitis, since children excrete the virus in their stools for several weeks after OPV immunization. Transmission can be prevented by appropriate hand washing, especially after diaper changing, and by immunization of child care providers.

Varicella-Zoster Virus, Herpes Simplex Virus, and Cytomegalovirus Infection

Children with varicella who have been excluded from child care may return on the sixth day after onset of rash or sooner if all lesions have dried and crusted. All staff members and parents should be notified when a case of varicella occurs; they should be informed concerning the greater likelihood of serious infection in susceptible adults and adolescents and of the potential for fetal damage if infection occurs during pregnancy. Approximately 5% to 10% of adults will be susceptible to varicella-zoster virus (VZV); susceptible child care staff who are pregnant and exposed to children with varicella should be referred to qualified physicians or other professionals for counseling and management within 24 hours of the exposure.

Exclusion of staff members or children with herpes zoster (shingles) whose lesions cannot be covered should be based on similar criteria to those for varicella. Lesions that can be covered pose little risk to susceptible persons, as transmission usually occurs because of direct contact with lesion fluid.

They should be covered by clothing or a dressing until lesions have crusted. Thorough hand washing is warranted whenever contact with lesion fluid has definitely or possibly occurred.

Children with herpes simplex virus (HSV) gingivostomatitis, who do not have control of oral secretions (drooling), should be excluded from child care during the time of active lesions. Although HSV can be transmitted from mother to fetus or newborn, maternal HSV infections that are a threat to off-spring are usually acquired by the infant during birth from genital infections of the mother; therefore, maternal exposure to HSV in a child care setting carries little risk for the fetus.

Care providers should be instructed in the importance of hand washing and other measures for limiting transfer of infected material from children with VZV or HSV infection (eg, saliva, tissue fluid, or fluid from a skin lesion).

Spread of cytomegalovirus (CMV) from asymptomatic infected children in child care to their mothers or to child care providers is the most important consequence of child-care-related CMV infection (see also Cytomegalovirus Infection, p 176). Children enrolled in child care programs are more likely to acquire CMV than those cared for primarily at home. The highest rates (eg, 70%) of viral excretion occur in children between 1 and 3 years of age, and excretion often continues for years. Studies of CMV seroconversion among child care providers have found annualized seroconversion rates of 8% to 20%. Exposure to CMV with the increased rate of acquisition that occurs in child care staff most likely leads to an increased rate of gestational CMV infection in seronegative staff and an increased risk of congenital CMV infection in their offspring. Women who are seropositive before pregnancy and who develop CMV infection have a small (about 1 in 500) risk of having an infant with congenital CMV infection; only about 5% of these infected infants have sequelae, which are mild and consist mostly of moderate hearing loss.

Transmission of CMV appears to require direct contact with virus-containing secretions. Therefore, careful attention to hygiene, specifically hand washing, is critical. Avoiding contact with secretions is recommended to prevent infection in child care providers. However, the effectiveness of these measures in an environment where CMV is ubiquitous has not been determined. Because CMV excretion is so prevalent, attempts at isolation or segregation of children who excrete CMV are impractical and inappropriate. Similarly, testing of children to detect CMV excretion is inappropriate because excretion is often intermittent, and results of testing can be misleading.

In view of the risk of CMV infection in child care staff and potential consequences of gestational CMV infection, child care staff should be counseled regarding risks. This counseling may include testing for serum antibody to CMV to determine the child care provider's immunity against CMV, but routine serologic testing is not currently recommended.

Blood-Borne Virus Infections — Hepatitis B Virus and Human Immunodeficiency Viruses

Hepatitis B Virus (HBV). Possible transmission of HBV in the child care setting is an increasing concern to public health authorities as the result of increasing numbers of children known to be HBV carriers (hepatitis B surface antigen [HBsAg] positive) in child care. Transmission of HBV in a child care setting is most likely to occur through direct exposure to blood after an injury or from bites or scratches that break the skin and introduce blood or body secretions from the HBV carrier into the victim. Indirect transmission through environmental contamination with blood or saliva is possible but has not been documented in the child care setting in the United States. Because saliva contains much less virus than blood, the potential infectivity of saliva is low. Infectivity of saliva has been demonstrated only when inoculated through the skin of gibbons and chimpanzees; it has not caused infection when administered by aerosol through the nose or mouth, ingestion through the mouth, or by toothbrush on the gums.

Based on limited data, the risk of disease transmission from an HBV carrier child or staff member with normal behavior and without injury, generalized dermatitis, or bleeding problems is small. This slight risk usually does not justify exclusion of an HBV carrier child from child care or the necessity for hepatitis B vaccination of their child care contacts. However, all children should receive hepatitis B vaccine as part of their routine immunization schedule. Immunization will not only further reduce the risk of transmission but it will also allay anxiety about transmission.

Routine screening of children for HBV carriage before admission to child care is not justified. The admission of each HBV carrier child with one or more risk factors (eg, biting, frequent scratching, generalized dermatitis, and bleeding problems) should be assessed by the child's physician, the program director, and the responsible public health authorities. Regular assessment of behavioral risk factors and medical conditions of enrolled HBV carrier children is necessary, and it requires that the child care director and primary care providers are informed about a known HBV carrier child.

Children who bite pose an additional concern. Existing data in humans suggest a small risk of HBV transmission from the bite of an HBV carrier. Several episodes and one outbreak have been reported in which the most likely pathway of HBV transmission was through bites by HBV carriers. For victims of bites by HBV carriers, hepatitis B immune globulin (HBIG) prophylaxis and HBV immunization is recommended in susceptible persons (see Hepatitis B, p 237).

The risk of HBV acquisition when a susceptible child bites an HBV carrier is not known. A theoretical risk exists if HBsAg-positive blood enters the oral cavity of the biter, but transmission by this route has not been reported. Although data on risks of transmission are limited, most experts would not give HBIG to the susceptible biting child who does not have oral mucosal disease when the amount of blood transferred is small.

In the common circumstance in which the HBsAg status of both the biting child and the victim is unknown, the risk of HBV transmission is extremely low because of the expected low seroprevalence of HBsAg in most groups of pre-school-aged children and the low efficiency of disease transmission from bites. Since all preschool children attending child care settings should receive hepatitis B vaccination, concern regarding bites and HBV transmission associated with breaks in the skin should be reduced. Serologic testing is not warranted for either the biting child or the recipient of the bite. Bites and other possible percutaneous exposures should serve to remind all parents of the need for routine hepatitis B vaccination.

Efforts to reduce risk of disease transmission in child care through hygienic and environmental standards in general, and particularly when a known HBV carrier child is enrolled, should focus primarily on precautions in blood exposures and limiting potential saliva contamination of the environment. Toothbrushes should not be shared among children. Accidents that lead to bleeding or contamination with blood-containing body fluids by any child should be handled as follows: (1) disposable gloves should be used to clean or remove all blood or blood-containing body fluid spills; (2) the area should be disinfected with a freshly prepared solution of 1:64 household bleach (1/4 cup diluted in 1 gallon of water); (3) persons involved in cleaning contaminated surfaces should avoid exposure of open skin lesions or mucous membranes to blood or blood-containing body fluids and to wound or tissue exudates; (4) hands should be washed thoroughly after exposure to blood or blood-containing body fluids; (5) optimally, disposable towels or tissues should be used and properly discarded, and mops should be rinsed in the disinfectant; and (6) blood- contaminated material and diapers should be disposed in a plastic bag with a secure tie.

HIV Infection (see also HIV Infection and AIDS, p 267). The risk of transmission of HIV infection to children in the child care setting appears to be neglible, although data directly addressing this issue are lacking. No need exists to restrict the placement of HIV-infected children in child care to protect other children or personnel in these settings. Caregivers need not be informed of the HIV status of a child to protect the health of personnel or other children. Since HIV-infected children whose status is unknown can be attending child care, routine procedures should be adopted for handling spills of blood and blood-containing body fluids and wound exudates of all children, as previously described.

The decision to admit HIV-infected children to child care is best made on an individual basis by qualified persons, including the child's physician, who are able to evaluate whether the child will receive optimal care in the program and whether an HIV-infected child poses a significant risk to others. Information regarding a child who has immunodeficiency, whatever its etiology, should be available to those caretakers who need to know how to help protect the child against other infections. For example, immunodeficient children exposed to measles or varicella should immediately receive postexposure immunoprophylaxis (see Measles, p 311, and Varicella-Zoster Infections, p 516).

Currently available data give no reason to believe that HIV-infected adults will transmit HIV to children in the course of their normal duties. Therefore, HIV-infected adults who do not have open and uncoverable skin lesions, other conditions that would allow contact with their body fluids, or a transmissible infectious disease may care for children in child care programs. However, immunosuppressed adults with AIDS or HIV may be more likely to acquire infectious agents from children and should consult with their physicians regarding the safety of their continuing child care work.

General Practices

The following practices are recommended to reduce the transmission of infectious agents in a child care setting without losing the developmentally desirable features of child care:

- Each day care facility should have **written policies** for managing child and employee illness in child care.
- **Toileting and toilet training equipment** should be maintained in a sanitary condition. **Diaper changing surfaces** should be nonporous and sanitized

between uses. Alternatively, the diaper changing surface should be covered with a paper pad, which is discarded after each use. If the surface becomes wet or soiled, it should be cleaned and sanitized.

- **Diaper changing procedures** should be posted at the changing area. Soiled disposable diapers or soiled disposable wiping cloths should be discarded in a secure, foot-activated, plastic-lined container. Diapers should be able to contain urine and stool and minimize fecal contamination of children, providers, and environmental surfaces and objects in the child care program. The diaper should have an absorbent inner lining completely contained within an outer covering made of waterproof material that prevents escape of feces and urine. The outer covering and inner lining must be changed as a unit and not reused unless both are cleaned and disinfected. The two types of diapers that meet these requirements are modern disposable paper diapers with absorbent gelling material or carboxymethyl cellulose, and single-unit reusable systems with an inner cotton lining attached to an outer waterproof covering. Reusable cloth diapers worn with a modern front-closure waterproof cover are acceptable only if the diaper and cover are removed simultaneously and not in two separate pieces, and they must not be reused until cleaned and disinfected. If these reusable diaper products are used in child care, the user should determine the waterproof characteristics of the covering material at frequent intervals. Reusable cloth diapers worn either without a covering or with pull-on pants made of waterproof material are not acceptable. Clothes should be worn over diapers while the child is in the day care facility. Fecal contents may be placed in a toilet, but diapers should not be rinsed.
- **Diaper changing areas should never be located in food preparation areas, and should never be used for temporary placement of food.**
- The use of **child-sized toilets**, or access to steps and modified toilet seats that provide for easier maintenance, should be encouraged in child care programs; the use of potty chairs should be discouraged. If potty chairs are used, they should be emptied into a toilet, cleaned in a utility sink, and disinfected after each use. Staff should sanitize potty chairs, flush toilets, and diaper changing areas with a freshly prepared solution of 1:64 household bleach (1/4 cup diluted in one gallon of water).
- **Written procedures for hand washing**, which is the single most important measure for preventing infection, should be established and enforced. Hand washing sinks should be adjacent to each diapering and toileting area. These sinks should be washed and disinfected at least daily and when soiled; they should not be used for food preparation; and they should not be used for rinsing soiled clothing or for cleaning potty chairs. Children should have access to height-appropriate sinks, soap dispensers, and disposable paper towels.
- Written **personal hygiene policies** for staff and children are necessary.
- Written **environmental sanitation policies and procedures** should include cleaning and disinfecting floors, covering sandboxes, cleaning and sanitizing play tables, and cleaning and disinfecting spills of blood, body fluids, and wound or tissue exudates. In general, routine housekeeping procedures using a freshly prepared solution of commercially available cleaner (detergents, disinfectant-detergents, or chemical germicides) compatible with

most surfaces are satisfactory for cleaning spills of vomitus, urine, and feces. For spills of blood or blood-containing body fluids, and of wound and tissue exudates, the previously described procedures should be used.

- Each item of **sleep equipment** should be used only by a single child while enrolled in the program, and should be cleaned and sanitized before assigning to another child. Crib mattresses should be cleaned and sanitized when soiled or wet. Sleeping mats should be stored so that contact with the sleeping surface of another mat does not occur. Bedding (sheets and blankets) should be assigned to each child and cleaned when soiled or wet.

- Optimally, **toys** that are placed in children's mouths or otherwise contaminated by body secretions should be cleaned with water and detergent, disinfected, and rinsed before handling by another child. All frequently touched toys in rooms that house infants and toddlers should be cleaned and disinfected daily. Toys in rooms for older children (nondiapered) should be cleaned weekly and when soiled. The use of soft, nonwashable toys in infant/toddler areas of child care programs should be discouraged.

- **Food** should be handled in a safe and careful manner to prevent the growth of bacteria, viruses, fungi, and parasites, and to prevent contamination by insects or rodents. Tables and counter tops used for food preparation and food service should be cleaned and sanitized between uses, and before and after eating. No one who has signs or symptoms of illness, including vomiting, diarrhea, and infectious skin lesions that cannot be covered, or who is infected with potential food-borne pathogens, should be responsible for food handling. Hands should be washed using soap and water before handling food. Because of their frequent exposure to feces and children with enteric diseases, staff who work with diapered children, whenever possible, should not prepare food for others. Caregivers who prepare food for infants should be especially aware of the importance of careful hand washing. No unpasteurized milk or milk products should be served.

- The living quarters of **pets** should be enclosed and kept clean of waste to reduce the risk of human contact with this waste. Hands should be washed after handling animals or animal wastes. Animals should be handled by children only under close staff supervision. Dogs and cats should be kept away from child play areas and should be handled only with staff supervision.

- Written policies, which comply with local and state regulations, for filing and regularly updating each child's **immunization records** should be maintained.

- Each child care program should use the services of a **health consultant** to assist in development and implementation of written policies for the prevention and control of communicable diseases and in providing related health education to children, staff, and parents.

- The child care program staff should, upon registering each child, **inform parents of the need to share information about illness**, which can be of a communicable nature, in the child or in any member of the immediate household to facilitate prompt reporting of disease. The program director, after consulting with the program's health consultant or the responsible public health authority, should follow the recommendations of the consultant or authority regarding **notification of parents of children** who attend the program about exposure of their child to a communicable disease.

• Local **health authorities should be notified** about cases of communicable diseases involving children or care providers in the child care setting.

Infection Control for Hospitalized Children

Isolation Precautions

Hospital-acquired infections are a major cause of morbidity and mortality in hospitalized children, particularly those in intensive care units. Procedures and policies for prevention of these infections include routine hygienic practices used in the care of all patients, such as hand washing and isolation precautions for patients suspected to be potential sources of transmission of infection. **Hand washing before and after each patient contact remains the single most important routine practice in the control of nosocomial infections.**

Recommendations for the isolation of hospitalized patients are based on the guidelines of the Centers for Disease Control and Prevention (CDC).[*,†] These guidelines recommend either of two systems of isolation—category-specific or disease-specific. Category-specific precautions are comprised of six categories, namely, (1) Strict, (2) Contact, (3) Respiratory, (4) Tuberculosis (AFB), (5) Enteric, and (6) Drainage/Secretion (see Categories of Isolation Precautions, p 93). The CDC has replaced the category of Blood/Body Fluids with Universal Precautions, which are recommended for all patients, irrespective of which system of isolation recommendations is used. The disease-specific recommendations constitute an alternative system that allows individualization of infection control measures for the disease in question, but the recommendations, as a result, are more complex for hospital personnel to implement.

Recommendations in the *Red Book* are primarily category-specific.

Universal precautions. Since medical history and examination cannot reliably identify all patients infected with the human immunodeficiency virus (HIV) or other blood-borne pathogens, such as the hepatitis B virus (HBV), the CDC recommends universal precautions for all patients to protect health care workers from infectious body fluids.[‡,§] These precautions apply to blood, certain other body fluids (amniotic fluid, pericardial fluid, peritoneal fluid, pleural fluid, synovial fluid, cerebrospinal fluid, and semen and vaginal secretions), or any other

---

[*]Garner JS, Simmons BP. Guidelines for isolation precautions in hospitals. *Infect Control*. 1983; 4(suppl):245-325.

[†]Centers for Disease Control. Update: Universal precautions for prevention of transmission of human immunodeficiency virus, hepatitis B virus, and other bloodborne pathogens in health-care settings. *MMWR*. 1988;37:377-382, 387-388.

[‡]Centers for Disease Control. Guidelines for prevention of transmission of human immunodeficiency virus and hepatitis B virus to health-care and public-safety workers. *MMWR*. 1989;38; (suppl 6):1-37.

[§]Centers for Disease Control. Recommendations for preventing transmission of human immunodeficiency virus and hepatitis B virus to patients during exposure-prone invasive procedures. *MMWR*. 1991;40(RR-8):1-9.

body fluid visibly contaminated with blood. Since HIV and HBV transmission has not been documented from exposure to other body fluids (feces, nasal secretions, sputum, sweat, tears, urine, and vomitus), universal precautions do not apply to these fluids. Universal precautions also do not apply to saliva, except in dental settings where saliva is likely to be contaminated with blood.

All hospitalized children's blood or blood-contaminated body fluids should be considered potentially infectious. Gloves should be worn for contact with blood or blood-containing fluids and for any procedures with potential exposure to blood, as listed in Table 2.4 (p 94). Exposure to non-blood-contaminated fluids, such as urine, nasal secretions, and stool, does not require gloves. However, if such an excretion contains blood, gloves are warranted. Barrier eye protection (goggles) should be used whenever splattering is likely.

Because contaminated needlestick injuries are the most likely route for acquisition of blood-borne infection by health care personnel in the workplace, careful education and compliance with the proper handling, disposal, or decontamination of needles and sharp instruments are required.

Categories of isolation precautions. The specifications for the categories of isolation precautions are summarized in Table 2.5 (p 95). Color-coded cards that give these specifications and help to draw attention to the precautions in effect have been designed (see sample instruction cards, pp 96-101). For patients in different categories of isolation, the appropriate card should be posted conspicuously in the immediate vicinity of the patient.

Intensive Care Units. Infection control practices in neonatal and pediatric intensive care units (ICUs) must be frequently modified to accommodate special circumstances, particularly those pertaining to isolation in a private room. Separate isolation rooms are often not available in ICUs, and newborn nurseries may not be desirable for the optimal care of critically ill patients. If airborne transmission is not likely, an isolation area can be defined within the ICU by curtains, partitions, or other markers. For newborn infants, separate isolation rooms are not necessary if the following conditions are met:

• The number of nursing and medical personnel is adequate, and sufficient time for appropriate hand washing is available.
• Sufficient space is available for a 4- to 6-foot aisle or area between newborn infant stations.
• An adequate number of sinks for hand washing are available in each nursery room and area.
• Continuing instruction is given to personnel about the mode of transmission of infections.

When a private room is mandated by the possibility of airborne transmission (eg, an infant with chickenpox), a forced-air incubator is not a substitute for a private room because such an incubator does not filter the air discharged into the environment. Another modification that may be necessary for newborn infants and children during outbreaks is the cohorting of patients and personnel. Decisions of this type should be made in conjunction with the hospital's infection control and nursery directors.* In all instances, appropriate hand washing between patient contacts is mandatory.

---

*See American Academy of Pediatrics and American College of Obstetricians & Gynecologists. Infection control. In: *Guidelines for Perinatal Care*. 3rd ed. Elk Grove Village, IL: American Academy of Pediatrics; 1992:141-175.

TABLE 2.4–Infection Control Recommendations for Exposure to Blood and Body Fluids

HAND WASHING IS NECESSARY AFTER
PHYSICAL CONTACT WITH ALL PATIENTS

Body fluids and procedures for which gloves are recommended (barrier eye protection should also be used whenever splattering is likely):

Body Fluids:
Blood
Blood-contaminated fluids
Cerebrospinal fluid
Peritoneal fluid
Amniotic fluid
Pleural fluid
Synovial fluid
Semen
Vaginal/cervical secretions

Procedures:
Intubation
Endoscopy
Dental procedures
Wound irrigation
Phlebotomy
Arterial puncture
Vascular catheter placement
Tracheostomy suctioning
Rinsing of used instruments
Lumbar puncture
Puncture of other cavities (eg, pleural or peritoneal)

Body fluids and procedures for which only hand washing is recommended unless the body fluid is grossly bloody:

Body Fluids:
Urine
Stool
Vomitus
Tears
Nasal secretions
Oral secretions

Procedures:
Diaper change

TABLE 2.5–Recommendations for Category-Specific Isolation Precautions for Hospitalized Patients*

Category of Precautions	Hand Washing for Patient Contact	Single Room	Masks	Gowns	Gloves	Other†
Strict isolation	Yes	Yes	Yes	Yes	Yes	—
Contact isolation	Yes	Yes‡	Yes, for those close to patient	Yes, if soiling is likely	Yes, for touching infective material	—
Respiratory isolation	Yes	Yes‡	Yes, for those close to patient	No	No	—
Tuberculosis (AFB) isolation	Yes	Yes, with negative-pressure ventilation	Yes, if patient is coughing and does not cover mouth	Only if needed to prevent gross contamination of clothing	No	—
Enteric precautions	Yes	Only if patient hygiene is poor‡	No	Yes, if soiling is likely	Yes, for touching infective material	—
Drainage/secretion precautions	Yes	No	No	Yes, if soiling is likely	Yes, for touching infective material	—
Universal precautions§	Yes (immediately after contact with blood or body fluids)	No	No	Yes, if soiling with blood or body fluids is likely	Yes, for touching blood or body fluids	Avoid needlestick injuries; clean up blood spills promptly with diluted bleach

*Based on recommendations of the Centers for Disease Control and Prevention (see p 92).
†In each case, articles contaminated with infective material should be discarded or bagged and labeled before they are sent for decontamination and reprocessing.
‡Cohorting allowed.
§Recommended for all patients (see p 92).

SAMPLE INSTRUCTION CARDS FOR CATEGORY-SPECIFIC ISOLATION PRECAUTIONS

(Front of Card)

Strict Isolation

Visitors—Report to Nurses' Station Before Entering Room

1. Masks are indicated for all persons entering room.
2. Gowns are indicated for all persons entering room.
3. Gloves are indicated for all persons entering room.
4. HANDS MUST BE WASHED AFTER TOUCHING THE PATIENT OR POTENTIALLY CONTAMINATED ARTICLES AND BEFORE TAKING CARE OF ANOTHER PATIENT.
5. Articles contaminated with infective material should be discarded or bagged and labeled before being sent for decontamination and reprocessing.

(Back of Card)

Diseases Requiring Strict Isolation*

Diphtheria, pharyngeal
Lassa fever and other viral hemorrhagic fevers, such as Marburg virus disease§
Plague, pneumonic
Smallpox§
Varicella (chickenpox)
Zoster, localized in immunocompromised patient, or disseminated

---

*A private room is indicated for Strict Isolation; in general, however, patients infected with the same organism may share a room. See Guideline for Isolation Precautions in Hospitals for details and for how long to apply precautions.
§A private room with special ventilation is indicated.

Contact Isolation

Visitors—Report to Nurses' Station Before Entering Room

1. Masks are indicated for those who come close to patient.
2. Gowns are indicated if soiling is likely.
3. Gloves are indicated for touching infective material.
4. HANDS MUST BE WASHED AFTER TOUCHING THE PATIENT OR POTENTIALLY CONTAMINATED ARTICLES AND BEFORE TAKING CARE OF ANOTHER PATIENT.
5. Articles contaminated with infective material should be discarded or bagged and labeled before being sent for decontamination and reprocessing.

Diseases or Conditions Requiring Contact Isolation*

Acute respiratory infections in infants and young children, including croup, colds, bronchitis, and bronchiolitis caused by respiratory syncytial virus, adenovirus, coronavirus, influenza viruses, parainfluenza viruses, and rhinovirus

Conjunctivitis, gonococcal, in newborns

Diphtheria, cutaneous

Endometritis, group A *Streptococcus*

Furunculosis, staphylococcal, in newborns

Herpes simplex, disseminated, severe primary or neonatal

Impetigo

Influenza, in infants and young children

Multiply-resistant bacteria, infection or colonization (any site) with any of the following:

1. Gram-negative bacilli resistant to all aminoglycosides that are tested. (In general, such organisms should be resistant to gentamicin, tobramycin, and amikacin for these special precautions to be indicated.)
2. *Staphylococcus aureus* resistant to methicillin (or nafcillin or oxacillin if they are used instead of methicillin for testing)
3. *Pneumococcus* resistant to penicillin
4. *Haemophilus influenzae* resistant to ampicillin (beta-lactamase positive) and chloramphenicol
5. Other resistant bacteria may be included in this isolation category if they are judged by the infection control team to be of special clinical and epidemiologic significance.

Pediculosis

Pharyngitis, infectious, in infants and young children

Pneumonia, viral, in infants and young children

Pneumonia, *Staphylococcus aureus* or group A *Streptococcus*

Rabies

Rubella, congenital and other

Scabies

Scalded skin syndrome (Ritter's disease)

Skin, wound, or burn infection, major (draining and not covered by a dressing or dressing does not adequately contain the purulent material), including those infected with *Staphylococcus aureus* or group A *Streptococcus*

Vaccinia (generalized and progressive eczema vaccinatum)

*A private room is indicated for Contact Isolation; in general, however, patients infected with the same organism may share a room. During outbreaks, infants and young children with the same respiratory clinical syndrome may share a room. See Guideline for Isolation Precautions in Hospitals for details and for how long to apply precautions.

(Front of Card)

Respiratory Isolation

Visitors—Report to Nurses' Station Before Entering Room

1. Masks are indicated for those who come close to patient.
2. Gowns are not indicated.
3. Gloves are not indicated.
4. HANDS MUST BE WASHED AFTER TOUCHING THE PATIENT OR POTENTIALLY CONTAMINATED ARTICLES AND BEFORE TAKING CARE OF ANOTHER PATIENT.
5. Articles contaminated with infective material should be discarded or bagged and labeled before being sent for decontamination and reprocessing.

(Back of Card)

Diseases Requiring Respiratory Isolation*

Epiglottitis, *Haemophilus influenzae*
Erythema infectiosum
Measles
Meningitis
    Bacterial, etiology unknown
    Haemophilus influenzae, known or suspected
    Meningococcal, known or suspected
Meningococcal pneumonia
Meningococcemia
Mumps
Pertussis (whooping cough)
Pneumonia, *Haemophilus influenzae*, in children (any age)

---

*A private room is indicated for Respiratory Isolation; in general, however, patients infected with the same organism may share a room. See Guideline for Isolation Precautions in Hospitals for details and for how long to apply precautions.

(Front of Card)

AFB Isolation

Visitors—Report to Nurses' Station Before Entering Room

1. Masks are indicated only when patient is coughing and does not reliably cover mouth.
2. Gowns are indicated only if needed to prevent gross contamination of clothing.
3. Gloves are not indicated.
4. HANDS MUST BE WASHED AFTER TOUCHING THE PATIENT OR POTENTIALLY CONTAMINATED ARTICLES AND BEFORE TAKING CARE OF ANOTHER PATIENT.
5. Articles should be discarded, cleaned, or sent for decontamination and reprocessing.

(Back of Card)

Diseases Requiring AFB Isolation*

This isolation category is for patients with current pulmonary TB who have a positive sputum smear or a chest X-ray appearance that strongly suggests current (active) TB. Laryngeal TB is also included in this category. In general, infants and young children with pulmonary TB do not require isolation precautions because they rarely cough and their bronchial secretions contain few AFB compared with adults with pulmonary TB. To protect the patient's privacy, this instruction card is labeled AFB (acid-fast bacilli) Isolation rather than Tuberculosis Isolation.

*A private room with special ventilation is indicated for AFB isolation. In general, patients infected with the same organism may share a room. See Guideline for Isolation Precautions in Hospitals for details and for how long to apply precautions.

(Front of Card)

Enteric Precautions

Visitors—Report to Nurses' Station Before Entering Room

1. Masks are not indicated.
2. Gowns are indicated if soiling is likely.
3. Gloves are indicated for touching infective material.
4. HANDS MUST BE WASHED AFTER TOUCHING THE PATIENT OR POTENTIALLY CONTAMINATED ARTICLES AND BEFORE TAKING CARE OF ANOTHER PATIENT.
5. Articles contaminated with infective material should be discarded or bagged and labeled before being sent for decontamintion and reprocessing.

(Back of Card)

Diseases Requiring Enteric Precautions*

Amebic dysentery
Cholera
Coxsackievirus disease
Diarrhea, acute illness with suspected infectious etiology
Echovirus disease
Encephalitis (unless known not to be caused by enteroviruses)
Enterocolitis caused by *Clostridium difficile* or *Staphylococcus aureus*
Enteroviral infection
Gastroenteritis caused by
    Campylobacter species
    Cryptosporidium species
    Dientamoeba fragilis
    Escherichia coli (enterotoxic, enteropathogenic, or enteroinvasive)
    Giardia lamblia
    Salmonella species

Shigella species
Vibrio parahaemolyticus
Viruses—including Norwalk agent and rotavirus
Yersinia enterocolitica
Unknown etiology but presumed to be an infectious agent
Hand, foot, and mouth disease
Hepatitis, viral, type A
Herpangina
Meningitis, viral (unless known not to be caused by enteroviruses)
Necrotizing enterocolitis
Pleurodynia
Poliomyelitis
Typhoid fever (*Salmonella typhi*)
Viral pericarditis, myocarditis, or meningitis (unless known not to be caused by enteroviruses)

*A private room is indicated for Enteric Precautions if patient hygiene is poor. A patient with poor hygiene does not wash hands after touching infective material, contaminates the environment with infective material, or shares contaminated articles with other patients. In general, patients infected with the same organism may share a room. See Guideline for Isolation Precautions in Hospitals for details and for how long to apply precautions.

Drainage/Secretion Precautions

Visitors—Report to Nurses' Station Before Entering Room

1. Masks are not indicated.
2. Gowns are indicated if soiling is likely.
3. Gloves are indicated for touching infective material.
4. HANDS MUST BE WASHED AFTER TOUCHING THE PATIENT OR POTENTIALLY CONTAMINATED ARTICLES AND BEFORE TAKING CARE OF ANOTHER PATIENT.
5. Articles contaminated with infective material should be discarded or bagged and labeled before being sent for decontamination and reprocessing.

Diseases Requiring Drainage/Secretion Precautions*

Infectious diseases included in this category are those that result in production of infective purulent material, drainage, or secretions, unless the disease is included in another isolation category that requires more rigorous precautions. (If you have questions about a specific disease, see the listing of infectious diseases in Guideline for Isolation Precautions in Hospitals, Table A, Disease-Specific Isolation Precautions.)

The following infections are examples of those included in this category provided they are *not* a) caused by multiply-resistant microorganisms, b) major (draining and not covered by a dressing or dressing does not adequately contain the drainage) skin, wound, or burn infections, including those caused by *Staphylococcus aureus* or group A *Streptococcus*, or c) gonococcal eye infections in newborns. See Contact Isolation if the infection is one of these 3.
Abscess, minor or limited
Burn infection, minor or limited
Conjunctivitis
Decubitus ulcer, infected, minor or limited
Skin infection, minor or limited
Wound infection, minor or limited

---

*A private room is usually not indicated for Drainage/Secretion Precautions. See Guideline for Isolation Precautions in Hospitals for details and for how long to apply precautions.

Employee Health

Prevention of the transmission of infectious agents between pediatric patients and health care personnel is particularly important in the care of children. Some infections pose increased risks for pregnant health care workers principally because of the possible adverse effect on the fetus (eg, parvovirus B19, cytomegalovirus, rubella, and herpes simplex) or because the worker may be immunocompromised (eg, infected with *Mycobacterium tuberculosis*, cytomegalovirus, or herpes simplex virus).

The consequences to pediatric patients of acquiring infections from infected adults are also significant. Since children often lack immunity to many common viruses and bacteria, they are a highly susceptible population. Mild and severe illness in adults, such as viral gastroenteritis, upper respiratory tract viral infection (eg, respiratory syncytial virus), varicella, pertussis, herpes simplex infection, and tuberculosis, can cause life-threatening disease in children. Those at greatest risk are premature infants, children who have heart disease or chronic pulmonary disease, and immunocompromised patients.

The transmission of infectious agents within hospitals is facilitated by the inevitable close contact between patients and health care providers. In addition, children do not routinely have good hygienic practices.

To limit the risks of infection to and from children and caretakers, hospitals should have established employee health policies and services. Employees born after 1956, should have measles immunity documented by receipt of two doses of live-virus measles vaccine on or after their first birthday, a positive serologic test, or a physician-documented illness. Individuals born before 1957 have generally been considered immune. However, measles has occurred in health care workers born before 1957. Therefore, health facilities should consider offering at least one dose of measles-containing vaccine to such workers who lack proof of immunity to measles, particularly in communities with ongoing measles transmission. All employees should also have evidence of immunity to (1) rubella by documented immunization after 1 year of age or by serologic test; (2) hepatitis B and mumps by documented immunization or history of disease; (3) varicella by history of disease; and (4) tetanus and diphtheria by history of immunization. Susceptible employees should be offered immunization against rubella, mumps, hepatitis B, tetanus, and diphtheria. Consideration should be given to offering serologic testing to employees with a negative or uncertain history for varicella, and, if susceptible, counseling about the risks of varicella. All employees should be offered annual influenza immunization (see Health Care Personnel, p 65). For non-vaccine-preventable infections, employees should be counseled about exposures and possible need for leave if they are exposed to, ill with, or a carrier of, a specific infectious agent, whether the exposure occurs in the home, community, or the medical setting.

Employees should be screened by skin testing for tuberculosis. Those with common infections, such as gastroenteritis, dermatitis, or upper respiratory infections, should be evaluated to determine the resulting risk of transmission to their patients or to other health care workers.

Pregnant personnel should be counseled about the risks of caring for children with potentially contagious diseases. Specific concerns include exposure to HIV, rubella, varicella, cytomegalovirus, and parvovirus B19 infection.

Employee education is of paramount importance in infection control. Pediatric health care providers should be knowledgeable about the modes of transmission of infectious agents, proper hand washing technique, and the potential serious risks to children of certain mild infections in adults.

Sibling Visits

Sibling visits to birthing centers, postpartum rooms, pediatric wards, and intensive care units are encouraged. Newborn intensive care, with its increasing sophistication in medical care, often results in long hospital stays for the sick newborn, making family visits an important part of neonatal care. Studies indicate that sibling visits in newborn intensive care units are favorably received by parents, and bacterial colonization or subsequent infection is not increased in either the sick or well newborn who has been visited by his or her brothers or sisters.

Guidelines for sibling visits should be established to maximize opportunities for visiting and to minimize the risks of nosocomial spread of pathogens brought into the hospital by these young visitors. They may need to be modified by local nursing, pediatric, obstetric, and infectious disease staffs to address specific issues in their hospital settings. Basic guidelines for sibling visits to pediatric patients are as follows:

- Sibling visits should be encouraged in both the healthy infant nursery and the newborn intensive care nursery, for chronically and critically ill children, and for other hospitalized children.
- Before the visit, a nurse or physician should interview the parents at a site outside the unit to assess the current health of each sibling visitor. No child with fever or symptoms of an acute illness, including an upper respiratory tract infection, gastroenteritis, or dermatitis, should be allowed to visit. Siblings who have recently been exposed to a known communicable disease (eg, chickenpox) should not be allowed to visit. These interviews should be documented in the patient's record, and approval for each sibling visit should be noted.
- Adequate observation and monitoring of all visitors by the medical and nursing staff should occur.
- The visiting sibling should visit only his or her sibling.
- Children should carefully wash their hands before patient contact, especially in the case of neonatal and immunocompromised siblings.
- Throughout the visit, sibling activity should be supervised by parents or a responsible adult and limited to the mother's or patient's private room and/ or other designated areas.

Sexually Transmitted Diseases

The incidence of sexually transmitted diseases (STDs), including HIV infection, is increasing in children, adolescents, and young adults. Among other factors, the increase has been associated with the declining age at first intercourse. Approximately 50% of American adolescents are sexually active by age 16 years. Sexually experienced adolescents have the highest rates of STDs of any age group.

Physicians should be aware of the increasing prevalence of STDs, the methods for their prevention, their myriad presentations and pathogenic agents, the potential seriousness of their sequelae for adolescents and their offspring, and the implications of the diagnosis of an acquired STD in a prepubescent child with regard to child abuse. In all 50 states, minors can be diagnosed and treated for STDs without parental consent or knowledge.

The traditional STDs (eg, syphilis, gonorrhea, chancroid, and lymphogranuloma venereum) presently account for only a fraction of the currently recognized sexually transmitted pathogens. For example, hepatitis B, *Chlamydia trachomatis*, and HIV are recognized as major STDs, as both heterosexual and homosexual activity are important modes of transmission of these agents.

Management

Physicians need to identify patients at risk for STD and to diagnose and appropriately treat infections caused by sexually transmitted pathogens. Adolescents with STDs, particularly females, are more likely to be asymptomatic than adults. Screening by history, physical examination, and appropriate laboratory tests, as well as patient education, are indicated for high-risk groups. These include the following:
- Adolescents who are heterosexually or homosexually active.
- Pregnant adolescents and their sexual contacts.
- Adolescents undergoing a therapeutic abortion.
- Adolescents with symptoms compatible with STD, such as cervical or urethral discharge, lower abdominal or right upper quadrant pain in a female, testicular tenderness, tenesmus, rectal pain, or rectal discharge.
- Prepubescent children with genital, anal, or perineal ulcers; perineal pruritus; condyloma acuminata; or vaginitis and dysuria.
- Adolescents living in group homes or in detention homes.
- Any child or adolescent suspected of being a victim of sexual abuse, rape, or incest.
- Adolescent prostitutes.
- Street youth.
- Drug and alcohol abusers.

Because more than one STD frequently coexist in the same patient, the detection of one infection should lead to a search for others, regardless of the presenting symptoms. A careful physical examination, including examination of the oropharynx, rectum, genitalia, and skin, should be performed. Relevant laboratory studies include urinalysis, appropriate serologic tests, Gram stains of cervical or urethral discharge, wet mounts of vaginal secretions, diagnostic tests for *C trachomatis* on cervical (vaginal in prepubertal girls) or urethral specimens, and gonococcal cultures of the oropharynx, rectum, and cervix, or penile urethra in individual circumstances. The detection of concurrent HIV infection may alter the management of STDs. For example, treatment of syphilis may need to be more prolonged in an HIV-infected patient (see Syphilis, p 453).

The diagnosis of a primary case of an STD incurs additional major responsibilities for public health reporting, evaluation for possible sexual abuse (see Sexual Abuse, p 107), contact tracing, and patient education. Patients who have an STD or who have multiple sexual partners (defined as two or more in 6 months) are at increased risk for hepatitis B and should be immunized (see Hepatitis B, p 233). The physician should explain to the patient the route of transmission of these infections and the importance of examining partners, and should report diseases to the responsible health department to facilitate partner notification. The potential long-term sequelae of disease(s) should be emphasized. Whereas control through partner notification and identification of secondary spread is frequently best coordinated by public health departments, the patient's physician is responsible for educating and appropriately treating the patient. In general, whereas health departments have been active in partner notification when the index patient has syphilis, they have been less so with other STDs, particularly chlamydial infection. Physicians should actively facilitate treatment of their patient's current partners.

The style and content of counseling should be adapted for adolescents, including the need for nonjudgmental approach and identification of other problem behaviors (eg, drug use, school failure, or depression).

Sequelae

Major sequelae of STDs in adolescent males and females include AIDS, chronic hepatitis, salpingitis, ectopic pregnancies, infertility, and carcinoma of the cervix. Although approximately 50% of adults with HIV infection acquired this disease during adolescence, sequelae often do not develop for 6 to 10 years. Sexually transmitted diseases also cause neonatal infections, and the risk of these infections is increased in adolescent pregnancies. Failure to consider the possibility of an STD in the mother can result in delay or omission of neonatal therapy with possibly serious consequences. Hence, screening and treatment in pregnancy and early diagnosis and treatment of the infant are essential. Neonatal consequences of certain maternal STDs are listed in Table 2.6 (p 106).

Prevention of STDs

Adolescents consider health care providers to be accurate and confidential sources of information about STD, including HIV infection. Physicians caring for adolescents not only need to be knowledgeable about the diagnosis and management of STDs, but they also need to educate adolescents about STDs and their prevention. Providing information about STDs, the role of abstinence, and the proper use of condoms (see Table 2.7, p 107) can help to overcome many myths and erroneous beliefs (see Table 2.8, p 108), and can reduce the patient's risk of acquiring a sexually transmitted pathogen. Condoms are classified as medical devices; consequently, their quality is regulated by the Food and Drug Administration. Condom failure usually results from inconsistent or incorrect use rather than from condom breakage. Condoms lubricated with spermicides are not likely to be more effective than other lubricated condoms since the amount of spermicide they contain is small.

Advice to abstain from sexual intercourse or always to use condoms, together with a discussion about ways to reach these goals, is the safest message. Advice to be monogamous may convey a false sense of security that works against the use of more reliable preventive strategies. Adolescents often interpret

TABLE 2.6–Neonatal Consequences of Certain Maternal Sexually Transmitted Pathogens

Maternal Infection	Infant Consequences	Prevention	Neonatal Treatment
Candida albicans	Thrush, dermatitis	None known	Nystatin, clotrimazole, miconazole
Chlamydia trachomatis	Conjunctivitis, pneumonia	Screen and treat mother and her sexual partner; neonatal ocular prophylaxis of some value	Erythromycin
Cytomegalovirus	Congenital infection	None known	None
Hepatitis B	Development of chronic infection and hepatitis	Screen mother	HBIG and HBV vaccine
Herpes simplex, type 2	Central nervous system disease, disseminated infection, spontaneous abortion, premature delivery	Cesarean section	Acyclovir, vidarabine
HIV	AIDS	Screen mother; if negative, counsel regarding prevention; if positive, consider abortion	Zidovudine
Neisseria gonorrhoeae	Conjunctivitis, arthritis, sepsis, meningitis, premature delivery	Screen and treat mother and her sexual partner; ocular silver nitrate, erythromycin, or tetracycline	Ceftriaxone
Syphilis	Stillbirth, low birth weight, premature delivery, congenital infection	Screen mother and her sexual partner and treat	Penicillin G

"monogamy" as having one sexual relationship at a time, which is not as effective a strategy to prevent STDs or HIV as abstinence or use of condoms.

Sexually transmitted diseases are a major and growing source of morbidity in children and adolescents. Active cooperation and involvement of both public and private sectors of medicine are necessary to control this significant problem. **Primary prevention is vastly more effective than treating STDs and their sequelae.**

TABLE 2.7–Recommendations for Use of Condoms*

1. Latex condoms should be used because they may offer greater protection against HIV and other viral STDs than natural membrane condoms.

2. Condoms should be stored in a cool, dry place out of direct sunlight.

3. Condoms in damaged packages or those that show obvious signs of age (eg, those that are brittle, sticky, or discolored) should not be used. They cannot be relied upon to prevent infection or pregnancy

4. Condoms should be handled with care to prevent puncture.

5. The condom should be put on before any genital contact to prevent exposure to fluids that may contain infectious agents. Hold the tip of the condom and unroll it onto the erect penis, leaving space at the tip to collect semen, yet ensuring that no air is trapped in the tip of the condom.

6. Only water-based lubricants should be used. Petroleum- or oil-based lubricants (such as petroleum jelly, cooking oils, shortening, and lotions) should not be used because they weaken the latex and may cause breakage.

7. Use of condoms containing spermicides may provide some additional protection against STDs. However, vaginal use of spermicides along with condoms is likely to provide still greater protection.

8. If a condom breaks, it should be replaced immediately. If ejaculation occurs after condom breakage, the immediate use of spermicide has been suggested. However, the protective value of postejaculation application of spermicide in reducing the risk of STD transmission is unknown.

9. After ejaculation, care should be taken so that the condom does not slip off the penis before withdrawal; the base of the condom should be held throughout withdrawal. The penis should be withdrawn while still erect.

10. Condoms should never be reused.

*From Centers for Disease Control and Prevention. 1989 Sexually transmitted diseases treatment guidelines. *MMWR*. 1989;38(S-8):ix.

Sexual Abuse

Some infections known to be sexually transmitted in adults are similarly spread to children. Recent studies suggest that approximately 20% of children will be sexually abused in some way before they reach adulthood. Child sexual abuse is defined as engaging a child in sexual activity for which the child is developmentally unprepared and cannot give informed consent. Sexual abuse is generally perpetrated by someone known to the child and frequently continues over a prolonged period.

TABLE 2.8–Barriers to Condom Use and Ways to Overcome Them*

Perceived Barrier	Intervention Strategy
Decreases sexual pleasure (sensation)	• Often perceived by those who have never used a condom. Encourage patient to try. • Try a thinner latex condom.
Decreases spontaneity of sexual activity	• Encourage incorporation of use of condom during time before actual intercourse. Peace of mind may actually enhance pleasure. • Demonstrates responsibility and respect.
Embarrassing, juvenile, "unmanly"	• This feeling is not shared by many in the population, especially now.
Poor fit, either too small or too big, slips off, uncomfortable (actually due to constriction of the urethra with subsequent painful ejaculation)	• Smaller and larger condoms are available. • Natural skin condoms are another alternative for "large" patients but are less reliable for prevention of STD.
Requires prompt withdrawal after ejaculation	• Reinforce the protective nature.
Fear of breakage may lead to less vigorous sexual activity	• With prolonged intercourse, lubricant wears off and the condom begins to rub. Have a water-soluble lubricant available to reapply.

*From Canadian Guidelines for the Prevention, Diagnosis, Management and Treatment of Sexually Transmitted Diseases in Neonates, Children, Adolescents and Adults. *CCDR*. 1992;18S1:8.

If sexual abuse is considered to be chronic or to have occurred more than 72 hours before evaluation, specimens can be collected for evaluation of sexually transmitted diseases (STDs). If the abuse was more recent, appropriate forensic specimens should be collected, but the collection of specimens for evaluation of STD may be delayed. Antimicrobial treatment should be considered if (1) the alleged perpetrator was known to be infected with an STD, (2) more than one assailant was involved, (3) the patient is unlikely to return for follow-up, or (4) the patient is very anxious about the possibility of acquiring an STD. When evaluating a child for possible sexual abuse, appropriate tests for gonorrhea, chlamydial infection, and syphilis (as well as for other infections in selected circumstances) should be considered, as described below (see also Table 2.9, p 109). Practitioners must assess which patients with suspected sexual abuse warrant laboratory evaluation for an STD. Some experts advise culturing all children examined for sexual abuse for *Chlamydia trachomatis* and *Neisseria gonorrhoeae* because many abused children do not disclose the extent of their abuse, and infection with these agents may be asymptomatic. Specimens must be properly evaluated, for both medical and legal reasons, given the implications of a positive test. Techniques of testing for *Neisseria gonorrhoeae*, *Chlamydia trachomatis*, and syphilis are as follows:

TABLE 2.9–Testing for Sexual Abuse

	Organism/Syndrome	Specimens
All children	Neisseria gonorrhoeae	Rectal, throat, urethral, vaginal, and/or endocervical culture(s)
	Chlamydia trachomatis	Throat, rectal, urethral, and/or vulvovaginal culture(s)
	Syphilis	Darkfield examination of chancre fluid, if present; blood for serologic tests
Selected cases	HIV	Serology of abuser (if possible), serology of child at time of abuse and 12 weeks later
	Hepatitis B	Serology of abuser
	Herpes simplex	Culture of lesion
	Bacterial vaginosis	Wet mount of vaginal discharge
	Papillomavirus	Biopsy of lesion
	Trichomonas vaginalis	Wet mount of vaginal discharge, culture of discharge

1. *Neisseria gonorrhoeae.* Swabs of the throat, rectum, urethra, and vagina should be obtained and placed immediately into commercially available transport media for *N gonorrhoeae* or plated immediately on a selective medium (eg, Thayer-Martin) and chocolate agar and incubated inactivated in a CO_2-enriched atmosphere. Isolates should be confirmed by biochemical and enzyme substrate or serologic techniques, preferably using at least two confirmatory techniques.

   Rapid detection techniques directly applied to patient specimens, such as Gram stain of discharge in a symptomatic child, should be used only to guide initial therapy pending culture results. They cannot be used as legal evidence of an STD. The presence of culture-proven *N gonorrhoeae* after a child is 1 year of age is the result of sexual contact in almost all cases (see Gonococcal Infections, p 196).

2. *Chlamydia trachomatis.* Specimens should be obtained from the throat, rectum, urethral meatus, and vagina for culture. Rapid-detection techniques should not be used since other flora may give a false-positive reaction. Vaginal chlamydial infection after a child is 2 years of age is usually due to sexual contact (see *Chlamydia trachomatis*, p 155).

3. *Syphilis.* Darkfield microscopy should be obtained to study fluid from a genital lesion, if present. Serology for syphilis (VDRL, rapid plasma reagin [RPR], or automated reagin test [ART]) should be obtained as part of an evaluation for sexual abuse (see Syphilis, p 446). Reactive nontreponemal tests should be confirmed by a treponemal test (eg, FTA-ABS, MHA-TP, or TPI). If not congenitally acquired, a confirmed reactive serology is highly suggestive of sexual contact.

Other infectious agents can be found in sexually abused children. In selected situations, screening for one or more of the following organisms may be desirable:

1. *Human immunodeficiency virus (HIV)*. If feasible, serologic evaluation of the alleged offender should be performed. The child should be tested serologically at the time of abuse and at 3 and 6 months after sexual contact with an assailant likely to be HIV infected. Counseling of the child and family should be provided. The risk of transmission of HIV is small.

2. *Hepatitis B*. If the alleged offender is a known or suspected carrier of hepatitis B surface antigen (HBsAg), the victim should be tested at that time and 3 months later for HBsAg. The victim should also receive hepatitis B immune globulin as soon as possible but within 14 days of sexual contact. In addition, the victim should be started on the hepatitis B vaccine series (see Hepatitis B, p 234).

3. *Herpes simplex virus (HSV)*. Type 1 HSV may be spread sexually or nonsexually, but type 2 HSV suggests sexual transmission. Viral culture of lesions should be done (see Herpes Simplex, p 244). Routine cultures in the absence of lesions are not recommended. The use of commercially available serologic tests is not recommended.

4. *Bacterial vaginosis (nonspecific vaginitis or Gardnerella-associated vaginalis)*. Bacterial vaginosis is more common in children who have had sexual contact. Clue cells may be seen in a wet preparation obtained from a vaginal discharge or a vaginal wash, and a fishy odor develops after 10% KOH is added to vaginal fluid (see Bacterial Vaginosis, p 136).

5. *Human papillomavirus (HPV)*. Genital or rectal warts (condyloma acuminata) that develop 3 months or later after sexual abuse may be biopsied. Perinatally acquired disease can appear as genital or rectal warts several years after birth (see Papillomaviruses, p 337).

6. *Trichomonas vaginalis*. A wet mount preparation of vaginal secretion or culture can be performed. Although infection has been reported to be spread from mother to infant, most infections in prepubertal girls are probably caused by sexual abuse (see *Trichomonas vaginalis* Infections, p 475).

Several organisms usually thought to be sexually transmitted can be seen in children where sexual abuse does not appear likely. Although infection with *Gardnerella vaginalis*, *Mycoplasma hominis*, and *Ureaplasma urealyticum* can be seen in sexually abused children, their presence in children who have not been abused suggests that acquisition may occur in other ways.

In addition to the medical evaluation, protecting the child, and reporting suspected abuse, counseling of the child and family is essential.

Child sexual abuse has been endemic for generations, but recognition of its prevalence and potentially devastating psychologic effects have only recently been recognized. Appropriate social service and law enforcement agencies must be involved whenever sexual abuse is suspected to ensure the child's protection, and counseling must be provided to the child and family.

Medical Evaluation of Internationally Adopted Children

More than 10,000 children from abroad are adopted each year by families in the United States. Asian nations (such as Korea, India, and the Philippines) and Central and South American countries account for nearly 90% of international adoptees. However, increasing numbers of adoptees are coming from Haiti, other areas in the Caribbean, African nations, and Eastern Europe. The diverse origins of these children, their unknown backgrounds before adoption, and inadequacy of health care in many developing countries make appropriate medical evaluation of internationally adopted children an important task.

Internationally adopted children differ from refugee children in several ways. International adoptees, regardless of country of origin, are seldom appropriately screened for medical illness. Preventive health care, such as immunizations, may be delayed or omitted. Although all internationally adopted children are required to have a medical examination performed by a physician designated by the United States Embassy in the country of origin before an immigrant visa is issued, the examination is limited to screening for certain communicable diseases and for serious physical defects. It is usually not a comprehensive assessment of the child's health status.

In prospective studies of internationally adopted children, infectious diseases have constituted most medical diagnoses and have been found in nearly 60% of international adoptees (see Table 2.10, p 212). Because these infections are often asymptomatic, the diagnosis must be made by screening tests rather than by history and physical examination. Use of screening tests for certain infections is cost-effective preventive health care for these children and their adoptive families.

Infectious diseases of special importance in internationally adopted children include the following:

1. *Viral hepatitis.* The prevalence of hepatitis B markers ranges from 5% to 50% in internationally adopted children, depending on the country of origin. These children should be tested for serum hepatitis B surface antigen (HBsAg), hepatitis B surface antibody (anti-HBs), and hepatitis B core antibody. The HBsAg and antibody testing alone will fail to identify children in the "window" period of acute hepatitis B virus (HBV) infection. They can be identified by the presence of antibodies to core antigens (anti-HbC) and the absence of HBsAg or anti-HBs.

   The prevalence of chronic hepatitis B (defined by the persistence of HBsAg for more than 6 months) is high. Serum transaminase and hepatitis e antigen testing should be obtained on HBsAg-positive patients, and susceptible household contacts should be immunized.

   Delta hepatitis, which occurs only in conjunction with hepatitis B, may be found in adoptees from Eastern Europe, Africa, South America, and the Middle East. Serologic tests for diagnoses are available (see Hepatitis Delta Virus, p 240).

   Since current diagnostic tests for hepatitis A detect antibodies formed in response to infection, and the child is usually not infectious once these anti-

TABLE 2.10–Infectious Diseases of Importance in International Adoptees and Refugees

Bacteria	Viruses	Protozoa	Helminths	Arthropoda
Campylobacter	Cytomegalovirus	Amebiasis	Ascariasis	Lice
Melioidosis*	Hepatitis A	Giardiasis	Filariasis*	Scabies
Salmonella	Hepatitis B	Malaria*	Hookworms	
Shigella	HIV		Liver flukes*	
Syphilis			Lung flukes*	
Tuberculosis*			Schistosomiasis*	
Typhoid fever*			Strongyloidiasis	
Yersinia			Tapeworms	
			Trichuriasis	

*More commonly encountered in refugee children than in international adoptees.

bodies are present, routine serologic screening for hepatitis A antibodies is not indicated. Many internationally adopted children acquire hepatitis A early in life; thus, acute infections after adoption are rare, and chronic hepatitis A does not occur.

Because presently available serologic tests for hepatitis C do not distinguish between acute and past infection, and because neither treatment nor immunoprophylaxis exists, screening for hepatitis C is not presently indicated.

2. *Cytomegalovirus.* Cytomegalovirus (CMV) is excreted by approximately one half of internationally adopted children, who typically acquired the virus perinatally and suffer no sequelae. Cytomegalovirus is readily transmitted to susceptible household members from infected children. Instructions on the value of good hand washing after contact with urine, diapers, and respiratory secretions should be given to the adoptive parents. Routine screening for CMV infection is not recommended. However, adoptive parents should be counseled about CMV infection, especially if an adoptive mother is not immune and is contemplating pregnancy.

3. *Intestinal pathogens.* Fecal examinations for ova and parasites by an experienced laboratory identify a pathogen in 20% to 30% of internationally adopted children. Because of the recognition of additional parasites after treatment of the primary infestation, follow-up stool examinations for ova and parasites should be obtained until all pathogens have been eliminated. In addition, children with diarrhea should have stool cultured for *Salmonella, Shigella, Yersinia,* and *Campylobacter.*

4. *Tuberculosis.* Although less common in international adoptees than in refugee children from Indochina, tuberculosis is still frequently encountered. Screening for tuberculosis should include the placement of the Mantoux test (5TU PPD) (see Tuberculosis, p 482). In addition, in children younger than 2 years and those of poor nutritional status, the simultaneous placement of a *Candida* skin test or other test of delayed hypersensitivity may be helpful in differentiating anergy from lack of exposure to *Mycobacterium*

tuberculosis. Routine chest roentgenograms are not warranted in asymptomatic children with negative PPD tests. A PPD should be placed even if a child has received BCG vaccine. A positive PPD test should not be attributed to BCG without further investigation (see Tuberculosis, p 498). In refugees and international adoptees found to have active tuberculosis, efforts to isolate the responsible organism and test it for drug sensitivities must be diligently pursued because of the high prevalence of drug resistance in many foreign countries.

5. *Syphilis.* Congenital syphilis, especially with involvement of the central nervous system, is sometimes undiagnosed and often inadequately treated in many developing nations. Each international adoptee should be screened for syphilis by a reliable serologic test (see Syphilis, p 446). Those found to be reactive should have appropriate supplemental testing, and those infected should be adequately treated (see Syphilis, p 450).

6. *HIV infection.* The risk of HIV infection in internationally adopted children depends on the country of origin. Because of the rapidly changing epidemiology of AIDS and because adoptees may come from subgroups at high risk for HIV infection, screening for HIV should be considered for internationally adopted children. Test results for HIV from the adoptee's country of origin should not be presumed reliable. Transplacentally acquired maternal antibody in the absence of infection in the child can be present in the child younger than 18 months. Hence, positive serologic tests in asymptomatic children of this age require follow-up testing and clinical evaluation (see HIV Infection and AIDS, p 258).

7. *Other infectious diseases.* Diseases such as typhoid fever or melioidosis are infrequently encountered in internationally adopted children, except those of southeast Asian origin. Routine screening for malaria is not indicated. However, malaria can occur. When children from countries where malaria is endemic develop fever of unknown etiology, anemia, or splenomegaly, Giemsa-stained thick smears of peripheral blood should be obtained (see Malaria, p 302).

Unsuspected problems may be detected by performing routine vision and hearing testing, developmental testing, and a test for anemia in all children. The use of other tests in specific groups of children may be warranted depending on ethnicity and country of origin. For example, screening for sickle hemoglobinopathies may be appropriate in children from India, Central America, or South America, and hemoglobin E can be found in children from Southeast Asia. Screening for glucose-6-phosphate dehydrogenase deficiency should be considered in children of Mediterranean or African origin before administering sulfa-containing antibiotics or primaquine.

International adoptees and refugees should be immunized according to recommended schedules for healthy US infants and children (see Tables 1.3 and 1.4, pp 23 and 24). Only written documentation should be accepted as evidence of prior immunization. Although some vaccines with inadequate potency have been produced in other countries, most vaccines used worldwide, including those in developing nations, are produced with adequate quality control standards and are reliable. In general, written immunization records that appear authentic may be considered valid if the vaccines, number of doses, interval between doses, and age of the patient at the time of vaccination would be appropriate for comparable

US-produced vaccines. The immunization schedules of other countries are acceptable if they meet the minimum requirements of the WHO schedule (see Table 1.5, p 25).

Control Measures for Prevention of Tick-Borne Infections

Tick-borne infectious pediatric diseases that can occur in the United States include diseases caused by spirochetes (Lyme disease, relapsing fever), rickettsia (Rocky Mountain spotted fever, ehrlichiosis), bacteria (tularemia), viruses (Colorado tick fever, California tick fever), and protozoa (babesiosis). The control of these and other tick-borne diseases requires preventing infected ticks from biting and engorging on humans, or at least minimizing opportunities for them to do so. Physicians should be aware of the epidemiology of tick-borne infections in their local area. Control of the tick population in the field is not always a practical public health measure. Specific control measures for prevention are as follows:

- Physicians, parents, and children, whenever possible, should be aware of ticks and the possibility of acquisition of disease.
- Tick-infested areas should be avoided whenever possible.
- If a tick-infested area is entered, protective clothing that covers the arms, legs, and other exposed areas should be worn. Other measures include tucking pants into boots or socks and buttoning long-sleeved shirts at the cuff. In addition, permethrin (a synthetic pyrethyroid) is effective in decreasing tick attachment and can be sprayed onto clothes. Permethrin toxicity includes itching, edema, erythema, temporary burning, stinging, numbness, and tingling of exposed skin. No systemic reactions have been reported.
- Tick and insect repellents*containing DEET[†] applied to the skin provide additional protection but require reapplication every 1 to 2 hours for effectiveness. Since seizures in young children have been reported coincident with application of DEET-containing insect repellents, they should be applied sparingly and only to exposed skin, not to a child's face, hands, or irritated or abraded skin. These preparations should be removed by washing after the child comes indoors.
- Persons should be taught to inspect themselves and their children's bodies and clothing daily after possible tick exposure. Special attention should be given to the exposed hairy regions of the body, including the head and neck in children, where ticks often attach.
- Ticks should be removed promptly. Care should be taken to avoid squeezing the body of the tick because transmission of infection can result. The tick should be grasped with a fine tweezer close to the skin and removed by gentle pulling. If fingers are used to remove ticks, they should be protected with facial tissue and washed afterwards.
- Daily inspection of pets and removal of ticks is indicated.

---

*For further information, see Insect repellents. *The Medical Letter.* 1989;31:45-47
[†]N,N-diethyl-m-toluamide

SECTION 3

SUMMARIES OF INFECTIOUS DISEASES

Actinomycosis

Clinical Manifestations: The three major types of clinical disease are cervicofacial, thoracic, and abdominal. Cervicofacial lesions frequently occur after tooth extraction or facial trauma, or are associated with carious teeth. Localized pain and induration progress to "woody hard," nodular lesions that can be complicated by draining sinus tracts. The infection usually spreads by direct invasion of adjacent tissues. Actinomyces infection may also contribute to chronic obstructive tonsillitis. Thoracopulmonary disease is most commonly secondary to aspiration of oropharyngeal secretions; it rarely occurs after esophageal disruption secondary to surgery or nonpenetrating trauma. Disease manifests as pneumonia, which can be complicated by the development of abscesses, empyema, and, rarely, pleurodermal sinuses. In abdominal infection, the appendix and cecum are the most frequent sites, and symptoms simulate those of appendicitis. Intra-abdominal abscesses and peritoneal-dermal draining sinuses eventually develop.

Etiology: *Actinomyces israeli* is the usual cause. *A israeli* and other *Actinomyces* and *Arachnia* (a related genus) species are slow-growing, Gram-positive, anaerobic bacteria that can be part of the normal oral flora.

Epidemiology: *Actinomyces* species are worldwide in distribution. Infection is rare in infants and children, and occurs sporadically. The organisms are components of the endogenous gastrointestinal tract flora. Disease results from penetrating trauma (including human bite wounds) and from nonpenetrating trauma. Actinomycosis is not contagious.

The **incubation period** is variable—probably many years after oral colonization and days to months after trauma.

Diagnostic Tests: A microscopic demonstration of beaded, branched, Gram-positive bacilli in pus suggests the diagnosis. A Gram stain of sulfur granules discloses a dense reticulum of filaments; the ends of individual filaments may project around the periphery of the granule, with or without radially arranged hyaline clubs. For recovery of the organism, specimens must be cultured anaerobically on selective media in the presence of carbon dioxide.

Treatment: Penicillin is the drug of choice. Erythromycin, clindamycin, chloramphenicol, and tetracycline (for children 9 years of age and older) are also usually effective. High doses of antimicrobial agents for periods of 6 months or longer are commonly required to effect a cure. Surgical drainage may be necessary.

Isolation of the Hospitalized Patient: No special precautions are recommended.

Control Measures: Good oral hygiene, adequate regular dental care, and careful cleansing of wounds (including human bite wounds) can prevent infection.

Adenovirus Infections

Clinical Manifestations: The major clinical syndromes caused by adenoviruses are upper respiratory tract symptoms accompanied by moderate systemic manifestations in children and adolescents. Severe pneumonia, which is occasionally fatal, can occur in younger infants and, less commonly, in older children and adolescents. Disease is often more severe in immunocompromised patients. Conjunctivitis is common, either alone or in combination with pharyngitis and other respiratory symptoms. Adenoviruses are infrequent causes of a pertussis-like syndrome, croup, bronchiolitis, and hemorrhagic cystitis. Adenoviruses have also been associated with gastroenteritis. The illness is similar to, although less common than, that caused by rotavirus.

Etiology: Adenoviruses are DNA viruses; 47 distinct serotypes cause human infections. Types 31, 40, and 41 have been incriminated as causes of gastroenteritis.

Epidemiology: Infection occurs throughout the pediatric age range. Adenoviruses causing respiratory infection are transmitted by person-to-person contact, usually through respiration. Enteric strains of adenoviruses can be transmitted by the fecal-oral route. Other routes have not been clearly defined and may vary with age, type of infection, and environmental or other factors. The eyes can provide a portal of entry; eg, infections have resulted from direct introduction of virus by the use of contaminated ophthalmologic instruments. Epidemics attributed to contaminated swimming pools have occurred. Shared towels and direct inoculation by fingers are involved in epidemic keratoconjunctivitis. Epidemics in military and educational institutions, or those resulting from a common source, have occurred. Nosocomial outbreaks of adenoviral respiratory and gastrointestinal infections have been documented. The incidence of adenovirus-induced respiratory disease is slightly increased in late winter, spring, and early summer. Enteric disease occurs during most of the year and primarily affects children younger than 4 years of age. Adenovirus infections are most communicable during the first few days of an acute illness. Asymptomatic infections are common.

The **incubation period** varies from 2 to 14 days. For gastroenteritis, it is 3 to 10 days.

Diagnostic Tests: Adenoviruses can be isolated from pharyngeal secretions, eye swabs, and feces by inoculation of specimens into a variety of cell cultures. A pharyngeal isolate is more suggestive of recent infection than a fecal isolate, which may indicate either prolonged carriage or recent infection. Adenovirus antigen has been detected in body fluids of infected patients by immunoassay techniques. These techniques are especially useful in the diagnosis of diarrheal disease, as the enteric adenovirus strains 40 and 41 usually cannot be isolated in standard tissue cultures. Enteric adenoviruses can also be identified by electron microscopy of stool specimens. Multiple serologic tests, including fluorescent antibody and enzyme immunoassay (EIA), are now commercially available for antigen and antibody testing. By complement fixation and EIA tests that detect antibody to the common adenovirus antigen (hexon), a fourfold or greater rise in antibody titer in paired acute and convalescent sera is diagnostic of recent infection. Type-specific antibodies are detectable by hemagglutination inhibition or neutralization techniques or, for types 40 and 41, by EIA.

Treatment: Supportive.

Isolation of the Hospitalized Patient: For young children with respiratory adenoviral infection, contact isolation is indicated for the duration of hospitalization. For patients with conjunctivitis, drainage/secretion precautions are recommended. Enteric precautions are indicated for patients with adenoviral gastroenteritis.

Control Measures: Children who participate in group child care, particularly those between the ages of 6 months and 2 years, are at increased risk of adenoviral respiratory infection and gastroenteritis. Measures for preventing spread of adenovirus infection in this setting have not been studied, but frequent hand washing is recommended.

Live enteric-coated adenovirus vaccines containing types 4, 7, and 21 have been used successfully to reduce acute respiratory disease among military personnel, but these vaccines are not available for civilian use.

Adequate chlorination of swimming pools is recommended to prevent pharyngoconjunctival fever. Appropriate hand washing before and after administering eye medications is required to prevent spread of keratoconjunctivitis. Ophthalmologic instruments should be decontaminated after use in infected patients.

Amebiasis

Clinical Manifestations: Persons with amebiasis are most commonly asymptomatic or have nonspecific or mild intestinal symptoms, such as abdominal distention, flatulence, constipation, and, occasionally, loose stools. Some infected persons have nondysenteric colitis with intermittent diarrhea and abdominal pain. Acute amebic colitis (dysentery) is associated with abdominal cramps, diarrhea containing blood and mucus, and tenesmus. The disease can progress to severe involvement of the colon with dilatation and paralysis resembling a toxic megacolon or ulcerative colitis. Rarely, perforation of the intestine with subsequent peritonitis occurs. An "apple core" deformity of the right colon, an ameboma, can be mistaken for colonic carcinoma. Extraintestinal disease occurs in a small percentage of infected patients. Although the lung, brain, genitalia, or kidneys can be involved, the liver is the most common site of infection. Onset of symptoms of an amebic liver abscess can be abrupt or insidious. Fever and localized abdominal pain are almost always present. Cough and right shoulder pain usually indicate diaphragmatic involvement. The liver is usually tender to palpation. Jaundice and impaired liver function rarely occur.

Etiology: *Entamoeba histolytica* is a protozoan that is excreted as cysts or trophozoites in the stool of infected patients. Trophozoites can cause invasive disease.

Epidemiology: Although the disease is occasionally transmitted through contaminated food and water, it is usually transmitted by the fecal-oral route, involving person-to-person spread, most commonly in the United States. Only cysts are infective by the fecal-oral route because trophozoites are fragile and destroyed by gastric acid. Transmission has also occurred from inappropriate reuse of enema equipment. Asymptomatic cyst passers are a major source of infection, as many infected persons are asymptomatic. Infection has a worldwide distribution. Infected patients excrete cysts intermittently and, if untreated, for years. In the United States, higher rates of infection have been found in southwestern and southeastern states and in male homosexuals. Invasive disease is found more commonly in tropical countries.

The **incubation period** is variable, ranging from a few days to months or years, but most commonly it is 2 to 4 weeks.

Diagnostic Tests: Colonic disease can be diagnosed by microscopic demonstration of trophozoites or cysts in the stool. *Entamoeba histolytica* must be differentiated from other nonpathogenic species (such as *Entamoeba hartmanni* and *Entamoeba coli*), which requires a laboratory technician skilled in the identification of protozoan parasites. Examination of serial stool samples increases the likelihood of demonstrating the parasite in the stool. To do so, three samples are collected on different days in kits containing both 10% formalin and polyvinyl alcohol fixatives. Samples may also be taken by direct touch preparations at the time of proctoscopy. Mucosa scrapings or rectal biopsies can be used.

Serologic tests are helpful in the diagnosis of extraintestinal amebiasis, particularly in patients with liver abscesses. Available tests include immunofluorescence, countercurrent immunoelectrophoresis, indirect hemagglutination, and enzyme immunoassay. These tests are sensitive and highly specific. Ultrasound and computed tomography can be effective in identifying liver abscesses and other extraintestinal sites of infection. Aspirates from a liver abscess may be examined for trophozoites but organisms are often not found.

Treatment: Treatment involves the elimination of the tissue-invading trophozoites as well as the cysts in the intestinal lumen. The following regimens are recommended:

- *Asymptomatic cyst passers*: iodoquinol; alternatively, paromomycin or diloxanide furoate.
- *Mild to moderate intestinal symptoms with no dysentery*: metronidazole followed by iodoquinol or paromomycin.
- *Dysentery or extraintestinal disease (including liver abscess)*: metronidazole followed by iodoquinol.

Some studies indicate that tinidazole, a drug similar to metronidazole but not available in the United States, is at least as effective as metronidazole and is better tolerated.

Patients for whom treatment of invasive disease has failed should be treated with dehydroemetine and chloroquine phosphate, followed by iodoquinol. Dehydroemetine is available from the Drug Service of the Centers for Disease Control and Prevention (see Directory of Telephone Numbers, p 601).

To prevent spontaneous rupture of the abscess, patients with large liver abscesses may benefit from percutaneous or surgical aspiration of the abscess.

Isolation of the Hospitalized Patient: Enteric precautions are recommended for patients with either symptomatic or asymptomatic infections.

Control Measures: Careful hand washing after defecation, sanitary disposal of fecal material, and treatment of drinking water will control the spread of infection. Sexual transmission may be controlled through the use of condoms.

Amebic Meningoencephalitis (Naegleria fowleri, Acanthamoeba)

Clinical Manifestations: *Naegleria fowleri* can cause a rapidly progressive, almost always fatal disease, primary amebic meningoencephalitis. Early symptoms include fever, headache, and sometimes disturbances of smell and/or taste. The illness rapidly progresses to signs of meningoencephalitis, including nuchal rigidity, lethargy, confusion, and altered level of consciousness. Seizures are common and death may occur soon after the onset of symptoms. No distinct clinical features differentiate this disease from bacterial meningitis except for the history of recent swimming in a warm body of water.

Granulomatous amebic encephalitis, caused by *Acanthamoeba* spp and leptomyxid amoebae, has a more insidious onset and progression of manifestations, occurring during weeks to months, and is more common in immuno– compromised persons. Signs and symptoms can include personality changes, seizures, headaches, nuchal rigidity, ataxia, cranial nerve palsies, hemiparesis, and other focal deficits. Fever is often low-grade and intermittent. Skin ulcers can be present. The course can resemble that of a bacterial brain abscess.

Etiology: *Naegleria fowleri*, *Acanthamoeba* species, and leptomyxid amoebae are small, free-living amoebae.

Epidemiology: *Naegleria fowleri* is found in warm, fresh water and moist soil. Most infections with *Naegleria* have been associated with swimming in warm, natural bodies of water, but other sources have included tap water, contaminated swimming pools, and baths. Small outbreaks associated with swimming in a lake and in a swimming pool have been reported. A few cases with no history of contact with water, however, have occurred. More than 160 cases, 68 from the United States, have been reported worldwide. Disease in the United States occurs primarily in the summer and usually affects children and young adults. The trophozoites of the parasite directly invade the brain from the nose along the olfactory nerves via the cribriform plate.

The **incubation period** of *N fowleri* infection is several days to a week.

The causative organisms of granulomatous amebic encephalitis are worldwide in distribution and are found in soil, fresh and brackish water, dust, hot tubs, and sewage. Infection occurs primarily in debilitated and immunocompromised persons. However, some patients have had no demonstrable underlying disease or defect. Acquisition probably occurs by inhalation or direct contact with contaminated soil or water. The primary focus of infection is probably the skin or respiratory tract, and spread to the brain is hematogenous.

Acanthamoeba also causes keratitis in contact lens wearers using contaminated saline solutions for lens care.

The **incubation period** is unknown.

Diagnostic Tests: *Naegleria fowleri* infection can be documented by microscopic demonstration of the motile trophozoites on a wet mount of centrifuged cerebrospinal fluid (CSF). The organism can also be cultured on 1.5% nonnutrient agar layered with enteric bacteria or in Page saline. Immunofluorescent tests to speciate the organism are available through the Centers for Disease Control and Prevention.

In *Acanthamoeba* infection, cysts can be seen in sections of brain or corneal tissue and may be present on brain biopsy, but they are never seen on CSF examination. The organism can also be cultured by the same method as that for *Naegleria*.

Treatment: If *Naegleria* meningoencephalitis is suspected because of the presence of organisms in the CSF, therapy should not be withheld while waiting confirmatory diagnostic tests. However, treatment is often unsuccessful. Amphotericin B is currently considered the drug of choice, although only one case of successful treatment in the United States has been documented. In this case, a 9-year-old girl was given intravenous and intrathecal amphotericin B and miconazole and oral rifampin. Early diagnosis and the institution of high-dose drug therapy may have contributed to the treatment success.

Effective treatment for *Acanthamoeba* central nervous infections has not been established. Only one case of partial recovery, an adult treated with sul-famethazine, has been reported. Experimental infections can be prevented or cured by sulfadiazone. Strains of *Acanthamoeba* isolated from patients with fatal encephalitis are usually sensitive in vivo to pentamidine, ketoconazole, 5-fluorocytosine, and, to a lesser degree, amphotericin B.*

Isolation of the Hospitalized Patient: No special precautions are recommended.

Control Measures: People should avoid swimming in hot springs and other bodies of warm, polluted fresh water. *Acanthamoeba* are resistant to freezing, drying, and the usual concentrations of chlorine found in drinking water and swimming pools.

Only sterile saline solutions should be used to clean contact lenses.

Anthrax

Clinical Manifestations: The spectrum of illness includes cutaneous (malignant pustule), inhalation (woolsorter's disease), gastrointestinal, septi-cemic, and meningeal anthrax. Cutaneous anthrax, which accounts for 95% of the cases of anthrax in the United States, is characterized by a painless lesion that progresses from a papule to a vesicle to necrosis and, eventually, to eschar formation. In inhalation anthrax, mild upper respiratory tract symp-toms occur initially; approximately 2 to 5 days later, severe dyspnea, cyano-sis, tachycardia, tachypnea, diaphoresis, fever, rales, and, usually, death occur. Gastrointestinal disease is characterized by abdominal pain and disten-tion, vomiting, bloody diarrhea, and, frequently, toxemia and shock. Pharyn-geal anthrax with profound submental swelling has also been reported. Septicemia and hemorrhagic meningitis are secondary manifestations of cuta-neous, inhalation, or gastrointestinal anthrax. Disease manifestations are sim-ilar in adults and children.

Etiology: *Bacillus anthracis* is a Gram-positive, encapsulated, spore-forming, nonmotile rod.

Epidemiology: Anthrax is a zoonotic disease endemic in many agricul-tural regions of the world. It is common in developing countries but is rarely reported in the United States. Human disease occurs after contact

---

Acanthamoeba keratitis has been treated with the investigational drug propamidine isethionate eye drops. Information is available from the Food and Drug Administration (see Directory of Telephone Numbers, p 601). Other treatment regimens have included a combination of propamidine isethionate with neosporin and/or clotrimazole 1%.

with infected animals or contaminated animal products. Spores of *B anthracis* are found on hides, carcasses, hair, wool, bone meal, and other animal byproducts of domesticated and wild animals such as goats, sheep, cattle, swine, horses, buffalo, and deer. Imported dolls and toys decorated with infected hair or hides have been a source of infection. Spore forms of the organism have been found in soil in rural farming regions in several areas of the United States. Spores can remain viable for 40 years or more. Although *B anthracis* has a soil growth cycle, human infections have not been reported to occur as a result.

Cutaneous anthrax, which occurs principally in agricultural and industrial employees, results from contact with infected animals, carcasses, hair (especially goat hair), wool, hides, or, rarely, soil. Inhalation anthrax is extremely rare, and has resulted from inhalation of spores aerosolized during industrial processing of animal by-products or laboratory work with *B anthracis*. In gastrointestinal anthrax, ingestion of contaminated, undercooked meat is the mode of acquisition. Biting flies and other insects may also serve as mechanical vectors. Discharges from cutaneous lesions are potentially infectious; accidental infections have occurred in laboratory workers. *Bacillus anthracis* is not known to be transmitted from person to person.

The **incubation period** is 1 to 7 days; most cases occur within 2 to 5 days of exposure.

Diagnostic Tests: The following procedures can be used for diagnosis: (1) microscopic visualization of *B anthracis* on direct Gram-stained smears and/or cultures on blood agar of lesions or discharges; (2) fluorescent antibody identification of the organisms in vesicle fluid, cultures, or tissue sections; (3) detection of antibody to *B anthracis* toxin by immunoblot.

Treatment: Penicillin is the antimicrobial of choice and is given for 5 to 7 days. Erythromycin, tetracycline (for children 9 years of age and older), chloramphenicol, and ciprofloxacin are also effective. High-dose penicillin combined with streptomycin, or, possibly, parenteral ciprofloxacin, should be used for treating meningitis or inhalation anthrax. Ciprofloxacin should not be used in patients younger than 18 years of age, however, unless the possible benefits are considered to be greater than the potential risks.

Isolation of the Hospitalized Patient: For patients with cutaneous or inhalation anthrax, drainage/secretion precautions are indicated until the patient has received 72 hours of antibiotic therapy. Gloves should be worn for touching infective material; gowns should be worn if soiling is likely. Contaminated dressings and bedclothes should be burned or steam sterilized to destroy spores.

Control Measures: A cell-free vaccine* is available for persons at significant ongoing risk of acquiring anthrax. The vaccine is effective in preventing

---

*Available from the Division of Biologic Products, Michigan Department of Public Health, Lansing, MI (see Directory of Telephone Numbers, p 601).

or significantly reducing the occurrence of cutaneous and inhalation anthrax in adults, and it produces minimal adverse effects. No data on vaccine effectiveness or reactogenicity in children are available and the vaccine is not currently licensed for use in children or pregnant women.

Surveillance and control of industrial and agricultural sources of *B anthracis* by public health authorities is important.

Arboviruses (Including Dengue, Japanese Encephalitis, and Yellow Fever)

Clinical Manifestations: Some arboviruses cause principally a central nervous system infection. Others produce an undifferentiated febrile illness, fever with rash, hemorrhagic manifestations, hepatitis, myalgia, or polyarthritis. Other organ systems can also be involved.

Etiology: Approximately 570 arthropod-borne viruses, commonly referred to as arboviruses, have been identified. Although originally they were grouped together because of a common mode of transmission, the viruses belong to a variety of taxonomic groups (Table 3.1, p 124). Most arboviruses are classified in the families *Bunyaviridae*, *Togaviridae*, or *Flaviviridae*. Of the more than 230 recognized arboviruses in the Western hemisphere, more than 30 have been demonstrated to be responsible for human disease.

Epidemiology: Most arboviruses are maintained in nature through cycles of transmission among birds or small mammals by arthropod vectors, such as mosquitoes, ticks, and phlebotomine flies. Humans and domestic animals are infected incidentally as "dead-end" hosts. Direct person-to-person spread does not occur; however, infected vectors may spread dengue, yellow fever, and chikungunya viruses from person to person. Colorado tick fever has been transmitted through transfusion. In the United States, mosquito-borne arboviral infections usually occur in late summer and early fall. During epidemics of arboviral encephalitis, persons of all ages may be infected, but most infections do not cause disease. St Louis encephalitis and Western equine encephalitis are more likely to produce clinical manifestations in the elderly than in children, whereas California encephalitis (eg, LaCrosse virus infection) occurs almost exclusively in children younger than 15 years of age. The prevalence of different arboviral diseases is related to ecologic conditions that affect the abundance of infected vectors.

The geographic distribution and **incubation periods** for the principal infections occurring in the Western hemisphere are given in Tables 3.2 and 3.3 (pp 125 and 126).

Diagnostic Tests: A definitive diagnosis can be made by serologic testing or by virus isolation techniques that are available in some state, research, and reference laboratories. In some infections, particularly dengue, yellow fever,

TABLE 3.1—Taxonomy of Major Arboviruses

Family	Genus	Representative Agents
Bunyaviridae	*Bunyavirus*	California serogroup viruses (Western hemisphere, Europe, Asia) Oropouche virus
	Phlebovirus	Sand fly fever virus
Togaviridae	*Alphavirus*	Western equine encephalitis virus Eastern equine encephalitis virus Venezuelan equine encephalitis virus Mayaro virus (South America) Chikungunya virus (Africa, Asia) Ross river virus (Oceania, Australia)
Flaviviridae	*Flavivirus*	St Louis encephalitis virus Japanese encephalitis virus (Asia) Dengue viruses (types 1-4) Yellow fever virus Tick-borne encephalitis virus (Europe) Russian summer-spring encephalitis virus (Asia) Murray Valley encephalitis virus (Australia) West Nile virus (Europe, Africa, Asia) Powassan virus
Reoviridae	*Orbivirus*	Colorado tick fever
Rhabdoviridae	*Rhabdovirus*	Vesicular stomatitis virus (Western hemisphere)

Colorado tick fever, sand fly fever, Chikungunya, epidemic polyarthritis, Oropouche fever, and Venezuelan equine encephalitis, virus can be isolated from blood obtained in the acute phase of illness. In cases of encephalitis, virus isolation should be attempted from biopsied or postmortem brain tissue. Viral-specific IgM antibodies appear in serum in the first week of illness. Although the presence of specific IgM can be suggestive of recent infection, serologic tests on paired serum samples are necessary to confirm the diagnosis. Identification of viral-specific IgM in cerebrospinal fluid is diagnostic.

Treatment: Supportive.

Isolation of the Hospitalized Patient: For patients with dengue, yellow fever, sand fly fever, oropouche fever, Venezuelan equine encephalitis, Chikungunya virus infection, epidemic polyarthritis, and Colorado tick fever, the routinely recommended universal precautions should be scrupulously followed.

TABLE 3.2—Arboviral Infections of the Central Nervous System Occurring in the Western Hemisphere

Diseases (Causal Agent*)	Geographic Distribution of Virus	Incubation Period (Days)
California encephalitis (primarily LaCrosse and several other California serogroup viruses)	Widespread in the US and Canada, including the Yukon and Northwest Territories, most prevalent in upper Midwest	5-15
Eastern equine encephalitis (Eastern equine encephalitis virus)	Central and eastern seaboard and Gulf states of the US; Canada; South and Central America (isolated inland foci)	3-10
Powassan encephalitis (Powassan virus)	Canada; northeastern, north central and western US	4-18
St Louis encephalitis (St Louis encephalitis virus)	Widespread: central, southern, northeastern, and western US; Manitoba and southern Ontario; Caribbean area; South America	4-21
Venezuelan equine encephalitis (Venezuelan equine encephalitis virus)	Texas, Florida, Mexico; Central and South America	2-5
Western equine encephalitis (Western equine encephalitis virus)	Central and western US; Canada; South America	5-10

*All are mosquito-borne except Powassan encephalitis, which is tick-borne.

Control Measures:

Active Immunization.

Yellow Fever Vaccine. The vaccine is a live attenuated virus (17D strain). Local health authorities should be contacted for information about vaccine availability. For immunization, a single dose of vaccine is given subcutaneously.

Immunization is recommended for all individuals 9 months or older living in or traveling to endemic areas. **Infants younger than 4 months should not be immunized** because they are more susceptible to encephalitis temporally associated with yellow fever vaccination. The decision to immunize infants between 4 and 9 months of age should be based upon estimates of the infant's risk of exposure (eg, infants older than 4 months who must travel to an area of ongoing endemic or epidemic activity may receive the vaccine if a high degree of protection against mosquito exposure is not feasible). If possible, cholera vaccine, when indicated, should not be given concurrently with yellow fever vaccine; ideally, administration of these vaccinations should be separated by at least 3 weeks.

TABLE 3.3—Acute, Febrile Diseases and Hemorrhagic Fevers Caused by Arboviruses in the Western Hemisphere That Are Not Characterized by Encephalitis

Disease (Causal Agent*)	Geographic Distribution of Virus	Clinical Syndrome	Incubation Period (Days)
Yellow fever (Yellow fever virus)	Tropical areas of South America and Africa	Febrile illness, hepatitis, hemorrhagic fever	3-6
Dengue fever/ dengue hemorrhagic fever (dengue virus types 1 to 4)	Tropical areas worldwide: Caribbean, Central and South America, Asia, Australia, Oceania, Africa	Febrile illness— may be biphasic with rash; hemorrhagic fever and shock	3-14
Mayaro fever (Mayaro virus)	Caribbean, Central and South America	Febrile illness and polyarthritis	4-11
Colorado tick fever (Colorado tick fever virus)	S Dakota, Rocky Mountain and Pacific states; Western Canada	Febrile illness— may be biphasic	3-6
Oropouche fever (Oropouche virus)	Central and South America	Febrile illness	2-6

*All are mosquito-borne except Colorado tick fever, which is tick-borne, and Oropouche fever, which is midge-borne.

Yellow fever vaccine is prepared in embryonated eggs and contains egg protein, which may cause allergic reactions. Persons who have experienced signs or symptoms of anaphylactic reaction after eating eggs should be excused from vaccination and issued a medical waiver letter to meet health regulations or they should be skin tested according to the package insert before vaccination. Pregnant women should not be vaccinated except in high-risk areas. The decision to immunize immunocompromised patients is based on assessment of the patient's risk of exposure and clinical status.

Japanese Encephalitis Vaccine. Japanese encephalitis (JE) vaccine* was licensed in the United States in 1992 to meet the needs of increasing travel by US citizens to endemic areas of Asia and to accommodate the needs of the US military. It is an inactivated vaccine derived from infected mouse brain.

---

*Produced in Japan and distributed in the United States by Connaught Laboratories, Inc, Swiftwater, PA.

In Japanese encephalitis endemic regions, the risk of disease for travelers to urban areas is low. Even in rural areas, the risk is low for travelers whose stay is brief (defined as fewer than 30 days). Travelers planning prolonged stays in rural areas and whose activities place them at increased risk of exposure, and persons who will be residing in endemic or epidemic areas should be advised to consider JE immunization.* Current information on locations of JE virus transmission and detailed information on vaccine recommendations can be obtained from the Centers for Disease Control and Prevention (see Directory of Telephone Numbers, p 601) and from the recommendations of the Advisory Committee on Immunization Practices.*

The recommended primary immunization series is three doses of 1.0 mL each, administered subcutaneously on days 0, 7, and 30. An abbreviated schedule can be used when the longer schedule is precluded by time constraints.* The schedule is the same for children as for adults except that the dosage for those 1 to 3 years of age is 0.5 mL. No data are available on vaccine safety and efficacy in infants (younger than 12 months of age).

Other Arboviral Vaccines. An inactivated vaccine for tick-borne encephalitis is licensed in various countries in Europe, where the disease is endemic, but it is not licensed in the United States.

Protection Against Vectors. Public health measures to control arthropod vectors are important. Individuals can help protect themselves by wearing long-sleeved shirts and trousers, and by using mosquito repellents. Permethrin applied to clothing kills adherent ticks and mosquitoes. Repellents containing DEET† should be applied to exposed skin only and used sparingly. Travelers to tropical countries should bring mosquito bed nets and aerosol insecticide sprays to reduce the risk of mosquito bites at night. The principal vectors of dengue and yellow fever bite during daytime hours, but many other vector and pest mosquitoes are most active in twilight hours.

Arcanobacterium haemolyticum Infections

Clinical Manifestations: The role of *Arcanobacterium haemolyticum* as a cause of pharyngitis has been suggested by several studies, but its pathogenicity has not been clearly defined. Acute pharyngitis associated with this organism is indistinguishable from that caused by group A streptococci. In nearly one half of reported cases, an exanthem that begins in the extensor surfaces of the distal extremities and spreads centripetally occurs. Pruritus is common, but palatal petechiae and strawberry tongue are absent. No postinfectious complications have been identified.

---

*Inactivated Japanese encephalitis virus vaccine. Recommendations of the Advisory Committee on Immunization Practices (ACIP). *MMWR.* 1993;42 (RR-1):1-15.
†N, N-diethyl-m-toluamide.

Skin infections, including chronic ulceration, cellulitis, wound infection, and paronychia, have been attributed to *A haemolyticum*. Invasive infections include sepsis, brain abscess, meningitis, endocarditis, osteomyelitis, sinusitis, and pneumonia.

Etiology: *Arcanobacterium haemolyticum* is a Gram-positive bacillus, formerly termed *Corynebacterium haemolyticum*.

Epidemiology: Humans are the primary reservoir of *A haemolyticum*. Disease is infrequently recognized. Pharyngitis occurs primarily in adolescents and young adults. Isolation of the bacteria from the nasopharynx or skin of asymptomatic persons is rare, although long-term pharyngeal carriage of *A haemolyticum* has been noted.

The **incubation period** is unknown.

Diagnostic Tests: The organism can be recovered on blood agar, the preferred medium. Its colonies cause beta hemolysis. Some growth on this medium is slow; hemolytic colonies may not be visible until 48 to 72 hours of inoculation. Culture on human or rabbit blood agar enhances the detection of the bacteria because the colonies and the zones of hemolysis are larger. Serologic tests for antibody to *A haemolyticum* have been used in epidemiologic investigations, but these tests have not been standardized and are not available commercially.

Treatment: Erythromycin is the drug of choice, but no prospective therapeutic trials have been performed. *Arcanobacterium haemolyticum* bacteria are susceptible in vitro to erythromycin, clindamycin, chloramphenicol, and tetracycline; susceptibility to penicillin is variable.

Isolation of the Hospitalized Patient: No special precautions are recommended.

Control Measures: None.

Ascaris lumbricoides Infections (Ascariasis, Roundworm)

Clinical Manifestations: Nonspecific gastrointestinal symptoms are reported in some patients, but their frequency is not known. During the larval migratory phase, an acute transient pneumonitis (Loeffler's syndrome) associated with fever and marked eosinophilia can occur. Acute intestinal obstruction can develop in patients with heavy infections. Children are more prone to this complication because they have smaller diameters of the intestinal lumen and often have large numbers of worms. Worm migration can cause peritonitis, secondary to intestinal wall penetration, and common bile duct obstruction with acute obstructive jaundice. The adult worms can be stimulated to migrate by stressful conditions (eg, fever, illness, or anesthesia) and by some antihelmintic drugs. *Ascaris* has been found in the appendiceal lumen in acute appendicitis, but an etiologic relationship is uncertain.

Etiology: *Ascaris lumbricoides* is a large roundworm of humans.

Epidemiology: The adult worms live in the small intestine; females produce 200,000 eggs per day. These eggs are excreted in the stool and must incubate in soil for 2 to 3 weeks to embryonate and become infectious. Infection results from ingestion of infective eggs from contaminated soil. Asymptomatic infections are common. Larvae hatch in the small intestine, penetrate the mucosa, and are passively transported by portal blood to the liver and subsequently to the lungs. They then ascend through the tracheo-bronchial tree to the pharynx, are swallowed, and mature into adults in the small intestine. The interval between ingestion of the egg and the development of egg-laying adults is approximately 8 weeks. *Ascaris* infection is cosmopolitan, but it is most common in the tropics, in areas of poor sanitation, and wherever human feces are used as fertilizer. If the infection is untreated, adult worms can live for as long as 12 to 18 months, resulting in daily excretion of large numbers of ova.

The **incubation period** is prolonged, as the life cycle of *Ascaris* is 4 to 8 weeks, and feces contain eggs about 2 months after ingestion of embryonated eggs.

Diagnostic Tests: Ova can be detected by microscopic stool examination. Occasionally, patients pass adult worms from the rectum or by vomiting.

Treatment: Pyrantel pamoate in a single dose or mebendazole for 3 days is recommended for treatment of asymptomatic and symptomatic infections (see Drugs for Parasitic Infections, p 574). Albendazole* is an alternative drug but is not yet approved by the Food and Drug Administration. In children younger than 2 years of age, in whom experience with these drugs is limited, the risks and benefits of therapy should be considered before drug administration. Re-examination of the stools 3 weeks after therapy to determine whether the worms have been eliminated is helpful in assessing therapy but is not essential.

In cases of partial or complete intestinal obstruction due to a heavy worm load, piperazine citrate solution (75 mg/kg/d, not to exceed 3.5 g) may be given through a gastrointestinal tube. Piperazine paralyzes the worms, allowing them to be excreted with intestinal peristalsis. Piperazine should not be used with pyrantel pamoate since the two drugs are antagonistic. Surgical intervention is occasionally necessary to relieve complete intestinal or biliary obstruction or for volvulus or peritonitis secondary to perforation. If surgery is performed for intestinal obstruction, massaging the worms to eliminate the obstruction is preferable to incision of the intestine.

---

*Available from SmithKline Beecham, Philadelphia, PA.

Isolation of the Hospitalized Patient: No special precautions are recommended.

Control Measures: Sanitary disposal of feces should be undertaken. Children's play areas should be given special attention. Vegetables cultivated in areas where human feces are used as fertilizer must be thoroughly cooked or soaked in a dilute iodine solution before eating. Bleach (hypochlorite) is ineffective.

Aspergillosis

Clinical Manifestations: Aspergillosis is manifested by the following types of disease:
- Allergic bronchopulmonary aspergillosis manifests as episodic wheezing, expectoration of brown mucus plugs, low-grade fever, eosinophilia, and transient pulmonary infiltrates.
- Aspergillomas are fungus balls that grow in pre-existing cavities or bronchogenic cysts and do not invade the lung tissue.
- Invasive aspergillosis occurs almost exclusively in immunocompromised patients with an underlying disease that causes neutrophil dysfunction (eg, chronic granulomatous disease or acute leukemia) or after cytotoxic chemotherapy or immunosuppressive therapy (eg, in organ transplantation).
- Paranasal sinusitis and otomycosis of the external canal occur as benign conditions in otherwise healthy patients in certain warm regions (eg, the Sudan).
- On rare occasion, endocarditis, osteomyelitis, meningitis, infection of the eye or orbit, and cutaneous aspergillosis occur.

Etiology: *Aspergillus fumigatus* and *Aspergillus flavus* are the most frequent etiologic agents. Other species can also cause aspergillosis.

Epidemiology: *Aspergillus* species are ubiquitous; they grow on decaying vegetation and in the soil. Most infected patients, other than those who develop otomycosis and allergic bronchopulmonary disease, have some impairment in host defenses. Nosocomial outbreaks of invasive pulmonary aspergillosis have occurred in which the probable source of the fungus was nearby construction sites or faulty ventilation systems. The principal route of transmission is inhalation of airborne conidiospores. Contact transmission through skin or wound is less likely. Person-to-person spread does not occur.
The **incubation period** is unknown.

Diagnostic Tests: Dichotomous branching, septate hyphae, identified by microscopic examination of 10% potassium hydroxide wet preparations or of Gomori methenamine silver nitrate stain of tissue specimens, are suggestive of the diagnosis. Isolation of an *Aspergillus* species in culture is required for definitive diagnosis. The organism is readily recovered from specimens other than blood on Sabouraud or brain-heart infusion media (without cycloheximide). *Aspergillus* species can also be found as laboratory contaminants, but when evaluating culture results from immunocompromised patients, recovery of this organism should be considered of possible or likely clinical significance. Biopsy of a lesion is usually required to confirm the diagnosis. Serologic antibody tests have no established value in the diagnosis of invasive aspergillosis, but assays for detecting circulating *Aspergillus* antigen are promising. In allergic aspergillosis, elevated serum immunoglobulin E, eosinophilia and serum antibody to *Aspergillus* are frequently present.

Treatment: Amphotericin B is the treatment of choice for systemic infection (see Systemic Treatment With Amphotericin B, p 562). Some experts recommend high doses of amphotericin B (1.0 to 1.5 mg/kg/d) and the addition of either flucytosine or rifampin. Itraconazole is an alternative drug, but it has not been adequately studied to warrant a recommendation. Surgical excision of a localized lesion is sometimes warranted. Allergic bronchopulmonary aspergillosis is usually managed with corticosteroid therapy.

Isolation of the Hospitalized Patient: No special precautions are recommended.

Control Measures: Outbreaks of invasive aspergillosis have occurred among hospitalized, immunosuppressed patients during construction in hospitals or at nearby sites. Environmental measures reported to be effective include erecting barriers between patient care areas and construction sites, cleaning of air handling systems with copper-8-quinolinolate, repair of faulty air flow, and replacement of contaminated air filters. High-efficiency particulate air filters and laminar flow rooms nearly eliminate the risk of airborne conidiospores in patient care areas. These measures, however, may be extremely expensive and difficult for patients to tolerate. Since immunosuppressed patients may be colonized and invasive disease may recur after therapy, studies of prophylactic use of antifungal agents are in progress.

Astroviruses

Clinical Manifestations: Illness is characterized by diarrhea, vomiting, fever, and malaise. Disease is recognized more frequently in young children and in the elderly. Illness in the healthy host is self-limited, lasting a median of 4 days.

Etiology: Astroviruses are nonenveloped, single-stranded, RNA viruses 28 to 30 nm in diameter, with a characteristic starlike appearance when visualized by direct electron microscopy.

Epidemiology: Human astroviruses probably have a worldwide distribution. Outbreaks of gastroenteritis have been detected in the young and the elderly. Multiple antigenic types cocirculate concurrently in the same region.

Astroviruses have been detected in as many as 10% of sporadic cases of gastroenteritis requiring hospitalization. Most astrovirus infections have been detected in children younger than 4 years of age.

Transmission is usually person to person via the fecal-oral route, although outbreaks associated with contaminated water and shellfish have been documented. Common-source outbreaks tend to occur in closed populations and have a high attack rate. Astrovirus infections in child care centers appear to be common.

Excretion lasts a median of 5 days after the onset of symptoms. The duration of asymptomatic excretion after illness is uncertain. Persistent excretion may occur in immunocompromised hosts. Asymptomatic infections also occur.

The **incubation period** is 1 to 2 days.

Diagnostic Tests: No tests are commercially available for diagnosis. Electron microscopy is the most widely available diagnostic tool in research laboratories for detection of viruses in stool specimens, but it is also fairly insensitive for this virus family. Paired serum samples for antibody testing can be helpful to confirm the diagnosis. Enzyme immunoassay for antigen or antibody detection are more sensitive than electron microscopy but are only available in reference and research laboratories. The virus can be cultured in tissue cultures.

Treatment: Supportive.

Isolation of the Hospitalized Patient: Enteric precautions are recommended.

Control Measures: No specific control measures are available. The spread of infection can be reduced by general measures for the control of diarrhea, such as training care providers about infection control, cleanliness of surfaces and food preparation areas, exclusion of ill or carrier care-providers or food handlers, adequate hand washing, and exclusion or cohorting of ill children.

Babesiosis

Clinical Manifestations: Gradual onset of malaise, anorexia, and fatigue typically occurs, followed by intermittent fever with temperatures as high as 40°C (104°F) and one or more of the following: chills, sweats, myalgias, arthralgias, nausea, and vomiting. Less common findings are emotional lability and depression, hyperesthesia, headache, sore throat, abdominal pain, conjunctival injection, photophobia, weight loss, and nonproductive cough. Findings on physical examination are generally minimal, often consisting only of fever, although mild splenomegaly, hepatomegaly, or both are noted occasionally. Many clinical features are similar to those of malaria. The illness lasts for a few weeks to several months with a prolonged recovery of as long as 18 months. Severe illness appears most likely to occur in persons older than 60 years of age, those who are asplenic, and those who are immunocompromised, such as persons with HIV infection. Some patients, especially those with splenectomy, can suffer fulminant illness lasting about a week and ending in death or a prolonged convalescence.

Etiology: The cause is *Babesia* species, an intraerythrocytic protozoa. In the United States, the species is *Babesia microti*; in Europe, *Babesia divergens* and *Babesia bovis* are the causes. Babesiosis caused by morphologically distinct organisms have been reported from California, Georgia, and Mexico.

Epidemiology: The primary reservoir for *B microti* is the white-footed mouse (*Peromyscus leucopus*). In the United States, the primary vector is the tick *Ixodes dammini*, which also transmits *Borrelia burgdorferi* (the etiologic agent of Lyme disease). Humans acquire the infection from bites of infected ticks. The white-tailed deer (*Odocoileus virginianus*) is an important host for the tick but is not a reservoir for *B microti*. An increase in the deer population during the past few decades is thought to be a major factor in the spread of *Ixodes dammini* and the resulting increase in human cases of babesiosis. Recent data indicate that the incidence of infection in children is much greater than previously recognized. Rarely, babesiosis is acquired through blood transfusions. Transplacental/perinatal transmission of babesiosis has also been described. Human cases of babesiosis have been reported in Connecticut, Massachusetts, New York, Rhode Island, Wisconsin, California, and Georgia. Most human cases of babesiosis occur in the summer or fall. In endemic areas, asymptomatic infections are common.

The **incubation period** ranges from 1 to 9 weeks.

Diagnostic Tests: Babesiosis can be diagnosed by microscopic identification of the organism on Giemsa or Wright-stained thick or thin blood smears. Multiple thick and thin blood smears should be examined. Diagnostic serologic tests for *Babesia* antibodies are available through the Centers for Disease Control and Prevention and several research and state reference laboratories.

Treatment: No reliably effective drug therapy has been developed. Since many patients have a mild clinical course and recover without specific antibabesial chemotherapy, therapy is reserved for patients who are seriously ill. The combination of clindamycin and quinine is the current therapy of choice (see Drugs for Parasitic Infections, p 574). Exchange blood transfusions have been used successfully in splenectomized patients with life-threatening *Babesia* species infections.

Isolation of the Hospitalized Patient: The routinely recommended universal precautions should be scrupulously followed.

Control Measures: Specific recommendations concern prevention of tick bites and are similar to those for Lyme disease and other tick-borne infections (see Control Measures for Prevention of Tick-Borne Infections, p 114).

Bacillus cereus Infections

Clinical Manifestations: Two clinical syndromes of *Bacillus cereus* food poisoning occur. One is a disease with a short incubation period, similar to that of staphylococcal food poisoning, characterized by nausea, vomiting, and abdominal cramps, with diarrhea in about one third of patients. The other has a longer incubation period, similar to that of *Clostridium perfringens* food poisoning, and is characterized predominantly by abdominal cramps and diarrhea, with vomiting in about one fourth of patients. In both syndromes, illness is mild, not associated with fever, and abates within 24 hours.

Bacillus cereus can also cause local skin and wound infections and invasive disease, including bacteremia, endocarditis, osteomyelitis, pneumonia, endophthalmitis, and meningitis.

Etiology: *Bacillus cereus* is an aerobic (facultative anaerobic), spore-forming, Gram-positive bacillus. The short-incubation disease is caused by a preformed, heat-stable toxin. The long-incubation disease is caused by the in vivo production of a heat-labile enterotoxin. This exotoxin also possesses tissue necrosis and cytotoxic properties, and it is probably the principal determinant of virulence in nongastrointestinal tract infections.

Epidemiology: *Bacillus cereus* is ubiquitous in the environment. It is frequently present in small numbers in raw, dried, and processed foods, but it is an uncommon cause of food poisoning in the United States. Spores of *B cereus* are heat resistant, and the organism can survive brief cooking or boiling. Vegetative forms can grow and produce enterotoxins over a wide range of temperatures (25° to 42°C; 77° to 107.6°F). The disease is acquired by ingestion of food containing heat-stable toxins or of inadequately cooked food contaminated with *B cereus* followed by toxin production in the gastrointestinal tract. The most common foods associated with illness are cooked rice (causing vomiting), and meat or vegetables (causing diarrhea). The disease is not transmissible from person to person.

Risk factors for invasive disease include history of injection drug use, presence of indwelling intravascular catheters or implanted devices, and immunosuppression. Fulminant *B cereus* endophthalmitis has occurred after penetrating ocular trauma and injection drug use.

The **incubation period** of short-incubation disease is 1 to 6 hours; for long-incubation disease it is 6 to 24 hours.

Diagnostic Tests: For food-borne illness, isolation of *B cereus* in a concentration of 10^5 or more per gram of epidemiologically incriminated food establishes the diagnosis. Since the organism can be recovered from some stool samples from well persons, the presence of *B cereus* in feces or vomitus of ill persons is not incriminating unless stool cultures from a comparable control group are negative.

In patients with risk factors for serious illness, isolation of *B cereus* from wounds or normally sterile body fluids can be significant and should not be dismissed as a contaminant. Repeat culture may help to confirm the diagnosis.

Treatment: Persons with *B cereus* food poisoning require only supportive treatment. Oral rehydration or, occasionally, intravenous fluid and electrolyte replacement for patients with severe dehydration, is indicated. Antibiotics are not indicated.

Patients with invasive disease, in contrast, require antibiotic therapy and prompt removal of any potentially infected foreign bodies (ie, catheters or implants). *Bacillus cereus* is usually susceptible *in vitro* to aminoglycosides, chloramphenicol, clindamycin, ciprofloxacin, erythromycin, imipenem, and vancomycin. Ciprofloxacin should not be given to patients younger than 18 years.

Isolation of the Hospitalized Patient: For patients with food poisoning, no special precautions are recommended. For patients with draining lesions, drainage/secretion precautions are indicated.

Control Measures: Proper cooking and storage of foods, particularly rice cooked for later use, will help to prevent food-borne outbreaks by limiting proliferation of *B cereus*. Hand washing and strict aseptic technique in caring for immunocompromised patients or patients with indwelling intravascular catheters are important to minimize invasive disease.

Bacterial Vaginosis

Clinical Manifestations: Bacterial vaginosis (BV) is a syndrome primarily occurring in sexually active adolescent and adult women. This syndrome is characterized by a profuse vaginal discharge, which is usually malodorous (having a fishy smell), nonviscous, homogenous, and white, and which adheres to the vaginal wall. Bacterial vaginosis may be asymptomatic and is not associated with abdominal pain, pruritus, or dysuria.

Vaginitis and vulvitis in prepubertal girls are rarely manifestations of BV and much more commonly have other causes, including foreign bodies and other infections (group A streptococci, *Shigella* spp, *Trichomonas vaginalis*, herpes simplex virus, *Neisseria gonorrhoeae*, or *Chlamydia trachomatis*). They may also be nonspecific in etiology.

Etiology: The microbiologic cause of BV has not been clearly delineated. Although the microbial flora of the vagina are significantly changed, little or no inflammation of the vaginal epithelium occurs. Instead of high concentrations of lactobacilli, anaerobes, *Gardnerella vaginalis*, and *Mycoplasma hominis* predominate.

Epidemiology: Bacterial vaginosis is the most prevalent vaginal infection in sexually active adolescents and adults. It may occur with other conditions associated with vaginal discharge, such as trichomoniasis or cervicitis. The evidence on the sexual transmissibility of BV is conflicting, although the condition is uncommon in sexually inexperienced females. Diagnosing BV in a prepubertal girl raises concern about, but does not prove, sexual abuse.

Bacterial vaginosis may be a risk factor for pelvic inflammatory disease. Pregnant women with BV are at increased risk for chorioamnionitis and premature delivery.

The **incubation period** of BV is unknown.

Diagnostic Tests: The clinical diagnosis of bacterial vaginosis requires the presence of three or more of the following signs:
• Homogenous, white, adherent discharge.
• Vaginal fluid pH >4.5.
• Release of a fishy amine odor from vaginal fluid mixed with 10% KOH.
• Presence of "clue cells" (squamous vaginal epithelial cells that are covered with many vaginal bacteria, causing a stippled or granular appearance). In BV, "clue cells" usually constitute at least 20% of vaginal epithelial cells.

Cultures for *Gardnerella* are not helpful since the organism may be found in females without BV, including those who are not sexually active.

Treatment: Patients should be treated with metronidazole (1.0 g/d, orally, in two divided doses) for 7 days. Alternative regimens are metronidazole 2 g, orally, in a single dose; clindamycin cream, 2%, one applicatorful (5 g), intravaginally, at bedtime for 7 days; metronidazole gel, 0.75%, one applicatorful (5 g), intravaginally, two times a day for 5 days; or clindamycin 600 mg/d, orally, in two divided doses for 7 days. For symptomatic pregnant women, topical therapy is preferred to oral therapy because of concern about possible teratogenicity of oral metronidazole. Routine follow-up visits on completion of therapy for BV are not necessary. Recurrences are common and can be treated with the same regimen given initially. Routine treatment of male sexual partners is not recommended since it does not influence relapse or recurrence rates. Clindamycin cream is oil-based and may weaken latex condoms for at least 72 hours after terminating therapy. Recommendations for treatment of BV in HIV-infected females are the same.

Isolation of the Hospitalized Patient: No special precautions are recommended.

Control Measures: None.

Bacteroides Infections

Clinical Manifestations: *Bacteroides* species of the oral cavity can cause chronic sinusitis, chronic otitis media, dental infection, peritonsillar abscess, cervical adenitis, retropharyngeal space infection, aspiration pneumonia, lung abscess, empyema, and necrotizing pneumonia. Species from the gastrointestinal tract flora are recovered in patients with peritonitis, intraabdominal abscess, pelvic inflammatory disease, postoperative wound infection, and vulvovaginal and perianal infections. Soft-tissue infections involving *Bacteroides* species include synergistic bacterial gangrene and necrotizing fasciitis. Invasion of the bloodstream by *Bacteroides* species from the oral cavity or intestinal tract can lead to brain abscess, meningitis, endocarditis, arthritis, or osteomyelitis. Skin involvement includes omphalitis in newborns, cellulitis at the site of fetal monitors, human bite wounds, infection of burns adjacent to the mouth or rectum, and decubitus ulcers. Neonatal infections, such as conjunctivitis, pneumonia, bacteremia, or meningitis, occur rarely. Most *Bacteroides* infections are polymicrobial.

Etiology: Most *Bacteroides* organisms associated with human disease are small, pleomorphic, non-spore-forming, obligately anaerobic, Gram-negative bacilli.

Epidemiology: *Bacteroides* infections are caused by endogenous organisms of patients' flora. Members of the *Bacteroides fragilis* group predominate in the gastrointestinal tract flora; members of the *Bacteroides melaninogenicus* and *Bacteroides oralis* groups are more common in the oral cavity. *Bacteroides* species cause infection as opportunists, usually in conjunction with other endogenous species. Encapsulation of organisms can enhance abscess formation. Endogenous transmission results from aspiration, spillage from the bowel, or damage to mucosal surfaces, such as from trauma or surgery. High concentrations of *Bacteroides* species in the vagina have been associated with an increased rate of preterm delivery. Peripartum transmission occurs when an infant is exposed during birth to organisms of the vagina or infected tissues. Deficiencies of normal immune mechanisms usually do not predispose to infection, but mucosal injury and granulocytopenia do. Except in infections resulting from human bites, no evidence for person-to-person transmission exists.

The **incubation period** is variable and depends on the concentration of organisms and the site of involvement, but generally it is 1 to 5 days.

Diagnostic Tests: Anaerobic cultures are necessary for recovery of *Bacteroides* species. Since infections are usually polymicrobial, aerobic cultures of infected clinical specimens are also indicated. A putrid odor of pus or other discharges is suggestive evidence of anaerobic infection; the Gram stain will show leukocytes and bacteria of differing morphology, but the morphologic features of *Bacteroides* species are not sufficiently distinctive to be diagnostic. Use of anaerobic transport tubes or a sealed syringe is recommended for clinical specimens unless specimens can be cultured immediately after collection. Collection of clinical materials, especially from the respiratory tract, must be performed so as to avoid contamination of the specimen with anaerobes normally present on mucosal surfaces. Rapid identification techniques including immunofluorescence and coagglutination are under development.

Treatment: Abscesses should be drained when feasible; those involving brain or liver sometimes resolve without drainage if appropriate antimicrobial agents are administered. Necrotizing lesions should be debrided surgically; the value of hyperbaric oxygenation is controversial.

The choice of antimicrobial agent(s) is based on anticipated (or proven, if available) in vitro susceptibility test results. *Bacteroides* species that cause infections of the mouth and respiratory tract are generally susceptible to penicillin G, ampicillin, broad-spectrum penicillins (such as ticarcillin), and cefuroxime. Some species (eg, members of the *B melaninogenicus* and *B oralis* groups) produce beta-lactamase and are resistant to those drugs. Other penicillins and first- and second-generation cephalosporins are less active in vitro. Clindamycin is active against virtually all mouth and respiratory tract *Bacteroides* isolates and is advocated by some experts as the drug of choice for anaerobic infections of the oral cavity and lungs. *Bacteroides* species of the gastrointestinal tract are usually resistant to penicillin G, but they are predictably susceptible to metronidazole, chloramphenicol, and, usually, clindamycin. Eighty percent or more of isolates are susceptible to cefoxitin, ceftizoxime, and imipenem. Cefuroxime, cefotaxime, and ceftriaxone are not reliably effective against *Bacteroides* species of the intestinal tract.

Isolation of the Hospitalized Patient: For draining wounds with *Bacteroides* species, drainage/secretion precautions are recommended.

Control Measures: None.

Balantidium coli Infections (Balantidiasis)

Clinical Manifestations: Acute infection is characterized by the rapid onset of nausea, vomiting, abdominal discomfort or pain, and bloody mucoid diarrhea. Infected patients can develop chronic, intermittent episodes of diarrhea. Since the organism causes inflammation of the gastrointestinal tract and of local lymphatics with resulting dilation, ulceration and secondary bacterial invasion can occur. Fulminant disease can occur in malnourished or otherwise debilitated patients.

Etiology: *Balantidium coli*, a ciliated protozoan, is the largest protozoan known to infect humans.

Epidemiology: Most human infections are asymptomatic. Pigs are believed to be the main reservoir of *B coli*. They excrete cysts in feces; the cysts can be transmitted directly from hand to mouth or indirectly through fecally contaminated water or food. The excysted trophozoites infect the colon. The patient is infectious as long as the cysts are excreted. The cysts can remain in the environment for months.

The **incubation period** is unknown; it may be only several days.

Diagnostic Tests: Prompt microscopic examination of fresh diarrheal stools for the rapidly motile trophozoites is necessary because of the rapid degeneration of trophozoites. Repeated stool examination may be necessary to identify infection, as shedding can be intermittent. Materials may also be obtained by scraping lesions during sigmoidoscopy.

Treatment: Tetracycline is the drug of choice; iodoquinol and metronidazole are alternative drugs. Tetracycline should not be given to children younger than 9 years of age unless the benefits of therapy are greater than the risks of dental staining.

Isolation of the Hospitalized Patient: No special precautions are recommended.

Control Measures: Control measures include sanitary disposal of human feces and avoidance of contamination of food and water with porcine feces.

Blastocystis hominis Infections

Clinical Manifestations: *Blastocystis hominis* has been associated with symptoms of bloating, flatulence, mild to moderate diarrhea without fecal leucocytes or blood, abdominal pain, and nausea. However, the importance of *B hominis* as a cause of gastrointestinal pathology is controversial. Hence, when *B hominis* is identified in stool from symptomatic patients, other etiologies of gastrointestinal disease should be investigated before assuming that it is the cause of the signs and symptoms.

Etiology: *Blastocystis hominis* is a protozoan parasite.

Epidemiology: *Blastocystis hominis* is recovered from 1% to 20% of stool samples examined for ova and parasites. The asymptomatic carrier state is well documented. Since transmission is believed to be via the fecal-oral route, however, the presence of the organism may be a marker for fecal contamination with other pathogens. Transmission from animals may also occur.

The **incubation period** is unknown.

Diagnostic Tests: Stool specimens should be preserved in polyvinyl alcohol and stained with hematoxylin or trichrome. The parasite occurs in varying numbers, and infections may be reported as light to very heavy. The presence of five or more organisms per high-powered field (400x magnification) is suggestive of heavy infection.

Treatment: Treatment should be reserved for immunocompromised patients who are symptomatic and in whom no other pathogen or process is found to explain the gastrointestinal symptoms. In anecdotal reports, metronidazole

(15 mg/kg/d in three daily doses, maximum 2.25 g/d) for 10 days has also been associated with improvement in symptoms. Iodoquinol (40 mg/kg/d divided in three doses, maximum 2 g/d) for 20 days has been effective in eliminating the organism and relieving symptoms in some patients. Controlled treatment trials are lacking.

Isolation of the Hospitalized Patient: No special precautions are indicated.

Control Measures: None.

Blastomycosis

Clinical Manifestations: Pulmonary, cutaneous, and disseminated diseases occur. Children commonly have pulmonary disease. Because blastomycosis can cause a wide variety of symptoms and radiographic appearances, the disease is often misdiagnosed as tuberculosis, other infections, sarcoidosis, or cancer. The infection may be asymptomatic or associated with acute, chronic, or fulminant disease. Skin lesions can be nodular, verrucous, or ulcerative, often with little inflammation. Abscesses are usually subcutaneous but may involve any organ. Disseminated blastomycosis usually begins with pulmonary infection and can involve the skin, bones, central nervous system, abdominal viscera, and kidney.

Etiology: The disease is caused by *Blastomyces dermatitidis*, a dimorphic fungus existing in the yeast form at 37°C and in infected tissues, and in a mycelial form at room temperature and in the soil.

Epidemiology: The source is probably the soil by inhalation of conidia (from the mycelial form), which are thought to be infectious for humans. Person-to-person transmission does not occur. Human infection is uncommon. The infection may be epidemic or sporadic and has been reported in the United States, Canada, Africa, and India. Endemic areas in the United States are the southeastern and central states and the midwestern states bordering the Great Lakes. Although blastomycosis may be associated with immunocompromised states, the disease has been infrequently reported in association with HIV infection.

The **incubation period** is unknown.

Diagnostic Tests: Thick-walled, figure-eight, broad-based, single-budding yeast forms may be seen in 10% potassium hydroxide preparations of sputum, cerebrospinal fluid (CSF), urine, or material from lesions. Organisms can be cultured on brain-heart infusion and Sabouraud's dextrose agar at room temperature. Chemiluminescent DNA probes are available for identification of *B dermatitidis*. The procedure can be applied to nonsporulating cultures, thereby reducing the risk of exposure to infectious forms. The skin test and serologic tests are not reliable for diagnosis but have been used for epidemiologic studies. A positive immunodiffusion test is a reliable indicator of infection, but a nonreactive test does not exclude the diagnosis.

Treatment: Amphotericin B is the treatment of choice for life-threatening infection (see Systemic Treatment with Amphotericin B, p 562). Oral itraconazole and ketoconazole are drugs for mild or moderately severe infections, but data on safety and efficacy of these drugs in children are limited. Itraconazole is highly effective in the treatment of nonmeningeal, non-life-threatening infections in adults, but it does not achieve effective CSF concentration. In a recent multicenter trial in adults, itraconazole was more effective and associated with less toxicity than ketoconazole. Mild pulmonary cases in otherwise healthy individuals with clinical improvement at the time of diagnosis may not require therapy.

Therapy is usually continued for at least 6 months for pulmonary disease and 12 months for patients with bone involvement.

Isolation of the Hospitalized Patient: No special precautions are recommended.

Control Measures: None.

Borrelia
(Relapsing Fever)

Clinical Manifestations: Illness is characterized by sudden onset of high fever, chills, headache, and myalgia, followed by splenomegaly and hepatomegaly. A fleeting macular rash on the trunk, which can become generalized and/or petechial, frequently occurs. Other possible findings include meningeal irritation, iridocyclitis, epistaxis, and myocarditis. An initial illness of 3 to 6 days is followed by an afebrile period of about 1 week, then a relapse. Relapses become progressively shorter and milder as the afebrile intervals lengthen. Infection during pregnancy is often clinically severe and can result in abortion or, rarely, severe infection in neonates.

Etiology: Relapsing fever is caused by motile spirochetes of the genus *Borrelia*. *Borrelia recurrentis* is the only species causing louse-borne infection. Among at least 15 species causing tick-borne infections, *Borrelia hermsii*, *Borrelia turicatae*, and *Borrelia parkeri* are the only species found in North America.

Epidemiology: Transmission is vector-borne. Infected lice (*Pediculus humanus*) and soft-bodied ticks (*Ornithodoros* species) are the source of human infections. Louse-borne infections are presently reported in Ethiopia and the Sudan; tick-borne infections are widely distributed in many countries. Most human cases in the United States occur in forested western mountain areas, including state and national parks, and result from tick bites. These bites often occur in rodent-infested mountain cabins. Because soft-bodied ticks have painless bites and feed briefly (10 to 30 minutes) and usually at night, many patients are unaware of having been bitten. Ticks become infected by feeding on rodents and other small mammals and transmit the organisms when they take blood meals. Infection is transmitted vertically in ticks, thereby establishing a reservoir. Lice become infected by feeding on spirochetemic humans and transmit organisms by contaminating a bite wound when they are crushed by the host's scratching. Infected lice and ticks remain contagious throughout their lives. All humans are susceptible. Human-to-human transmission does not occur.

The **incubation period** is 5 to 11 days or more.

Diagnostic Tests: Spirochetes can be observed in darkfield preparations or Wright-stained thin and thick smears of peripheral blood, or Giemsa or acridine orange stains of dehemoglobinized thick smears or buffy-coat preparations. Blood is cultured by inoculating special medium or by intraperitoneal inoculation of immature laboratory mice. Serum agglutinins against *Proteus* OX-K (Weil-Felix reaction) in convalescent sera support the diagnosis. Serum antibodies to *Borrelia* can be detected by enzyme immunoassay, but the tests are limited by species and phase variations in the *Borrelia* antigenic content. Serologic cross-reactions with *Borrelia burgdorferi* can occur.

Treatment: Tetracycline, penicillin, chloramphenicol, and erythromycin are each effective in producing prompt defervescence and preventing relapses. For children younger than 9 years and for pregnant women, penicillin or erythromycin are the preferred drugs. The first dose of penicillin should be lower than those subsequently given to prevent or modify the Jarisch-Herxheimer reaction. Because this reaction can be life threatening, the patient should be monitored closely during the first 8 hours of therapy. For a febrile patient, oral phenoxymethyl penicillin, 7.5 mg/kg, in a single dose (or intravenous penicillin G, 10,000 U/kg, infused during 30 minutes for those unable to take oral medication) is recommended as initial therapy, to be followed by a 10-day course of an effective antibiotic.

Louse infestation, if present, should be treated.

Isolation of the Hospitalized Patient: Other than the routinely recommended universal precautions, no special precautions are indicated unless louse infection is present (see Pediculosis, p 350).

Control Measures: Limitation of contact with vectors (lice and ticks) through use of protective clothing, insecticides, insect repellents, and good personal hygiene is indicated. Persons in tick-infested areas should check frequently for attached ticks after possible exposure and remove them promptly (see Control Measures for Prevention of Tick-Borne Infections, p 114). Prevention of rodent access to the foundations or attics of homes or vacation cabins also reduces tick exposure. Case reporting is important for public health control.

Brucellosis

Clinical Manifestations: In children, brucellosis is frequently a mild, self-limited disease, especially when caused by *Brucella abortus*. However, in areas where *Brucella melitensis* is the endemic species, the disease can be severe. Onset of illness can be acute or insidious. Complaints are nonspecific, such as fever, sweats, weakness, malaise, anorexia, weight loss, arthralgias, myalgias, and backache. Abnormal physical findings include fever, lymphadenopathy, and, occasionally, hepatosplenomegaly, but they are often minimal. Serious complications include meningitis, endocarditis, and osteomyelitis.

Etiology: *Brucella* species are small, nonmotile, Gram-negative coccobacilli. The species that infect humans are *B abortus*, *B melitensis*, *Brucella suis*, and, rarely, *Brucella canis*.

Epidemiology: Brucellosis is a disease primarily of wild and domestic animals. Humans are accidental hosts, contracting the disease by direct contact with infected animals, their carcasses, and their secretions, or by ingesting unpasteurized milk or milk products. Persons in occupations such as farming, ranching, and veterinary medicine, as well as abattoir workers, meat inspectors, and laboratory personnel, are at increased risk. Infection is transmitted by inoculation through cuts and abrasions in the skin, by inhalation of contaminated aerosols, by contact with the conjunctival mucosa, or by oral ingestion. Brucellosis is unusual in children in the United States, with fewer than 10% of reported cases occurring in persons younger than 19 years of age. Human-to-human transmission has rarely been documented.

The **incubation period** varies from less than 1 week to several months, but most patients become ill within 3 to 4 weeks of exposure.

Diagnostic Tests: A definitive diagnosis is made by recovering *Brucella* organisms from blood, bone marrow, or other tissues. A variety of media will support the growth of *Brucella* species, but some require 5% to 10% CO_2 for primary isolation. The laboratory should be alerted to the possibility of brucellosis so that cultures can be incubated for a minimum of 4 weeks. Lysis-centrifugation techniques may shorten the time to *Brucella* isolation. A presumptive diagnosis can be made by demonstrating elevated serum titers of specific antibodies. The serum agglutination test (SAT) using killed *B abortus* cells as antigen is the most commonly used serologic test for brucellosis. This test will detect antibodies against *B abortus*, *B suis*, and *B melitensis*; detection of antibodies against *B canis* requires the use of specific *B canis* antigen. In human brucellosis, although no single titer is always diagnostic, most patients with active infection will have SAT titers of 1:160 or less. Since lower titers can be found early in the course of infection, repeat tests are recommended in order to demonstrate a rising titer. Since low titers of IgM agglutinins can persist in the serum for months and even years after infection, the 2-mercaptoethanol (2ME) agglutination test is useful. Elevated concentrations of IgG agglutinins are found in acute infection, chronic infection, and relapse. In interpreting SAT titers the possibility of cross-reactions of

Brucella antibodies with those against other Gram-negative bacteria, such as a *Yersinia enterocolitica* serotype, *Francisella tularenis*, and *Vibrio cholerae*, should be considered. In addition, the prozone phenomenon can give false-negative results in the presence of high titers of antibody. To avoid this problem, serum should be routinely diluted to 1:320 or higher. Rarely, negative agglutination occurs from the presence of so-called blocking antibodies. These substances can be detected by the Coombs test or by a blocking antibody test, but they rarely interfere with the diagnosis.

Treatment: Prolonged therapy is imperative in achieving a cure. Relapses are generally not caused by development of resistance but from premature discontinuation of oral antibiotics.

Oral tetracycline (30 to 40 mg/kg/d, maximum 2 g/d, in four divided doses) or, preferably, oral doxycycline (5 mg/kg/d, maximum 200 mg/d, in two divided doses) should be administered for 4 to 6 weeks.

Tetracyclines should not be given routinely to children younger than 9 years of age or to pregnant women after the sixth month of gestation. Hence, in children that are younger than 9 years of age, oral trimethoprim-sulfamethoxazole (trimethoprim 10 mg/kg/d, maximum 480 mg/d; sulfamethoxazole 50 mg/kg/d, maximum 2.4 mg/d) for 4 to 6 weeks is acceptable alternative therapy.

For treatment of serious infection including endocarditis, and in order to decrease the incidence of relapse, streptomycin* (20 mg/kg/d, maximum 1 g/d, intramuscularly) or gentamicin (5 mg/kg/d) is often given for the first 7 to 14 days of therapy in conjunction with doxycycline or tetracycline.

For life-threatening complications of brucellosis, such as meningitis or endocarditis, the duration of therapy is often extended for several months. In addition, rifampin (20 mg/kg/d) can be used in conjunction with a tetracycline and an aminoglycoside as adjunctive therapy. Because of the potential emergence of rifampin-resistance, rifampin is not recommended as monotherapy.

Prednisone has been given with antibiotics in culture-proven meningitis, but benefits of steroids in neurobrucellosis are unproven at this time. Occasionally, a Herxheimer-like reaction occurs shortly after beginning antibiotics, but it is rarely severe enough to require steroids.

Isolation of the Hospitalized Patient: Other than contact isolation precautions for patients with draining wounds, no special precautions are indicated.

Control Measures: The control of human brucellosis depends on eradication of brucellosis in cattle, goats, swine, and other animals. Pasteurization of milk and milk products for human consumption is especially important to prevent disease in children. The certification of raw milk does not eliminate the risk of *Brucella* transmission.

---

*As of December 1993, available from Pfizer Streptomycin Program, Pfizer Pharmaceuticals, New York, NY (800/254-4445).

Caliciviruses and Calici-like Viruses Causing Gastroenteritis

Clinical Manifestations: Diarrhea and vomiting, frequently accompanied by fever, headache, malaise, myalgia, and abdominal cramps, are characteristic. Infection in the healthy host is self-limited, lasting 1 to 4 days.

Etiology: Caliciviruses are nonenveloped RNA viruses and include the Norwalk virus and hepatitis E virus. Most agents are named for the site of the outbreak where they were identified (eg, Norwalk, Snow Mountain, or Hawaii). Hepatitis E virus may represent a distinct genus of caliciviruses.

Epidemiology: Human caliciviruses probably have a worldwide distribution. Outbreaks of gastroenteritis have been detected in all age groups. Multiple antigenic types cocirculate simultaneously in the same region. Caliciviruses cause 0.2% to 6.6% of sporadic cases of gastroenteritis requiring hospitalization. Most calicivirus infections have been detected in children younger than 4 years of age. Norwalk is more likely than other strains to cause disease after the first decade of life in developed countries.

Transmission presumably is person to person via the fecal-oral route. Outbreaks tend to occur in closed populations and have a high attack rate. Calicivirus infections in child care centers have been reported. Common-source outbreaks occur in association with the ingestion of contaminated water and food, particularly shellfish and salads. Airborne transmission has been implicated in one institutional outbreak.

Excretion lasts 5 to 7 days after the onset of symptoms in half the infected persons and can extend to 13 days. Virus excretion may continue as long as 4 days after symptoms cease. Persistent excretion can occur in immunocompromised hosts. Asymptomatic, persistent virus excretion has been detected for months after primary calicivirus infections in animals.

The **incubation period** is 12 hours to 4 days.

Diagnostic Tests: No tests are commercially available for diagnosis. Electron microscopy is the most widely available diagnostic tool in research laboratories for detection of viruses in stool specimens (which should be stored at 4°C until testing), but it is also fairly insensitive for this virus family. Paired serum samples for antibody testing can help establish the diagnosis. Enzyme immunoassays for antigen or antibody detection are more sensitive than electron microscopy, but they are only available in reference and research laboratories and for only some strains.

Treatment: Supportive.

Isolation of the Hospitalized Patient: Enteric precautions are recommended.

Control Measures: No specific control measures are available. The spread of infection can be reduced by generic measures for the control of diarrhea, such as training care providers about infection control, cleanliness of surfaces and food preparation areas, exclusion of ill or carrier care-providers or food handlers, adequate hand washing, and exclusion or cohorting of ill children.

Campylobacter Infections

Clinical Manifestations: Predominant symptoms are diarrhea, abdominal pain, malaise, and fever. Stools frequently contain visible blood. In neonates, bloody diarrhea can be the only manifestation of infection. Abdominal pain can mimic that produced by appendicitis. Mild infection can last even 1 or 2 days and resembles viral gastroenteritis. Most patients recover in less than 1 week, but 20% have a relapse or a prolonged or severe illness. Severe or persistent infection can mimic acute inflammatory bowel disease. Convulsions develop in some young children in association with high fever. Bacteremia is uncommon, but neonatal septicemia occasionally occurs. Immunoreactive complications such as reactive arthritis, Guillain-Barré syndrome, Reiter syndrome, and erythema nodosum can occur during convalescence.

Etiology: *Campylobacter jejuni* (formerly *Campylobacter fetus* subspecies *jejuni* or *Vibrio fetus*) is a motile, comma-shaped, Gram-negative bacilli that causes gastroenteritis. *Campylobacter fetus* (formerly *C fetus* subspecies *intestinalis*), a related organism, is an infrequent cause of systemic illness in neonates and debilitated hosts.

Epidemiology: The gastrointestinal tract of domestic and wild birds and animals is the reservoir of infection. *Campylobacter jejuni* has been isolated from the feces of 30% to 100% of chickens, turkeys, and water fowl. Poultry carcasses are usually contaminated with the organism. Many farm animals and meat sources can harbor the organism, and pets such as dogs and cats (especially young animals) are potential sources. Transmission of *C jejuni* occurs by ingestion of contaminated food, including unpasteurized milk and water, or by direct contact with fecal material from infected animals or persons. Improperly cooked poultry, untreated water, and unpasteurized milk have been the main vehicles. Outbreaks in schoolchildren have occurred after field trips to dairy farms during which children drank unpasteurized milk. Person-to-person spread appears to occur particularly among young children with fecal incontinence and in families. Outbreaks of *Campylobacter* diarrhea in child care have been reported but appear to be uncommon. Person-to-person transmission has also occurred in neonates of infected mothers and has resulted in nosocomial nursery outbreaks. In perinatal infection, *C jejuni* usually causes neonatal gastroenteritis, whereas *C fetus* usually results in neonatal septicemia or meningitis. Enteritis occurs in persons of all ages. Communicability is uncommon but is greatest during the acute phase of the illness. Convalescent excretion is usually brief, typically 2 to 3 weeks, and is shortened by treatment to 1 to 2 days. Asymptomatic carriage is uncommon.

The **incubation period** is usually 1 to 7 days but can be longer.

Diagnostic Tests: Rapid, presumptive diagnosis is possible in laboratories experienced in examining stool smears by darkfield microscopic or Gram staining techniques. *Campylobacter jejuni* can be cultured from the feces and occasionally from the bloodstream. Because laboratory identification of the organism from stool specimens requires special techniques, the physician should be aware of whether the laboratory routinely attempts *Campylobacter* isolation or whether it requires special notification.

Treatment:

- When given early in the course of infection, erythromycin shortens the duration of illness and prevents relapse. Treatment with erythromycin usually eradicates the organism from stool within 2 or 3 days. Ciprofloxacin is an alternative agent but is not approved by the Food and Drug Administration for persons younger than 18 years of age.
- Antimicrobials for resistant or bacteremic strains should be selected on the basis of laboratory susceptibility tests. Bacteremic strains are usually susceptible to aminoglycosides, chloramphenicol, and cefotaxime.
- If antimicrobial therapy is given, the recommended duration is 5 to 7 days.

Isolation of the Hospitalized Patient: Enteric precautions are indicated until *Campylobacter* can no longer be isolated from stool specimens.

Control Measures:

- Hand washing after handling raw poultry, washing cutting boards and utensils with soap after contact with raw poultry, and thorough cooking of poultry are critical.
- Pasteurization of milk and chlorination of water supplies are also important.
- Infected food handlers and hospital employees who are asymptomatic pose no known hazard for disease transmission and need not be excluded from work if proper personal hygiene measures are carefully maintained.
- Outbreaks of campylobacteriosis are uncommon in child care centers, and specific strategies for controlling infection in these settings have not been evaluated. General measures for interrupting enteric transmissions in child care centers are recommended (see Children in Out-of-Home Child Care, p 83). Infants and children in diapers with symptomatic *Campylobacter* infection should be excluded from child care or cared for in a separate protected area until the diarrhea has subsided. In addition, they should receive at least 2 or 3 days of erythromycin treatment.
- Stool cultures of asymptomatic exposed children generally are not recommended.

Candidiasis
(Moniliasis, Thrush)

Clinical Manifestations: Mucocutaneous infection results in oral (thrush) or vaginal candidiasis; intertriginous lesions of the gluteal folds, neck, groin, and axilla; paronychia; and onychia. Chronic mucocutaneous candidiasis can be associated with endocrinologic diseases or progressive immunodeficiency, particularly T-lymphocyte deficiency, and can be the presenting symptom of HIV infection. Granulomas of the scalp and face are rare. Disseminated candidiasis occurs in very-low-birth-weight newborns and in immunocompromised or debilitated hosts. It may involve the lungs, kidneys, spleen, heart, liver, brain, eye, esophagus, meninges, skin, and/or mucous membranes, and it may be rapidly fatal. Transient candidemia can occur with or without systemic disease in patients with indwelling catheters or in those receiving prolonged intravenous infusions. Other types of *Candida* infection include cystitis, endocarditis, and enteritis.

Etiology: *Candida albicans* causes most of the infections. Other species, such as *Candida tropicalis*, can also cause serious infections in compromised hosts. Yeast forms and pseudohyphae can be found in infected tissues.

Epidemiology: *Candida albicans* is ubiquitous. Like other *Candida* species, it is present in the intestinal tract, vagina, and mucous membranes of healthy individuals. Person-to-person transmission occurs. Vulvovaginal candidiasis is associated with pregnancy. Newborns can acquire the organism in utero, during passage through the vagina, or postnatally. Mild mucocutaneous infection is common in healthy infants. Invasive disease occurs almost exclusively in persons with impaired resistance to infection. Individuals with HIV infection or those who are immunodeficient for other reasons, such as neutropenia, diabetes mellitus, or treatment with corticosteroids or antimetabolites, are unusually susceptible. Patients receiving prolonged intravenous hyperalimentation or broad-spectrum antimicrobials also have increased susceptibility.

The **incubation period** is unknown. Most infections are of endogenous origin.

Diagnostic Tests: The presumptive diagnosis of mucocutaneous candidiasis or thrush can usually be made by physical examination, but thrush-like lesions can also be caused by other organisms or trauma to the mucous membranes. Typical yeast and pseudohyphal forms are identified by microscopic examination of scrapings suspended in 10% potassium hydroxide. Gram stains of smears from skin and mucous membrane lesions can identify these forms, but isolation in culture is required for specific diagnoses. Barium studies and endoscopy are useful in the diagnosis of esophagitis.

A definitive diagnosis of invasive candidiasis requires the isolation of the organism from an otherwise sterile body fluid or tissue (eg, blood, cerebrospinal fluid, bone marrow, or biopsy specimen) or the demonstration of organisms in a tissue biopsy specimen. Negative cultures, however, do not necessarily exclude invasive infection. Positive cultures from urine or other potentially contaminated sites are more difficult to interpret but may be helpful in diagnosis. Tests for antibody, antigen, and metabolite detection are investigational. None of the current commercially available tests have been accepted as dependable diagnostic aids. Other tests are in development.

Treatment:

Mucous Membrane and Skin Infections. Oral candidiasis is treated with oral nystatin suspension or clotrimazole troches. However, the safety and effectiveness of clotrimazole have not been established in children younger than 3 years of age. In immunocompromised patients with oropharyngeal candidiasis, both ketoconazole and fluconazole (in patients 14 years of age and older) have therapeutic benefit but may not eradicate the organism.

Mild *Candida* esophagitis can be treated with high-dose oral nystatin; more severe disease is treated with ketoconazole for 14 days or with low-dose (10 to 20 mg/d) intravenous amphotericin B for at least 5 to 7 days. Fluconazole is also approved for the treatment of oropharyngeal and esophageal candidiasis. Although the safety profile of the drug is generally excellent, the number of children younger than 14 years treated with fluconazole is insufficient to establish its safety in infants and children.

Skin infections are treated with topical nystatin, miconazole, clotrimazole, amphotericin B, ketoconazole, econazole, or ciclopirox (see Topical Drugs for Superficial Fungal Infections, p 565). Nystatin is usually effective and is the least expensive of these drugs.

Vaginal candidiasis is effectively treated with many topical formulations, including clotrimazole, miconazole, butaconazole, terconazole, and tioconazole. Such topically applied azole drugs are more effective than nystatin. Oral agents (eg, ketoconazole, fluconazole, and itraconazole), although not specifically approved by the Food and Drug Administration for vulvovaginal candidiasis, are effective. Their use should be considered for recurrent or refractory cases.

For chronic mucocutaneous candidiasis, ketoconazole and clotrimazole are effective drugs. Amphotericin B, given intravenously, with or without oral flucytosine, is also effective. Relapses are common when therapy with any of these agents is terminated, but systemic infection is rare. Keratomycosis is treated with corneal baths of amphotericin B, 1 mg/mL. Some patients with *Candida* cystitis may be successfully treated with bladder irrigations with amphotericin B, 50 μg/mL in distilled water, or short courses (3 to 5 days) of low-dose amphotericin B (0.3 mg/kg/d).

Systemic Infections. Amphotericin B is the drug of choice in systemic candidiasis (see Systemic Treatment With Amphotericin B, p 562). Usually a 4- to 6-week course of treatment is necessary, but the length will vary with the clinical response and presence or absence of neutropenia. Longer courses may be required in persistently neutropenic patients with hepatosplenic candidiasis. A shorter course of therapy may be successful for catheter-associated infection, provided the catheter is removed.

Flucytosine (150 mg/kg/d in four divided doses, given orally) should be given to supplement amphotericin B if the infection is severe and in patients with central nervous system involvement, as in vitro and clinical studies suggest synergism of flucytosine and amphotericin B against *C albicans*. Susceptibility testing, if available, should be performed because some strains of *C albicans* and other *Candida* species are resistant to flucytosine. Peak plasma concentrations should be maintained between 40 and 60 µg/mL; higher concentrations lead to toxicity. The dose of flucytosine must be decreased in patients with renal insufficiency. Adverse side effects include thrombocytopenia, leukopenia, hepatic dysfunction, rash, and diarrhea, especially in azotemic patients. The imidazole derivatives miconazole, ketoconazole, and fluconazole, administered systemically, can be beneficial in the treatment of systemic candidiasis, but data for recommending these drugs are limited.

Isolation of the Hospitalized Patient: No special precautions are recommended.

Control Measures: Prolonged, broad-spectrum, antimicrobial therapy in susceptible patients predisposes to *Candida* colonization and infection, and should be avoided whenever possible. Meticulous care of the venous catheter site is recommended in any patient requiring long-term intravenous alimentation; such care should include dry gauze dressing changes every 48 hours and the application of a povidone-iodine solution, which is fungistatic as well as bacteriostatic. Transparent dressings are associated with an increased incidence of catheter-related infections.

Cat Scratch Disease

Clinical Manifestations: The predominant sign is regional lymphadenopathy in an otherwise healthy person. Fever and mild systemic symptoms occur in 30% of patients. A skin papule is often found at the presumed site of bacterial inoculation and usually precedes development of lymphadenopathy by 1 to 2 weeks. Occasionally, infection can produce Parinaud's oculoglandular syndrome, involving the conjunctiva and a unilateral preauricular lymph node. Rare complications include encephalitis, osteolytic lesions, hepatitis, thrombocytopenia purpura, erythema nodosum, or chronic, systemic disease.

Etiology: *Rochalimaea henselae* (or other closely related *Rochalimaea* species) is considered, as of December 1993, to be responsible for most cases of cat scratch disease (CSD). This conclusion is based primarily on serologic, epidemiologic, and molecular probe rather than culture data, although *R henselae* has been isolated from a few patients with classic signs of CSD as well as from domestic cats. *Rochalimaea henselae* is a fastidious, slow-growing, Gram-negative organism that is a rickettsia. Recently, it has also been identified as the etiologic agent of bacillary angiomatosis and peliosis hepatitis, two infections that have been reported in HIV-infected patients, and it is closely related to *Rochalimaea quintana*, the rickettsial agent of trench fever. Previously, *Afipia felis*, formerly known as the "cat scratch bacillus," was isolated from lymph nodes of patients with CSD. Further studies will be needed to fully define the roles of *Rochalimaea* species and *A felis* in CSD.

Epidemiology: Cat scratch disease is believed to be a relatively common infection, although its true incidence is not known. Approximately 80% of cases occur in patients younger than 20 years of age. More than 90% of patients have a history of recent contact with a cat, often a kitten. The cat is usually healthy. Other animals, such as dogs and monkeys, and inanimate objects have been implicated in transmission. No evidence for person-to-person transmission exists. However, multiple cases have been observed in families, presumably resulting from contact with the same animal. Infection occurs more frequently in the fall and winter.

The **incubation period**, from the scratch to the appearance of the primary cutaneous lesion, is 7 to 12 days and 5 to 50 days (median of 12 days) from appearance of the primary lesion to appearance of lymphadenopathy.

Diagnostic Tests: The cat scratch antigen skin test, which has been used in the past by some investigators to establish the diagnosis, is an investigational test. The antigen that is prepared from aspirated pus from suppurative lymph nodes of patients with apparent CSD is not standardized, and the skin test is of unproven safety and is not commercially available.

The indirect fluorescent antibody test for detection of antibody to *Rochalimaea* species antigens may be useful in serologic diagnosis of CSD. It is available through the Centers for Disease Control and Prevention.

If lymph node, skin, or conjunctival tissue is available, the putative agent of the disease may be identified by the Warthin-Starry silver impregnation stain. Pathologic and microbiologic examinations are also useful to exclude other diseases. Histologic findings in lymph node sections are characteristic but not pathognomic for CSD. Early histologic changes consist of lymphocytic infiltrates with epithelioid granuloma formation, similar to changes in lymphomas and sarcoidosis. Later changes consist of polymorphonuclear leukocyte infiltrates with granulomas that become necrotic and resemble those of tularemia, brucellosis, and mycobacterial infections.

Treatment: Management is primarily symptomatic since the disease is usually self-limited, resolving spontaneously in 2 to 4 months. Painful, suppurative nodes can be treated with needle aspiration for relief of symptoms; surgical excision is generally unnecessary.

Antibiotic therapy should be considered only for acutely or severely ill patients with systemic symptoms, particularly those with hepatosplenomegaly. Recent anecdotal reports have suggested that several oral antibiotics (rifampin, trimethoprim-sulfamethoxazole, and ciprofloxacin) or intravenous gentamicin may be effective, but no controlled antimicrobial trials have been performed.

Isolation of the Hospitalized Patient: No special precautions are recommended.

Control Measures: None are known. Disposing of cats believed to transmit infection does not appear to be indicated.

Chlamydial Infections

Chlamydia pneumoniae

Clinical Manifestations: Severe pharyngitis, hoarseness, fever, productive cough, and cervical adenopathy are frequent symptoms. Illness is prolonged and can have a biphasic course. In some patients, sore throat precedes the onset of cough by a week or more. Pharyngitis without exudate and cough without rales are present on physical examination. Patients may be asymptomatic or mildly to moderately ill. Bronchospasm is common. An infiltrate in any part of the lung may be present on chest roentgenogram. Usually the white blood cell count is normal but the sedimentation rate is elevated.

Etiology: *Chlamydia pneumoniae* (formerly termed the TWAR strain) is a species of *Chlamydia* that is antigenically, genetically, and morphologically distinct from other *Chlamydia* species.

Epidemiology: *Chlamydia pneumoniae* infection is assumed to be transmitted from person to person. No animal or bird reservoir is known. The disease occurs worldwide. *Chlamydia pneumoniae*-specific serum antibody is present in most adults but is uncommon in children younger than 8 years. The peak age of initial infection is between the years of 5 and 20. Recurrent infection is common, especially in adults after middle age. Clusters of infection have been reported in groups of children and young adults.

The **incubation period** averages about 30 days but may be as short as 5 days.

Diagnostic Tests: The organism can be isolated from posterior oropharyngeal swabs inoculated into tissue culture. A fluorescent antibody research test using monoclonal antibody specific for *C pneumoniae* is available. Complement-fixing antibodies are present in children but are often absent in adolescents. Microimmunofluorescent antibody is the most sensitive indicator of infection. A fourfold serum antibody titer rise, a specific IgM titer of 1:16 or greater, or an IgG titer of 1:512 or greater is evidence of current infection.

Treatment: Erythromycin or tetracycline is recommended. Tetracycline should not be given routinely to children younger than 9 years of age. Adolescents and older patients have been treated with erythromycin for 5 to 10 days, but longer courses of therapy may be needed, as prolonged or recurrent symptoms are common. For adolescents and adults, tetracycline for 21 days or doxycycline for 7 to 10 days is also appropriate. In vitro data suggest that *C pneumoniae* is not susceptible to the sulfonamides. The new macrolide drugs, azithromycin and clarithromycin, may prove effective.

Isolation of the Hospitalized Patient: No special precautions are recommended.

Control Measures: None.

Chlamydia psittaci (Psittacosis, Ornithosis)

Clinical Manifestations: Psittacosis (ornithosis) is an acute febrile respiratory tract infection with systemic symptoms and signs that often include headache and rash. Extensive pneumonia can occur. Endocarditis, superficial thrombophlebitis, hepatitis, and encephalopathy are rare complications.

Etiology: *Chlamydia psittaci* is the cause. It is antigenically and genetically distinct from other *Chlamydia* species.

Epidemiology: Birds are the major reservoir of *C psittaci*. In the United States, imported birds, especially those smuggled into the country, pigeons, and turkeys are important sources. Both healthy and sick birds harbor and transmit the organism, usually via the airborne route. Excretion of *C psittaci* can be intermittent or continuous for weeks or months. Those in the environment of the infected bird, such as workers at poultry slaughter plants, poultry farms, and pet shops, or pet owners, are at special risk. Laboratory workers are also at high risk. Psittacosis is worldwide in distribution and tends to occur sporadically in any season. Infections are rare in children. Person-to-person transmission from acutely ill patients, presumably via the respiratory route, has been documented infrequently.

The **incubation period** is usually 7 to 14 days but may be longer.

Diagnostic Tests: The usual method of diagnosis is serologic, with demonstration of a fourfold increase in complement fixation (CF) antibody titer between acute and convalescent specimens collected 2 to 3 weeks apart. The CF test is not species specific and, therefore, cannot distinguish between *C psittaci*, *Chlamydia pneumoniae*, and *Chlamydia trachomatis* antibodies. Isolation of the agent from the respiratory tract should be attempted only by experienced laboratories where strict measures to prevent spread of the organism are used in the collection and handling of specimens.

Treatment: A tetracycline is the preferred therapy, except in children younger than 9 years, and it should be administered for at least 10 to 14 days after defervescence. Erythromycin is an alternative drug and is recommended for younger children.

Isolation of the Hospitalized Patient: Drainage/secretion precautions are prudent for the duration of the illness.

Control Measures: Epidemiologic investigation to determine the source of infection is indicated. Suspect birds should be killed and immersed in 2% phenol or a similar disinfectant to prevent spread of the organism from feathers. The specimen should be sealed in an impermeable container and transported on dry ice to the appropriate laboratory. All potentially contaminated caging and housing areas should be thoroughly disinfected and aired before reuse because these areas contain infectious organisms. When cleaning cages and other bird housing areas, care should be taken to avoid scattering the contents. Persons exposed to common sources of infection should be observed for development of fever or respiratory symptoms; early diagnostic tests should be performed and therapy started if these manifestations develop.

Chlamydia trachomatis

Clinical Manifestations: In neonatal chlamydial conjunctivitis, congestion, edema, and discharge develop a few days to several weeks after birth and last for 1 to 2 weeks, occasionally much longer. In contrast to trachoma, scars and pannus formation are rare.

Pneumonia in young infants caused by *Chlamydia trachomatis* is usually an afebrile illness that presents between 3 and 19 weeks after birth. A repetitive, staccato cough and tachypnea are characteristic but not always present. Rales can be present; wheezing is rare. Hyperinflation on a chest roentgenogram is prominent. Untreated disease can linger or recur. Severe chlamydial pneumonia has occurred in infants and some immunocompromised adults.

Trachoma is a chronic follicular keratoconjunctivitis with neovascularization of the cornea that results from repeated and chronic infection. Blindness secondary to extensive local scarring and inflammation occurs in 1% to 15% of trachoma patients.

Chlamydia trachomatis as a sexually transmitted pathogen can cause asymptomatic infection, urethritis in both sexes, vaginitis in prepubertal females, cervicitis in postpubertal females, and epididymitis in males. Infection can persist for months or years. Reinfection is common. In postpubertal females, chlamydial infection can progress to acute or chronic pelvic inflammatory disease and result in ectopic pregnancy or infertility.

Lymphogranuloma venereum (LGV) is an invasive lymphatic infection with an initial local lesion on the genitalia accompanied by regional lymphadenitis. The disease has a chronic, low-grade course.

Etiology: *Chlamydia trachomatis* is a bacterial agent with at least 15 serologic variants (serovars) divided between the following two biologic variants (biovars): oculogenital (serovars A-K) and LGV (serovars L_1-L_3). Trachoma is usually caused by serovars A-C, and genital infections are caused by B and D-K.

Epidemiology: *Chlamydia trachomatis* is currently the most common sexually transmitted infection in the United States. Oculogenital serovars of *C trachomatis* can be transmitted from the genital tract of infected mothers to their newborn infants. Acquisition occurs in about 50% of infants born vaginally of infected mothers and in some infants delivered by cesarean section with intact membranes. Of infants acquiring *C trachomatis*, the risk of conjunctivitis is 25% to 50% and the risk of pneumonia is 5% to 20%. The nasopharynx is the most commonly infected anatomic site. Asymptomatic infection of the conjunctiva, pharynx, rectum, or vagina of the infant can persist for more than 2 years. Prevalence in pregnant women varies between 6% and 12% in most populations, but it can be as low as 2% or as high as 37% in adolescents. Sexually active adolescents and young adults are at very high risk for *C trachomatis* infection.

Lymphogranuloma venereum biovars are worldwide in distribution, but are particularly prevalent in tropical and subtropical areas. Lymphogranuloma venereum is often asymptomatic in women. Perinatal transmission is rare.

Genital infection in adolescents and adults is sexually transmitted. In prepubertal children beyond infancy who have vaginal, urethral, or rectal chlamydial infection, possible sexual abuse must be considered. In infants and children, infection is not known to be communicable. The degree of contagiousness of pulmonary disease is unknown but appears to be low. Lymphogranuloma venereum is infective during active clinical disease, which may last from weeks to many years.

The **incubation period** is variable, depending on the type of infection, but is usually at least 1 week.

Diagnostic Tests: Definitive diagnosis can be made by isolating the organism in tissue culture. Conjunctival specimens must contain conjunctival cells, not exudate alone.

Currently available tests for rapid detection of antigen are useful for evaluating urethral specimens from symptomatic males, cervical specimens from both symptomatic and asymptomatic females, and eye and nasopharyngeal specimens from infants. These tests should not be used for testing rectal, vaginal, or urethral specimens from children, since fecal bacterial flora cross-react with *C trachomatis* antisera. When evaluating a child for possible sexual abuse, rapid antigen tests are not appropriate, as culture of the organism is the only acceptable method for diagnosis at this time.

Available tests for rapid detection of antigen include (1) direct fluorescent staining for elementary bodies in clinical specimens using monoclonal antibody (DFA); (2) enzyme immunoassay (EIA); and (3) a DNA probe. This latter test has been evaluated primarily in adult females at high risk for chlamydial infection. In this population, its sensitivity and specificity is similar to that of EIA and DFA tests. Its utility in other populations has not been as well documented.

Diagnostic tests based on polymerase chain reaction (PCR) and related technologies are currently being evaluated.

Serum antibody determinations are difficult and not generally available. In children with pneumonia, an elevated serum titer of *Chlamydia*-specific immunoglobulin M (IgM) is diagnostic of infection, but this test is available in only a few laboratories.

Indirect laboratory evidence of chlamydial pneumonia includes hyperinflation and bilateral diffuse infiltrates on roentgenographs, eosinophilia of 300 to 400/mm^3 or more in peripheral blood counts, and elevated total serum IgG (500 mg/dL or more) and IgM (110 mg/dL or more) concentrations. However, the absence of these findings does not exclude the diagnosis.

Treatment:

- **Chlamydial conjunctivitis and pneumonia** in young infants are treated with oral erythromycin (50 mg/kg/d in four divided doses) for 14 days. Oral sulfonamides may be used after the immediate neonatal period for infants who do not tolerate erythromycin. Topical treatment of conjunctivitis is ineffective and unnecessary. Since the efficacy of erythromycin therapy is approximately 80%, a second course is sometimes required. A specific diagnosis of *C trachomatis* infection in an infant should prompt treatment of the mother and evaluation of her sex partner(s).
- Infants born to mothers known to have untreated chlamydial infection should be treated with oral erythromycin (or a sulfonamide) after the immediate neonatal period.
- Treatment of **trachoma** is more difficult and recommendations for therapy differ. The most widely used therapy is topical treatment with erythromycin, tetracycline, or sulfacetamide ointment twice daily for 2 months or twice daily for the first 5 days of the month for 6 months. Oral erythromycin or doxycycline for 40 days is also given.
- For *C trachomatis* **genital tract infection** in adolescents, oral doxycycline (200 mg/d in two divided doses) for 7 days or azithromycin in a single 1-g oral dose is recommended. The alternatives are oral erythromycin base (2.0 g/d in four divided doses) for 7 days or erythromycin ethylsuccinate (3.2 g/d in four divided doses) for 7 days, either of which is also the recommended therapy for pregnant patients and young children. Because the efficacy of erythromycin regimens is approximately 80%, a second course of therapy may be required. If a pregnant woman cannot tolerate erythromycin, alternate but less effective regimens are oral amoxicillin (1.5 g/d in three divided doses) for 7 to 10 days or sulfisoxazole (2.0 g/d in four divided doses) for 10 days. Sulfisoxazole is contraindicated in pregnant women near term and in nursing mothers. Azithromycin is not licensed for use in pregnant or lactating women.
- For **LGV**, azithromycin, a tetracycline (for children 9 years of age and older), sulfonamide, or erythromycin may be given for 3 to 6 weeks.

Follow-up testing: Patients do not need to be retested for *Chlamydia* after completing treatment with doxycycline or azithromycin unless symptoms persist or reinfection is suspected. Retesting may be considered 2 weeks after completing regimens with erythromycin, sulfisoxazole, or amoxicillin.

Isolation of the Hospitalized Patient: Drainage/secretion precautions for the duration of the illness are recommended for patients with conjunctivitis or genital tract disease. Patients with pneumonia or LGV need not be isolated.

Control Measures:

Pregnancy. The identification and treatment of women with *C trachomatis* genital tract infection during pregnancy can prevent disease in the infant. Pregnant women at high risk for *C trachomatis* infection, in particular those younger than 25 years of age and those with new or multiple sex partners, should be targeted for screening. Some experts advocate universal testing of pregnant women in the third trimester.

Neonatal Chlamydial Conjunctivitis. The recommended topical prophylaxis with silver nitrate, erythromycin, or tetracycline for all newborns for the prevention of gonococcal ophthalmia will not reliably prevent neonatal chlamydia conjunctivitis or extraocular infection (see Prevention of Neonatal Ophthalmia, p 533).

Contacts of Infants With C trachomatis Conjunctivitis and/or Pneumonia. Mothers (and their sexual partners) of infected infants should also be treated for *C trachomatis*.

Gynecologic Examination. Sexually active adolescents should be routinely tested for *Chlamydia* infection during gynecologic examination even if no symptoms are present. Screening of young adult women aged 20 to 24 years is also desirable, particularly those who do not consistently use barrier contraceptives and who have multiple partners.

Management of Sexual Partners. Sexual contacts of patients with *C trachomatis* infection, nongonococcal urethritis, mucopurulent cervicitis, epididymitis, or pelvic inflammatory disease should be evaluated for exposure to *C trachomatis*. Contacts should be treated if the last sexual contact was within 30 days of a symptomatic index patient's onset of symptoms or within 60 days of an asymptomatic index patient's diagnosis.

LGV. Nonspecific, preventive measures for LGV are those for sexually transmitted diseases in general, and include education, case reporting, and avoidance of contact with infected patients.

Cholera

Clinical Manifestations: Most persons infected with *Vibrio cholerae* have no symptoms, some have mild to moderate diarrhea, and fewer than 5% have severe watery diarrhea, vomiting, and dehydration (cholera gravis). Cholera is characterized by painless, voluminous diarrhea without abdominal cramps or fever. Dehydration, hypokalemia, metabolic acidosis, and, occasionally, hypovolemic shock can occur in 4 to 12 hours if fluid losses are not replaced. Coma, convulsions, and hypoglycemia can also occur, particularly in children. Typical stools are colorless, with small flecks of mucus ("rice-water"), and contain high concentrations of sodium, potassium, chloride, and bicarbonate.

Etiology: *Vibrio cholerae* is a Gram-negative, curved, motile bacillus with many serogroups. Until recently, only enterotoxin-producing organisms of serogroup 01 have caused epidemics. *Vibrio cholerae* 01 is divided into two serotypes, Inaba and Ogawa, and two biotypes, classical and E1 Tor. The current predominant biotype is E1 Tor. Serotype 0139 (a non-01, toxigenic strain) has recently caused widespread illness in India and Bangladesh. Non-toxigenic strains of *V cholerae* can cause sporadic diarrhea disease but do not cause epidemics.

Epidemiology: In the last three decades, *V cholerae* 01, biotype E1 Tor has spread from India and Southeast Asia to Africa, the Middle East, Southern Europe, and the Western Pacific Islands (Oceania). In 1991, epidemic cholera caused by toxigenic *V cholera* 01, serotype Inaba, biotype E1 Tor, appeared in Peru. It has spread to most countries in South and North America. In the United States, cases associated with travel to Latin America or Asia and with ingestion of contaminated food transported from Latin America or Asia have been reported. In addition, in the United States, the Gulf Coast of Louisiana and Texas has an endemic focus of a unique strain of toxigenic *V cholerae* 01. Most cases of disease from this strain have resulted from consumption of raw or undercooked shellfish. Humans are the only documented natural host, but free-living *V cholerae* organisms can exist in the aquatic environment. The usual mode of infection is ingestion of contaminated water or food (particularly raw or undercooked shellfish), moist grains held at ambient temperature, and raw or partially dried fish. Boiling of water or treating it with chlorine or iodine, and adequate cooking of food kills the organism. Direct person-to-person spread by contact has not been documented. Persons with low gastric acidity are at increased risk for cholera infection. The period of communicability is unknown but presumably is related to the duration of carriage.

The **incubation period** is usually 1 to 3 days, with a range of a few hours to 5 days.

Diagnostic Tests: *Vibrio cholerae* can be cultured from stool or a rectal swab that is placed in transport media and plated on appropriate selective media. Suspect colonies are serologically confirmed by agglutination with specific antisera. Since most laboratories in the United States do not routinely culture for *V cholerae* or other vibrios, clinicians should request appropriate cultures for clinically suspected cases. Isolated specimens of *V cholerae* 01 should be confirmed at a state health department and then sent to the Centers for Disease Control and Prevention for testing for production of cholera toxin. A fourfold rise in vibriocidal antibody titers between acute and convalescent serum samples or a fourfold decline in vibriocidal titers between early and late convalescent (more than a 2-month interval) sera can confirm the diagnosis.

Treatment: Oral or parenteral rehydration therapy to correct dehydration and electrolyte abnormalities is the most important modality of therapy.* Antimicrobial therapy results in prompt eradication of vibrios, reduces the duration of diarrhea, and reduces the requirements for fluid replacement. It should be considered for persons who are moderately to severely ill. Oral

---

*For further information and detailed recommendations, see Duggan C, Santosham M, Glass RI. The management of acute diarrhea in children: oral rehydration, maintenance, and nutritional therapy. *MMWR*. 1992;41(RR-16):1-20.

tetracycline (50 mg/kg/d, maximum 2 g/d, in four divided doses) for 3 days or doxycycline (6 mg/kg, maximum 300 mg) as a single dose are the drugs of choice for cholera. If strains are resistant to tetracyclines, trimethoprim-sulfamethoxazole (8 mg/kg/d of trimethoprim and 40 mg/kg/d of sulfamethoxazole), erythromycin (40 mg/kg/d, maximum 1,000 mg), or furazolidone (5 to 8 mg/kg/d, maximum 400 mg) may be used. The use of tetracyclines is not generally recommended for children younger than 9 years of age, but in severe cholera infections the benefits may offset the risks of staining of developing teeth. Ciprofloxacin or ofloxacin are effective but should only be used in individuals 18 years and older. Antimicrobial susceptibility of newly isolated organisms should be determined.

Isolation of the Hospitalized Patient: Enteric precautions are indicated for the duration of illness.

Control Measures:
Hygiene. Because cholera spreads by contaminated food or water, and infection frequently requires ingestion of large numbers of organisms, disinfection or boiling of water will prevent transmission. Thoroughly cooking crabs, oysters, and other shellfish from the Gulf Coast before eating is also recommended to reduce the likelihood of transmission. Foods such as fish, rice, or grain gruels should be refrigerated. Appropriate hand washing after defecating and before preparing or eating food is important in preventing transmission.

Treatment of Contacts. The administration of tetracycline, doxycycline, or trimethoprim-sulfamethoxazole within 24 hours of identification of the index case may be effective in preventing coprimary and secondary cases of cholera among household contacts if the household secondary rate is high. The use of tetracyclines is not recommended for children younger than 9 years of age. Prophylactic treatment in the United States is not recommended unless unusual sanitary and hygienic conditions indicate that the rate of secondary transmission may be high.

Vaccine. The only currently available vaccine in the United States is of limited value. It protects about 50% of those immunized for only 3 to 6 months, does not prevent *Vibrio* excretion or inapparent infection, and is serologically unrelated to the new serotype causing cholera (see Etiology, p 157). Furthermore, travelers using standard tourist accommodations are at virtually no risk of infection in countries with cholera. Cholera vaccination is not required for travelers entering the United States from cholera-affected areas, and the World Health Organization no longer recommends vaccination for travel to or from cholera-infected areas. No country currently requires cholera vaccine for entry. The vaccine should not be administered to contacts of patients with cholera or used to control the spread of infection, and it is not generally recommended for international travelers. Several experimental, orally administered vaccines have demonstrated improved efficacy with fewer side effects than the currently available parenterally administered vaccine.

Reporting. Cholera is an internationally notifiable disease.

Clostridial Infections

Botulism and Infant Botulism
(Clostridium botulinum)

Clinical Manifestations: Botulism is a neurologic disorder with onset of symptoms either occurring abruptly within a few hours or evolving gradually during several days. A symmetric descending flaccid paralysis occurs, typically involving the bulbar musculature initially and later affecting the somatic musculature. Patients with rapidly evolving illness may have generalized weakness and hypotonia initially. Signs and symptoms in older children or adults can consist of diplopia, blurred vision, dry mouth, dysphagia, dysphonia, and dysarthria. Infant botulism, which occurs predominantly in infants younger than 6 months of age, is usually preceded by constipation and is accompanied by lethargy, poor feeding, weak cry, diminished gag reflex, subtle ocular palsies, and generalized weakness and hypotonia ("floppy infant").

Etiology: Human botulism is caused by the neurotoxins A, B, E, and, rarely, F and G of *Clostridium botulinum* (and occasionally by those of other clostridia).

Epidemiology: Food-borne botulism results when a food contaminated with spores of *C botulinum* is preserved improperly and stored under anaerobic conditions that permit germination, multiplication, and toxin production. Almost all food-borne botulism currently results from ingestion of improperly prepared home-canned foods. Illness occurs when the unheated food is eaten and preformed botulinum toxin is ingested. Food-borne botulism rarely occurs in infants or children because they are less likely to be exposed to foods that might contain botulinum toxin. Botulism is not transmitted from person to person.

Infant botulism results after ingested species of *C botulinum* have germinated, multiplied, and produced botulinum toxin in the intestine. Infant botulism is not transmitted from person to person. In most cases of infant botulism, the source of spores remains unknown; however, honey is one identified source. Light and dark corn syrups have also been reported to contain botulinum spores, but at lower rates than honey.

Wound botulism, although rarely reported, results when *C botulinum* grows in traumatized tissue and produces its toxin. Of the nearly 50 cases of documented wound botulism, approximately half have occurred in children and teenagers.

The usual **incubation period** for food-borne botulism is 12 to 36 hours (range, 6 hours to 8 days); for wound botulism, it is 4 to 14 days between the time of injury and the onset of symptoms. In infant botulism, the incubation period is unknown.

Diagnostic Tests: A toxin neutralization bioassay in mice is used to identify botulinum toxin in serum, stool, or suspect foods. Enriched and selective media are used to culture *C botulinum* from stool and foods. In infant botulism, the diagnosis is made by demonstrating *C botulinum* organisms or toxin in feces. Toxin has been demonstrated in serum in only about 10% of infants with botulism. To increase the likelihood of diagnosis, both serum and stool should be obtained from all persons with suspected botulism. Serum specimens collected more than 3 days after ingestion of toxin are frequently negative; at this time, stool culture is the best diagnostic test. When obtaining a stool specimen is difficult because of constipation, an enema using sterile, nonbacteriostatic water can be given. Electromyography can be helpful in diagnosis; an incremental response of evoked muscle potentials at high-frequency nerve stimulation (more than 20 cycles per second) can occur, and in infant botulism a characteristic pattern of brief, small, abundant motor action potentials (BSAP) is often found.

Treatment:

Meticulous Supportive Care. The most important aspect of therapy in all forms of botulism is meticulous supportive care, particularly nutritional and respiratory.

Antitoxin. For food-borne and wound botulism, botulinum antitoxin should be administered to symptomatic persons as soon as possible after testing for hypersensitivity to equine sera. This antitoxin is of equine origin. Approximately 20% of treated persons experience some degree of hypersensitivity reaction. Trivalent Antitoxin (ABE)* can be obtained by contacting the state health department. If contact cannot be made with the state health department, the physician should call the Centers for Disease Control and Prevention (CDC) directly.

Equine antitoxin rarely has been used in infant botulism because of the risk of inducing lifelong hypersensitivity to equine antigens and lack of evidence of its benefit. However, a human-derived botulism antitoxin, formerly termed botulism immune globulin, has been prepared, and a clinical trial of its efficacy when given early in the course of the illness is in progress in California.†

Antimicrobial Agents. In infant botulism, antibiotics are used only to treat secondary infections. Aminoglycosides may potentiate the effects of the toxin. Some physicians give penicillin to eradicate bowel carriage of *C botulinum*, but the resulting benefit is uncertain.

Isolation of the Hospitalized Patient: No special precautions are recommended.

---

*Prepared by Connaught Laboratories, Inc, Swiftwater, PA, and distributed in the United States through the Drug Service of the Centers for Disease Control and Prevention (see the Directory of Telephone Numbers, p 601).

†For possible enrollment of patients in California, call the Infant Botulism Prevention Program, Health and Human Services (510/540-2646).

Control Measures:

- Prophylactic antitoxin for asymptomatic persons who have ingested a food known to contain botulinum toxin is not recommended. Because of the danger of hypersensitivity reactions, the decision to administer antitoxin requires careful consideration. Consultation in this regard may be obtained from the state health department or the CDC (see Treatment, p 161).

- Elimination of ingested toxin may be facilitated by inducing vomiting and/ or by gastric lavage, rapid purgation (eg, with magnesium sulfate, 15 to 30 g in children and 30 to 45 g in adults), and high enemas. The value of these measures in infant botulism is not clear. Enemas should not be administered to persons with illness except perhaps to obtain a stool specimen for diagnostic purposes.

- Exposed persons should have close medical observation.

- Contacts of persons with wound or infant botulism are not at an increased risk of acquiring botulism. Botulinum toxoid (types A, B, C, D, and E) is available from the CDC for immunization of laboratory workers whose regular exposure places them at high risk.

- Education to improve home canning methods should be promoted. Use of a pressure cooker (at 116°C or 240.8°F) is necessary to kill spores of *C botulinum*. Boiling for 10 minutes will destroy the toxin. Time-temperature-pressure requirements vary with the product being heated.

- Most sources of spores for infant botulism are unavoidable; however, honey is a source and should not be given to infants, ie, children younger than 12 months of age, and it should not be placed on nipples before breast-feeding. Although cases of infant botulism have not been linked to corn syrup, prudence indicates that infants should not be fed this nonessential food, which also has been reported to contain *C botulinum*.

Clostridium difficile

Clinical Manifestations: Infections include pseudomembranous colitis and antimicrobial-associated diarrhea. Pseudomembranous colitis generally is characterized by diarrhea, abdominal cramps, fever, systemic toxicity, abdominal tenderness, and passage of stool with blood, mucus, and pus. The colonic mucosa often contains small (2 to 5 mm), raised, yellowish plaques. Characteristically, the disease begins while the patient is in a hospital receiving antimicrobial therapy, but it may occur weeks after discharge from the hospital, after discontinuation of therapy, or unassociated with hospitalization or antimicrobial therapy. Severe or fatal disease has been described in severely neutropenic children with leukemia, in infants with Hirschsprung's disease, and in patients with inflammatory bowel disease. *Clostridium difficile* may also be associated with mild diarrhea or asymptomatic carriage.

Etiology: *Clostridium difficile* is a spore-forming, obligately anaerobic, Gram-positive bacillus. It is the cause of pseudomembranous colitis and of a high percentage of cases of antimicrobial-associated diarrhea. Disease is related to the action of toxin(s) produced by vegetative organisms. Two toxins (A and B) have been characterized.

Epidemiology: *Clostridium difficile* can be isolated from soil and is frequently present in the hospital environment. Spores of *C difficile* are acquired from the environment or by fecal-oral transmission from colonized individuals. Intestinal colonization rates in healthy neonates and young infants can be as high as 50% but are usually less than 5% in children older than 2 years of age and in adults. Hospitals are major reservoirs for *C difficile*, and child care facilities may be a source. Risk factors for the disease are those that increase exposure to organisms and those that diminish the barrier effect of the normal intestinal flora, allowing *C difficile* to proliferate and elaborate toxin(s) in vivo. Among these factors are repeated enemas, prolonged nasogastric tube insertion, and gastrointestinal tract surgery. Penicillins, clindamycin, and cephalosporins are the agents most frequently received by patients who subsequently develop pseudomembranous colitis, but colitis can be associated with almost any antimicrobial agent. Although *C difficile* toxin is rarely recovered from stools of asymptomatic adults, it is recovered frequently from stools of neonates who have no gastrointestinal tract illness. This finding confounds interpretation of positive toxin assays in patients younger than 6 months of age.

The **incubation period** is unknown.

Diagnostic Tests: Endoscopic findings of pseudomembranes and hyperemic, friable rectal mucosa suggest pseudomembranous colitis. In the diagnosis of *C difficile* disease, the organism is cultured using a selective medium, latex agglutination, cell culture assays, and enzyme immunoassay (EIA) for toxin detection. Isolation of *C difficile* from stool and testing fecal specimens by latex agglutination do not distinguish between toxigenic and nontoxigenic isolates. If these methods are used, testing for toxin either by cell culture or EIA should be performed to confirm the presence of toxigenic *C difficile*. Several commercially available EIAs that detect either toxin A or both toxins A and B are available. The EIAs are sensitive and easy to perform.

Treatment:
- Antimicrobial therapy should be discontinued in patients who develop significant diarrhea or colitis.
- In patients with severe toxicity or in whom diarrhea persists after antimicrobial therapy is discontinued, antimicrobial therapy is indicated. Orally administered vancomycin (40 mg/kg/d in four divided doses) is the drug of choice. Vancomycin is poorly absorbed from the gastrointestinal tract but can accumulate in the serum of patients with renal failure. Orally or intravenously administered metronidazole (35 mg/kg/d in four divided doses) is also effective and is less expensive. However, its safety has not been established in children, and the drug is not currently approved by the Food and Drug Administration for this indication. The efficacy of intravenously administered vancomycin is uncertain for this indication.
- Antimicrobial agents are usually given for 10 days.

- As many as 10% to 20% of patients relapse after discontinuing therapy, but they usually respond to a second course of treatment. Intravenous immune globulin has been successfully used in a few patients with chronic relapsing colitis.
- Cholestyramine, which binds toxin, can relieve symptoms.* However, its effect has not been evaluated in children with disease caused by *C difficile*. Because cholestyramine also binds vancomycin, the two drugs should not be administered concurrently.
- Drugs that decrease intestinal motility should not be given.

Isolation of the Hospitalized Patient: Enteric precautions are recommended until diarrhea subsides.

Control Measures:
- Infants and children with *C difficile* colitis should be in a separate, protected area or excluded from child care for the duration of diarrhea.
- Meticulous hand washing techniques, proper handling of contaminated waste (including diapers) and fomites, and limiting the use of antibiotics are the best currently available methods for the control of *C difficile* disease.
- Cleaning procedures that kill *C difficile* spores are under study.

Clostridial Myonecrosis (Gas Gangrene)

Clinical Manifestations: The onset is heralded by acute pain at the site of the wound, followed by edema, tenderness, exudate, and progression of pain. Systemic findings, which occur in conjunction with severe local toxicity, initially include tachycardia disproportionate to the degree of fever, pallor, diaphoresis, hypotension, renal failure, and, later, alterations in mental status. Crepitus (which is not always present) is not pathognomic of *Clostridia* infection. Diagnosis is based on clinical manifestations, including the characteristic appearance of the necrotic muscle at surgery. Untreated gas gangrene can lead to death within hours.

Etiology: Gas gangrene is caused by *Clostridium* species, most commonly *C perfringens*, which are large, Gram-positive, anaerobic bacilli with blunt ends. Mixed infection with other Gram-positive and/or Gram-negative bacteria is frequent.

Epidemiology: Gas gangrene usually results from contamination of traumatic wounds involving muscle injury. The sources of *Clostridia* species are soil, contaminated objects, and human and animal feces. Contamination of wounds can occur as long as open lesions are present. Dirty surgical or traumatic wounds with significant devitalized tissue and foreign bodies predis-

---

*Use for this indication is not currently approved by the Food and Drug Administration.

pose to disease. Nontraumatic gas gangrene occurs occasionally from *Clostridia* in the patient's intestinal tract.

The **incubation period** is 6 hours to 3 weeks, usually 2 to 4 days.

Diagnostic Tests: Anaerobic cultures of wound exudate, affected soft tissue and muscle, and blood should be performed. Because *Clostridia* species are ubiquitous, their recovery from a wound is not diagnostic unless the appropriate clinical manifestations are present. A Gram-stained smear of wound discharge demonstrating characteristic Gram-positive bacilli and absent or sparse polymorphonuclear leukocytes is indicative of clostridial infection. Tissue samples and aspirates, but not swabs, are appropriate specimens for anaerobic culture; rapid transport of samples to the laboratory is essential to insure recovery of anaerobic organisms. A roentgenogram of the affected site may demonstrate gas in the tissue.

Treatment:
- Early and complete surgical excision of necrotic infected tissue and removal of foreign material is the most important therapeutic measure.
- Supportive management of shock, fluid and electrolyte imbalance, hemolytic anemia, and other complications is essential.
- High-dose penicillin G (250,000 to 400,000 U/kg/d) should be given intravenously. Chloramphenicol, clindamycin, and metronidazole are alternative drugs for penicillin-sensitive patients.
- Hyperbaric oxygen may be beneficial.
- Treatment with antitoxin is of no value. Equine gas gangrene polyvalent antitoxin is no longer available commercially in the United States.

Isolation of the Hospitalized Patient: Drainage/secretion precautions are indicated for as long as the lesion drains.

Control Measures: Prompt and careful debridement, flushing of contaminated wounds, and removal of foreign material with standard aseptic surgical techniques should be done.

Penicillin G (50,000 U/kg/d) or clindamycin (20 to 30 mg/kg/d) may be of prophylactic value in patients with grossly contaminated wounds.

Clostridium perfringens Food Poisoning

Clinical Manifestations: *Clostridium perfringens* food poisoning is characterized by watery diarrhea and moderate to severe, crampy, midepigastric pain. Vomiting is uncommon. Symptoms usually resolve within 24 hours. The absence of fever in most patients differentiates *C perfringens* food-borne disease from shigellosis and salmonellosis, and the infrequency of vomiting and longer incubation period contrast with the clinical features of staphylococcal and food-borne disease of chemical origin. Diarrheal illness caused by *Bacillus cereus* enterotoxin may be clinically indistinguishable from that caused by *C perfringens*.

Etiology: Disease is caused by a heat-labile toxin produced in vivo by type A *C perfringens*.

Epidemiology: *Clostridium perfringens* is ubiquitous in the environment and is frequently present in raw meat and poultry. The organism survives initial cooking by sporulation. The spores germinate and multiply during cooling; an enterotoxin produced by the organisms in the lower intestine is responsible for symptoms. Beef, poultry, gravies, and Mexican-style food are common sources. Infection is usually acquired at banquets or institutions (eg, schools and camps), or from food caterers or restaurants where food is prepared in large quantities and kept warm for prolonged periods. Illness is not transmissible from person to person.

The **incubation period** is 6 to 24 hours, usually 8 to 12 hours.

Diagnostic Tests: Because the fecal flora of healthy persons frequently includes *C perfringens*, counts of at least 10^6 *C perfringens* spores per gram of feces obtained within 48 hours of onset of illness are required to support the diagnosis in ill persons. The diagnosis can be established by detection of *C perfringens* enterotoxin in stool; kits are available commercially for this purpose. To confirm *C perfringens* as the etiology, the concentration of organisms should be at least 10^5 per gram in the epidemiologically implicated food. Although *C perfringens* is an anaerobe, special transport conditions are not necessary because the spores are durable. Stool rather than rectal swabs should be collected because the former permit enumeration of spores.

Treatment: Usually no treatment is required. Oral rehydration or, occasionally, intravenous fluid and electrolyte replacement may be indicated for patients with unusually severe dehydration. Antibiotics are not indicated.

Isolation of the Hospitalized Patient: No special precautions are recommended.

Control Measures: Preventive measures depend on limiting proliferation of *C perfringens* in foods by maintaining food warmer than 60°C (140°F) or cooler than 7°C (45°F). Meat dishes should be served hot shortly after cooking. Foods should never be held at room temperature to cool; they should be refrigerated after removal from warming devices or serving tables. They should be reheated to at least 74°C (165.2°F) or higher before serving. Roasts, stews, and similar dishes should be divided into small quantities for cooking and refrigeration to limit the time such foods are at temperatures at which *C perfringens* replicates.

Coccidioidomycosis

Clinical Manifestations: The primary pulmonary infection is usually asymptomatic and inapparent. Symptomatic disease may resemble influenza, with cough, fever, and chest pain. Chronic pulmonary lesions are rare in children. A diffuse erythematous maculopapular rash, erythema multiforme, erythema nodosum, and/or arthralgias frequently occur.

Primary extrapulmonary lesions include cutaneous lesions, which usually follow trauma or can result from dissemination. The progressive disease is similar to tuberculosis; lungs, lymph nodes, bones, joints, abdominal organs, the central nervous system, and the skin are frequently affected sites. Meningitis is a particularly serious common manifestation of disseminated disease and can be fatal if untreated. Hydrocephalus is a common complication of central nervous system infections. Limited dissemination to one or more sites is common in children.

Etiology: *Coccidioides immitis* is a dimorphic fungus. In soil, it exists in the mycelial phase, the mature hyphal forms of which are termed arthroconidia. From these structures, spores and, later in the infected host, spherules develop.

Epidemiology: *Coccidioides immitis* is found extensively in the soil of southwestern United States and California, northern Mexico, and certain areas of Central and South America. Climatic conditions (hot summers, little winter frost) combine with soil conditions (alkaline, dry) and local characteristics (moderate to low rainfall) to produce ideal circumstances for preservation of arthroconidia and their dissemination by aerosols. Persons are infected by inhalation of dust-borne arthroconidia. Person-to-person transmission of coccidioidomycosis does not occur because the fungal form that exists in patients is the spherule, which is less infectious. One episode of multiple infections from a plaster cast that was contaminated with arthroconidia has been reported. The rate of disseminated disease is increased in blacks, Hispanics, Filipinos, pregnant women, and immunocompromised patients.

The **incubation period** is 10 to 16 days; the range is from less than 1 week to approximately 1 month, depending on the quantity of arthroconidia inhaled.

Diagnostic Tests: Skin tests can be useful in diagnosis. A reactive coccidioidin or spherulin skin test is characteristic of a hypersensitivity reaction of the delayed type. The spherule skin test is now the one preferred for general use and its conversion from negative to positive in a patient with a clinically compatible syndrome strongly suggests coccidioidomycosis. A positive skin test usually appears 10 to 21 days after infection, but it is characteristically absent in progressive disease. Therefore, overreliance on skin test results can lead to errors in diagnosis, particularly since dissemination can occur in patients whose skin tests are nonreactive.

Serologic tests are useful to confirm diagnoses and provide prognostic information. Immunoglobulin M response can be detected by latex agglutination, tube precipitin, or immunodiffusion. Latex agglutination is a rapid, very sensitive test that lacks specificity. Positive tests should be confirmed by other tests. Tube precipitins are detectable 1 to 3 weeks after symptoms appear and last 3 to 4 months in most cases.

Immunoglobulin G response can be detected by immunodiffusion or complement fixation. Complement fixation antibodies in serum usually are of low titer and transient if the disease is asymptomatic or mild. Higher and persistent complement fixation titers are observed when the disease is severe, and almost always when infection is disseminated. Cerebrospinal fluid (CSF) antibodies are detectable by complement fixation. The concentration and persistence of complement fixation antibody titers in serum in patients with disseminated, severe disease and in CSF in those with meningitis are useful prognostically and in guiding treatment. Rising titers in serum and CSF indicate progressive disease, and decreasing titers suggest improvement.

Spherules as large as 80 micrometers in diameter may be visualized in appropriate clinical specimens in selected instances, such as tracheal aspirates, biopsies of skin lesions or organs, urine, or CSF. A chemiluminescent DNA probe (called "Accuprobe"*) can identify cultures of *C immitis*. The procedure can be applied to nonsporulating cultures, thereby reducing the risk of exposure to infectious forms of the fungi. Culture of the organism is possible but is a potential infectious hazard to laboratory personnel since conversion of spherules to arthroconidial-bearing mycelium can take place. Suspect cultures should be sealed at the outset and thereafter handled cautiously by trained persons.

Treatment: Antifungal therapy is not indicated in uncomplicated primary infection and is only required in fewer than 5% of cases of coccidioidomycosis.

Amphotericin B is the recommended therapy in severe progressive pulmonary disease, disseminated infection, central nervous system (CNS) infections, and in immunocompromised patients, such as those with AIDS (see Systemic Treatment With Amphotericin B, p 562).

Experience with agents other than amphotericin B is limited. Ketoconazole has effectively suppressed symptoms and arrested progression of infection in most patients with pulmonary or disseminated coccidioidomycosis, but the relapse rate after treatment is high. Efficacy in comparison to that of amphotericin B has not been evaluated. Ketoconazole should not be used in place of amphotericin B in patients with severe disease or those who are immunocompromised.

In CNS infections, intravenous amphotericin B therapy is augmented by repetitive instillation of this drug into the lumbar, cisternal, or ventricular spaces, frequently by the use of a subcutaneous reservoir (see Systemic Treatment With Amphotericin B, p 562). High doses of ketoconazole, given orally, with intraventricular miconazole, have also been used successfully. Some recent studies indicate that fluconazole is a promising agent in the treatment of coccidioidal meningitis.

---

*Available from Gene-Probe, Inc, San Diego, CA.

In some localized infections (eg, mandibular), local instillation of amphotericin B has been used with occasional success.

The duration of amphotericin B therapy is variable and depends on the site(s) of involvement, clinical response, and mycologic and immunologic tests. In general, therapy is continued until clinical and laboratory evidence indicates that the active infection has subsided. Minimum treatment for invasive coccidioidomycosis is 1 month, and treatment for 1 year or longer is frequently necessary for CNS disease.

Surgical debridement or excision of lesions in bone and lung has been advocated for localized, symptomatic, persistent, resistant, or progressive lesions. Surgical treatment by shunt procedures of hydrocephalus in CNS infections is frequently necessary.

Isolation of the Hospitalized Patient: No special precautions are recommended. Care should be exercised in handling, changing, and discarding dressings, casts, and similar materials in which arthroconidial contamination could occur.

Control Measures: None.

Coronaviruses

Clinical Manifestations: Coronaviruses are a common cause of upper respiratory tract infection in adults and children and have occasionally been implicated in lower respiratory tract disease. Enteric coronaviruses have been identified by electron microscopy in the feces of infants and children with gastroenteritis, but their etiologic significance is unproven. Coronavirus-like agents have also been associated with several outbreaks of diarrhea in nurseries and, rarely, with neonatal necrotizing enterocolitis in infants.

Etiology: Coronaviruses are RNA viruses that are large (80 to 160 nm), enveloped with lipid-soluble coats, and pleomorphic (spherical or elliptical). At least two distinct antigenic groups of respiratory coronaviruses are recognized.

Epidemiology: Human coronaviruses are most likely transmitted by the respiratory route, possibly by aerosols and large droplets, and facilitated by close contact. Because of prolonged carriage of enteric coronaviruses in the stool, fecal-oral transmission may also occur. Although several animal coronaviruses have antigens in common with human strains, no evidence implicates animals as reservoirs or vectors for human disease. Coronaviruses are worldwide in distribution. In temperate climates, outbreaks occur in the winter. Young children have the highest infection rate in outbreaks. The period of communicability is unknown but probably persists for the duration of respiratory symptoms.

The **incubation period** is usually 2 to 4 days.

Diagnostic Tests: Diagnostic tests for human coronaviruses are not commercially available. Most strains cannot be isolated by the methods commonly used in diagnostic virology laboratories. Viral particles have been visualized by immune electron microscopy and viral antigens detected by immunoassay techniques. Antibody to coronaviruses can be determined by several assay methods, such as neutralization, complement fixation, indirect hemagglutination, hemagglutination-inhibition, fluorescent antibody, enzyme immunoassay, and electron microscopy, but these tests are not routinely available.

Treatment: Supportive.

Isolation of the Hospitalized Patient: For infants and young children with possible coronavirus infection, contact isolation is recommended for the duration of symptoms.

Control Measures: None.

Cryptococcus neoformans Infections (Cryptococcosis, Torulosis)

Clinical Manifestations: Infection can involve primarily the central nervous system (meningoencephalitis), lungs (pneumonia), lymph nodes (adenopathy), heart (endocarditis), skin (ulcers), bones and joints, and mucous membranes. Usually, several sites are infected, but manifestations of the involvement of one site predominate. Cryptococcal meningitis is the most common and most serious form of cryptococcal disease. Cryptococcal fungemia, without apparent organ involvement, occurs in patients with AIDS.

Etiology: *Cryptococcus neoformans* is an encapsulated yeast.

Epidemiology: *Crytococcus neoformans* var *neoformans* is worldwide in distribution, primarily in association with bird droppings, and causes most human infections. *Cryptococcus neoformans* var *gattii* occurs mainly in tropical and subtropical regions. Acquisition is by inhalation of particles containing the organism. The fungus is not transmitted from person to person. Cryptococcus infects 5% to 10% of adults with AIDS but is less common in HIV-infected children.

The **incubation period**, although not well defined, is probably a few weeks from the time of exposure.

Diagnostic Tests: Encapsulated yeast cells can be demonstrated in wet mounts of sputum or pus or in India ink preparations of cerebrospinal fluid (CSF) sediment in some cases. Precise diagnosis depends on the isolation and identification of the organism by culture. The lysis-centrifugation method for the culture of blood is the most sensitive and rapid method for culture. Media containing cycloheximide, which inhibits growth of *C neoformans*, should not be used as the only fungal isolation medium. Few organisms may be present in the CSF, and large quantities of fluid may need to be cultured to recover the organism. The latex particle agglutination test for detection of cryptococcal antigen in serum or CSF is a useful and rapid diagnostic tool. Skin testing with the antigen cryptococcin is of no value.

Treatment: Amphotericin B in combination with flucytosine is indicated for meningeal and other serious cryptococcal infections. Combination antifungal therapy is probably superior to amphotericin B alone but the toxicities of combined therapy can limit its use. Flucytosine often induces cytopenias, which necessitate discontinuation of the medication. Amphotericin B is administered intravenously (see Systemic Treatment With Amphotericin B, p 562) and flucytosine is given orally. Meningitis in most patients is treated for at least six weeks. Patients with AIDS require maintenance therapy, for which fluconazole is the drug of choice.

Fluconazole may be an alternative drug for the primary treatment of cryptococcosis in HIV-infected patients. Data on its use in children are limited.

Isolation of the Hospitalized Patient: No special precautions are recommended.

Control Measures: None.

Cryptosporidiosis

Clinical Manifestations: Frequent, watery diarrhea and low-grade fever are the most common presenting symptoms. Other symptoms include abdominal pain, anorexia, and weight loss. In infected immunocompetent individuals, including children, the diarrheal illness is self-limited, usually lasting 1 to 20 days (average, 10 days). Immunocompromised patients, especially those with AIDS, can develop chronic, severe diarrhea with malnutrition, dehydration, and death. Although infection is usually limited to the gastrointestinal tract, pulmonary, biliary tract, or disseminated infection has occurred in immunocompromised patients.

Etiology: *Cryptosporidium parvum* is a coccidian protozoan.

Epidemiology: Cryptosporidia have been found in a variety of hosts, including mammals, birds, and reptiles. Transmission of *Cryptosporidium* from farm livestock or pets to humans can occur. In experimental studies, *Cryptosporidium* has been transmitted from humans to various species of animals. Person-to-person transmission occurs and can cause outbreaks in child care centers, with high rates (30% to 60%) of infection. Waterborne outbreaks have occurred. Infection can be asymptomatic as well as symptomatic. Peak infection rates occur in the young and decrease progressively with age.

The parasite is resistant to chlorine; therefore, appropriately functioning water filtration systems are critical for the safety of public water supplies. Sand filters used for swimming pools are effective in removing oocysts from contaminated water.

The estimated **incubation period** is 2 to 14 days.

Diagnostic Tests: Oocysts on microscopic examination of stool specimens is diagnostic. To do so, either the sucrose flotation method or formalin-K is used to concentrate the oocysts in stool, followed by staining with a modified Kinyoun acid-fast stain. Since shedding can be intermittent, at least two stool specimens should be examined before considering the test to be negative. Oocysts are small (4 to 6 micrometers in diameter) and can be missed in a rapid scan of the slide. The organism can also be identified on intestinal biopsy tissue. A monoclonal antibody-based fluorescein conjugated stain for oocysts in stool and an enzyme immunoassay for detecting antigen in stool are available commercially.

Treatment: Other than rehydration and correction of electrolyte abnormalities, definitive treatment has not been established. Paromomycin or azithromycin may be beneficial in some cases. In HIV-infected patients with cryptosporidiosis, orally administered hyperimmune immunoglobulin therapy with bovine colostrum or bovine serum has been successful, often in combination with zidovudine therapy. Somatostatin analogues have been used with variable success in controlling secretory diarrhea in patients with AIDS, but controlled trials are needed.

Isolation of the Hospitalized Patient: Enteric precautions are recommended.

Control Measures: None.

Cutaneous Larva Migrans (Creeping Eruption)

Clinical Manifestations: Nematode larvae produce itching, reddish papules at the site of skin entry. As the larvae migrate through the skin and advance several millimeters to a few centimeters a day, they leave intensely pruritic, serpiginous tracks. Larval activity can continue for several weeks or months but eventually is self-limiting. The clinical picture of an advancing serpiginous tunnel in the skin with an associated intense pruritus is virtually pathognomonic.

Etiology: Infective larvae of cat and dog hookworms, ie, *Ancylostoma brasiliensis* and *Ancylostoma caninum*, are the usual causes. Other skin-penetrating nematodes are occasional causes.

Epidemiology: Cutaneous larva migrans is a disease of children, utility workers, gardeners, sunbathers, and others who come in contact with sandy soil contaminated with cat and dog feces. In the United States, the disease is most prevalent in the Southeast.

Diagnostic Tests: Since the diagnosis is usually made clinically, biopsies are not usually indicated. Biopsy specimens typically demonstrate an eosinophilic inflammatory infiltrate, but the migrating parasite is not visualized. Eosinophilia occurs in some cases.

Treatment: The disease is usually self-limited, with spontaneous cure after several weeks or months. Thiabendazole given orally and/or topically relieves cutaneous symptoms (see Drugs for Parasitic Infections, p 574). Oral albendazole* has also been reported to be effective, but is not yet approved by the Food and Drug Administration.

Isolation of the Hospitalized Patient: No special precautions are recommended.

Control Measures: Skin contact with moist soil contaminated with animal feces should be avoided.

Cytomegalovirus Infection

Clinical Manifestations: The manifestations of acquired cytomegalovirus (CMV) infection vary with the age and immunocompetence of the host. Asymptomatic infections are the most common, particularly in children. Hepatosplenomegaly are occasionally associated with acquired infection in childhood. An infectious mononucleosis-like syndrome with prolonged fever and mild hepatitis, occurring in the absence of heterophile antibody production, can occur in adults. Pneumonia and retinitis are common in immunocompromised hosts, particularly those receiving treatment for malignancies, those infected with human immunodeficiency virus (HIV), or those receiving immunosuppressive therapy for organ transplantation.

Congenital infections also have a spectrum of manifestations. Usually, infection is asymptomatic, but some congenitally infected infants who appear to be asymptomatic at birth are found in infancy or childhood to have a hearing loss or learning disability. Profound involvement, with intrauterine growth retardation, neonatal jaundice, purpura, hepatosplenomegaly, microcephaly, brain damage, intracerebral calcifications, and chorioretinitis, occurs in approximately 5% of infants with CMV infections.

Infection acquired at birth or shortly thereafter from maternal cervical secretions or human milk is usually not associated with clinical illness. Infection resulting from transfusion from CMV seropositive donors to preterm infants has been associated with lower respiratory tract disease.

---

*Available from SmithKline Beecham, Philadelphia, PA.

Etiology: Human CMV, a DNA virus, is a member of the herpesvirus group.

Epidemiology: Infection in humans is caused almost entirely by human CMV; simian CMV is very rarely a cause. Human CMV is ubiquitous and is transmitted both horizontally (by direct person-to-person contact with virus-containing secretions) and vertically (from mother to infant before, during, or after birth). Infections have no seasonal predilection. Cytomegalovirus persists in latent form after a primary infection, and reactivation can occur years later, particularly under conditions of immunosuppression.

Horizontal transmission is probably the result of salivary contamination or sexual transmission, but contact with infected urine can also play a role. Although the virus is not highly contagious, spread of CMV in households and child care centers is well documented. Excretion rates in child care centers can reach 70% in 1- to 3-year-old children. Young children can transmit CMV to their parents and other caregivers, such as child care staff (see also Children in Out-of-Home Child Care, p 86). In adolescents and adults, sexual transmission also occurs, as evidenced by virus in seminal and cervical fluids.

Seropositive healthy persons carry latent CMV in white blood cells and tissues; hence, blood transfusions and organ transplantation can result in viral transmission. Severe CMV disease is more likely to occur if the recipient is seronegative or is a premature infant. Latent CMV will frequently reactivate in immunosuppressed individuals, and can result in disease if the immunosuppression is severe (eg, AIDS patients, solid-organ-transplant recipients, and bone marrow transplant recipients).

Vertical transmission of CMV to the infant occurs (1) in utero by transplacental passage of maternal blood-borne virus, (2) at birth by passage through an infected maternal genital tract, or (3) postnatally by ingestion of CMV-positive human milk. Approximately 1% of all infants are infected in utero and excrete CMV at birth. In utero fetal infection can occur regardless of whether the mother had primary infection or reactivation during pregnancy. However, infants infected in utero during maternal reactivation are much less frequently affected than those infected in utero after maternal primary infection, presumably because of immunity in the mother. Of infants whose infection resulted from maternal primary infection, 10% to 20% will have mental retardation or sensorineural deafness. Severe disease with manifestations at birth occurs in about 5% of infants infected in utero.

Maternal cervical infection is common, resulting in exposure of many infants to CMV at birth. Cervical excretion rates are higher among young mothers in lower socioeconomic groups. Although interstitial pneumonia caused by CMV can develop in the early months of life, most infected infants remain asymptomatic. Similarly, although symptomatic disease can occur in seronegative infants fed CMV-infected milk from milk banks, most infants infected from human milk do not develop clinical illness, most likely because of the presence of passively transferred maternal antibody. For infants who acquire infection from maternal cervical secretions or human milk, premature infants are at greater risk of symptomatic disease and sequelae than term infants.

The **incubation period** for horizontally transmitted CMV infections in households is unknown. Infection usually manifests 3 to 12 weeks after blood transfusions, and between 4 weeks and 4 months after tissue transplantation.

Diagnostic Tests: The diagnosis of CMV is frequently confounded by the ubiquity of the virus, the high rate of asymptomatic excretion, the frequency of reactivated infections, the development of immunoglobulin M (IgM) CMV antibody in some episodes of reactivation, and the simultaneous presence of other pathogens.

Virus can be isolated in tissue culture from urine, pharynx, peripheral blood leukocytes, human milk, semen, cervical secretions, and other tissues and body fluids. Virus present in large quantity can also be identified by electron microscopic examination of urine or tissue. Examination of cells shed in the urine for intranuclear inclusions is an insensitive test.

Only recovery of virus from a target organ provides unequivocal evidence that the disease is caused by CMV infection. However, a presumptive diagnosis can be made on the basis of a fourfold antibody titer rise in paired sera or by virus excretion. DNA hybridization techniques are available from specialty laboratories for detection of CMV in tissues and some fluids, especially cerebrospinal fluid.

Complement fixation is the least sensitive serologic method for the diagnosis of CMV infection and should not be used to establish previous infection or passively acquired maternal antibody. Various fluorescence assays, indirect hemagglutination, latex agglutination, and enzyme immunoassays are preferred for this purpose.

Proof of congenital infection requires obtaining specimens within 3 weeks of birth. Viral isolation or a strongly positive test for serum IgM anti-CMV antibody is considered diagnostic. Later in infancy, differentiation between intrauterine and perinatal infection is difficult unless clinical signs of the former, such as chorioretinitis or ventriculitis, are present. Special serologic tests that are available only in reference laboratories may help to differentiate between these two possibilities in the first 2 or 3 months of life.

Treatment: The drug ganciclovir (see Antiviral Drugs, p 567) is beneficial in the treatment of retinitis caused by acquired or recurrent CMV infection in patients with AIDS. This drug is approved in the United States for the treatment of severe retinitis in immunocompromised adults. Limited data in children suggest that efficacy is similar to that in adults, but available data are insufficient to establish safety in children. The drug may be useful in other types of CMV organ involvement. The combination of CMV Immune Globulin, given intravenously, and ganciclovir has been reported to be synergistic in the treatment of CMV infections in bone marrow transplant recipients. Foscarnet has also been approved for the treatment of CMV retinitis and is an alternative drug (see Antiviral Drugs, p 567). This drug is more toxic but may be advantageous for some patients with HIV infection, such as those with disease caused by ganciclovir-resistant disease or those unable to tolerate ganciclovir.

Isolation of the Hospitalized Patient: No special precautions are recommended. Hospitalized patients do not need separate rooms. However, since CMV is spread by intimate contact with infectious secretions, hand washing after exposure to secretions is particularly important for pregnant personnel.

Control Measures:

Care of Exposed Persons.
- In caring for all children, hand washing, particularly after changing diapers, is advised to reduce transmission of CMV and other infectious agents. Since asymptomatic infection and excretion of CMV is common in newborn infants, children, and adults, the child with congenital CMV infection should not be given special handling and should not be excluded from schools or institutions. Institution-sponsored screening programs for CMV-excreting children are also not justified. The intermittent and prolonged shedding of CMV in the urine makes screening programs impractical and prohibitively costly.
- Although unrecognized exposure to individuals asymptomatically shedding CMV is likely to be frequent, concern arises when immunocompromised or pregnant patients or health care workers are exposed to patients with clinically recognizable CMV infection. Many exposed adults and children are already immune, but because most infections are asymptomatic, the history is of no value in assessing susceptibility. Serologic testing can be used to identify nonimmune individuals, although as yet no prophylactic agent can be offered. Follow-up serologic testing will establish whether infection has occurred. However, routine serologic screening of personnel is not currently recommended.
- Prevention of exposure of severely immunocompromised patients to recognized cases of CMV infection is prudent. Since unrecognized exposure may occur, infection control procedures as warranted for these patients should be used.
- Pregnant personnel who may be in contact with CMV-infected patients should be counseled about the potential risks of acquisition and urged to practice good hygiene, particularly hand washing. Approximately 1% of infants in most newborn nurseries, and a higher percentage of older children, excrete CMV without clinical manifestations. Fetal risks are greatest in the first half of gestation. Amniocentesis has been used in several small series of patients to establish the presence of intrauterine infection.

Child Care (see also Children in Out-of-Home Child Care, p 87). Educational programs about the epidemiology of CMV, its potential risks, and appropriate hygienic measures to minimize occupationally acquired infection should be provided for female child care workers. The prevalence of CMV in urine or saliva of apparently healthy children can be high, and spread to their mothers and child care workers has been documented. Risk appears to be greatest for child care personnel who care for children younger than 2 years. Routine serologic screening for antibody to CMV in staff at child care centers is not currently recommended.

Immunoprophylaxis. Cytomegalovirus Immune Globulin has been developed for prophylaxis of disease in seronegative transplant patients. It appears to be moderately effective in kidney transplant recipients who receive 150 mg/kg every other week. Results of studies of its use in prevention of CMV transmission to newborn infants, to date, are inconclusive. Evaluation of an investigational live-virus vaccine in healthy volunteers and renal transplant patients is in progress.

Prevention of Transmission by Blood Transfusion. Transmission of CMV by blood transfusion to preterm infants or others has been virtually eliminated by the use of CMV antibody-negative donors, by freezing blood in glycerol before administration, by removal of the buffy coat, or by filtration to remove the white blood cells.

Prevention of Transmission by Human Milk. Pasteurization or freezing of donated human milk can reduce the likelihood of CMV transmission. If fresh donated milk is provided to infants born to CMV antibody-negative mothers, providing these infants with milk from CMV antibody-negative women only should be considered. For further information on breast-feeding, see Human Milk (pp 74 and 76).

Prevention of Transmission in Transplant Patients. Cytomegalovirus antibody-negative donors who receive tissue from CMV seropositive persons are at high risk for CMV disease. High doses of acyclovir or ganciclovir in transplant patients shedding CMV may prevent serious CMV disease.

Diphtheria

Clinical Manifestations: Diphtheria usually occurs as membranous nasopharyngitis and/or obstructive laryngotracheitis. These local infections are associated with a low-grade fever and the gradual onset of manifestations during 1 to 2 days. Less commonly, the disease presents as cutaneous, vaginal, conjunctival, or otic infections. Cutaneous diphtheria is more common in tropical areas and among the homeless. Life-threatening complications of diphtheria include thrombocytopenia, myocarditis, and neurologic problems such as vocal cord paralysis and ascending paralysis similar to that of Guillain-Barré syndrome.

Etiology: *Corynebacterium diphtheriae* is an irregularly staining, Gram-positive, nonmotile, pleomorphic bacillus with three colony types (mitis, gravis, and intermedius). The *C diphtheriae* strains may be either toxigenic or nontoxigenic. The ability to produce toxin is mediated by infection of the bacterium by a bacteriophage and is not related to colony type.

Epidemiology: Humans are the only known reservoir of *C diphtheriae*. Sources of infection include discharges from the nose, throat, eye, and skin lesions of infected persons. Transmission results primarily from intimate contact with a patient or carrier. Rarely, fomites can serve as vehicles of transmission, and food-borne outbreaks have occurred. Illness is most common in low socioeconomic groups living in crowded conditions. Infection can occur in immunized and partially immunized persons as well as in the unimmunized; disease is most common and most severe in unimmunized or inadequately immunized individuals. The incidence of disease is greatest in the fall and winter, but summer epidemics can occur in warmer climates in which skin infections are prevalent. Communicability in untreated persons usually lasts for 2 weeks or less, but occasionally it persists for several months. In patients treated with appropriate antibiotics, communicability usually lasts less than 4 days. Occasionally, chronic carriage occurs, even after antimicrobial therapy.

The **incubation period** is usually 2 to 5 days but occasionally longer.

Diagnostic Tests: Specimens for culture should be obtained from the nose and throat and from any lesions. Material should be obtained from beneath the membrane, or a portion of the membrane itself should be submitted for culture. Because special media are required, the laboratory should be notified that *C diphtheriae* is suspected. In remote areas, throat swabs can be placed in silica gel packs and sent to reference laboratories for culture, as *C diphtheriae* survive drying. Direct-stained smears and fluorescent antibody-stained smears are unreliable. When *C diphtheriae* is recovered, the strain should be tested for toxigenicity.

Treatment:

Antitoxin. Because the condition of patients with diphtheria may deteriorate rapidly, a single dose of equine antitoxin should be administered on the basis of clinical diagnosis, even before culture results are available. The site and size of the diphtheritic membrane, the degree of toxicity, and the duration of the illness are guides for estimating the dose of antitoxin; the presence of soft, diffuse cervical lymphadenitis suggests moderate to severe toxin absorption. Suggested dose ranges are the following: pharyngeal or laryngeal disease of 48 hours' duration, 20,000 to 40,000 U; nasopharyngeal lesions, 40,000 to 60,000 U; extensive disease of 3 or more days' duration or diffuse swelling of the neck, 80,000 to 100,000 U. To neutralize toxin as rapidly as possible, the preferred route of administration is intravenous. Before intravenous administration, however, tests for sensitivity with 1:10 antitoxin dilution for conjunctival testing or 1:100 dilution for intradermal testing should be performed (see Sensitivity Tests for Reactions to Animal Sera, p 46). If the patient is sensitive to equine antitoxin, desensitization (see "Desensitization" for Animal Sera, p 47) is necessary. Antitoxin can be obtained from Connaught Laboratories or from the National Immunization Program of the Centers for Disease Control and Prevention (see Directory of Telephone Numbers, p 601). Antitoxin is probably of no value for cutaneous disease, but some authorities use 20,000 to 40,000 U of antitoxin because toxic sequelae have been reported. Although intravenous immunoglobulin preparations contain antibodies to diphtheria toxin, their use for therapy of cutaneous or respiratory diphtheria has not been approved and optimal dosages have not been established.

Antimicrobial Therapy. Erythromycin given orally or parenterally (40 to 50 mg/kg/d, maximum 2 g/d) for 14 days; or penicillin G daily, intramuscularly (aqueous crystalline, 100,000 to 150,000 U/kg/d, in four divided doses, or procaine, 25,000 to 50,000 U/kg/d, in two divided doses) for 14 days, comprises acceptable therapy. Antimicrobial therapy is required to eradicate the organism and prevent spread; **it is not a substitute for antitoxin**. Elimination of the organism should be documented by two consecutive negative cultures after completion of treatment.

Cutaneous diphtheria. Thorough cleansing of the lesion with soap and water and administration of antimicrobials for 10 days is recommended.

Carriers. If unimmunized, carriers should receive active immunization promptly, and measures should be taken to ensure completion of the immunization schedule. If a carrier has been previously immunized but has not received a booster within 1 year, a booster dose of a preparation containing diphtheria toxoid (DTP, DTaP, DT, or Td) should be given. Carriers should be given antimicrobial therapy, specifically oral erythromycin or penicillin G for 7 days, or a single, intramuscular dose of benzathine penicillin G (600,000 U for those weighing less than 30 kg and 1,200,000 U for larger children and adults). Follow-up cultures should be obtained at least 2 weeks after the completion of therapy; if they are positive, an additional 10-day course of oral erythromycin should be given. Erythromycin-resistant strains have been identified but their epidemiologic significance has not been determined.

Isolation of the Hospitalized Patient: For pharyngeal diphtheria, patients and carriers of toxigenic strains should be placed in strict isolation until two cultures from both the nose and the throat are negative for *C diphtheriae*. Patients with cutaneous diphtheria should be placed in contact isolation until two cultures of skin lesions are negative. Material for these cultures should be taken at least 24 hours apart after cessation of antimicrobial therapy.

Control Measures:

Care of Exposed Persons. Whenever the diagnosis of diphtheria is strongly suspected or proven, local public health officials should be notified promptly. Management of exposed persons is based on individual circumstances, including immunization status and the likelihood of surveillance and adherence to prophylaxis.

- Identification of close contacts of a suspected patient should be promptly initiated. Contact tracing should begin in the household and can usually be limited to household members and other persons with history of habitual, close contact with the suspected case.
- Close contacts, *irrespective of their immunization status*, should be (1) kept under surveillance for 7 days for evidence of disease, (2) cultured for *C diphtheria*, and (3) given antimicrobial prophylaxis with oral erythromycin (40 to 50 mg/kg/d for 7 days, maximum 2 g/d) or benzathine penicillin G (600,000 to 1,200,000 U, intramuscularly; the lower dose is for patients weighing less than 30 kg). The efficacy of antimicrobial prophylaxis is presumed but not proven. Repeat pharyngeal cultures should be obtained from

contacts proven to be carriers at a minimum of 2 weeks after completion of their therapy (see Carriers, p 179).

- Asymptomatic, previously immunized, close contacts should receive a booster dose of a preparation containing diphtheria toxoid (DTP, DTaP, DT, or Td) if they have not received a booster dose of diphtheria toxoid within 5 years. Children in need of their fourth dose should be vaccinated.
- For asymptomatic close contacts who are not fully immunized (defined as having had fewer than 3 doses of diphtheria toxoid) or whose immunization status is not known, active immunization should be undertaken with DTP, DT, or Td, depending on age.
- Contacts who cannot be kept under surveillance should receive (1) benzathine penicillin G, but not erythromycin for reasons of compliance; and (2) a dose of DTP, DTaP, DT, or Td, depending on age and the person's immunization history.
- The use of equine diphtheria antitoxin in unimmunized close contacts is not recommended because no evidence demonstrates any additional benefit of diphtheria antitoxin use for contacts who have received antimicrobial prophylaxis and because of the risk of allergic reactions to horse serum. If antitoxin is used, the usual recommended dose is 5,000 to 10,000 U, injected intramuscularly at a site separate from the site of the toxoid injection, after appropriate testing for sensitivity.

Immunization. Universal immunization with diphtheria toxoid is the only effective control measure. Its value is proven by the rarity of the disease in countries in which high rates of immunization with diphtheria toxoid have been achieved. Fewer than five cases have been reported annually in the United States in recent years. As a result of high immunization rates, exposure to persons with diphtheria or to carriers is less frequent now than in the past. However, the decreased frequency of exposure to the organism implies decreased maintenance of immunity secondary to community contact. Therefore, assurance of continuing immunity requires regular booster injections of diphtheria toxoid (as Td) every 10 years after completion of the initial immunization series.

Immunization for children from age 2 months to the seventh birthday (see Tables 1.3 and 1.4, pp 23 and 24) should consist of five doses of diphtheria vaccine. The initial three doses are given as DTP vaccine, administered intramuscularly, at 2-month intervals commencing at 2 months of age. A fourth dose either of DTaP or DTP is recommended 6 to 12 months after the third dose, usually at 15 to 18 months of age; if given before 15 months, DTP is given since DTaP is not currently licensed for use in children of that age. A fifth dose of DTaP or DTP is given before school entry (kindergarten or elementary school) at 4 to 6 years of age, unless the fourth dose was given after the fourth birthday. Doses may be given concurrently with other vaccines (see Simultaneous Administration of Multiple Vaccines, p 25).

Haemophilus influenzae conjugate vaccines containing diphtheria toxoid (PRP-D) or CRM_{197} protein (HbOC), a nontoxic variant of diphtheria toxin, are not substitutes for diphtheria toxoid immunization with DTP, DT, or DTaP. HbOC vaccine is available in the United States both as a single vaccine and in combination with DTP (HbOC-DTP) (see *Haemophilus influenzae* Infections, p 207).

Immunization against diphtheria for children in whom pertussis immunization is contraindicated (see Pertussis, p 364) should be accomplished with DT vaccine instead of DTP, as follows:

- For children who are younger than 1 year, three doses of DT are given at 2-month intervals; a fourth dose should be given approximately 1 year after the third dose; and the fifth dose should be given before school entry at 4 to 6 years of age.
- For children aged 1 through 6 years who have not received prior doses of DT or DTP, two doses of DT approximately 2 months apart should be given, followed by a third dose 6 to 12 months later to complete the initial series. DT vaccine can be given concurrently with other vaccines. An additional dose is necessary before school entry at 4 to 6 years of age, unless the preceding dose was given after the fourth birthday.
- For children aged 1 through 6 years (ie, less than 7 years) who have received one or two doses of DTP (or DT) in the first year of life and for whom further pertussis vaccination is contraindicated, additional doses of DT should be given until a total of five doses of diphtheria and tetanus toxoids are received by the time of school entry. The fourth dose is administered 6 to 12 months after the third dose. The preschool (fifth) dose is omitted if the fourth dose was given after the fourth birthday.
- For children after their seventh birthday (see Table 1.4, p 24), diphtheria immunization should consist of Td, ie, adult-type tetanus and diphtheria toxoids. The Td preparation contains not more than 2 flocculating units (Lf) of diphtheria toxoid per dose, as compared with 6.7 to 12.5 Lf in the DTP, DTaP, and DT preparations for use in infants and younger children. Td vaccine is less likely than DTP, DTaP, or DT to produce reactions in older children and adults. Two doses are given 1 to 2 months apart; a third dose should be given 6 to 12 months after the second. Complete immunization requires three doses followed by booster doses every 10 years.
- When children and adults require tetanus toxoid for wound management (see Tetanus, p 460), the use of preparations containing diphtheria toxoid (DTP, DTaP, DT, or Td as appropriate for age or specific contraindications) will help ensure continuing diphtheria immunity.
- DT and Td may be given concurrently with other vaccines (see Simultaneous Administration of Multiple Vaccines, p 25).
- Active immunization against diphtheria should be undertaken during convalescence from diphtheria in every patient because this exotoxin-mediated disease does not necessarily confer immunity.

Precautions and Contraindications: see Pertussis (p 364) and Tetanus (p 463).

Ehrlichiosis (Human)

Clinical Manifestations: Human ehrlichiosis is an acute, systemic febrile illness clinically similar to Rocky Mountain spotted fever but with more frequent occurrence of leukopenia and less frequent occurrence of rash. The febrile illness is often accompanied by headache, chills, malaise, myalgia, arthralgia, nausea, vomiting, anorexia, and acute weight loss. Rash is variable in appearance and location. It typically develops about 1 week after onset of illness but only occurs in approximately 40% of reported cases. Diarrhea, abdominal pain, and change in mental status are noted less frequently. Reported complications include pulmonary infiltrates, bone marrow hypoplasia, respiratory failure, encephalopathy, meningitis, and renal failure. Leukopenia, lymphopenia, anemia, hyponatremia, thrombocytopenia, elevated liver function tests, and cerebrospinal fluid abnormalities (pleocytosis with a predominance of lymphocytes and elevated total protein concentration) are common. The disease typically lasts 1 to 2 weeks, and recovery generally occurs without sequelae. Fatal as well as asymptomatic infections have been reported.

Etiology: The cause is *Ehrlichia chaffeensis*, a rickettsial species closely related to *Ehrlichia canis*, the causative agent of canine ehrlichiosis.

Epidemiology: Most human cases have been reported from southeastern and south central United States, but cases have been reported as far west as Washington state. The disease appears to be transmitted by ticks. Which tick transmits the infection to humans is not known. Compared to those with Rocky Mountain spotted fever, patients with ehrlichiosis have been somewhat older but similar regarding gender, race, and recognized tick exposures. Most human infections occur from May through July. The incidence of reported cases appears to be increasing. Epidemiologic data are limited.

The **incubation period** appears to be 1 to 3 weeks; the median has been 11 to 12 days.

Diagnostic Tests: The diagnosis of *E chaffeensis* infection can be established by demonstrating a fourfold or greater increase or decrease in antibody titer between acute and convalescent sera, preferably obtained 2 to 4 weeks apart, using an indirect fluorescent antibody test with *E chaffeensis* as antigen. The test is available only through state health departments and the Centers for Disease Control and Prevention. Isolation of *Ehrlichia* from a human patient has been accomplished.

Treatment: The decision to initiate antibiotic therapy is based on clinical findings and epidemiologic considerations. Tetracycline appears to be effective therapy for human ehrlichiosis. Limited data suggest that chloramphenicol is also effective. Tetracycline drugs ordinarily should not be given to children younger than 9 years of age in view of the risk of dental staining. However, in deciding which antibiotic to give a patient with presumed ehrlichiosis who is younger than 9 years of age, the benefits and risks of a single course of tetracycline therapy should be compared with those of chloramphenicol.

Isolation of the Hospitalized Patient: No special precautions are recommended.

Control Measures: Specific measures concern prevention of contact with ticks and are similar to those for Rocky Mountain spotted fever and other tick-borne diseases (see Control Measures for Prevention of Tick-Borne Infections, p 114).

Enterovirus (Nonpolio) Infections (Coxsackieviruses, Group A and Group B; Echoviruses; and Enteroviruses)

Clinical Manifestations: Nonpolio enteroviruses are responsible for significant and frequent illnesses in infants and children and result in protean clinical manifestations. The most common presentation is nonspecific febrile illness, which in infants frequently leads to suspicion of bacterial sepsis. Other manifestations include the following: (1) respiratory—common cold, pharyngitis, herpangina, stomatitis, pneumonia, and pleurodynia; (2) gastrointestinal—vomiting, diarrhea, abdominal pain, and hepatitis; (3) eye—acute hemorrhagic conjunctivitis; (4) heart—myopericarditis; (5) skin—exanthem; and (6) neurologic—aseptic meningitis, encephalitis, and paralysis. Although each of these findings can be caused by several different enteroviruses, some associations between virus and disease are particularly noteworthy, including the following: coxsackievirus A16 in the hand, foot, and mouth syndrome; coxsackievirus A24 and enterovirus 70 in acute hemorrhagic conjunctivitis; enterovirus 71 in encephalitis and polio-like paralysis; echovirus 9 in petechial exanthem and meningitis; coxsackieviruses B1-B5 in myopericarditis and in fulminating neonatal encephalomyocarditis; and echovirus 11 in fulminating neonatal hepatic necrosis.

Etiology: The nonpolio enteroviruses are RNA viruses, which include 23 group A coxsackieviruses (types A1-A24, except type A23), 6 group B coxsackieviruses (types B1-B6), 31 echoviruses (types 1-33, except types 10 and 28), and 4 enteroviruses (types 68-71).

Epidemiology: Enteroviruses are ubiquitous in humans, and humans are their only known natural host. Enteroviruses are spread by fecal-oral and possibly oral-oral (respiratory) routes. Attack rates are highest in young children, and infections occur more frequently in lower socioeconomic groups and in tropical areas where hygiene is poor. In temperate climates, enteroviral infections are most common in the summer and fall. In contrast, no seasonal pattern is evident in the tropics. Fecal viral excretion and transmission can continue for several weeks after the onset of infection.

The **incubation period** is usually 3 to 6 days.

Diagnostic Tests: Specimens for viral isolation should be obtained from the throat and rectum and any sites of clinical involvement, such as the cerebrospinal fluid, blood, and biopsy material. Attempts to recover virus are particularly important in patients with serious illnesses during epidemics. Viral isolation from any specimen except feces can usually be considered causally related to the patient's illness. Because enteroviruses can persist in the lower gastrointestinal tract for as long as 8 to 12 weeks, fecal isolates may not be causally related to the patient's illness. Most viral diagnostic laboratories use only tissue culture techniques that are capable of recovering echoviruses, group B coxsackieviruses, and some group A coxsackieviruses. Suckling mouse inoculation, which is not a routine procedure, is required for the recovery of some group A coxsackieviruses. Sera for antibody testing should be collected at the onset of illness and 4 weeks later and stored frozen. The demonstration of a rise in titer of neutralizing antibody to a virus recovered from the feces suggests a causal role for the isolated virus. Because no common enterovirus antigen is available for laboratory use, serologic screening without viral isolation is generally not performed.

Treatment: No specific therapy for enteroviral infections exists. Intravenous immune globulin with a high antibody titer to the infecting virus may be of benefit in immunocompromised patients and has been used in life-threatening neonatal infections.

Isolation of the Hospitalized Patient: Enteric precautions are indicated for the duration of hospitalization.

Control Measures: Particular attention should be given to hand washing and personal hygiene, especially after diaper changing.

Escherichia coli and Other Gram-Negative Bacilli

Septicemia and Meningitis in Neonates

Clinical Manifestations: Neonatal septicemia or meningitis caused by *Escherichia coli* and other Gram-negative bacilli cannot be differentiated clinically from serious infections caused by other infectious agents. Moreover, the first signs of sepsis may be minimal and similar to those observed in noninfectious processes. Clinical signs of sepsis include fever, temperature instability, apnea, cyanosis, jaundice, hepatomegaly, lethargy, irritability, anorexia, vomiting, abdominal distention, and diarrhea. Meningitis may be concomitant with sepsis without overt signs attributable to the central nervous system.

Etiology: *Escherichia coli* strains with the K1 capsular polysaccharide antigen cause about 41% of cases of septicemia and 75% of cases of meningitis caused by *E coli*. Other important Gram-negative bacilli responsible for neonatal sepsis include non-K1 strains of *E coli*, *Klebsiella*, *Enterobacter*, *Proteus*, *Citrobacter*, and *Salmonella* species. Anaerobic Gram-negative bacilli are infrequent causes. *Haemophilus influenzae* infection can occur in the newborn period. In contrast to invasive *H influenzae* infections occurring after the newborn period, invasive infections in neonates can be caused by nonencapsulated strains.

Epidemiology: The source of *E coli* and other Gram-negative pathogens in early-onset neonatal infections is usually the maternal gastrointestinal tract. In addition, nosocomial acquisition of Gram-negative flora through person-to-person transmission among nursery personnel and from nursery environmental sites, such as fluid reservoirs of incubators, has been documented, especially in preterm infants requiring prolonged intensive care management. Predisposing host factors in neonatal Gram-negative infection include maternal perinatal infection, low birth weight, prolonged rupture of membranes, and septic or traumatic delivery. Metabolic abnormalities such as galactosemia, fetal hypoxia, and acidosis have also been implicated as predisposing factors. Neonates with immunologic defects, defects in the integrity of the skin or mucosa (eg, meningomyelocele), or asplenia can also be at increased risk for Gram-negative infection. In intensive care nurseries, the sophisticated systems for respiratory and metabolic support, invasive procedures (eg, umbilical catheters), and the frequent use of antimicrobial agents enable proliferation and selection for multiply antimicrobial-resistant strains of Gram-negative pathogens, and, thus, predispose infants to colonization and infection.

The **incubation period** is highly variable; time of onset of the infection ranges from birth to several weeks of age.

Diagnostic Tests: Blood, urine, cerebrospinal fluid, and other fluids or tissues that might be infected should be stained and examined for bacteria and cultured in any neonate who is to be treated for septicemia. Techniques for detection of bacterial antigens, such as latex particle agglutination, are not commercially available for Gram-negative pathogens implicated in neonatal sepsis, with the exception of *H influenzae* type b and *E coli* K1 (whose capsular antigen cross-reacts with that of group B *Neisseria meningitidis*, thus affecting the interpretation of a positive test).

Treatment:
- Initial empiric treatment for a neonate with suspected septicemia and/or meningitis entails a combination of a penicillin (usually ampicillin) and an aminoglycoside. An alternative regimen of a penicillin (usually ampicillin) and a cephalosporin (such as cefotaxime or ceftazidime) active against most etiologic Gram-negative bacilli can be used, but rapid emergence of cephalosporin-resistant strains, especially *Enterobacter cloacae* and *Serratia* species, can occur as a result of frequent cephalosporin use in a nursery. Hence, routine use of cephalosporins in newborn units for empiric treatment of infections is not recommended, unless Gram-negative meningitis is strongly suspected.
- Once the etiologic agent has been identified and the susceptibility pattern defined, cefotaxime, an aminoglycoside, or both may be used. Definitive therapy should be based on in vitro susceptibility studies of the pathogen.

- Duration of therapy is based on the patient's response; the usual duration of therapy in uncomplicated septicemia is 10 to 14 days, and in meningitis the minimum is 21 days.
- Data on the efficacy of granulocyte transfusions in septic, neutrophil-depleted neonates are limited and remain controversial; some experts recommend this therapy in neonates with bacteriologically proven Gram-negative sepsis and severe neutropenia.
- A therapeutic role for immunoglobulin therapy in septicemia or meningitis caused by *E coli* or other Gram-negative organisms has not been established, although its use may be warranted in very-low-birth-weight (less than 1,500 g) infants.

Isolation of the Hospitalized Patient: The infant with septicemia or meningitis caused by *E coli* or other enteric Gram-negative bacilli usually does not require isolation or special precautions. Exceptions include infants with *Salmonella* meningitis, for whom enteric precautions are indicated, and nursery outbreaks. In outbreaks, gowns should be used if soiling is likely, gloves are indicated if caretakers are handling feces, and cohorting of ill and colonized infants may be warranted. Contact isolation for infants with infection caused by multiply antibiotic-resistant Gram-negative bacilli, such as those resistant to the aminoglycosides (including amikacin) or to cefotaxime and ceftazidime, should also be considered.

Control Measures:
- The physician in charge of the nursery and infection control personnel should be aware of pathogens causing infections in all sick infants and the nature of infections in personnel, so that clusters of infections are recognized and appropriately investigated. They should be notified by other physicians in the community of serious infections in infants recently discharged from the nursery, as nursery-acquired infections can become apparent only several weeks to a month after discharge.
- Several cases of infection caused by the same genus and species of bacteria occurring in infants in close physical proximity or caused by an unusual pathogen can indicate an epidemic, in which case an epidemiologic investigation should be initiated. The decision to perform culture surveys of personnel or the environment to identify the source should be based on epidemiologic data.
- The routine performance of ongoing surveillance cultures of the environment or personnel, infants, or families is not recommended.
- An ongoing, in-service educational program for nursery personnel to review and reinforce concepts of infection control, especially hand washing between all patient contacts, is recommended.
- Periodic review of antimicrobial susceptibility patterns of clinically important bacterial isolates from newborns, especially those in the intensive care nursery, can provide useful epidemiologic and therapeutic information.

Escherichia coli **Diarrhea**

Clinical Manifestations: At least five different classes of diarrhea-producing *Escherichia coli* have been identified. Clinical features of disease caused by each class are summarized as follows (see also Table 3.4, p 188):

- Diarrhea caused by enteropathogenic *E coli* (EPEC) typically occurs in neonates and children younger than 2 years of age in developing countries, either sporadically or in epidemics. Illness is characterized by watery diarrhea that is often severe and can result in dehydration. Enteropathogenic *E coli* is an important cause of chronic diarrhea that can cause failure to thrive.
- Diarrhea caused by enterotoxigenic *E coli* (ETEC) is a self-limited illness of moderate severity with watery stools and abdominal cramps. It occurs in persons of all ages but is an important cause of diarrhea in infants in developing countries. Outbreaks have occurred in adults, usually from ingestion of contaminated food or water. Enterotoxigenic *E coli* is the major cause of travelers' diarrhea.
- Enteroinvasive *E coli* (EIEC) causes dysentery, similar to that caused by *Shigella*, characterized by fever, diarrhea, vomiting, crampy abdominal pain, and tenesmus. Stools often contain blood and leukocytes.
- Enterohemorrhagic *E coli* (EHEC) strains are associated with diarrhea, hemorrhagic colitis, hemolytic-uremic syndrome (HUS), and postdiarrheal thrombotic thrombocytopenic purpura. *Escherichia coli* 0157:H7 is the prototype for this class of organisms and is the only one for which extensive epidemiologic and clinical information is available. *Escherichia coli* 0157:H7 infections can occur sporadically or in outbreaks. The illness usually begins as nonbloody diarrhea and may progress to grossly bloody diarrhea. Fever occurs in one third of cases; severe abdominal pain is typical.
- The clinical manifestations of infection with enteroaggregative *E coli* (EAggEC) are not fully defined.

Etiology: Each class of *E coli* has a distinct group of somatic (O) and flagellar (H) antigens and has specific virulence characteristics that are usually plasmid-mediated. Microbiologic characteristics are as follows:

- The EPEC class is defined as specific *E coli* serotypes that have been epidemiologically incriminated as causes of infantile diarrhea and include the following somatic (O) serogroups: 044, 055, 086, 0111, 0114, 0119, 0125, 0126, 0127, 0128, 0142, and 0158. Most EPEC strains have been demonstrated to adhere to intestinal mucosa and produce a characteristic lesion in the gastrointestinal tract termed an attaching and effacing lesion. Enteropathogenic *E coli* do not produce enterotoxins and are not invasive.
- The ETEC strains produce either or both heat-labile and heat-stable enterotoxins.
- The EIEC strains include specific serotypes of *E coli* that are different from EPEC serotypes. The EIEC strains resemble *Shigella* biochemically and have the capacity to invade intestinal epithelial cells.
- Hemorrhagic colitis is caused by *E coli* 0157:H7 and, less frequently, by other serotypes of *E coli* that produce cytotoxins resembling those found in

TABLE 3.4—Classification of *Escherichia coli* Associated With Diarrhea

Types of *E coli*	Epidemiology	Type of Diarrhea	Mechanism of Action
Enteropathogenic	Acute and chronic endemic and epidemic diarrhea in infants	Watery	Adherence, effacement
Enterotoxigenic	Infantile diarrhea in developing countries and travelers' diarrhea	Watery	Adherence, enterotoxin production
Enteroinvasive	Diarrhea with fever in all ages	Bloody or nonbloody	Adherence, invasion of mucosa
Enterohemorrhagic	Hemorrhagic colitis and hemolytic uremic syndrome in all ages and thrombotic thrombocytopenic purpura in adults	Bloody or nonbloody	Cytotoxin production, adherence, effacement
Enteroaggregative	Incompletely defined	Watery	Adherence

Shigella dysenteriae, type 1. These toxins are referred to as Shiga-like toxins or verotoxins.

- Enteroaggregative *E coli* are defined by their adherence pattern in tissue-culture-based assays. Unlike EPEC, which demonstrates localized adherence, these strains exhibit aggregative adherence patterns in HE-2 or HeLa cells.

A sixth category of *E coli* that adhere diffusely to these cell lines needs further clarification.

Epidemiology: Transmission of most diarrhea-associated *E coli* strains is from infected symptomatic persons or carriers or from food or water contaminated with human or animal feces. *E coli* 0157:H7 has a bovine reservoir and is transmitted by undercooked meat and unpasteurized milk; it also spreads easily from person to person. Outbreaks from contaminated apple cider have been reported. Diarrhea caused by *E coli* strains other than 0157:H7 is common in areas of the world where food and water supplies are contaminated and facilities for hand washing are suboptimal. Three decades ago, nursery epidemics caused by EPEC strains were common in the United States; currently, epidemic diseases in newborn infants from these strains are uncommon. Enteropathogenic *E coli* and *E coli* 0157:H7 have caused outbreaks of diarrhea in child care settings. The role of enteroaggregative *E coli* as a cause of disease needs to be defined, although these *E coli* appear to be associated with persistent diarrhea in infants and young children. The period of communicability is for the duration of excretion of the specific pathogen.

The **incubation period** for most strains is from 10 hours to 6 days; for *E coli* 0157:H7 it is usually 3 to 4 days but can extend to 10 days.

Diagnostic Tests: Diagnosis of infection caused by diarrhea-associated *E coli* is a problem for clinicians. Except for *E coli* 0157:H7 and EIEC, in which case presumptive identification can be established, clinical laboratories cannot differentiate diarrhea-associated *E coli* from the normal *E coli* stool flora. Isolates suspected to be associated with diarrhea need to be sent to reference or research laboratories for definitive identification.

Stool specimens from all children with bloody diarrhea should be cultured for *E coli* 0157:H7. Clinical laboratories can screen for *E coli* 0157:H7 by using MacConkey agar base with sorbitol substituted for lactose. Most (approximately 90%) human intestinal *E coli* strains rapidly ferment sorbitol, whereas *E coli* 0157:H7 strains do not. These sorbitol-negative *E coli* can then be serotyped, using commercially available antisera to determine if they are 0157:H7.

Serotyping is recommended only for outbreaks when diarrhea-associated *E coli*, such as EPEC, is suspected; for identification of EHEC strains such as 0157:H7; and in epidemiologic studies. Probes are available in research laboratories for identification of strains in each class of diarrhea-associated *E coli*.

Suggested indications for EHEC confirmation include the following: bloody diarrhea, HUS, postdiarrheal thrombotic thrombocytopenic purpura, and any type of diarrhea in contacts of patients with HUS. Persons with presumptive diagnosis of intussusception, inflammatory bowel disease, and ischemic colitis are sometimes found to have disease caused by *E coli* 0157:H7. Methods for detection of EHEC that are used in reference or research laboratories include testing strains or stool specimens for shiga-like toxin and use of DNA probes, polymerase chain reaction assays, and enzyme immunoassay (EIA). Serologic diagnosis using an EIA to detect serum antibodies to *E coli* 0157:H7 lipopolysaccharide is available in reference laboratories.

Treatment: Dehydration and electrolyte abnormalities should be corrected. Orally administered solutions are usually adequate.* Antimotility agents should not be administered to children or adolescents with inflammatory or bloody diarrhea.

Antimicrobial Therapy. For infants with mild EPEC diarrhea, nonabsorbable antibiotics such as neomycin or gentamicin, given orally, in three to four divided doses for 5 days can be administered, although resistance can develop. These agents should not be used in infants with inflammatory or bloody diarrhea because of potential toxicity if absorbed. Trimethoprim-sulfamethoxazole should be considered if diarrhea is moderate to severe or intractable, and the organism is susceptible. If systemic infection is suspected, parenteral antimicrobial therapy should be given. For dysen-tery caused by EIEC strains and for chronic diarrhea caused by EPEC strains, antimicrobial agents such as trimethoprim-sulfamethoxazole can be given. Antimicrobial selection should be based on susceptibility of the isolates.

---

*For further information and detailed recommendations, see Duggan C, Santosham M, Glass RI. The management of acute diarrhea in children: oral rehydration, maintenance, and nutritional therapy. *MMWR*. 1992;41(RR-16):1-20.

The role of antimicrobial therapy in patients with hemorrhagic colitis caused by EHEC is uncertain. Antibiotic therapy does not appear to prevent progression to HUS.

Late Sequelae. Hemolytic-uremic syndrome is a sequela of enteric infection with shiga-like, toxin-producing *E coli* strains, such as *E coli* 0157:H7. This syndrome is defined by the triad of microangiopathic hemolytic anemia, thrombocytopenia, and acute renal dysfunction. Many children with hemorrhagic colitis caused by *E coli* 0157:H7 develop mild, self-limited, microangiopathic hematologic changes and/or nephropathy in the week after the onset of diarrhea. Close follow-up of patients with hemorrhagic colitis is recommended during this period to detect pallor, edema, or oliguria. The frequency of developing HUS as a complication of *E coli* 0157:H7 infection has been estimated to be 5% to 10%. Patients with HUS should be cultured for enteric pathogens, including *E coli* 0157:H7, and enteric precautions should be instituted to avoid nosocomial spread. The absence of EHEC in feces does not preclude the diagnosis of EHEC-associated HUS, since HUS is typically diagnosed a week after the onset of diarrhea when the organism no longer may be detectable in stool. Thrombotic thrombocytopenic purpura (TTP) is considered part of a spectrum often designated as TTP-HUS. This condition occurs in adults and may follow EHEC infection.

Isolation of the Hospitalized Patient: Enteric precautions are indicated for patients with all types of *E coli* diarrhea for the duration of illness. During outbreaks, enteric precautions for infants with diarrhea caused by EPEC strains should be maintained until cultures of stool taken after cessation of antimicrobial therapy are negative for the infecting strain. For patients with HUS, precautions should be continued until stool cultures are negative for *E coli* 0157:H7, or, if these tests are not available, for at least 10 days.

Control Measures:

Nursery and Other Institutional Outbreaks. Strict attention to hand washing techniques is essential in limiting spread. Exposed patients should be observed closely and their stools cultured for the causative organism. Unexposed patients should be separated from infants who have been exposed.

In a newborn nursery, management of EPEC infection is based on the number of cases. If a single case occurs, the infant should be isolated in a unit away from the nursery area. If multiple cases occur, the nursery room should be closed to admissions and not reopened until all infants in the room have been discharged and the room has been cleaned. Infants should be discharged home and not transferred to other infant wards. Personnel caring for infants in the closed nursery cohort should not have duties in other open nursery rooms. If epidemic disease involves more than one room in a nursery, the entire nursery should be closed and not reopened until a strict cohort system has been established in each room of the nursery for the duration of the epidemic. Admissions to a room should be limited to infants born in a 1- to 2-day period. The room should then be closed to admissions until all infants have been discharged and the room has been cleaned. Personnel should be cohorted with the infants.

Travelers' Diarrhea. This condition is a significant problem for persons traveling in developing countries. Travelers' diarrhea has been associated with many enteropathogens and is usually acquired by ingestion of contaminated food or water. Travelers should be advised to drink only boiled or carbonated water or carbonated beverages; they should avoid ice, salads, and fruit they have not peeled themselves. Foods should be eaten hot. Antimicrobial drugs are not recommended for prevention of travelers' diarrhea in children. Although several antimicrobial agents, such as trimethoprim-sulfamethoxazole, doxycycline, and ciprofloxacin, are effective prophylactically in decreasing the incidence of travelers' diarrhea, the benefit is usually outweighed by potential risks, including allergic drug reactions, infections induced by antimicrobial therapy (eg, antibiotic-associated colitis), and the selective pressure of wide-spread use of antimicrobial agents leading to antimicrobial resistance. Instead of prophylaxis, empiric treatment with an antimicrobial agent at the onset of symptoms is recommended; this approach is effective and can shorten the disease duration to 30 hours or less in most patients.

E coli 0157:H7 Infection. In a child care outbreak of *E coli* 0157:H7 diarrhea and HUS, immediate involvement of public health authorities is recommended. Ill children should not be permitted to reenter the classroom until diarrhea has stopped and a stool culture is negative for *E coli* 0157:H7. Strict attention to hand washing and hygiene is important but may not be sufficient to prevent continued transmission. The center should be closed to new admissions and particular care should be exercised to prevent transfer of children to other child care centers. Most *E coli* 0157:H7 infections are likely to be caused by eating contaminated ground beef. Ground beef should be thoroughly cooked until no pink meat remains. Raw milk should not be ingested. Rapid reporting of cases of *E coli* 0157:H7 infection to public health authorities can lead to action to prevent further disease.

Filariasis
(Bancroftian, Malayan, and Timorian)

Clinical Manifestations: Most filarial infections cause no symptoms. Symptoms are caused either by acute inflammation or, most commonly, by inflammation and obstruction of the lymphatic channels where the adult worms develop. In the former, patients develop fever, headache, myalgia, and lymphadenitis. In lymphatic disease, manifestations usually occur 3 months to 1 year after acquisition. Occasionally, moderate lymphadenopathy, particularly involving the inguinal lymph nodes, occurs. Inflammation of the lymphatics of the extremities and genitalia leads to retrograde lymphangitis, epididymitis, orchitis, and funiculitis. Fever, chills, and other nonspecific systemic symptoms also occur. Death of adult worms can result in localized abscesses. Obstructive lymphatic disease with resulting chronically progressive edema of the limbs and genitalia is relatively infrequent in children. In a few individuals, elephantiasis can result from fibrosis caused by chronic obstruction of the lymphatic channels. Chyluria can occur as a manifestation of Bancroftian filariasis.

Patients with the tropical pulmonary eosinophilia syndrome present with cough, fever, marked eosinophilia, and high serum IgE concentrations.

Etiology: Filariasis is caused by the following three filarial nematodes: *Wuchereria bancrofti*, *Brugia malayi*, and *Brugia timori*.

Epidemiology: The disease is transmitted by the bite of infected species of various genera of mosquitoes, including *Culex*, *Aedes*, *Anopheles*, and *Mansonia*. *Wuchereria bancrofti* is found in many scattered areas of the Caribbean, Venezuela, Columbia, the Guianas, Brazil, Central America, sub-Saharan Africa, North Africa, Turkey, and Asia, extending into a broad zone from Saudi Arabia through the Indonesian archipelago into Southern China and Oceania. *Brugia malayi* is found mostly in India, Southeast Asia, and the Far East. *Brugia timori* is restricted to certain islands at the eastern end of the Indonesian archipelago. Microfilariae infective for mosquitoes are in the patient's blood for as long as 1.5 years after the death of the adult worms and several years after the original infection. The infection is not transmissible from person to person or by blood transfusion.

The **incubation period** is not well established; the period from acquisition to the appearance of microfilariae in blood can be 2 to 12 months, depending on the nematode.

Diagnostic Tests: Microfilariae can be detected microscopically, either on routine blood smears obtained at night (10 pm to 2 am) after concentration of blood preserved in formalin or by membrane filtration. Adult worms can be identified in tissue specimens obtained at biopsy. Serologic enzyme immunoassay tests are available, but interpretation of results is affected by cross-reactions of filarial antibodies with those against other helminths. Lymphatic filariasis must often be diagnosed clinically because dependable serologic assays are not available and in elephantiasis the microfilariae may no longer be present. Eosinophilia of 25% frequently occurs in the early, inflammatory phase of the disease.

Treatment: Diethylcarbamazine citrate* is the drug of choice. Because allergic reactions caused by disintegrating worms occur in heavy infections, beginning treatment with low doses for the first 4 to 5 days may be advantageous. Some experts advise pretreatment with antihistamines or corticosteroids. The late obstructive phase of the disease is not affected by chemotherapy. Ivermectin, an investigational drug in the United States, is effective against the microfilariae and may become the drug of choice for most filarial infections. It is currently available primarily for patients unable to tolerate diethylcarbamazine and may be obtained through the Drug Service of the Centers for Disease Control and Prevention (see Directory of Telephone Numbers, p 601). Resection of the severely enlarged tissues, particularly plastic surgical repair of the genitalia, gives variable results. Chyluria originating in the bladder responds to fulguration; chyluria originating in the

---

*Available from Lederle, Pearl River, NY.

kidney cannot be corrected. Prompt identification and treatment of superinfections, particularly streptococcal and staphylococcal infections, are important aspects of therapy.

Isolation of the Hospitalized Patient: No special precautions are recommended.

Control Measures: The mosquito population should be controlled. Treatment of those with asymptomatic infection, ie, carriers or an entire community if a substantial percentage are infected, should be considered.

Giardia lamblia Infections (Giardiasis)

Clinical Manifestations: *Giardia* infections have a broad spectrum of manifestations. Patients with clinical illness may develop acute watery diarrhea with abdominal pain, or they may experience a protracted, intermittent, often debilitating disease, which is characterized by passage of foul-smelling diarrheal or soft stools associated with flatulence, abdominal distention, and anorexia. Anorexia combined with malabsorption can lead to significant weight loss, failure to thrive, and anemia.

Etiology: *Giardia lamblia* is a flagellate protozoan that exists in trophozoite and cyst forms; the infective form is the cyst. Infection is limited to the small intestine and/or biliary tract.

Epidemiology: Giardiasis has a worldwide distribution. Humans are the principal reservoir of infection, but *Giardia* organisms can infect dogs, cats, beavers, and other animals. These animals can contaminate water with feces containing cysts that are infectious for humans. Persons become infected either directly (by hand-to-mouth transfer of cysts from feces of an infected individual) or indirectly (by ingestion of fecally contaminated water or food). Most community-wide epidemics result from contaminated water supplies. Epidemics resulting from person-to-person transmission occur in child care centers, especially those that care for children who are not toilet trained, and in institutions for mentally retarded persons. Staff and family members in contact with these individuals occasionally become infected. *Giardia* transmission has also been documented among male homosexuals. Humoral immunodeficiencies predispose to chronic symptomatic *Giardia* infections. Patients with cystic fibrosis have an increased frequency of giardiasis. Surveys conducted in the United States have demonstrated prevalence rates of *Giardia* in stool specimens that range from 1% to 20%, depending on geographic location and age. Infection is frequently asymptomatic. Duration of cyst excretion is variable and may persist for months. The disease is communicable as long as the infected person excretes cysts.

The **incubation period** is usually 1 to 4 weeks.

Diagnostic Tests: Identification of either trophozoites or cysts on direct smear examination of stool specimens or duodenal fluid, or detection of *Giardia* antigens in these specimens by enzyme immunoassay (EIA) is diagnostic. A single stool microscopic examination detects 50% to 75% of infections; sensitivity is increased to approximately 95% by testing three specimens. Examination of duodenal contents obtained by direct aspiration or by using a commercially available string test (Enterotest*) is a more sensitive procedure than a single stool examination. Rarely, biopsy of the small intestine is used. To enhance detection, microscopic examination of stool specimens or duodenal fluid should be performed soon after they are obtained, or stool should be mixed, placed in fixative, concentrated, and examined by both wet mount and permanent stain. Commercially available stool collection kits containing a vial of 10% formalin and a vial of polyvinyl alcohol fixative in childproof containers are convenient for preserving specimens collected at home. Enzyme immunoassay techniques for detection of *G lamblia* antigens in stool specimens are commercially available and have greater sensitivity than microscopy.

Treatment: Quinacrine hydrochloride is the most effective drug for treatment of symptomatic infections; cure rates range from 85% to 95%. However, compliance and, consequently, cure rates may be lower in children because of the bitter taste of quinacrine. Furazolidone is 80% effective, but since it is the only drug available in liquid suspension, it is more acceptable to children. Metronidazole is an alternative drug that is 90% effective in adults, but its safety and effectiveness for children with giardiasis have not been established. If therapy fails, a course of any of these drugs can be repeated. Paromomycin, a nonabsorbable aminoglycoside that is 50% to 70% effective, is recommended for treatment of symptomatic infection in pregnant women. Relapse is common in immunocompromised patients and may require continuous therapy for long periods of time.

Treatment of asymptomatic carriers is not recommended except possibly for prevention of household transmission by toddlers to pregnant women and in patients with hypogammaglobulinemia or cystic fibrosis.

Isolation of the Hospitalized Patient: Enteric precautions for the duration of illness are recommended.

Control Measures:
- In child care centers improved sanitation and personal hygiene should be emphasized (see also Children in Out-of-Home Child Care, p 80). Hand washing by staff and children should be stressed, especially after using the toilet or handling soiled diapers. When an outbreak is suspected, an epidemiologic investigation should be undertaken to identify and treat all symptomatic children, child care workers, and family members infected with *Giardia*. Persons with diarrhea should be excluded from the child care center until they become asymptomatic. Treatment of asymptomatic carriers

---

*Available from Hedeco, Palo Alto, CA.

has not been demonstrated to be effective in outbreak control. Exclusion of carriers from child care is not recommended.

- Prevention of waterborne outbreaks requires adequate filtration of municipal water obtained from surface water sources since concentrations of chlorine used to disinfect drinking water are not effective against cysts.
- Backpackers, campers, and persons likely to be exposed to contaminated water should avoid drinking directly from streams. Boiling of water will eliminate the infective cysts.

Gonococcal Infections

Clinical Manifestations: Gonococcal infections in children occur in three distinct age groups.

- Infection in the **newborn infant** usually involves the eye. Other types of involvement include scalp abscess (which can complicate fetal monitoring), vaginitis, and systemic disease with bacteremia, arthritis, meningitis, or endocarditis.
- In **prepubertal children** beyond the newborn period, gonococcal infection usually occurs in the genital tract. Vaginitis is the most common manifestation; pelvic inflammatory disease (PID) and perihepatitis can occur but are uncommon, as is gonococcal urethritis in the prepubertal male. Anorectal and tonsillopharyngeal colonization can also occur in prepubertal children.
- In **sexually active adolescents**, as in adults, gonococcal infection of the genital tract in females is most frequently asymptomatic or manifest by urethritis, endocervicitis, and PID. In adolescent males, the infection is often symptomatic, and the primary site is the urethra. Asymptomatic infection of the urethra, endocervix, rectum, and pharynx can occur. Extension from primary genital mucosal sites results in epididymitis, bartholinitis, PID, and perihepatitis. Even asymptomatic infection can progress to PID with tubal scarring that can result in ectopic pregnancy or infertility. Infection involving other mucous membranes can produce conjunctivitis, pharyngitis, or proctitis. Hematogenous spread can involve skin and joints (arthritis-dermatitis syndrome); meningitis and endocarditis occur rarely.

Etiology: *Neisseria gonorrhoeae* organisms are Gram-negative diplococci.

Epidemiology: *Neisseria gonorrhoeae* infections occur only in humans. The source of the organism is exudate and secretions of infected mucous surfaces. Transmission results from intimate contact, such as sexual acts, parturition, and, very rarely, household exposure in prepubertal children. Sexual abuse should be strongly considered when genital, rectal, or oral infections are diagnosed in children beyond the newborn period and before puberty, and in non-sexually-active adolescents. Approximately 1,000,000 new cases of gonococcal infection are reported annually in the United States. Young men, 20 to 24 years of age, have the highest reported incidence of infection, followed by those 15 to 19 years of age. In females, the highest rates are in adolescents 15 to 19 years old. Concurrent infection with *Chlamydia trachomatis* is very common. *Neisseria gonorrhoeae* is communicable as long as an individual harbors the organism.

The **incubation period** is usually 2 to 7 days.

Diagnostic Tests: Microscopic examinations of Gram-stained smears of exudate from the eyes, the endocervix of postpubertal females, the vagina of prepubertal girls, male urethra, skin lesions, synovial fluid, and, when clinically warranted, cerebrospinal fluid are useful in the initial evaluation. These smears occasionally contain Gram-negative intracellular diplococci; this finding is particularly helpful when the organism is not recovered in culture. Gram stains of material obtained from the endocervix of pubertal and postpubertal females are less sensitive than culture in the detection of infection, but they can be of immediate help in the differential diagnosis of a patient with an acute abdomen or when immediate therapy is indicated. Other *Neisseria* species and Gram-negative cocci may be present in the female genital tract, but these organisms are seldom observed on smear within polymorphonuclear leukocytes. In prepubertal girls, vaginal specimens are adequate for diagnosis, and endocervical specimens are unnecessary.

Culture from normally sterile sites, such as blood, cerebrospinal fluid, or synovial fluid, can be accomplished on nonselective chocolate agar with incubation in 5% to 10% CO_2. Selective *N gonorrhoeae* culture media, such as Thayer-Martin (chocolate agar supplemented with antibiotics), inhibit most normal flora and nonpathogenic *Neisseria* found on mucosal surfaces. These selective media are used for culture from nonsterile sites, such as the cervix, vagina, rectum, urethra, and pharynx. Specimens for *N gonorrhoeae* culture from mucosal sites should be inoculated immediately onto the selective medium before transport to the laboratory because *N gonorrhoeae* is extremely sensitive to drying and temperature changes. Transport systems containing selective medium are available commercially; these allow satisfactory shipment of inoculated media if they have been preincubated for 24 hours.

Sexual Abuse. In all prepubertal children beyond the newborn period and in nonsexually-active adolescents who have gonococcal infection, sexual abuse must be considered. Genital, rectal, and pharyngeal cultures should be obtained from all patients before antibiotic treatment and gonococcal isolates should be preserved. Nonculture gonococcal tests, including Gram stain, DNA probes, or enzyme immunoassay tests of oropharyngeal, rectal, or genital tract specimens in children are not appropriate for diagnosis. Caution should be exercised in interpreting the significance of the isolation of *Neisseria* organisms, as *N gonorrhoeae* can be confused with other *Neisseria* species. At least two confirmatory bacteriologic tests involving different principles, eg, biochemical, enzyme substrate or serology, should be performed. Culture results of *N gonorrhoeae* from the pharynx of young children necessitate particular caution because of the high carriage rate of nonpathogenic *Neisseria* species. Appropriate cultures should be obtained from persons who have had contact with the abused child. Children in whom sexual abuse is suspected should undergo tests for other sexually transmitted diseases, such as *Chlamydia* infection, syphilis, and HIV (for further information, see Sexual Abuse, p 107).

Treatment: Because of the increased prevalence of penicillin-resistant *N gonorrhoeae*, an extended spectrum (third-generation) cephalosporin, such as ceftriaxone, is now recommended as initial therapy for persons of all ages. High-level resistance to tetracycline is becoming more common. Resistance to spectinomycin is still rare.

Only parenteral cephalosporins are recommended for use in young children; ceftriaxone is approved for all gonococcal indications in children, and cefotaxime for gonococcal ophthalmia only. Oral cephalosporins (cefixime, cefuroxime, and cefpodoxime) have not received adequate evaluation in the treatment of gonococcal infections in children to recommend their use. The pharmacokinetic activity of these drugs in adults cannot be extrapolated to children. Nonetheless, in unusual circumstances, oral therapy can be considered for uncomplicated gonococcal infections in children. Data from adults suggest that cefixime (8 mg/kg in a single oral dose, maximum 400 mg) and an appropriate antimicrobial for *Chlamydia* may prove to be an acceptable, oral alternative regimen, provided follow-up, including test of cure cultures, can be ensured.

All patients with presumed or proven gonorrhea should be evaluated for concurrent syphilis and *Chlamydia* infection. Patients beyond the neonatal period should be treated presumptively for this infection (see *Chlamydia trachomatis*, p 156), particularly if testing for *Chlamydia* is not available.

Patients with uncomplicated gonorrhea who are asymptomatic after treatment with one of the recommended antibiotic regimens need not be cultured for a test of cure.

Specific recommendations for management and antimicrobial therapy are as follows:

Neonatal Disease. Infants with clinical evidence of ophthalmia, scalp abscess, or disseminated infections should be hospitalized. Appropriate cultures should be obtained from the mother. Cultures of blood, cerebrospinal fluid, and eye discharge should be obtained from the infant to confirm the diagnosis and determine antimicrobial susceptibility. Tests for concomitant infection with *C trachomatis* should also be done.

Nondisseminated infections: Recommended antimicrobial therapy, including for ophthalmia neonatorum caused by *N gonorrhoeae*, is ceftriaxone (25 to 50 mg/kg/d, intravenously or intramuscularly, not to exceed 125 mg) given once. Ceftriaxone is not routinely indicated in hyperbilirubinemic infants, especially premature infants. Cefotaxime (50 to 100 mg/kg/d, given intravenously or intramuscularly in two divided doses) for 7 days is an alternative.

Infants with gonococcal ophthalmia should have their eyes irrigated with saline immediately and at frequent intervals until the discharge is eliminated. Topical antibiotic treatment alone is inadequate, and it is unnecessary when recommended systemic antibiotic treatment is given.

Disseminated infections: Ceftriaxone (25 to 50 mg/kg, intravenously or intramuscularly, given once daily) for 10 to 14 days, or cefotaxime (50 to 100 mg/kg/d, given intravenously or intramuscularly, in two divided doses) for 10 to 14 days, is recommended, including for meningitis, arthritis, and septicemia.

Since most neonates with gonorrhea acquire the organism from their mothers, both the mother and her sexual partner(s) should be evaluated and treated appropriately.

Gonococcal Infections in Children Beyond the Neonatal Period and in Adolescents. Recommendations for treatment of gonococcal infections, by age and weight, are given in Tables 3.5 and 3.6 (pp 199 and 200).

Two newer antimicrobials that have been demonstrated to be effective for treating gonococcal urethritis and cervicitis in adults and older adolescents are cefixime (400 or 800 mg, orally, in a single dose) and ofloxacin (400 mg, orally, in a single dose). Data to support the use of these newer agents to treat gonorrhea in young children are not available. Quinolones are not approved by the Food and Drug Administration for use in persons younger than 18 years of age or in pregnant or nursing women.

Presumptive Treatment for Chlamydia Infection. Children 9 years or older with uncomplicated gonococcal endocervical, urethral, or rectal infection should also be treated for presumptive *Chlamydia* infection with oral doxycycline (200 mg/d in two divided doses) for 7 days or oral azithromycin (1 g), given as a single dose. Tetracycline (2.0 g/d in four divided doses) can be substituted for doxycycline and should be given between meals. Compliance, however, may be poorer because each dose must be taken four times daily and between meals. Children younger than 9 years and pregnant women should also be treated but not with a tetracycline drug; erythromycin is recommended (40 mg/kg/d in four divided doses) for 7 days. Patients should also be evaluated for coinfection with syphilis.

Approximately one half of recurrent infections after treatment with the recommended schedules are caused by reinfection and indicate the need for improved contact tracing and patient education.

Special Problems in Treatment of Children (Beyond the Neonatal Period) and Adolescents.

- Patients with uncomplicated endocervical infection, urethritis, or proctitis, who are allergic to cephalosporins, should be treated with spectinomycin (40 mg/kg, maximum 2 g, given intramuscularly). In patients in whom doxycycline, tetracycline, and azithromycin are contraindicated or not tolerated, erythromycin base or stearate (2 g/d, orally, in four divided doses for adults) or erythromycin ethyl succinate (2.4 g/d, orally, in three divided doses for adults) can be substituted for the concurrent treatment of presumptive *Chlamydia* infection.
- Patients with uncomplicated pharyngeal gonococcal infection should be treated with ceftriaxone (125 mg, intramuscularly) in a single dose.
- Patients who are incubating syphilis (seronegative, without clinical signs) may be cured by regimens that include ceftriaxone, or a 7-day course of either doxycycline for those 9 years of age and older, or erythromycin, but few data are available. Quinolones are not active against *Treponema pallidum*. All patients who are treated for gonorrhea should undergo serologic testing for syphilis at the initial visit and 6 to 8 weeks later.

Acute Pelvic Inflammatory Disease (PID). *Neisseria gonorrhoeae* and *C trachomatis* are implicated in most cases, and many cases have a polymicrobial etiology. No reliable clinical criteria distinguish gonococcal from nongonococcal PID. Hence, broad-spectrum treatment regimens are recommended (see Pelvic Inflammatory Disease, p 353).

Acute Epididymitis. Sexually transmitted organisms, such as *N gonorrhoeae* or *C trachomatis*, can cause acute epididymitis in sexually active adoles-

TABLE 3.5—Uncomplicated Gonococcal Infection: Treatment in Children Beyond the Newborn Period and in Adolescents. Recommended Antimicrobial Regimens Include Therapy for Presumed Concomitant Infection With *Chlamydia trachomatis*

Disease	Prepubertal Children Who Weigh <100 lb (45 kg)	Disease	Patients Who Weigh ≥100 lb (45 kg) and Are 9 Years or Older
Uncomplicated vulvovaginitis, urethritis, proctitis, or pharyngitis[a]	Ceftriaxone, 125 mg, IM,[b] in a single dose OR Spectinomycin[c] 40 mg/kg (max 2 g), IM, in a single dose PLUS Erythromycin[d] 40 mg/kg/d in divided doses for 7 d	Uncomplicated endocervicitis or urethritis	Ceftriaxone, 125 mg, IM,[b] in a single dose OR Ciprofloxacin,[e] 500 mg, orally, in a single dose OR Cefixime, 400 mg, orally, in a single dose OR Ofloxacin,[e] 400 mg, orally, in a single dose OR Spectinomycin,[c] 2 g, IM, in a single dose PLUS Doxycycline, 100 mg, orally, twice daily for 7 d[f] OR Azithromycin, 1 g, orally, in a single dose

[a] Hospitalization should be considered, especially for patients who have been treated as outpatients and have failed to respond, and for those who are unlikely to adhere to treatment regimens.
[b] Some clinicians believe the discomfort of an IM injection can be reduced by using 1% lidocaine as a diluent.
[c] Spectinomycin is not recommended for treatment of pharyngeal infections; in persons who cannot take a cephalosporin, a quinolone, or spectinomycin, a 5-day oral regimen of trimethoprim-sulfamethoxazole may be given.
[d] Doxycycline can be given instead of erythromycin if the child is 9 y or older.
[e] Quinolones are contraindicated for persons younger than 18 y, pregnant women, and nursing women.
[f] Tetracycline, 500 mg, 4 times daily, can be substituted for doxycycline.

TABLE 3.6—Complicated Gonococcal Infection: Treatment for Children Beyond the Newborn Period and for Adolescents[a]

Disease[b]	Prepubertal Children Who Weigh <100 lb (45 kg)	Disease	Patients Who Weigh ≥100 lb (45 kg) and Are 9 Years or Older
Ophthalmia, peritonitis, bacteremia, or arthritis	Ceftriaxone, 50 mg/kg/d (max 1 g/d), IV or IM,[c] once daily for 7 d	Gonococcal pharyngitis	Ceftriaxone 125 mg, IM,[c] in a single dose
Meningitis or endocarditis	Ceftriaxone, 50 mg/kg/d (max 2 g/d), IV or IM,[c] once or twice daily: for meningitis, duration is 10-14 d; for endocarditis, duration is at least 28 d	Pelvic inflammatory disease	See Table 3.35 (p 354)
		Disseminated gonococcal infections[d,e]	Ceftriaxone, 1 g/d, IV or IM, given once daily for 7 d[f] OR Cefotaxime, 1 g, IV, given three times daily for 7 d[f] OR Spectinomycin, 2 g, IM, every 12 h for 7 d[f] for persons allergic to β-lactam drugs
		Meningitis or endocarditis[b]	Ceftriaxone, 1-2 g, IV, given twice daily: for meningitis, duration is 10-14 d; for endocarditis, duration is at least 28 d

[a]In all cases, in addition to the recommended treatment for gonococcal infection, **doxycycline (100 mg, orally, twice daily for 7 d), tetracycline (500 mg, 4 times daily for 7 d), or azithromycin (1 g, orally, in a single dose) is recommended on the presumption that the patient has concomitant infection with *Chlamydia trachomatis*; for children younger than 9 years and pregnant women, erythromycin is recommended (see p 198).**

[b]Hospitalization is required; follow-up cultures are necessary to ensure that treatment has been effective.

[c]Some clinicians believe the discomfort of IM injection can be reduced by using 1% lidocaine as a diluent.

[d]Such as the arthritis-dermatitis syndrome.

[e]Spectinomycin is not recommended for treatment of pharyngeal gonococcal infection. For patients who cannot take a cephalosporin, spectinomycin, or a quinolone, a 5-day oral regimen of trimethoprim-sulfamethoxazole may be given.

[f]Alternatively, parenteral therapy can be discontinued 24 to 48 h after improvement begins and a 7-d course is completed with an appropriate oral antimicrobial. Some experts advise a 10- to 14-d course of therapy.

cents and young adults. (Its pathogenesis can also be related to infection in the urinary tract, usually caused by Enterobacteriaceae or *Pseudomonas. Haemophilus influenzae* type b and meningococci are rare causes in infants and young children.)

The recommended regimen is a single dose of ceftriaxone (250 mg, intramuscularly) **plus** azithromycin (1 g orally) in a single dose, or doxycycline (200 mg/d, orally, in two divided doses) for 7 days; tetracycline (2 g/d, orally, in four divided doses) for 7 days is an acceptable alternative. Children younger than 9 years should receive a single dose of ceftriaxone (250 mg, intramuscularly) **plus** erythromycin (50 mg/kg/d, maximum 2 g, orally, in four divided doses).

Isolation of the Hospitalized Patient: All newborn infants (including those with ophthalmia) and prepubertal children with gonococcal infections should be managed with contact isolation precautions until effective parenteral antimicrobial therapy has been administered for 24 hours. Special precautions are not indicated for other patients with gonococcal infection.

Control Measures:

Neonatal Ophthalmia. For routine prophylaxis of infants immediately after birth, a 1% solution of silver nitrate, 1% tetracycline, or 0.5% erythromycin ophthalmic ointment is instilled into each eye; subsequent irrigation should not be performed (see Prevention of Neonatal Ophthalmia, p 533). Prophylaxis may be delayed for as long as 1 hour after birth to facilitate maternal-infant bonding.

These prophylactic regimens are ineffective for prevention of chlamydial eye disease.

Infants Born to Mothers With Gonococcal Infections. When prophylaxis is correctly administered, infants born to mothers with gonococcal infection infrequently develop gonococcal ophthalmia. However, an occasional case of gonococcal ophthalmia or disseminated gonococcal infection can occur in infants born to mothers with gonococcal disease at parturition. Hence, infants born to mothers with active gonorrhea should receive a single dose of ceftriaxone, 125 mg, intravenously or intramuscularly; for low-birth-weight infants, the dose is 25 to 50 mg/kg.

Children and Adolescents With Sexual Exposure to a Patient Known to Have Gonorrhea. Patients should be examined, cultured, and treated the same as those known to have gonorrhea.

Education. **Effective sustained educational efforts are necessary** to control sexually transmitted diseases among adolescents (see Sexually Transmitted Diseases, p 103).

Other Infections. Patients with gonococcal infection should be evaluated for other sexually transmitted diseases, specifically *Chlamydia*, syphilis, and HIV. Hepatitis B vaccination is indicated (see Hepatitis B, p 230).

Pregnancy. All pregnant females should have an endocervical culture for gonococci as an integral part of the prenatal care at the first visit. A second culture late in the third trimester should be done for women at high risk of exposure to gonococcal infection. Recommended therapeutic regimens for patients found to be infected are those previously described for uncomplicated gonorrhea, except that a tetracycline should not be used because of the potential toxic effects on the fetus. Women who are allergic to penicillin or probenecid should be treated with spectinomycin.

Case Reporting. All cases of gonorrhea must be reported. Cases in prepubertal children must be investigated to determine the source of infection. Ensuring that sexual contacts are treated and counseled is essential for community control, prevention of reinfection, and prevention of complications in the contact.

Granuloma inguinale (Donovanosis)

Clinical Manifestations: Initial lesions are single or multiple subcutaneous nodules that progress to cutaneous ulceration and granuloma(s). Lesions usually involve the genitalia; anal lesions occur in 5% to 10% of the patients, and lesions at distant sites are rare. Extension into the inguinal area results in subcutaneous induration that mimics inguinal adenopathy—the pseudobubo of granuloma inguinale. Fibrosis manifests as sinus tracts, adhesions, and lymphedema, resulting in extreme genital deformity.

Etiology: The disease is caused by *Calymmatobacterium granulomatis*, a Gram-negative bacillus.

Epidemiology: Granuloma inguinale is extremely rare in the United States and most developed countries, but it is common in New Guinea and parts of India, Africa, and the Caribbean. The highest incidence of disease occurs in tropical and subtropical environments. Studies suggest a strong correlation between the incidence of infection and sustained high temperatures and high relative humidity. The source of infection is persons with active infection, possibly including those with asymptomatic rectal infection. Transmission is usually by sexual intercourse. Infection is only mildly contagious and repeated exposure may be necessary for the development of disease. Young children can acquire infection by contact with infected secretions. The period of communicability extends throughout the duration of active lesions or rectal colonization.

The **incubation period** is 8 to 80 days.

Diagnostic Tests: The microscopic demonstration of Donovan bodies on Wright's or Giemsa's stain of a crush preparation from a lesion is diagnostic. The microorganism can also be detected by histologic procedures on biopsy specimens. Lesions should be cultured for *Haemophilus ducreyi* to exclude pseudogranuloma inguinale (chancroid). Granuloma inguinale is frequently misdiagnosed as carcinoma, which can be excluded by histologic examination of the tissue or by the response of the lesion to antibiotics.

Treatment: Tetracycline (which ordinarily should not be given to children younger than 9 years of age) and trimethoprim-sulfamethoxazole have been reported to be effective. Gentamicin and chloramphenicol are reserved for resistant cases. Erythromycin has been used in pregnant patients. Antimicrobial therapy is continued for at least 3 weeks or until the lesions have resolved. If antimicrobial therapy is effective, some healing is usually noted within 7 days. Patients should be evaluated for concomitant infection with other sexually transmitted diseases, such as gonorrhea, syphilis, and *Chlamydia trachomatis* infection.

Isolation of the Hospitalized Patient: No special precautions are recommended.

Control Measures: Sexual partners should be examined, counseled to use condoms, and probably given prophylactic antimicrobial therapy.

Haemophilus influenzae Infections

Clinical Manifestations: In infants and young children, *Haemophilus influenzae* can cause meningitis, otitis media, sinusitis, epiglottitis, septic arthritis, occult febrile bacteremia, cellulitis, pneumonia, and empyema; occasionally this organism causes neonatal meningitis and septicemia. Other *H influenzae* infections include purulent pericarditis, endocarditis, conjunctivitis, osteomyelitis, peritonitis, epididymo-orchitis, glossitis, uvulitis, and septic thrombophlebitis.

Etiology: *Haemophilus influenzae* organisms are small, pleomorphic, Gram-negative coccobacilli, consisting of six antigenically distinct capsular types (a to f) as well as nonencapsulated, nontypable strains. Invasive diseases in infants and children are caused by encapsulated strains, nearly always type b. An exception is neonatal septicemia, which can be caused by nonencapsulated organisms. Nontypable strains are frequent constituents of the normal upper respiratory tract flora. These organisms can cause local respiratory tract disease, including otitis media, sinusitis, and bronchitis.

Epidemiology: The source of the organism is the upper respiratory tract of humans. The mode of transmission is presumably person to person, by direct contact, or through inhalation of droplets of respiratory tract secretions containing the organism. Asymptomatic colonization by nonencapsulated strains is frequent; organisms are recovered from the throat of 60% to 90% of children. Colonization by type b organisms, however, is usually infrequent, ranging from 2% to 5% of children, and has been reported to be even lower since the introduction of conjugate vaccination. The exact period of communicability is unknown but may be for as long as the organism is present in the upper respiratory tract.

The incidence of invasive disease caused by *H influenzae* type b has declined dramatically since introduction of conjugate vaccination in the United States. Disease is most common in children 3 months to 3 years of age. Before introduction of vaccination, about half the cases in this country occurred in infants younger than 12 months. However, the age-specific incidence of disease varies in different populations and countries. The proportion of disease in infants younger than 12 months tends to be greatest in populations with the highest total incidence, resulting in lower median age of cases. In contrast to meningitis and most other invasive *H influenzae* type b disease, epiglottitis is rare in infants younger than 12 months, has a peak occurrence at 2 to 4 years of age, and appears to be relatively more common in populations with the lowest total incidence of *H influenzae* type b diseases. *Haemophilus influenzae* type b disease has been more frequent in boys, urban dwellers, blacks, Alaskan Eskimos, Apache and Navajo Indians, and child care center attendees. Unvaccinated children, particularly those younger than 4 years of age who are in prolonged, close contact (such as in a household) with a child who has developed invasive disease caused by *H influenzae* type b, are at increased risk for serious infection from this organism. Other factors predisposing to invasive *H influenzae* type b disease include sickle-cell disease, asplenia, certain immunodeficiency syndromes including HIV infection, and malignancies. Infants younger than 1 year who have not been vaccinated and who have had episodes of documented invasive infection are at an approximate 1% risk for recurrence.

The **incubation period** is unknown and probably is widely variable.

Diagnostic Tests: Cerebrospinal fluid (CSF), blood, synovial fluid, pleural fluid, and middle ear aspirates should be cultured on a medium such as chocolate agar, enriched with X and V co-factors. A Gram stain of an infected body fluid can disclose the organism and allows a presumptive diagnosis to be made. Latex particle agglutination for detection of capsular antigen in CSF or serum can aid in rapid diagnosis and can be helpful to patients in whom antimicrobial therapy was initiated before culture. However, detection of antigen in urine can be unreliable for diagnosis since antigenuria can result from asymptomatic nasopharyngeal carriage of *H influenzae* type b, recent vaccination with *H influenzae* conjugate vaccine, or contamination of urine specimens by cross-reacting fecal organisms. Antimicrobial susceptibility testing should be performed on all clinically important isolates.

Treatment:
- Initial therapy for children with meningitis possibly caused by *H influenzae* type b can be cefotaxime, ceftriaxone, or ampicillin in combination with chloramphenicol. Ampicillin alone should not be used as initial therapy since, depending on the locality, 12% to 40% of *H influenzae* isolates (type b and nontypable strains) produce beta-lactamase and, therefore, are resistant to ampicillin. Chloramphenicol resistance is also common in some countries but, as of December 1993, has rarely been reported in the United States. Isolates resistant to both ampicillin and chloramphenicol are also rare in the United States.
- For patients with uncomplicated meningitis who respond rapidly, therapy for 7 to 10 days with an appropriate antimicrobial agent (ie, to which the organism is susceptible by in vitro testing), administered intravenously in a high dose, is usually satisfactory. In selected cases, oral therapy with chloramphenicol may be used, particularly if monitoring of serum concen-

trations of drug can be readily performed. Therapy for more than 10 days may be indicated in complicated cases of meningitis caused by *H influenzae* type b.

- For treatment of other invasive *H influenzae* infections, recommendations are similar but are primarily based on empiric experience.
- Chloramphenicol pharmacokinetics are unpredictable. Moreover, concurrent treatment with certain drugs such as phenobarbital, phenytoin, carbamazepine, and rifampin can alter chloramphenicol metabolism. Conversely, chloramphenicol can interfere with the metabolism of drugs such as phenytoin, tolbutamide, and dicumarol. Hence, if testing is available, serum chloramphenicol concentrations should be monitored in patients receiving chloramphenicol.
- Dexamethasone therapy is recommended for infants and children 2 months and older with *H influenzae* type b meningitis (see Dexamethasone Therapy for Bacterial Meningitis in Infants and Children, p 558).
- **Epiglottitis is a medical emergency. An airway must be established promptly by endotracheal tube or tracheostomy.**
- Infected synovial, pleural, or pericardial fluid should be drained.
- For otitis media, many experts recommend oral treatment with amoxicillin for initial therapy. Effective alternative drugs, especially for ampicillin-resistant strains of *H influenzae*, include trimethoprim-sulfamethoxazole, erythromycin-sulfisoxazole, amoxicillin-clavulanic acid, cefaclor, cefixime, cefuroxime axetil, and other extended spectrum oral cephalosporins and related drugs that have Food and Drug Administration (FDA) approval for the treatment of otitis media.

Isolation of the Hospitalized Patient: Respiratory isolation for 24 hours after initiation of effective antimicrobial therapy is indicated.

Control Measures (for invasive *H influenzae* type b infections):
Care of Exposed Persons.
- Careful observation of exposed household, child care, or nursery contacts is essential. Exposed children who develop a febrile illness should receive prompt medical evaluation, irrespective of *Haemophilus* vaccination status. If indicated, antimicrobial therapy appropriate for invasive *H influenzae* type b infection should be administered.
- **Rifampin chemoprophylaxis.** The risk of invasive *H influenzae* type b disease among unvaccinated household contacts younger than 4 years is increased. Asymptomatic colonization with *H influenzae* type b is also more frequent in household contacts of all ages than in the general population. Rifampin eradicates *H influenzae* type b from the pharynx in approximately 95% of carriers. Limited data indicate that rifampin prophylaxis also decreases the risk of secondary invasive illness in exposed household contacts. Nursery and child care center contacts may also be at increased risk of secondary disease, but experts disagree regarding the magnitude of the risk. The risk of secondary disease in children attending child care centers is probably lower than that observed for age-susceptible household contacts, and secondary disease in child care contacts is rare when all contacts are older than 2 years. Moreover, the efficacy of rifampin in prevent-

ing disease in child care groups is not well established and the difficulties in delivering prophylaxis are considerable.

Indications and guidelines for chemoprophylaxis in different circumstances are as follows:

1. *Household.* Rifampin prophylaxis is recommended for all household contacts, irrespective of age, in those households with at least one unvaccinated contact younger than 48 months.* Based on the high efficacy of conjugate vaccination, rifampin prophylaxis is not required when all of the household contacts younger than 48 months have completed their immunization. Complete immunization is defined as having had at least one dose of conjugate vaccine at 15 months or older; two doses between 12 and 14 months; or two or more doses when younger than 12 months with a booster/reinforcing dose at 12 months or older (see Recommendations, p 210). All members of a household with a child younger than 12 months of age (ie, with a child who has not yet received the booster/reinforcing vaccine dose) should receive rifampin prophylaxis, irrespective of the vaccination status of the child, although the risk of secondary disease is very low in a child of this age who has completed the primary two- or three-dose series.

The exception to these recommendations is that all members of households with a fully vaccinated but immunocompromised child, regardless of age, should receive rifampin because of concern that the vaccination may not have been effective.

When prophylaxis is indicated, it should be initiated as soon as possible because the majority of secondary cases in households occur in the first week after hospitalization of the index patient. The time of occurrence of the remaining secondary cases after the first week suggests that prophylaxis of household contacts initiated 7 days or more after hospitalization of the index patient, although not optimal, may still be of benefit.

Index Case. In families receiving prophylaxis, the index patient should also receive rifampin prophylaxis. It should be initiated during hospitalization, usually just before discharge.

2. *Child Care and Nursery School.* When a single case has occurred, the advisability of rifampin prophylaxis in exposed child care groups with unvaccinated or incompletely vaccinated children is controversial. The following guidelines should be considered:

(a) In child care homes attended by unvaccinated or incompletely vaccinated children younger than 2 years, and where contact is 25 hours per week or more, rifampin prophylaxis can be used in the same regimen as recommended for household contacts. Unvaccinated or incompletely vaccinated children should also be given a dose of conjugate vaccine, and their immunizations should be brought up to date by administration of the recommended doses (see Immunization, p 207).

---

*A household contact is defined in these circumstances as an individual residing with the index patient, or a nonresident who spent 4 or more hours with the index patient for at least 5 of the 7 days preceding the day of hospital admission of the index patient.

(b) In child care facilities where all contacts are older than 2 years, rifampin prophylaxis need not be given, irrespective of vaccination status. Unvaccinated or incompletely vaccinated children should be given a dose of conjugate vaccine.

When two or more cases of invasive disease have occurred among attendees within 60 days, and unvaccinated or incompletely vaccinated children attend the child care, administering rifampin to all attendees and supervisory personnel is recommended. The success of rifampin prophylaxis in child care groups appears to depend on strict, prompt compliance by attendees and supervisory personnel.

3. *Other Generic Recommendations*:

(a) *Vaccinated children*. Children who have been vaccinated with any *Haemophilus influenzae* vaccine as well as susceptible, unvaccinated children should receive prophylaxis; and only children who have been age-appropriately vaccinated should be permitted to enter the group during the time prophylaxis is given and for 2 months after onset of the case (see Recommendations, p 210). For children younger than 12 months, only those who have completed their primary vaccination series (see Immunization, below) should be permitted to enroll in the group.

(b) *Dosage*. Rifampin should be given orally once daily for 4 days (in a dose of 20 mg/kg; maximum dose, 600 mg). The dose for infants younger than 1 month is not established; some experts recommend lowering the dose to 10 mg/kg. For adults, each dose is 600 mg. Rifampin is available in 150- and 300-mg capsules. Patients unable to swallow capsules may be given aliquots of rifampin powder, preweighed by a trained individual. The rifampin dose can then be mixed with a small amount of applesauce immediately before administration. Although rifampin suspension is not commercially available, a liquid suspension (1% in simple syrup) can be prepared (see rifampin package insert). If a suspension is used, it must be freshly prepared for administration to each contact group, shaken vigorously before each administration, and not used for more than 1 week.

(c) *Pregnancy*. Prophylaxis is not recommended for pregnant women who are contacts of cases because the effect of rifampin on the fetus has not been established.

Immunization. As of December 1993, four *H influenzae* type b conjugate vaccines and one combination H influenzae type b conjugate-DTP vaccine are licensed in the United States (see Table 3.7, p 208). These vaccines consist of the *H influenzae* type b capsular polysaccharide (PRP) or PRP oligomers covalently linked to a carrier protein directly, or via an intervening spacer molecule (see Table 3.7). Protein carriers include diphtheria toxoid, CRM_{197} (a nontoxic mutant diphtheria toxin), an outer membrane protein complex of *Neisseria meningitidis*, and tetanus toxoid. Protective antibodies are directed against PRP. Conjugate vaccines differ in composition and immunogenicity, and, as a result, recommendations for their use differ. For example, PRP-D is recommended only for children 12 months and older, whereas the other three vaccines, HbOC, PRP-T, and PRP-OMP, are recommended for infants beginning at 2 months of age. Currently, three doses given at 2, 4, and 6 months of age are recommended as a primary series for HbOC or PRP-T, whereas two

TABLE 3.7—*Haemophilus influenzae* type b Conjugate Vaccines*

Manufacturer	Abbreviation	Trade Name	Carrier Protein
Connaught Laboratories, Inc	PRP-D	ProHIBit	Diphtheria toxoid
Lederle Laboratories	HbOC†	HIBTITER	CRM_{197} (a nontoxic mutant diphtheria toxin)
Merck & Co	PRP-OMP	PedvaxHIB	OMP (an outer membrane protein complex of *Neisseria meningitidis*)
Pasteur Mérieux Vaccins(Distributed by Connaught Labor-atories, Inc, and by SmithKline Beecham)	PRP-T‡	ActHIB OmniHIB	Tetanus toxoid

*PRP-D is recommended by the Academy only for infants 12 mo or older. HbOC, PRP-OMP, and PRP-T are recommended for infants beginning at approximately 2 mo of age.

†HbOC is also available from Lederle Laboratories as a combination vaccine with DTP (TETRAMUNE, referred to here as HbOC-DTP).

‡PRP-T may be reconstituted with DTP, manufactured by Connaught Laboratories. Other licensed formulations of DTP have not been approved by the FDA for reconstitution and may not be used for this purpose.

doses given at 2 and 4 months of age are recommended for PRP-OMP (see Recommendations, p 210). In infants scheduled to receive separate injections of HbOC and DTP, a single injection of the combination vaccine HbOC-DTP can be substituted. PRP-T may be reconstituted with DTP, manufactured by Connaught Laboratories; other licensed formulations of DTP may not be used for this purpose. HbOC, PRP-T, and PRP-OMP vaccines are likely to be equivalent in the protection achieved after completing the recommended primary series of three or two doses, and all four vaccines are likely to be equivalent in the protection achieved in children vaccinated at 12 months of age or older.

Until recently, immunogenicity studies conducted in infants younger than 12 months of age used the same conjugate vaccine product for all doses. Since conjugate vaccines differ chemically and immunologically, studies are necessary to determine the responses of infants given sequential doses of different vaccines. Until data from current studies addressing this question are available, when feasible, the same conjugate vaccine that was used for the initial dose should be used for subsequent doses for infants younger than 12 months. However, for infants who receive different conjugate vaccines, giving more than a total of three doses of any vaccine to complete the primary series is not necessary.

Following administration of the initial two recommended doses of PRP-OMP at 2 and 4 months of age, or three doses of HbOC or PRP-T at 2, 4, and 6 months, serum antibody concentrations decline rapidly. At 12 months of age, the antibody concentrations have decreased approximately three- to six-fold compared to the respective peak concentrations. Therefore, an additional booster dose of conjugate vaccine is recommended at 12 to 15 months of age. For this dose, any conjugate vaccine, PRP-D, HbOC, PRP-OMP, or PRP-T, is acceptable, regardless of which vaccine was used for the primary series. For children scheduled to receive HbOC and DTP, a single injection of the HbOC-DTP combination vaccine may be substituted. For those scheduled to receive PRP-T and DTP, PRP-T may be reconstituted with DTP, manufactured by Connaught Laboratories.

For children whose initial vaccination is given at 12 to 14 months of age, the Academy considers that any conjugate vaccine, PRP-D, HbOC, PRP-OMP, or PRP-T, is acceptable. However, the FDA has approved labeling for PRP-D for use beginning at 15 months of age.

Children in Whom DTP or DT Vaccination is Deferred. The carrier proteins used in PRP-T, PRP-D, and HbOC (but not PRP-OMP) are chemically and immunologically related to toxoids contained in DTP vaccine (see Table 3.7, p 208). Earlier or simultaneous vaccination with diphtheria or tetanus toxoids may be required to elicit an optimal anti-PRP antibody response to PRP-T, PRP-D, or HbOC. In contrast, the immunogenicity of PRP-OMP is not affected by vaccination with DTP. Thus, in infants in whom DTP or DT vaccination is deferred, PRP-OMP may be advantageous for *H influenzae* type b vaccination.

Children with Immunologic Impairment. Children with chronic illnesses associated with increased risk of *H influenzae* type b disease may have impaired anti-PRP antibody responses to conjugate vaccination. Examples of such children include those with HIV infection, immunoglobulin deficiency, anatomic or functional asplenia, and sickle-cell disease, as well as recipients of bone marrow transplants and recipients of chemotherapy for malignancy. Some children with immunologic impairment may benefit from more doses of conjugate vaccine than normally indicated (see Recommendations, p 210).

Vaccine Failure. Despite receiving conjugate vaccination, *H influenzae* type b disease can still occur. Since serum antibody responses do not occur for 1 to 2 weeks after vaccination, recipients are not expected to be protected during this immediate postvaccination period. Current data do not indicate that the risk of disease is increased during the 1 to 2 weeks after conjugate vaccination.

Adverse Reactions. Adverse reactions to the four licensed *H influenzae* type b conjugate vaccines are few. Pain, redness, and/or swelling at the injection site occur in about 25% of recipients, but these symptoms typically are mild and last less than 24 hours. Systemic reactions such as fever and irritability are infrequent. When conjugate vaccines are administered during the same visit that DTP vaccine is given, the rates of systemic reactions do not differ from those observed when only DTP vaccine is administered.

Recommendations

Dosage and Route of Administration. The dose of each *Haemophilus influenzae* type b conjugate vaccine is 0.5 mL, given intramuscularly.

Indications and Schedule

1. All children should be immunized with an *H influenzae* type b conjugate vaccine beginning at approximately 2 months of age or as soon as possible thereafter (see Table 3.8, p 211). Only HbOC, PRP-OMP, or PRP-T should be given to children younger than 12 months of age.

   (a) The *H influenzae* type b conjugate immunization can be initiated as early as 6 weeks of age.

   (b) When DT or DTP vaccination is deferred, use of PRP-OMP may be advantageous (see Deferring DTP or DT Vaccination, p 213).

   (c) *Haemophilus influenzae* type b conjugate vaccination may be given during visits when vaccines for diphtheria, tetanus, pertussis (DTP or DTaP), polio, hepatitis B, and/or measles, mumps, and rubella (MMR) are given (see Simultaneous Administration of Multiple Vaccines, p 25).

   (d) HbOC, PRP-T, or PRP-OMP should be given in a separate syringe and at a separate site from DTP or other vaccinations unless specific combinations are approved by the FDA. Those approved are as follows:

      (i) In infants scheduled to receive both HbOC and DTP, a single injection of the combination vaccine, HbOC-DTP, can be substituted for the two injections.

      (ii) PRP-T may be reconstituted with DTP, manufactured by Connaught Laboratories, to give the two vaccines in a single injection. Other licensed formulations of DTP have not been approved for reconstitution and may not be used for this purpose.

2. The following schedule should be followed for routine immunization of children younger than 7 months of age:

   (a) *Primary series.* Either a three-dose series of HbOC or PRP-T, or a two-dose series of PRP-OMP should be administered (see Table 3.8, p 211). Doses are given at approximately 2-month intervals. When feasible, the conjugate vaccine product used for the first dose should be used for subsequent doses in children younger than 12 months of age. When sequential doses of different vaccine products are given, more than three doses of any conjugate vaccine to complete the primary series is not considered necessary. For those scheduled to receive HbOC or PRP-T and DTP, a single injection can be substituted, as described in 1(d) above. The safety and efficacy of the different vaccines given in their recommended schedules appear to be equivalent.

   (b) *Reinforcing/booster vaccination at 12 to 15 months of age.* For children who have completed a primary series, an additional dose of conjugate vaccine is recommended at 12 to 15 months of age, or as soon as possible thereafter. Any conjugate vaccine (PRP-D, HbOC, PRP-OMP, or PRP-T) is acceptable for this dose regardless of the vaccine used previously. For infants scheduled to receive HbOC or

TABLE 3.8—Recommendations for *Haemophilus influenzae* type b Conjugate Vaccination in Children Immunized Beginning at 2 to 6 Months of Age

Vaccine Product at Initiation*	Total Number of Doses to Be Administered	Currently Recommended Vaccine Regimens*
HbOC or PRP-T	4	3 doses at 2-mo intervals When feasible, same vaccine for doses 1-3 Fourth dose at 12 to 15 mo of age Any conjugate vaccine for dose 4†
PRP-OMP	3	2 doses at 2-mo intervals When feasible, same vaccine for doses 1 and 2 Third dose at 12-15 mo of age Any conjugate vaccine for dose 3†

*See text. The HbOC, PRP-T, or PRP-OMP should be given in a separate syringe and at a separate site from other immunizations unless specific combinations are approved by the FDA. HbOC is also available as a combination vaccine with DTP (HbOC-DTP). This combination can be used in infants scheduled to receive separate injections of DTP and HbOC. PRP-T may be reconstituted with DTP, made by Connaught Laboratories; other licensed formulations of DTP may not be used for this purpose.

†The safety and efficacy of PRP-OMP, PRP-D, PRP-T, and HbOC are likely to be equivalent in children 12 mo and older.

PRP-T and DTP, a single injection can be substituted. However, as previously described, for this dose in children 15 months or older, separate injections of *H influenzae* conjugate and DTaP vaccines are acceptable because of the lower frequency of local and systemic reactions associated with use of acellular pertussis vaccine.

Measles-mumps-rubella vaccination can be given at the same time as *H influenzae* type b conjugate vaccine, but it should be given at a separate site and in a separate syringe. Some physicians may choose to give these injections in more than one visit. In this circumstance, for patients who have not been immunized previously against measles, priority should be given to administering MMR vaccine at the appropriate age.

3. Children younger than 5 years of age who did not receive *H influenzae* conjugate vaccine in the first 6 months of life should be immunized according to the following recommended schedules (see Table 3.9):

(a) For children in whom immunization is initiated at 7 to 11 months of age, the recommended schedules for HbOC, PRP-OMP, and PRP-T are identical and require three doses. The first two doses are given at 2-month intervals using the same vaccine product, when feasible, for both doses. The third (booster) dose should be

TABLE 3.9—Recommendations for *Haemophilus influenzae* type b Conjugate Vaccination in Children in Whom Initial Vaccination Is Delayed Until 7 Months of Age or Older

Age at Initiation of Immunization (mo)	Vaccine Product at Initiation	Total Number of Doses to Be Administered	Currently Recommended Vaccine Regimens[a]
7-11	HbOC, PRP-T, or PRP-OMP	3	2 doses at 2-mo intervals[b] When feasible, same vaccine for doses 1 and 2 Third dose at 12-18 mo, given at least 2 mo after dose 2 Any conjugate vaccine for dose 3[c]
12-14	HbOC, PRP-T, PRP-OMP, or PRP-D	2	2-mo interval between doses[b] Any conjugate vaccine for dose 2[c]
15-59	HbOC, PRP-T, PRP-OMP, or PRP-D	1[d]	Any conjugate vaccine
60 and older[e]	HbOC, PRP-T, PRP-OMP, or PRP-D	1 or 2[d]	Any conjugate vaccine

[a]See text. HbOC, PRP-T, or PRP-OMP should be given in a separate syringe and at a separate site from other immunizations unless specific combinations are approved by the FDA. HbOC is also available as a combination vaccine with DTP (HbOC-DTP). This combination can be used in infants scheduled to receive separate injections of DTP and HbOC. PRP-T may be reconstituted with DTP, made by Connaught Laboratories; other licensed formulations of DTP may not be used for this purpose. In children 15 mo or older eligible to receive DTaP (containing acellular pertussis vaccine), however, separate injections of conjugate vaccine and DTaP are acceptable because of the lower rate of febrile, minor local and systemic reactions associated with DTaP.

[b]For "catch up," a minimum of a 1-mo interval between doses may be used.

[c]The safety and efficacy of PRP-OMP, PRP-D, PRP-T, and HbOC are likely to be equivalent for use as a booster dose in children 12 mo or older.

[d]Two doses separated by 2 mo are recommended by some experts for children with certain underlying diseases associated with increased risk of disease and impaired antibody responses to *H influenzae* type b conjugate vaccination (see text).

[e]Only for children with chronic illness known to be associated with an increased risk for *H influenzae* type b disease (see text).

given at 12 to 18 months of age, preferably 2 months after the second dose. For the third dose, any licensed conjugate vaccine is acceptable.

(b) For children in whom immunization is initiated at 12 to 14 months of age, the recommended regimens for PRP-D, HbOC, PRP-OMP, or PRP-T are identical and require two doses given at a 2-month interval.

(c) For children in whom immunization is initiated at 15 months or older, and who have not yet reached their fifth birthday (ie, 59 months or younger), the recommended regimen is a single dose of any licensed conjugate vaccine.

(d) Circumstances may suggest a need for more rapid "catch-up" immunization, in which case a 1-month interval between doses is the minimum.

(e) For infants in whom immunization with both DTP and conjugate vaccination is initiated late, the HbOC-DTP combination or PRP-T reconstituted with Connaught DTP can be substituted for separate injections of the two vaccines. However, additional doses of DTP alone will be necessary to complete the primary DTP immunization since, in contrast to *H influenzae* type b vaccination, delay in DTP vaccination does not decrease the total number of required injections.

4. Special circumstances to be noted are as follows:

(a) *Lapsed immunizations.* Recommendations for vaccination of children who have had a lapse in the schedule of immunizations are based on limited data. The current recommendations are summarized in Table 3.10 (p 214).

(b) *Premature infants.* For infants born prematurely, immunization should be based on chronologic age and initiated at 2 months of age according to recommendations in Table 3.8. Data are needed on responses of these infants to *H influenzae* conjugate vaccines. However, experiences with other antigens that are T-cell dependent, such as diphtheria and tetanus toxoids, justify this interim recommendation.

(c) *Deferring DTP or DT vaccination.* In infants with certain neurologic disorders, DTP and DT vaccination may be deferred until the first birthday (see Pertussis, p 364). Use of PRP-OMP may be advantageous in this circumstance. In infants in whom a decision has been made to use DT vaccine instead of DTP, however, any *H influenzae* type b conjugate vaccine may be used.

(d) *Pertussis vaccine contraindications and precautions.* In infants and children in whom pertussis vaccination is contraindicated, HbOC-DTP should not be used. Similarly, precautions about the use of pertussis vaccination also apply to the use of HbOC-DTP (see Pertussis, p 364).

(e) *Immunologic impairment associated with increased risk of invasive H influenzae type b disease.* Patients with HIV infection, IgG2 subclass deficiency, bone marrow transplants, sickle-cell disease, and splenectomy, and those receiving chemotherapy for malignancies

TABLE 3.10—Recommendations for *Haemophilus influenzae* type b Conjugate Vaccination in Children With a Lapse in Vaccination

Age at Presentation (mo)	Previous Vaccination History	Recommended Regimen
7-11	1 dose*	1 dose of conjugate at 7 to 11 mo, with a booster dose given at least 2 mo later, at 12 to 15 mo†
	2 doses of HbOC or PRP-T	Same as above
12-14	2 doses before 12 mo*	A single dose of any licensed conjugate‡
12-14	1 dose before 12 mo*	2 additional doses of any licensed conjugate, separated by 2 mo‡
15-59	Any incomplete schedule	A single dose of any licensed conjugate‡

*PRP-OMP, PRP-T, or HbOC. HbOC is also available as a combination vaccine with DTP (HbOC-DTP), which may be used in infants scheduled to receive separate injections of DTP and HbOC. PRP-T may be reconstituted with DTP, made by Connaught Laboratories; other licensed formulations of DTP may not be used for this purpose. In children 15 mo or older eligible to receive DTaP (containing acellular pertussis), however, separate injections of conjugate vaccine and DTaP may be given because of the lower rate of febrile, minor local and systemic reactions associated with DTaP.

†For the dose given at 7 to 11 mo, when feasible, the same vaccine should be given as was used for the dose given at 2 to 6 mo. For the dose given at 12 to 15 mo, any licensed conjugate can be used.

‡The Academy considers that safety and efficacy of PRP-OMP, PRP-D, PRP-T, or HbOC are likely to be equivalent when used in children 12 mo or older.

are at increased risk for invasive *H influenzae* type b disease. When children with splenectomy or sickle-cell disease have completed a primary series of immunizations and have received a booster/reinforcing dose at 12 months of age or older, additional doses are not needed. For children with malignancies, some experts recommend an additional dose of conjugate vaccine before chemotherapy and/or splenectomy. Whether children with HIV infection or IgG2 deficiency will benefit from additional doses if they have completed a primary series of immunizations and have received a booster dose at 12 months or later is not known.

For those children 12 to 59 months of age with one of these underlying conditions predisposing to *H influenzae* type b disease who are unvaccinated or have received only one dose of conjugate vaccine before 12 months of age, two doses of any conjugate vaccine, separated by 2 months, are recommended. For those in this age group who received two doses before 12 months of age, one additional dose of conjugate vaccine is recommended.

Unvaccinated children with underlying diseases predisposing to *H influenzae* type b disease who are older than 59 months of age should be vaccinated with any licensed conjugate vaccine. One dose appears sufficient in this age group for children with sickle-cell disease or asplenia. Two doses separated by 1 to 2 months are suggested, based on limited data, for children with HIV infection, IgG2 deficiency, bone marrow transplants, or malignancies. Because DTP vaccination is not routinely recommended for persons 7 years or older, HbOC-DTP is also not recommended for use at this age.

No known contraindications exist to simultaneous administration of *H influenzae* conjugate vaccine with pneumococcal vaccine or meningococcal vaccine when given in separate syringes at different sites.

(f) *H influenzae type b disease.* Children who had invasive *H influenzae* type b disease when younger than 24 months of age frequently have low anticapsular antibody concentrations in convalescent sera and may remain at risk of developing a second episode of disease. Any conjugate vaccination given before disease developed should be ignored, and conjugate vaccination in these patients should be readministered according to the age-appropriate schedule for unvaccinated children (see Tables 3.8, 3.9, and 3.10, pp 211, 212, and 214). Revaccination should be initiated one month after onset of disease or as soon as possible thereafter.

Children whose disease occurred at age 24 months or older do not need immunization, irrespective of previous vaccination status, because the disease most likely induced a protective immune response and second episodes of disease at this age are rare.

Immunized children who experience invasive *H influenzae* type b disease after receiving a dose of a conjugate vaccine at 15 months or older have a high incidence of IgG2 deficiency and, therefore, should be considered for immunologic evaluation. Children who completed the recommended vaccination schedule before 15 months of age (ie, final dose given at 12 to 14 months of age) and who develop invasive disease should also be considered for immunologic evaluation. Whether immunologic evaluation should be performed for children who experience invasive *H influenzae* type b disease after conjugate immunization given earlier than 12 months of age is uncertain. Nevertheless, evaluation of immunoglobulin concentrations in such patients, particularly those with a history of recurrent infection, should be considered.

5. *H influenzae* type b disease and adverse reactions after immunization should be reported. All important adverse reactions occurring at any time after immunization, including cases of disease occurring in fully or partially immunized children, should be reported promptly to the Vaccine Adverse Event Reporting System (VAERS) (see Vaccine Safety and Contraindications: Reporting of Adverse Events, p 30). In addition, all cases of invasive *H influenzae* type b disease, including those in fully or partially vaccinated children, should be reported to the Centers for Disease Control and Prevention through the state and

local public health department. The time after immunization when protection can be anticipated is not known with precision and probably differs depending on the number of previous doses. Providers should be aware of this uncertainty and should not expect protection simultaneously with vaccine administration.

Helicobacter pylori Infections

Clinical Manifestations: Acute infection may be manifest by epigastric pain, nausea, vomiting, hematemesis, and guaiac positive stools. Symptoms usually resolve within a few days, but a minority of infected persons can develop duodenal or gastric ulceration. Long-term infection (ie, lasting decades) increases the risk for gastric adenocarcinoma. *Helicobacter pylori* is not associated with autoimmune or chemical gastritis.

Etiology: *Helicobacter pylori* (formerly *Campylobacter pylori*) are Gram-negative, spirally curved or U-shaped microaerophilic bacilli that have a tuft of flagella at one end.

Epidemiology: *Helicobacter pylori* have been isolated from humans and other primates only. No animal reservoir for human transmission has been found. The routes by which organisms are transmitted from the reservoir of infected humans are unknown. Infection rates are low in children but rise until age 60 years, at which time serologic studies indicate that 25% to 50% of the population have been infected. Most carriage is asymptomatic, but essentially all infected persons have chronic gastritis. Infection is acquired at a younger age in developing countries and in those in lower socioeconomic groups.

The **incubation period** is unknown.

Diagnostic Tests: *Helicobacter pylori* infection can be diagnosed by culture from gastric biopsy tissue on nonselective media (eg, chocolate agar) or selective media (eg, Skirrow's) at 37°C under microaerobic conditions for 2 to 5 days. Organisms can usually be visualized easily on histologic sections with Gram, hematoxylin-eosin, silver, Giemsa, or acridine orange staining. Because of the production of urease by the organisms, urease testing of a gastric specimen can give a rapid and specific microbiologic diagnosis. All of these tests require endoscopy and biopsy to obtain tissue. Noninvasive, commercially available tests include detection of labeled CO_2 in expired air after oral administration of isotopically labeled urea and serology for the presence of antibody to *H pylori*. Each of the diagnostic tests is greater than 95% accurate.

Treatment: *Helicobacter pylori* is susceptible to a wide variety of antimicrobial agents including ampicillin, tetracycline, metronidazole, clindamycin, erythromycin, and bismuth salts, but none have been proved effective in vivo as single agents. Combination therapy of amoxicillin, metronidazole, and bismuth subsalicylate is often effective in eliminating the organism, healing duodenal ulceration, and avoiding ulcer relapse, but recurrences occur. Eradication rates with triple therapy are 60% to 90%.

Isolation of the Hospitalized Patient: No special precautions are currently recommended.

Control Measures: Disinfection of gastroscopes will prevent transmission of the organism between patients.

Hemorrhagic Fevers Caused by Arenaviruses

Clinical Manifestations: These diseases range from mild infections to severe acute febrile illnesses in which shock is a prominent feature. Fever, headache, myalgia, conjunctival suffusions, and abdominal pain are common early symptoms in all infections. Axillary petechiae are usual in Argentine, Bolivian, and Venezuelan hemorrhagic fevers, and exudative pharyngitis often occurs in Lassa fever. Mucosal bleeding occurs in severe cases as a consequence of thrombocytopenia and platelet dysfunction. Proteinuria is common, but renal failure is unusual. Elevated serum concentrations of aspartate aminotransferase can be an indicator of adverse or fatal outcome in Lassa fever. Serum alpha interferon concentrations are markedly elevated in Argentine hemorrhagic fever; higher concentrations correlate with poorer prognoses. Shock develops 7 to 9 days after onset of the illness in more severely ill patients. Upper and lower respiratory symptoms can develop in Lassa fever. Encephalopathic signs with tremor, alterations in consciousness, and seizures can occur in the South American hemorrhagic fevers as well as in severe cases of Lassa virus infections. Sensorineural hearing loss is a common sequela of Lassa fever.

Etiology: Arenaviruses contain RNA. Argentine hemorrhagic fever (AHF), Bolivian hemorrhagic fever (BHF), and Venezuelan hemorrhagic fever (VHF), the arenavirus diseases occurring in the Western hemisphere, are caused by Junin, Machupo, and Guanarito viruses, respectively. Lassa fever, a disease occurring in West Africa, is caused by Lassa virus.

Epidemiology: Inhalation or skin contact (eg, through cuts, scratches, or abrasions) with urine and salivary secretions from persistently infected rodents are the principal routes of infection. All arenaviruses are infectious as aerosols; those causing hemorrhagic fever should be considered highly hazardous to laboratory workers. The geographic distribution and habitats of the specific rodents that serve as reservoir hosts largely determine the endemic area and groups of persons at risk. Several hundred cases of AHF occur yearly in agricultural workers and inhabitants of Argentina. Other than a large epidemic from 1962 to 1964, few cases of BHF have been reported. Venezuelan hemorrhagic fever has only recently been recognized in rural north-central Venezuela. Lassa fever is highly endemic in most of West Africa, where its rodent host lives commensally with man, causing thousands of infections annually. Lassa fever virus (and, rarely, BHF or AHF) can be transmitted from person to person, typically through intimate contact, including within hospitals. Lassa fever has been imported by travelers from West Africa.

The **incubation period** is from 6 to 17 days.

Diagnostic Tests: Diagnosis is made by demonstrating virus-specific IgM in blood, an increase in virus-specific serum IgG antibody titers in serial serum specimens, virus isolation, or by identifying viral antigen in blood or tissues. Circulating antibody detected by immunofluorescence occurs earlier in Lassa fever (7 to 10 days) than in South American diseases (14 to 21 days). Neutralizing antibodies occur later and are difficult to detect in Lassa fever. These viruses may be recovered from the blood of acutely ill patients as well as from various tissues obtained postmortem.

Treatment: Plasma from convalescent patients has proved effective in reducing the mortality of AHF from 15% to 30% in untreated patients to less than 1% in those receiving appropriate quantities (based on neutralizing antibody content) within the first 8 days of illness. Intravenous ribavirin reduces mortality significantly in high-risk Lassa fever patients, particularly if treated in the first week of illness.

Isolation of the Hospitalized Patient: Strict isolation precautions are recommended for Lassa fever, including scrupulous adherence to universal precautions and prevention of needlestick injuries. Although nosocomial infections are rare with South American diseases, scrupulous adherence to universal precautions is prudent for these diseases as well.

Control Measures:

Care of Exposed Persons. No specific measures are warranted for persons exposed to Lassa fever unless direct contamination with patient blood, excretions, or secretions has occurred. If such contamination has occurred, daily temperature recordings for 21 days and prevention of intimate contact with other individuals during this interval are recommended. Recommendations are similar for those who have had sexual contact (both immediately before illness and for several weeks afterward) with patients who have AHF or BHF.

Rodent Control. In the village-based outbreaks of BHF, rodent control has proved successful. Rodent control is not practical for AHF because the reservoirs are sylvatic and ubiquitous. Rodent control has reduced Lassa fever infections but has not eliminated infection in household members because the rodents are also peridomestic and eventually return to the human dwellings.

Vaccine. An investigational live-attenuated Junin vaccine developed by the US Army protects against AHF and probably BHF. The vaccine is associated with minimal side effects in adults.

Hemorrhagic Fevers Caused by Bunyaviruses, Including Hantaviruses

Clinical Manifestations: These infections are severe, febrile diseases in which shock and bleeding can be significant, and multisystem involvement can occur. Recently in the United States, these infections have caused an illness marked by acute respiratory failure.

Hemorrhagic fever with renal syndrome (HFRS) is a complex, multiphasic disease characterized by vascular instability and varying degrees of renal insufficiency. Fever, flushing, conjunctival injection, abdominal pain, and lumbar pain are followed by hypotension, oliguria, and, subsequently, polyuria. Axillary petechiae are common. Shock and acute renal insufficiency may require intensive care and dialysis. Nephropathia epidemica, the clinical syndrome of HFRS in Europe, is a milder disease characterized by a grippe-like illness with abdominal pain and proteinuria. Acute renal dysfunction also occurs, which may require hospitalization, but hypotensive shock or a requirement for dialysis are infrequent.

Recently in the United States, an acute febrile illness that progresses to noncardiogenic pulmonary edema (NCPE), causing acute respiratory failure and shock, has been attributed to a new hantavirus. Clinical findings during the prodrome are nonspecific, but hemoconcentration, hypoalbuminemia, leukocytosis, thrombocytopenia, arterial oxygen desaturation, and interstitial or alveolar pulmonary edema are often present when patients are admitted to the hospital. Unlike other hantaviral diseases, renal failure has been mild or absent.

Crimean-Congo hemorrhagic fever (CCHF) is a multisystem disease characterized by hepatitis and, often, profuse bleeding. Fever, headache, and myalgia are followed by signs of a diffuse capillary leak syndrome, such as facial suffusion, conjunctivitis, and proteinuria. Bradycardia is common, and petechiae and purpura frequently appear on the skin and mucous membranes. A hypotensive crisis often occurs after the appearance of frank hemorrhage from the gastrointestinal tract, nose, mouth, or uterus.

Rift Valley fever (RVF), in most cases, is a self-limited, febrile illness. Occasionally, patients develop hepatitis, hemorrhagic fever with shock and bleeding, encephalitis, or retinitis.

Etiology: *Bunyaviridae* are RNA viruses with different geographic distributions and vectors of transmission. Hantaviruses cause HFRS. The prototype Hantaan virus is responsible for severe disease in Asia and the Balkans, and Puumala virus causes the milder disease occurring in Europe. A hantavirus is the cause of the recently recognized NCPE syndrome in North America.

Epidemiology: Hemmorrhagic fever with renal syndrome occurs throughout much of Asia, Eastern and Western Europe, and the Balkans. Hantaan and related viruses cause chronic infections in various species of field mice, voles, peridomestic rats, and other small mammals. Disease in humans is acquired by contact, most frequently from inhalation of aerosols, of infectious secreta and excreta of these animals. The most severe forms of disease are acquired in rural areas of Asia and the Balkan nations; urban-acquired cases that occur in Europe are generally milder. Numerous infections have occurred in the laboratory by contact with chronically infected rodents, either captured wild rodents or colonies of laboratory rats. Hantaviruses have been isolated from rodents in the United States but the only association with acute disease is the syndrome of NCPE and shock. This syndrome was initially identified in the southwestern United States in 1993 but has occurred in several other states. Crimean-Congo hemorrhagic fever occurs in much of sub-Saharan Africa, the Middle East, areas in West and Central Asia, and Eastern Europe. The CCHF virus is transmitted by ticks, and, occasionally, at the slaughter of domestic animals. Nosocomial transmission of CCHF is a serious hazard. Rift Valley fever occurs throughout sub-Saharan Africa and has extended into Egypt. The virus is mosquito-borne, and is transmitted from domestic livestock to humans (or from person to person) by mosquito bites. It can also be transmitted by aerosol, and by direct contact with infected fresh animal carcasses.

The **incubation periods** for CCHF and RVF range from 2 to 10 days; for HFRS they are usually longer, ranging from 9 to 40 days. For hantaviral infection causing NCPE, the incubation period may be 1 to 3 weeks, but has not been definitively established.

Diagnostic Tests: The CCHF and RVF viruses are readily recovered from blood and tissues of infected patients; recovery of hantaviruses is difficult and infrequent. Detection of viral antigen is a useful alternative for the diagnosis of CCHF and RVF, but it has been unsuccessful for HFRS. Serologic virus-specific IgM and IgG antibodies typically develop early in convalescence in CCHF and RVF. In HFRS, IgM and IgG antibodies are usually detectable at the time of onset of the illness or within 48 hours. IgM antibodies or rising IgG titers, as demonstrated by enzyme immunoassay (EIA), establish a diagnosis. Neutralizing antibody tests provide greater virus-strain specificity. Immunofluorescent and complement-fixing antibody tests are also used for serologic diagnosis. Tests for the laboratory diagnosis of hantaviral NCPE are in development. These tests include IgM antibodies detected by EIA, polymerase chain reaction for viral RNA on fresh or frozen tissue, and immunohistochemistry performed on formalin-fixed lung tissue.

Treatment: Ribavirin given intravenously to patients with HFRS is effective in reducing renal dysfunction, vascular instability, and mortality when given in the first 4 days of illness. Supportive therapy for HFRS should include (1) avoidance of transporting patients, (2) supportive care for shock, (3) prevention of overhydration (particularly with crystalloid solutions), (4) dialysis for complications of renal failure, and (5) control of hypertension during the oliguric phase.

The treatment of hantaviral NCPE is careful supportive management to prevent severe hypoxemia and maintain adequate tissue perfusion without exacerbation of the pulmonary capillary leak syndrome by excess fluid administration.

Ribavirin given to patients with CCHF has resulted in clinical responses, although no controlled studies have been performed. Experimental animal data suggest the potential for use of ribavirin in treatment of hemorrhagic RVF as well.

Isolation of the Hospitalized Patient: Patients with CCHF are potentially contagious. Strict isolation precautions, with particular attention to the hazards posed by laboratory specimens and needlesticks, are indicated. Rift Valley fever has not been demonstrated to be contagious, but since virus is present in blood, universal precautions should be scrupulously followed. Hemorrhagic fever with renal syndrome is not transmitted from person to person, and no special precautions are needed. Hantaviral NCPE has not been associated with nosocomial or person-to-person transmission.

Control Measures:

Care of Exposed Persons: Persons having direct contact with blood or other secretions from patients with CCHF should be monitored for fever daily for 14 days and precluded from intimate contact with other persons during this time. For those with parenteral exposure to contaminated objects or extensive blood exposure, oral ribavirin should be considered after consultation with appropriate experts.

Other Measures:
- *HFRS.* Monitoring of laboratory rat colonies and urban rodent control may be effective for rat-borne disease.
- *Hantaviruses.* Control of sylvatic reservoirs of rurally acquired hantaviruses, including the newly recognized hantaviruses causing NCPE in the United States, is not practical. However, reduction of human contact with rodents and their excreta through targeted rodent elimination programs is prudent.
- *CCHF.* Insecticides for tick control have limited benefit, but personal protective measures (eg, physical tick removal and protective clothing with permethrin sprays) are effective.
- *RVF.* Mosquito control measures may be effective in certain areas. Vaccination of domestic animals is important in limiting or preventing RVF outbreaks. An effective experimental vaccine for humans has been developed by the US Army.

Hepatitis A

Clinical Manifestations: Hepatitis A is characteristically an acute febrile illness with jaundice, anorexia, nausea, and malaise. In infants and preschool-aged children, most infections are either asymptomatic or cause mild nonspecific symptoms without jaundice. Fulminant hepatitis A is rare, and chronic infection does not occur.

Etiology: Hepatitis A virus (HAV) is an RNA virus that is classified as a member of the picornavirus group.

Epidemiology: The most common mode of transmission is person to person, resulting from fecal contamination and oral ingestion (ie, the fecal-oral route). Infection is endemic in developing countries. Spread occurs readily in households and in child care centers. In the United States, these centers have become an important source for HAV infection in the community and for epidemics. In contrast to most other infectious diseases in child care settings, symptomatic (icteric) illness occurs primarily among adult contacts of day care children; most day care attendees with HAV are asymptomatic or have nonspecific manifestations. Hence, spread of HAV infection in and from a child care center frequently occurs before recognition of the index case(s). The risk of spread and of an outbreak occurring in a child care center increases with the number of children enrolled who are younger than 2 years and who wear diapers.

Common-source food-borne and waterborne epidemics, including several caused by shellfish contaminated by human sewage, have occurred. Transmission by blood transfusion or from mother to newborn infant (ie, vertical) is rare, but both have been responsible for nosocomial outbreaks among infants and staff in neonatal intensive care units as the result of asymptomatic shedding of virus from infected neonates. On rare occasion, infection has been contracted from nonhuman primates.

Age of infection varies with socioeconomic status and resulting living conditions. In developing countries, infection in the first decade of life is common; in developed countries, infection occurs at an older age. In the United States, infection is most common in young adults. Cases of hepatitis A among intravenous drug users have increased. No appreciable seasonal variation in the incidence of infection has been noted. Viral shedding and probably the contagious period last 1 to 3 weeks. The highest titers of HAV in stool of infected patients occur in the 1 to 2 weeks before the onset of illness, during which time patients probably are most likely to spread infection. The risk subsequently diminishes and is minimal in the week after the onset of jaundice. No HAV carrier state exists. The presence of serum anti-HAV antibody (IgM and/or IgG) in unvaccinated persons indicates lifelong immunity to HAV.

The **incubation period** is 15 to 50 days, with an average of 25 to 30 days.

Diagnostic Tests: Serologic tests for anti-HAV and IgM-specific anti-HAV antibodies are commercially available. The presence of IgM anti-HAV antibodies usually indicates recent infection. These antibodies are present at the onset of illness and usually disappear within 4 months, but in some persons they may persist for 6 months or longer. IgG anti-HAV antibodies develop shortly after IgM anti-HAV antibodies. The presence of IgG without IgM anti-HAV antibodies indicates past infection.

Treatment: Supportive.

Isolation of the Hospitalized Patient: Enteric precautions should be observed. Patients who are not toilet trained or who have diarrhea, stool incontinence, or poor personal hygiene require private rooms and enteric precautions for 1 week after the onset of jaundice. Others do not require a private room. Patients with acute viral hepatitis of unknown type should be managed with enteric as well as universal precautions.

Control Measures:

Care of Household and Sexual Contacts. All household and sexual contacts should receive 0.02 mL/kg of immune globulin (IG) as soon as possible after exposure. Serologic testing of contacts usually is not recommended because it adds unnecessary cost and may delay the administration of IG. The use of IG more than 2 weeks after the last exposure is not indicated.

Newborn Infants of Infected Mothers. Since vertical transmission has been the source of hepatitis A transmission in neonatal nurseries, contact isolation is indicated for the infant. Breast-feeding should be allowed. Some experts have advised giving the infant IG (0.02 mL/kg) if the mother has onset of symptoms in the period from 2 weeks before to 1 week after delivery. However, efficacy in this circumstance has not been established. In the absence of immunoprophylaxis, severe disease in infants has not been reported. The need for proper hygiene should be emphasized to the mother.

Child Care Employees, Children, and Their Household Contacts.

Prevention. Prevention of spread of HAV in a child care facility necessitates education of the employees and families about the importance of hygienic measures in preventing fecal-oral spread of HAV and other enteric pathogens. Careful hand washing is imperative, particularly after changing diapers and before preparing or serving food. Because HAV may survive on objects in the environment for weeks, environmental hygiene is also important (see also Children in Out-of-Home Child Care, p 89).

Surveillance. Prompt reporting to local public health officials of hepatitis A cases, especially child-care-associated cases, is encouraged.

Case Identification. Testing for anti-HAV IgM antibody should be done to confirm the existence of infection in suspect cases in employees, enrolled children, and in those who are household contacts of a patient with hepatitis.

Uses of Immune Globulin (IG):

• In child care facilities with all children older than 2 years or all toilet trained, when a case of hepatitis A is identified in an employee or enrolled child, IG (0.02 mL/kg) is recommended for employees in contact with the index case and for children in the same room as the index case.

• In child care facilities with children not yet toilet trained, when one case of HAV infection is identified in either an employee or a child, or in the household contacts of two of the enrolled children, IG (0.02 mL/kg) is recommended for all employees and enrolled children in the facility. During the 6 weeks after the last case is identified, new employees and children should also receive IG.

• If recognition of the child care outbreak is delayed by 3 or more weeks from the onset of the index case or if illness has occurred in three or more families, the disease is likely to have already spread widely. In this situation, IG should be considered for use in all the child care staff and children and for the household contacts of all enrolled children in diapers.

Exclusion. Children and adults with acute hepatitis A should be excluded from the child care facility until 1 week after the onset of the illness or until

IG has been administered to appropriate children and staff in the program, as directed by the responsible health department.

Schools. Schoolroom exposure generally does not pose a significant risk of infection and IG is not indicated. However, IG may be given to those who have close personal contact with infected persons. Children and adults with acute hepatitis A should be excluded for 1 week after the onset of the illness.

Institutions and Hospitals. In institutions for custodial care, HAV infection can be transmitted easily. If an outbreak occurs, residents and staff in close personal contact with the patients should receive IG (0.02 mL/kg). Administration of IG to hospital personnel caring for patients with HAV infection is not routinely indicated, unless an outbreak is occurring. Emphasis should be placed on hand washing and proper hygienic procedures in the management of patients.

Food- or Waterborne Outbreaks. The source is usually recognized too late for IG to be effective. Immune globulin may be effective if it can be administered to exposed individuals within 2 weeks of the last exposure to the HAV-contaminated water or food.

Pre-exposure Prophylaxis for Foreign Travel. Immune globulin prophylaxis is recommended for all susceptible travelers to developing countries. For stays of less than 3 months, travelers should receive IG (0.02 mL/kg). For longer stays, 0.06 mL/kg should be given every 5 months. For persons who require repeated immunoprophylaxis, screening for anti-HAV antibody before travel can reduce the need for IG by identifying immune persons. Travelers should be counseled to avoid potentially contaminated food or water.

General Measures. Good sanitation and personal hygiene, particularly careful hand washing and sanitary disposal of feces, are important general measures.

Vaccines. Experimental inactivated and live vaccines have been developed. Data from several studies indicate that the inactivated vaccines are highly effective in preventing HAV infection and illness. Licensure of one or more of these vaccines in the United States may occur in the near future. These vaccines are already licensed in at least eight other countries.

Hepatitis B

Clinical Manifestations: Hepatitis B virus (HBV) causes a wide spectrum of infections, ranging from asymptomatic seroconversion, subacute illness with nonspecific symptoms (anorexia, nausea, malaise) or extrahepatic symptoms, and clinical hepatitis with jaundice, to fulminant fatal hepatitis. Anicteric or asymptomatic infection is most common in young children. Arthralgias, arthritis, or macular rashes can occur early in the course of the illness. Chronic HBV infection with persistence of hepatitis B surface antigen (HBsAg) occurs in as many as 90% of infants who become infected by perinatal transmission, and in 6% to 10% of older children, adolescents, and adults who acquire HBV infection. Chronically infected persons are at increased risk for developing chronic liver disease (cirrhosis, chronic active hepatitis, chronic persistent hepatitis) or primary hepatocellular carcinoma in later life.

Etiology: Hepatitis B virus is a DNA-containing, 42-nm hepadnavirus. Important components include HBsAg, hepatitis B core antigen (HBcAg), and hepatitis B e antigen (HBeAg).

Epidemiology: Hepatitis B virus is transmitted through blood or body fluids such as wound exudates, semen, cervical secretions, and saliva. Blood and serum contain the highest quantities of virus; saliva contains the lowest titers. The HBV chronic carrier (defined as an individual who is HBsAg-positive for 6 months or who is immunoglobulin M (IgM) anti-HBc-negative and HBsAg-positive) is the primary reservoir for infection. Modes of transmission include transfusion of blood or blood products (now rare in the United States as the result of current donor screening practices), sharing or reusing unsterilized needles or syringes, percutaneous or mucous membrane exposure to blood or body fluids, and homosexual and heterosexual activity. Hepatitis B virus can survive in the dried state for 1 week or longer and percutaneous contact with contaminated inanimate objects may transmit infection. Hepatitis B virus is not transmitted by the fecal-oral route.

A substantial proportion of individuals chronically infected with HBV ultimately die from chronic liver disease (ie, chronic active hepatitis or cirrhosis) or primary hepatocellular carcinoma. Persons infected as infants or young children appear to be at higher risk of death from liver disease than those infected as adults. The risk of chronic infection with HBV is related inversely to the age at the time infection occurs. Transmission from mother to infant during the perinatal period occurs in infants born to HBsAg-positive mothers. Among those who are also HBeAg-positive, 70% to 90% of their infants become chronically infected. If not infected during the perinatal period, infants of HBsAg-positive mothers remain at high risk of acquiring chronic HBV infection by person-to-person (horizontal) transmission during the first 5 years of life. Horizontal transmission during early childhood occurs frequently where the prevalence of HBV infection is high. It has been documented among infants of Alaskan natives, Pacific Islanders, and first-generation immigrant mothers from parts of the world (most of Asia, parts of the Middle East, Africa, the Amazon Basin, and eastern Europe) where HBV infection is highly endemic.

Other children at risk for infection include (1) residents in institutions for the developmentally disabled, (2) patients with clotting disorders and others receiving blood products, (3) hemodialysis patients, and (4) household contacts of HBV carriers. In child care facilities in the United States, the risk of transmission appears to be negligible from the limited available information. In some circumstances, however, school contacts of deinstitutionalized, developmentally disabled HBV carriers may be at increased risk for infection.

Most infected persons in the United States acquire their infection as adolescents or adults. Groups at highest risk include users of intravenous drugs, persons with multiple heterosexual partners, and homosexual men. Others at increased risk include those with occupational exposure to blood or body fluids, staff of institutions and nonresidential child care programs for the developmentally disabled, patients receiving hemodialysis, and sexual or household contacts of persons with an acute or chronic infection. However, more than one third of infected persons do not have a readily identifiable risk factor. The prevalence of infection among adolescents and adults in the general population is three to four times greater for blacks than for whites. Infection with HBV in adolescents and adults is associated with other sexually transmitted diseases, including syphilis.

The frequency of HBV infection and patterns of transmission vary markedly throughout the world. In the United States, Canada, Western Europe, Australia, and southern South America, infection is of low endemicity and occurs primarily in adulthood; 5% to 8% of the population have been infected and 0.2% to 0.9% are chronically infected. In contrast, HBV infection is highly endemic in China, Southeast Asia, the Central Asian republics, parts of the Middle East, Africa, the Amazon Basin, some Caribbean islands, and the Pacific Islands. In these areas, most infections occur in infants or children younger than 5 years of age, 70% to 90% of the adult population has been infected, and 8% to 15% are chronically infected. In the rest of the world, HBV infection is of moderate endemicity with chronic HBV carriage occurring in 2% to 7% of the population. Worldwide, HBV is a major cause of chronic liver disease and primary hepatocellular carcinoma.

The **incubation period** of acute infection is 45 to 160 days with an average of 120 days.

Diagnostic Tests: Commercial serologic antigen tests are available to detect HBsAg and HBeAg. Assays are also available for detection of antibody to HBsAg (anti-HBs), total antibody to hepatitis B core antigen (anti-HBc), IgM anti-HBc, and antibody to HBeAg (anti-HBe) (see Table 3.11, p 227). Hepatitis B surface antigen is detectable during acute infection, except during the period of resolution when anti-HBs has not yet appeared ("window phase"). Immunoglobulin M anti-HBc is highly specific in establishing the diagnosis of acute infection; it is present early in the infection as well as during the "window phase" in older children and adults. However, IgM anti-HBc is usually not present in perinatal HBV infection. Persons with chronic HBV infection have circulating HBsAg and anti-HBc. Only anti-HBs and anti-HBc are detected in persons with resolved infection, whereas anti-HBs alone is present in persons immunized with hepatitis B vaccine.

Treatment: No specific therapy for acute HBV infection is available. In chronic liver disease from adult-acquired HBV infection, alpha-interferon has been demonstrated to have limited efficacy in resolving the chronic infection, but the drug has been less effective for chronic infections acquired during early childhood.

Isolation of the Hospitalized Patient: Universal precautions should be scrupulously followed for patients with acute or chronic HBV infection. Patients with jaundice caused by a hepatitis virus yet to be identified should also be managed with enteric precautions in view of possible hepatitis A or hepatitis E viral infection.

TABLE 3.11—Diagnostic Tests for Hepatitis B Virus (HBV) Antigens and Antibodies

Abbreviation	Hepatitis B Virus Antigen or Antibody	Use
HBsAg	Surface antigen	Detection of acutely or chronically infected persons
Anti-HBs	Antibody to surface antigen (HBsAg)	Identification of persons who have had infections with HBV; determination of immunity after vaccination
HBeAg	e antigen	Identification of infected persons at increased risk for transmitting HBV
Anti-HBe	Antibody to HBe	Identification of HBsAg carriers with low risk for transmitting HBV
Anti-HBc	Antibody to core antigen (HBcAg)*	Identification of persons with acute or past HBV infection (not immunization)
IgM Anti-HBc	IgM antibody to core antigen	Identification of acute or recent HBV infections (including those in HBsAg-negative persons)

*No test is commercially available to measure core antigen (HBcAg).

For infants born to HBsAg-positive mothers, no special care other than removal of maternal blood by a gloved attendant is necessary. Blood of these infants should be handled with universal precautions since 1% to 3% are HBsAg positive due to in utero infection.

Control measures:

Hepatitis B Immunoprophylaxis. Pre-exposure immunization of susceptible persons with hepatitis B vaccine is the most effective means to prevent HBV transmission. To reduce transmission of HBV as soon as possible and, eventually, to eliminate it, universal immunization is necessary. Accordingly, hepatitis B vaccination is recommended for all infants as part of the routine childhood immunization schedule (see Tables 1.3 and 1.4, pp 23 and 24).

To accomplish universal vaccination most rapidly, immunization of all children during or before adolescence is necessary and recommended. If resources are insufficient to allow concurrent immunization of both infants and adolescents or preadolescents, infants should be preferentially immunized before all adolescents are routinely vaccinated. However, resources should be sought so that immunization of all children before or at adolescence can be accomplished. Immunization of adolescents can be accomplished by vaccination at an earlier age than 11 years, which has the advantage of less cost because of the lower recommended dose for younger children.

Postexposure immunoprophylaxis with hepatitis B vaccine and hepatitis B immune globulin (HBIG) can effectively prevent infection after exposure to virus. Serologic testing of all pregnant women for HBsAg identifies infants who require postexposure treatment beginning at birth to prevent perinatal HBV infections. Routine screening of blood donors and terminal inactivation of certain blood products has almost eliminated HBV transmission in the United States by administration of blood products.

Two types of products are available for immunoprophylaxis. Hepatitis B Immune Globulin (HBIG) provides temporary protection and is indicated only in specific postexposure circumstances (see Care of Exposed Persons, p 234). Hepatitis B vaccine is used for both pre-exposure and postexposure protection and provides long-term protection.

Hepatitis B Immune Globulin.* Hepatitis B Immune Globulin is prepared from plasma known to contain a high titer of anti-HBs and to be negative for antibodies to human immunodeficiency virus (HIV). The process used to prepare HBIG inactivates and eliminates HIV from the final product. The concentration of anti-HBs in immune globulin (IG) has declined as the result of current blood donor screening practices, and IG no longer has a role in postexposure prophylaxis of hepatitis B.

Hepatitis B Vaccines. Two types of hepatitis B vaccine have been licensed in the United States. The original vaccine prepared from the plasma of HBsAg carriers is no longer produced in the United States, but plasma-derived vaccines are available in other countries. The vaccines currently available in the United States are produced by recombinant DNA technology, using common bakers' yeast genetically modified to synthesize HBsAg. Vaccines contain 5 to 40 µg HBsAg protein per milliliter adsorbed to aluminum hydroxide, and thimerosal (1:20,000) as a preservative. Both plasma-derived and recombinant vaccines are highly effective and safe.

The concentration of HBsAg protein differs in the two recombinant vaccines currently licensed in the United States. However, equal rates of seroconversion are achieved with both vaccines when given to healthy infants, children, adolescents, or young adults in the dose recommended according to the person's age and other host factors (see Table 3.12, p 229).

Three intramuscular doses are required to induce a protective antibody response (anti-HBs $\geq$ 10 milli-international units [mIU] per milliliter) in more than 90% of healthy adults and in more than 95% of infants, children, and adolescents.

Vaccine Interchangeability. The immune response using one or two doses of a vaccine produced by one manufacturer, followed by one or more subsequent doses from a different manufacturer, has been demonstrated to be comparable to a full course of vaccination with a single product.

Routes and Sites of Administration. Vaccine can be given in the deltoid muscle to persons of any age or in the anterolateral thigh muscle of neonates and infants. If more than one injection must be given in a single limb, the thigh is the preferred site, and the injections are sufficiently separated so that

---

*Dosages recommended for postexposure prophylaxis are for products licensed in the United States. Since the concentration of anti-HBsAg in other products may vary, different dosages may be recommended in other countries.

TABLE 3.12—Recommended Dosages of Hepatitis B Vaccines[a]

	Vaccine[b,c]			
	Recombivax HB[d] Dose: µg	(mL)	Energix-B[e,f] Dose: µg	(mL)
Infants of HBsAg-negative mothers and children <11 y	2.5	(0.5)[g]	10	(0.5)
Infants of HBsAg-positive mothers (HBIG [0.5 mL] should also be given)	5	(0.5)[h] (1.0)[g]	10	(0.5)
Children and adolescents 11-19 y	5	(0.5)[h]	20	(1.0)
Adults ≥ 20 y	10	(1.0)[h]	20	(1.0)
Dialysis patients and other immunosuppressed adults	40	(1.0)[i]	40	(2.0)[j]

[a]Heptavax B (available from Merck & Co), a plasma-derived vaccine, is also licensed but no longer produced in the US.
[b]Vaccines should be stored at 2°C to 8°C. Freezing destroys effectiveness.
[c]Both vaccines are administered in a 3-dose schedule.
[d]Available from Merck & Co.
[e]The Food and Drug Administration has approved this vaccine for use in an optional 4-dose schedule at 0, 1, 2, and 12 mo.
[f]Available from SmithKline Beecham.
[g]Pediatric formulation.
[h]Adult formulation.
[i]Special formulation for dialysis patients.
[j]Two 1.0-mL doses given at one site in a 4-dose schedule at 0, 1, 2, and 6-12 mo.

four-dose local reactions are unlikely to overlap. Immunogenicity of hepatitis B vaccine in adults is diminished when given in the buttock. In patients with a bleeding diathesis, the risk of bleeding after intramuscular vaccine injection can be minimized by administration immediately after the patient's receipt of replacement factor, use of a 23-gauge (or less) needle, and application of direct pressure to the vaccination site for at least 2 minutes.

Low doses of hepatitis B vaccine given by the intradermal route result in lower seroconversion rates and serologic titers of anti-HBs. Intradermal vaccination should not be used in infants or children, and is not recommended for adults.

Efficacy and Booster Doses. Hepatitis B vaccines licensed in the United States have a 90% to 95% efficacy in preventing HBV infection and clinical hepatitis among susceptible children and adults. Among young adults, the incidence of loss of detectable serum antibody after 10 years of follow-up has ranged from 13% to 60%. Long-term studies of adults and children indicate that immune memory remains intact for 10 years or more and protects against chronic HBV infection, even though anti-HBs concentrations may become low or undetectable. Follow-up studies of children immunized at birth to prevent perinatal HBV infection have demonstrated continued high vaccine efficacy for at least 5 years.

For children and adults with normal immune status, routine booster doses of vaccine are not currently recommended. The possible need for booster doses will be assessed as additional information becomes available. For hemodialysis patients, the need for booster doses should be assessed by annual anti-HBs testing; a booster dose should be given when the antibody concentrations decline to less than 10 mIU/mL.

Adverse Reactions. Pain at the injection site and temperature higher than 37.7°C are the most frequently reported side effects in adults and children, occurring in 1% to 6% of recipients. Children receiving both hepatitis B vaccine and diphtheria-tetanus-pertussis (DTP) vaccine do not have a greater frequency of these mild side effects than children receiving DTP vaccine alone.

Allergic reactions after hepatitis B vaccination have been reported but appear to occur infrequently. Anaphylaxis appears to be exceedingly rare and has only been reported in adults.

Postvaccination surveillance for 3 years after licensure of the plasma-derived vaccine suggested an association in adults of borderline significance between Guillain-Barré syndrome (GBS) and receipt of the first vaccine dose. No association has been demonstrated in postvaccination surveillance for the recombinant hepatitis B vaccines. The Vaccine Safety Committee of the Institute of Medicine concluded in 1993 that the evidence was inadequate to accept or reject a causal relationship between hepatitis B vaccine and GBS. Early concerns that infectious agents, such as HIV, present in the donor plasma pools might contaminate the plasma-derived final product have proven to be unfounded.

Vaccination During Pregnancy. No adverse effect on the developing fetus has been observed when pregnant women have been vaccinated. Since HBV infection may result in severe disease for the mother and chronic infection in the newborn, pregnancy should not be considered a contraindication to vaccination of women. Lactation is also not a contraindication.

Serologic Testing. Susceptibility testing before vaccination is not routinely indicated for children or adolescents. Because of the higher cost of vaccine, testing for previous infection should be considered for risk groups with high rates of HBV infection, such as users of intravenous drugs, homosexual men, and household contacts of HBV carriers.

Postvaccination testing for immunity is not necessary after routine immunization. Postvaccination testing for anti-HBs is advised 1 to 3 months after the third vaccine dose for persons whose subsequent management depends on knowing their immune status. Such persons include (1) hemodialysis patients, (2) those with HIV infection, (3) those at occupational risk of exposure from sharp injuries, and (4) infants born to HBsAg-positive mothers. Testing for anti-HBs and HBsAg will identify those few infants who did not respond or who become chronically infected despite immunoprophylaxis, and will aid, thus, in their long-term medical management (see Management of Infants Born to HBsAg-Positive Mothers, p 235).

Pre-exposure Vaccination. High seroconversion rates and protective concentrations of anti-HBs (≥10 mIU/mL) are achieved when hepatitis B vaccine is administered in a variety of three-dose schedules, including those begun soon after birth in term infants. The preferred schedule for vaccinating adolescents and adults has been three doses, given at 0, 1, and 6 months, but alternative schedules, including those recommended for infants (see Universal Vaccination of Infants, below) are acceptable. The minimal interval between the first and second dose is 1 month. For the second and third doses, the minimal interval is 2 months. High response rates have been demonstrated with intervals of as long as 1 year between the second and third doses. Age-specific vaccine dosages are given in Table 3.12 (p 229).

Lapsed Immunizations. For infants with lapsed immunization (ie, the interval between doses is longer than that in one of the recommended schedules), the three-dose series can be completed, regardless of the interval from the last dose of vaccine (see Lapsed Immunizations, p 26). The series does not need to be restarted, and routine serologic testing for anti-HBs is not indicated (unless the child's mother is HBsAg-positive). Sufficient doses to complete the three-dose series should be administered at appropriate intervals.

Hepatitis B vaccine can be given to infants concurrently with other vaccines (see Simultaneous Administration of Multiple Vaccines, p 25).

Special Considerations. Larger vaccine doses or an increased number of doses have been required to induce protective antibody concentrations in a high proportion of adult hemodialysis patients (Table 3.12, p 229). Additional or larger doses may be necessary for immunocompromised persons, including HIV-seropositive individuals. Insufficient data are available to make specific recommendations at this time.

Universal Vaccination of Infants. Hepatitis B vaccination is recommended for all infants born to HBsAg-negative mothers. Three doses of vaccine before 18 months of age should be given. Special efforts should be made to ensure that infants are completely vaccinated by 6 to 9 months of age in populations with high rates of childhood hepatitis B infection, such as Alaskan Natives, Pacific Islanders, and infants of immigrants from countries in which HBV is endemic.

The recommended three-dose schedule is initiated during the newborn period or by 2 months of age; the second dose is given 1 to 2 months later; and the third dose is given at 6 to 18 months of age (see Table 3.13, p 232). The vaccines, however, are highly immunogenic in multiple schedules. Although the highest titers of anti-HBs are achieved when the last two doses of vaccine are spaced 4 months apart or longer, schedules with 2-month intervals between doses have been demonstrated to produce high rates of seroconversion. Some pediatricians have adopted other three-dose schedules in order to minimize the numbers of simultaneous injections (see Pre-exposure Vaccination, p 230, for the minimal intervals between doses). Vaccine dosages are given in Table 3.12 (p 229).

Preterm Infants. The optimal time to initiate hepatitis B immunization in premature infants with birth weight less than 2 kg has not been determined. Seroconversion rates in very-low-birth-weight infants in whom vaccination was initiated shortly after birth have been reported in some studies to be lower than those in preterm infants vaccinated at an older age or in term infants vaccinated shortly after birth. Therefore, for preterm infants weighing less than 2 kg at birth and born to HBsAg-negative women, initiation of vaccination should be delayed until just before hospital discharge if the infant weighs 2 kg or more, or until approximately 2 months of age when other rou-

TABLE 3.13—Recommended Schedules of Hepatitis B Vaccination for Infants Born to HBsAg-Negative Mothers.* (These guidelines may not apply to preterm infants; see p 231.)

Hepatitis B vaccine	Timing†
Dose 1	Birth (ie, preferably before hospital discharge) to 2 mo of age
Dose 2	1 to 2 mo after dose 1
Dose 3	6 to 18 mo of age‡

*Hepatitis B vaccine can be given concurrently with other vaccines, including DTP, *Haemophilus influenzae* type b conjugate, MMR, and/or oral poliovirus vaccine.
†See p 231for further explanation of possible variations in the schedule.
‡Infants in populations with high rates of childhood infections should complete the 3-dose series by 6 to 9 mo of age (see text).

tine immunizations are given. These infants do not need to have serologic testing for anti-HBs performed routinely after the third dose.

However, all premature infants born to HBsAg-positive mothers should receive immunoprophylaxis (HBIG and vaccine) beginning as soon as possible after birth, followed by appropriate postvaccination testing (see Prevention of Perinatal HBV Infection, p 234).

Vaccination of Adolescents. All adolescents should be immunized against HBV infection (see Hepatitis B Immunoprophylaxis, p 227). Implementation of hepatitis B immunization recommendations for adolescents can be initiated before adolescence, which has the advantage of lower cost per dose for children younger than 11 years of age (see Table 3.12, p 229). Special efforts should be made to vaccinate adolescents who (1) have sexually transmitted disease(s), (2) have had more than one sexual partner in the previous 6 months, (3) are intravenous drug users, (4) are sexually active homosexual or bisexual males, (5) are sexual contacts of high risk individuals, or (6) have tasks as employees, volunteers, or trainees that involve contact with blood or blood-contaminated body fluids (see also Table 3.14, p 234).

For users of intravenous drugs and male homosexual or bisexual teenagers, prevaccination serologic screening should be considered. Those known to have HIV infection should be tested for anti-HBs response after completion of the vaccine series. The choice of vaccination schedule should take into account compliance and resulting feasibility of delivering three doses of vaccine.

Immunization Between Infancy and Adolescence. A large number of children and adolescents will remain at risk for HBV infection for several decades after the initiation of universal immunization of infants. For most children in the United States, the risk of HBV infection is low until adolescence. Immunization of teenagers and children as, or before, they reach adolescence will provide age-appropriate protection from HBV infection (see Vaccination of Adolescents, above). However, children of certain ethnic groups (eg, Alaskan Natives, Pacific Islanders, and children of immigrants from countries with high rates of HBV infection) are at high risk for HBV infection resulting from person-to-person (horizontal) transmission. Because the highest risk of chronic HBV infection is in the first 5 years of life, "catch-up" vaccination of this age cohort is a high priority. In addition, immunization of other children before adolescence should be encouraged.

Immunization of High-Risk Groups (see Table 3.14, p 234, for complete listing).

Health Care Workers and Others With Occupational Exposure to Blood. The risk to a health care worker for HBV exposure depends on the tasks that he or she performs. If those tasks involve contact with blood or blood-contaminated body fluids, such workers should be vaccinated.

The risks for occupational HBV infection are often highest during the training of health care professionals. For this reason, when possible, vaccination should be completed during training and before contact with blood.

Children and Staff of Institutions for the Developmentally Disabled. Susceptible children in institutions for the developmentally disabled should be vaccinated. Staff who work closely with children should also be vaccinated. Susceptible children and staff who live or work in smaller (group) residential settings with known HBV carriers should also be vaccinated. Children discharged from residential institutions into community programs should be screened for HBsAg so that appropriate measures can be taken to prevent HBV transmission.

Staff of nonresidential child care programs (eg, schools and sheltered workshops) attended by known HBV carriers have a risk of infection comparable to that of health care workers, and they should be vaccinated. Vaccination of attendees in these programs should be considered and is strongly encouraged if a classmate who is an HBV carrier behaves aggressively or has special medical problems (eg, exudative dermatitis or open skin lesions) that increase the risk of exposure to his or her blood or serous secretions.

Hemodialysis Patients. Vaccination is recommended for susceptible, hemodialysis patients. Identification of patients with renal disease for vaccination early in the course of their disease is encouraged since the immunologic response to vaccine in patients with uremia who are vaccinated before they require dialysis is better than that when the vaccine is given after dialysis is required.

Patients With Bleeding Disorders Who Receive Certain Blood Products. Vaccination is recommended as soon as the specific clotting disorder is diagnosed. Prevaccination testing for HBsAg and anti-HBc is recommended for patients who have already received multiple infusions of these products.

Household Contacts and Sexual Partners of HBV Carriers. When HBV carriers are identified through prenatal screening, donor screening, or diagnostic or other serologic testing, their household and sexual contacts should be vaccinated.

Adoptees From Countries Where HBV Infection Is Endemic. Adoptees from countries where HBV infection is endemic should be screened for HBsAg. If the adoptee is HBsAg positive, other family members should be vaccinated.

International Travelers. Vaccination should be considered for persons who plan to spend more than 6 months in areas with high rates of HBV infection

TABLE 3.14—Persons Who Should Receive Hepatitis B Immunization

All Infants - Infants of HBsAg-positive mothers require postexposure immuno-prophylaxis with HBIG and vaccine.

Infants and children at risk of acquisition of HBV by person-to-person (horizontal) transmission should be immunized by 6-9 mo of age.

Adolescents* - Special efforts should be made to vaccinate those adolescents in the categories of high risk for hepatitis B virus (HBV) infection (see p 232).

Users of intravenous drugs.

Sexually active heterosexual persons with more than 1 sex partner in the previous 6 mo or with a sexually transmitted disease.

Sexually active homosexual or bisexual males.

Health care workers at risk of exposure to blood or body fluids.

Residents and staff of institutions for developmentally disabled persons.

Staff of nonresidential child care and school programs for developmentally disabled persons if attended by a known HBV carrier.

Hemodialysis patients.

Patients with bleeding disorders who receive certain blood products.

Household contacts and sexual partners of HBV carriers.

Members of households with adoptees from countries where HBV infection is endemic who are HBsAg positive.

International travelers who will live for more than 6 mo in an area of high HBV endemicity and who otherwise will be at risk.

Inmates of long-term correctional facilities.

*Implementation can be initiated before children reach adolescence.

and who will have close contact with the local population. Short-term travelers likely to have blood or sexual contact with residents of these areas should be vaccinated. Vaccination should begin at least 6 months before travel, although a partial series will offer some protection. The alternative four-dose schedule of 0, 1, 2, and 12 months (see Table 3.12, p 229) should provide protection if the first three doses can be delivered before travel.

These and additional indications for immunization of high-risk persons are given in Table 3.14, above.

Care of Exposed Persons (Postexposure Immunoprophylaxis) (see also Table 3.15, p 235). After exposure to HBV, appropriate immunoprophylactic treatment prevents infection.

Prevention of Perinatal HBV Infection. Transmission of perinatal HBV infection can be prevented in approximately 95% of infants born to HBsAg-positive mothers if HBIG is given within 12 hours after birth in conjunction with active immunization shortly after birth, and completed in the first 6 months of life. Hepatitis B vaccination given alone is 70% to 95% effective in preventing perinatal HBV infections.

TABLE 3.15—Guide to Postexposure Immunoprophylaxis for Hepatitis B Infection

Type of Exposure	Immunoprophylaxis	Refer to:
Perinatal	HBIG + vaccination	pp 234-236
Sexual - acute infection	HBIG + vaccination	p 237
Sexual - chronic carrier	Vaccination	p 233
Household contact - chronic carrier	Vaccination	p 233
Household contact - acute case with identifiable blood exposure	HBIG + vaccination	p 237
Infant (<12 mo) - acute case in primary caregiver	HBIG + vaccination	p 236
Accidental - percutaneous/ permucosal	HBIG ± vaccination	p 237 and Table 3.17, p 238

Serologic Screening of Pregnant Women. Prenatal HBsAg testing of all pregnant women is recommended to identify newborns who require immediate postexposure prophylaxis and because selective testing has failed to detect more than 50% of women who were HBsAg positive. Testing should be done during an early prenatal visit in each pregnancy, and it should be repeated late in pregnancy for HBsAg-negative women who are at high risk for HBV infection (eg, intravenous drug users and those with other intercurrent sexually transmitted diseases) or who have had clinical hepatitis. Household contacts and sexual partners of HBsAg-positive women identified through prenatal screening should be vaccinated if susceptible or judged likely to be susceptible to infection.

Management of Infants Born to HBsAg-Positive Women. Infants born to HBsAg-positive mothers should receive HBIG (0.5 mL) within 12 hours of birth and the initial dose of hepatitis B vaccine (see Table 3.12, p 229, for appropriate dosages) should be given concurrently at a different site. Subsequent doses of vaccine should be given as indicated in Table 3.16 (p 236). Preterm infants should also receive HBIG at birth, and the vaccine schedule should be initiated as soon as feasible (preferably also at birth) and always within the first month of life.

Infants born to HBsAg-positive women should be tested for anti-HBs and HBsAg 1 to 3 months after completion of the vaccination series. Testing for HBsAg will identify those few infants who become chronically infected and will aid in their long-term medical management. Infants who are anti-HBs and HBsAg-negative should receive 1 to 3 additional doses of vaccine, followed by testing for anti-HBs 1 month after each dose. Alternatively, a second three-dose series of vaccine can be administered at 1- to 2-month intervals, followed by testing for anti-HBs.

TABLE 3.16—Recommended Schedule of Hepatitis B Immuno-prophylaxis to Prevent Perinatal Transmission

Infant born to mother known to be HBsAg-positive:

Vaccine Dose* and HBIG	Age
First	Birth (within 12 h)
HBIG†	Birth (within 12 h)
Second	1 mo
Third	6 mo

Infant born to mother not screened for HBsAg:

Vaccine Dose	Age
First‡	Birth (within 12 h)
HBIG†	If mother is found to be HBsAg positive, give 0.5 mL as soon as possible, not later than 1 wk after birth
Second	1-2 mo§
Third	6-18 mo‖

*See Table 3.12 (p 229) for appropriate vaccine dose.
†HBIG (0.5 mL) given intramuscularly at a site different from that used for vaccine.
‡First dose is same as that for infant of HBsAg-positive mother (see Table 3.12, p 229). Subsequent doses and schedules are determined by maternal HBsAg status (see p 235 and Table 3.12, p 229).
§Infants of HBsAg-positive mothers should be vaccinated at 1 mo of age.
‖Infants of HBsAg-positive mothers should be vaccinated at 6 mo.

Infants Born to Mothers Not Tested for HBsAg. Pregnant women presenting for delivery whose HBsAg status is unknown should have their blood drawn for testing. While awaiting results, the infant should receive hepatitis B vaccine within 12 hours of birth in the dose recommended for infants born to HBsAg-positive mothers (see Table 3.12, p 229). If the woman is HBsAg-positive, the infant should receive HBIG as soon as possible and within 7 days of birth. If HBIG is unavailable, the infant, nevertheless, should continue to receive the subsequent two doses of hepatitis B vaccine at 1 and 6 months of age (Table 3.16, above). If the mother is HBsAg-negative, the infant should complete hepatitis B vaccination in the dose and schedule recommended for infants born to HBsAg-negative women (see Tables 3.12 and 3.13, pp 229 and 232).

Breast-feeding. Breast-feeding poses no additional risk for acquisition of HBV infection by the infant (see Human Milk, p 73).

Household Contacts of Persons With Acute HBV Infection. Since infants (younger than 12 months of age) have close contact with primary caregivers and have a higher risk for becoming HBV carriers after acute HBV infection, prophylaxis of an infant younger than 12 months of age with HBIG (0.5 mL) and hepatitis B vaccine in the recommended three-dose schedule is indicated if the mother or primary caregiver has acute HBV infection, unless the infant has already been fully vaccinated.

Prophylaxis for other household contacts of persons with acute HBV infection is not immediately indicated unless they have identifiable blood exposure to the index patient, such as by sharing of toothbrushes or razors. Such exposures should be treated like sexual exposures. If the index patient becomes an HBV carrier, all household contacts should receive hepatitis B vaccine. However, the routine immunization of these contacts is encouraged in view of the possibility of future household exposures and in accordance with the national goal of universal immunization.

Sexual Partners of Persons With Acute HBV Infection. Sexual partners of persons with acute HBV infection are at increased risk for infection, and HBIG is 75% effective in preventing these infections. The period after sexual exposure during which HBIG is effective is unknown, but it is unlikely to exceed 14 days. Susceptible sex partners should receive a single dose of HBIG (0.06 mL/kg) and should begin the hepatitis B vaccine series.

Acute Exposure to Blood That Contains (or Might Contain) HBsAg. For inadvertent percutaneous (needlestick, laceration, or bite), or permucosal (ocular or mucous membrane) exposure to blood, the decision to give HBIG prophylaxis and to vaccinate the patient, must include consideration of (1) whether the HBsAg status of the person who was the source of the exposure is available, and (2) the hepatitis B vaccination and vaccine-response status of the exposed person. For any exposure of a person not previously vaccinated, hepatitis B vaccination is recommended.

If possible, a blood sample should be tested for HBsAg from the person who was the source of the exposure and appropriate prophylaxis administered according to the hepatitis B vaccination status and anti-HBs response status (if known) of the exposed person (see Table 3.17, p 238).

Detailed advice on the management of health care workers and other persons exposed to blood that is or might be HBsAg positive is provided in the recommendations of the Advisory Committee of the Immunization Practices (ACIP) of the United States Public Health Service.*

Child Care. Children in out-of-home child care should receive hepatitis B vaccine as part of their routine immunization schedule. Immunization will not only reduce the potential for transmission after bites but will also allay anxiety about transmission from attendees who may be HBV carriers.

Children who are HBV carriers and who have no behavioral or medical risk factors, such as unusually aggressive behavior (eg, biting), generalized dermatitis, or a bleeding problem, should be admitted to child care without restrictions. The risk of HBV transmission in child care appears to be negligible. Routine screening for HBsAg is not warranted. Admission of HBV carrier children with risk factors such as those mentioned above should be assessed on an individual basis by the child's physician, the program director, and the responsible public health authorities. For further discussion, see Children in Out-of-Home Child Care (p 87).

---

*Centers for Disease Control and Prevention. Hepatitis B virus: a comprehensive strategy for eliminating transmission in the United States through universal childhood vaccination: recommendations of the Immunizations Practices Advisory Committee (ACIP). *MMWR.* 1991;40(RR-13):21-25

TABLE 3.17—Recommendations for Hepatitis B Prophylaxis After Percutaneous Exposure to Blood That Contains (or Might Contain) HBsAg*

Exposed Person	Treatment when source is found to be		
	HBsAg-Positive	HBsAg-Negative	Unknown or Not Tested
Unvaccinated	Administer HBIG x 1† and initiate hepatitis B vaccine‡	Initiate hepatitis B vaccine‡	Initiate hepatits B vaccine‡
Previously vaccinated			
Known responder	Test exposed person for anti-HBs§ 1. If adequate, no treatment 2. If inadequate, hepatitis B vaccine booster dose‡	No treatment	No treatment
Known nonresponder	HBIG x 2 or HBIG x 1, plus 1 dose of hepatitis B vaccine‡	No treatment	If known high-risk source, may treat as if source were HBsAg-positive
Person for whom response is unknown	Test exposed person for anti-HBs§ 1. If inadequate, HBIG x 1, plus hepatitis B vaccine booster dose‡ 2. If inadequate, no treatment	No treatment	Test exposed person for anti-HBs§ 1. If inadequate, hepatitis B vaccine booster dose 2. If adequate, no treatment

*Reproduced from Centers for Disease Control and Prevention. Hepatitis B virus: a comprehensive strategy for eliminating transmission in the United States through universal childhood vaccination: recommendations of the Immunization Practices Advisory Committee (ACIP). *MMWR.* 1991:40(RR-13):22
†Hepatitis B immune globulin (HBIG) dose 0.06 mL/kg, intramuscularly.
‡Hepatitis B vaccine dose—see Table 3.12 (p 229).
§Adequate anti-HBs is ≥10 mIU.

Hepatitis C (Parenterally Transmitted Non-A, Non-B Hepatitis)

Clinical Manifestations: Hepatitis C is characterized by mild or asymptomatic infection with an insidious onset of jaundice and malaise. In some cases, the course is remittent. An average of 50% of the patients develop chronic liver disease, including cirrhosis. Hepatocellular carcinoma may be associated with hepatitis C as well as chronic hepatitis B infections.

Etiology: The hepatitis C virus (HCV) is a single-stranded RNA virus classified as a separate genus in the *Flaviviridae* family.

Epidemiology: Transmission of HCV can occur by parenteral administration of blood or blood products, but most hepatitis C cases in the United States are not associated with blood transfusions. Approximately 70% to 90% of cases of parenterally transmitted non-A, non-B hepatitis in the United States are caused by HCV. Some evidence indicates that HCV is also sexually transmitted, but the role of person-to-person contact is not well defined. Groups at high risk include parenteral drug users, persons transfused with blood or blood components, health care workers with frequent blood exposure, persons with sexual or household contact with an infected person, and persons with multiple sexual partners. No source or risk factor can be identified in a substantial number of cases. Perinatal transmission probably occurs, but the risks and consequences have not been defined. Disease is most frequently recognized in adults; reported cases are infrequent in children younger than 15 years of age. Like hepatitis B virus infection, HCV can result in chronic infection. The period of communicability is not known.

The average **incubation period** is 7 to 9 weeks, with a range of 2 to 24 weeks.

Diagnostic Tests: Serologic tests for anti-HCV have been commercially available since 1990, and improved screening tests became available in 1992. The screening test is positive in most patients infected with HCV; however, anti-HCV may be absent during the acute illness. In populations with a low prevalence of HCV infection, the rate of false positivity for anti-HCV with the screening enzyme immunoassay is high. Although no confirmatory tests have been developed, supplemental tests for specificity are available.

Treatment: Alpha interferon has been approved by the Food and Drug Administration for the treatment of chronic hepatitis C. It is beneficial in a small proportion of cases.

Isolation of the Hospitalized Patient: The routinely recommended universal precautions are indicated for the duration of the illness. Patients with acute viral hepatitis of unknown type should be managed with enteric as well as universal precautions.

Control Measures:
Care of Exposed Persons:
- Results of studies evaluating the prophylactic value of IG have been equivocal. Now that screening of plasma donors for anti-HCV and exclusion of anti-HCV positive persons from the donor pool is recommended in the United States, IG manufactured in this country does not contain antibodies to HCV. Therefore, IG is unlikely to prevent hepatitis C.
- Screening donors of blood, organs, tissue, and semen for anti-HCV antibody is recommended. When screening is done in low-prevalence populations, a high percentage of the positive results are false positives.

Hepatitis Delta Virus

Clinical Manifestations: Hepatitis delta virus (HDV) infection causes hepatitis, but only in conjunction with hepatitis B virus (HBV) infection. Infection in a person with acute or chronic HBV infection can result in acute, possibly fulminant hepatitis, or in chronic hepatitis that may progress to cirrhosis.

Etiology: Hepatitis delta virus has been characterized as a 35- to 37-nm particle consisting of an RNA fragment and a delta protein antigen (HDAg), both of which are coated with hepatitis B surface antigen (HBsAg). Hepatitis delta virus requires HBV as a "helper virus" and cannot produce infection in the absence of HBV.

Epidemiology: Hepatitis delta virus can cause an infection at the same time as the initial hepatitis B infection (coinfection), or it can infect an individual already chronically infected with HBV (superinfection). Transmission is similar to that of HBV, ie, by parenteral, percutaneous, or mucous membrane inoculation. Hepatitis delta virus can be transmitted by blood or blood products, injecting drug use, or sexual contact, as long as HBsAg is present in the patient's blood. Transmission from mother to newborn infant is uncommon. Intrafamilial spread can occur among HBsAg carriers. Some chronic HBV infections can be accompanied by chronic HDV infection. High-prevalence areas include southern Italy and parts of Eastern Europe, South America, Africa, and the Middle East. In contrast to HBV infection, HDV is uncommon in the Far East. In the United States, HDV infection is found most frequently in parenteral drug abusers, hemophiliacs, and persons immigrating from endemic areas.

The **incubation period** for HDV superinfection, estimated from inoculation of animals, is about 2 to 8 weeks. When HBV and HDV coinfect, the incubation period is similar to that of HBV infection (45 to 160 days; average 120 days).

Diagnostic Tests: A test for anti-HDV antibody is commercially available. Tests for IgM-specific anti-HDV antibody and delta antigen (HDAg) are research procedures at present. If markers of HDV infection exist, coinfection with hepatitis B virus can usually be differentiated from superinfection of an established HBsAg carrier by testing for IgM hepatitis B core antibody (IgM anti-HBc). Absence of markers of acute hepatitis B infection in a patient with HDV infection suggests that the person is an HBsAg carrier.

Treatment: Supportive.

Isolation of the Hospitalized Patient: The same precautions as for HBV infection, ie, the routinely recommended universal precautions for all patients, should be followed (see Hepatitis B, p 226).

Control Measures: The same control and preventive measures as for HBV infection are indicated, since HDV cannot be transmitted in the absence of HBV infection. Carriers of HBsAg should take extreme care to avoid exposure to HDV since no currently available immunobiologic exists for prevention of HDV superinfection.

Hepatitis E
(Enterically Transmitted
Non-A, Non-B Hepatitis)

Clinical Manifestations: Hepatitis E is an acute illness with jaundice, malaise, anorexia, fever, abdominal pain, and arthralgia.

Etiology: The hepatitis E virus (HEV) is a single-stranded RNA virus that is structurally similar to a calicivirus.

Epidemiology: Transmission of HEV is by the fecal-oral route. Disease is more common in adults than in children, and it has an unusually high incidence of mortality in pregnant women. Cases have been reported in epidemics or sporadically in parts of Asia, Africa, and Mexico, and have usually been related to contaminated water. Endemic HEV transmission has not been recognized in Western Europe or the United States, but cases have occurred in travelers to endemic areas. The period of communicability after acute infection is unknown, but chronic infection appears not to occur.

The mean **incubation period** is approximately 40 days, with a range of 15 to 60 days.

Diagnostic Tests: No serologic test is commercially available. The diagnosis is established by exclusion of acute hepatitis A, B, C, D, and other viral causes of acute hepatitis. Research laboratories have developed serologic assays (enzyme immunoassay, Western blot, and fluorescent antibody blocking assay) that detect antibody to HEV; virus RNA can be identified in stool and serum by the polymerase chain reaction.

Treatment: Supportive.

Isolation of the Hospitalized Patient: Enteric precautions should be observed for the duration of the illness, in addition to the routinely recommended universal precautions.

Control Measures: Good sanitation and not ingesting potentially contaminated food and water are the most effective measures. Passive immunoprophylaxis against hepatitis E with immune globulin prepared in the United States has not been demonstrated to be effective.

Herpes Simplex

Clinical Manifestations:

Neonatal. In newborn infants, herpes simplex virus (HSV) infection can manifest as (1) generalized, systemic infection involving the liver and other organs, occasionally including the central nervous system (CNS) (encephalitis); (2) localized CNS disease; or (3) localized infection that may involve the skin, eyes, and mouth (SEM). Ocular manifestations include conjunctivitis, keratitis, and chorioretinitis. Typical vesicular skin lesions are helpful diagnostically, if present. In about one third of the patients, SEM involvement is the first indication of the infection. In another third, other evidence of systemic or CNS disease can occur before the appearance of SEM lesions. In another third, infants with systemic or localized encephalitis will not have SEM involvement. In the absence of the more characteristic SEM lesions (such as keratitis), the differential diagnosis of respiratory distress, sepsis, and convulsions in newborn infants must include HSV infection. Although common in older children, asymptomatic HSV infection probably occurs rarely, if at all, in neonates.

Neonatal herpetic infections are frequently severe, with a high mortality rate and significant neurologic and/or ocular impairment of survivors, particularly in the absence of antiviral therapy. Recurrent skin lesions are frequently noted in surviving infants and are associated with sequelae if they occur more than three times in the first 6 months.

Initial symptoms can occur shortly after birth or as late as 4 to 6 weeks after birth. Disseminated disease usually occurs during the first 2 weeks of life; disease localized to the CNS or to the SEM more often occurs during the second or third week.

Children and Infants Beyond the Neonatal Period. Gingivostomatitis is the most commonly recognized manifestation of primary HSV infection. Gingivostomatitis is characterized by fever, irritability, and an ulcerative enanthem involving the gingiva and the mucous membranes of the mouth. Most HSV infections at this age are asymptomatic.

Genital herpes is characterized by vesicular or ulcerative lesions of the male or female genital organs and/or perineum. It is most common in adolescents and adults.

Patients with eczematoid dermatitis who are infected with HSV can develop eczema herpeticum with vesicular lesions concentrated in the areas of eczematous involvement.

In immunocompromised patients, severe local lesions and less commonly disseminated HSV infection with generalized vesicular skin lesions and visceral involvement can occur.

Herpes simplex virus persists in a latent form after primary infection. Reactivation of latent virus most often is manifested by "cold sores" (herpes labialis). These lesions appear as single or grouped vesicles in the perioral region, usually on the vermilion border of the lips. Reactivation of genital HSV on the penis, scrotum, vulva, cervix, buttocks, and perianal areas, or on the thighs or back can also occur.

Eye infections can be a primary manifestation of HSV infection or a recurrence; they vary in severity from a superficial conjunctivitis to involvement of the deeper layers of the cornea.

Herpes simplex virus encephalitis can result from primary or recurrent infection and is associated with fever, alterations in the state of consciousness, personality changes, convulsions, and usually focal neurologic findings. Encephalitis frequently has an acute onset with a fulminant course, leading to coma and death in untreated patients. Cerebrospinal fluid (CSF) pleocytosis with both lymphocytes and red blood cells is usual. Herpes simplex virus can also cause meningitis with nonspecific clinical manifestations that are usually mild and self-limited. Meningitis is usually associated with primary HSV-2 genital infection.

An herpetic whitlow consists of single or multiple vesicular lesions on the distal parts of fingers.

Etiology: Herpes simplex viruses are large, enveloped viruses containing DNA. The two types have major genomic and antigenic differences. Type 1 (HSV-1) usually involves the face and skin above the waist. Type 2 (HSV-2) usually involves the genitalia and skin below the waist in adults and is the most common cause of disease in the neonate. However, either type of virus can be found in either site, depending on the source of the infection.

Epidemiology:

Neonatal. The incidence of neonatal HSV infection is low; estimates range from 1 per 3,000 to 1 per 20,000 live births. Infants who develop HSV infection are significantly more likely to have been born prematurely and/or to be of low birth weight. Herpes simplex virus is most frequently transmitted to an infant during passage through an infected maternal lower genital tract during birth or by an ascending infection, sometimes through apparently intact membranes. Thus, most neonatal infections are caused by HSV-2, but 15% to 20% are HSV-1 infections. Late intrauterine infections that manifest soon after birth are not infrequent. Intrauterine infections causing congenital malformations have been implicated in rare cases. Other less common sources of neonatal infection include the following: (1) postnatal transmission from the mother or father, most often from a nongenital infection (eg, mouth, hands, or around the nipples); or (2) postnatal transmission in the nursery from another infected infant, probably via the hands of personnel attending the infants. Postnatal transmission from personnel with fever blisters to neonates has been extremely rare.

The risk of HSV infection in an infant born vaginally to a mother with a first-episode, primary genital infection is high and has been estimated to be at least 33% to 50%. The risk to an infant born to a mother with recurrent HSV infection at delivery is much lower—at most 3% to 5%. **Distinguishing between primary and recurrent HSV infection in women by history or physical examination may not be possible.** Surveys suggest that 0.01% to 0.39% of American women shed HSV at delivery. Either primary or recurrent infection can be present without signs or symptoms or with nonspecific findings (eg, vaginal discharge, genital pain, or shallow ulcers). Most infants who develop HSV infection have been born to women without history or clinical findings suggestive of active infection during pregnancy.

Incubation period: see Clinical Manifestations.

Children and Infants Beyond the Neonatal Period. Herpes simplex virus infections are ubiquitous and are transmitted from person to person throughout the year. Infection with HSV-1 results primarily from direct contact with infected oral secretions or lesions. Infection with HSV-2 usually results from direct contact with infected genital secretions or lesions through sexual activity. Type 1 strains can be recovered from the genital tract; type 2 strains probably can be recovered from the pharynx as a result of oral-genital sexual activity. Herpes simplex virus type 1 genital infections in children can also result from autoinoculation of virus from the mouth. Nevertheless, sexual abuse must always be considered in prepubertal children with genital herpes.

Herpes simplex virus type 1 is usually contracted during the first few years of life in infected individuals in lower socioeconomic groups; in higher socioeconomic groups, more than one half of infected individuals do not contract HSV-1 until after they reach adulthood. Children in child care centers may have high rates of HSV-1 acquisition. The frequency of HSV-2 infection correlates with sexual activity, and HSV infections can occur in association with other sexually transmitted diseases.

Direct inoculation can cause herpetic whitlows of the fingers, usually from hand contact with HSV-containing oral or genital secretions. Direct inoculation of skin can also occur, particularly among wrestlers (eg, herpes gladiatorum).

The period of time that patients with primary gingivostomatitis or genital HSV can transmit infection is difficult to define. Virus can usually be isolated for at least 1 week, and occasionally for several months. Herpes simplex virus may be shed intermittently from the mouth or genital tract in the absence of clinical manifestations years after infection. Most primary infections and recurrences are asymptomatic or are associated with minor intraoral or genital lesions. In recurrent lesions, virus is present in the highest concentrations in the first 24 hours after the appearance of vesicles. The amount of virus decreases rapidly in the next 24 hours and usually cannot be recovered after 5 days. Herpes simplex virus can be transmitted during primary infections or during recurrences, regardless of whether signs or symptoms are present.

Genital HSV-2 and HSV-1 infections are commonly transmitted during sexual intercourse and by oral-genital sexual activity. Many primary infections are asymptomatic. Some individuals may not have recurrences; in others, recurrences can occur as often as every month. Genital HSV-2 infections are more likely to recur than those caused by HSV-1. Viral shedding during recurrences can also occur in the absence of clinical signs.

The **incubation period** of genital infection, although not well defined, has been estimated to be 2 to 14 days. For gingivostomatitis, it is estimated to be 2 to 12 days.

Diagnostic Tests: Herpes simplex virus can be cultured relatively easily. Special transport media are available for specimens that cannot be inoculated immediately. Viral detection usually requires 1 to 3 days after tissue culture inoculation. Newer diagnostic techniques, such as direct fluorescent antibody staining of vesicle scrapings or enzyme immunoassay detection of HSV antigens, offer more rapid diagnosis. These techniques are as specific but less sensitive than culture. A variety of techniques are available for distinguishing HSV-1 from HSV-2 isolates.

For the diagnosis of neonatal HSV infection, specimens for culture are obtained from skin vesicles, mouth or nasopharynx, eyes, urine, blood, stool or rectum, and CSF. Positive swab cultures obtained from the conjunctiva, nasopharynx, mouth, stool, or rectum of infants more than 24 to 48 hours after birth are more likely to indicate viral replication and infection than transient colonization from intrapartum exposure. The most sensitive technique for detecting genital HSV infection in symptomatic pregnant women is culture of labial or cervical lesions or, in the absence of lesions, culture of the cervix and vulva. The presence of multinucleated giant cells and eosinophilic intranuclear inclusions in Papanicolaou-stained smears of the cervix indicates probable HSV infection, but this method is less sensitive than viral isolation.

Acute and convalescent sera can be tested for rises in HSV antibody to confirm acute primary infection, but serologic diagnosis is frequently less helpful than viral isolation, as "acute" sera are often obtained late in the course of the illness. Rises in antibody titer are not usually demonstrable during recurrences. Tests available in research laboratories are reliable in differentiating antibodies to HSV-1 from HSV-2 antibodies.

In children with suspected HSV encephalitis, a brain biopsy is useful before (or soon after) therapy is initiated, as it may identify other treatable causes of encephalitis or confirm a diagnosis of HSV infection. Cerebrospinal fluid cultures are rarely positive for virus in patients with encephalitis. Herpes simplex virus DNA in the CSF of patients with HSV encephalitis may be detected by the polymerase chain reaction (PCR), obviating the need for a brain biopsy. However, this test is currently available only in research laboratories.

Treatment: In children, acyclovir and vidarabine have been used primarily for potentially serious infections, as occur in neonates and immunocompromised children. The use of these drugs in less serious conditions has been limited primarily to adults, and information on children with these conditions is limited. For recommended antiviral dosages and duration of therapy, see Antiviral Drugs (p 567).

Neonatal. Acyclovir and vidarabine are both effective in the treatment of neonatal HSV infection localized to the skin, eyes, and mouth. Antiviral treatment is also beneficial in the treatment of localized CNS disease and, to a lesser extent, in the treatment of generalized, systemic infection. Initiation of therapy early in the course of the disease may enhance its efficacy. For reasons of less toxicity and ease of administration, acyclovir (30 mg/kg/d in three divided doses, given intravenously) is the preferred drug. Some experts give higher doses (45 to 60 mg/kg/d). The optimal duration of therapy has not been established; the recommended minimal duration is 14 days. Courses as long as 21 days may be indicated in some cases. A collaborative, multi-institution trial to determine whether 21 days of therapy improves outcome is in progress. Relapse of disease after cessation of treatment can occur and most often appears to be related to host factors. The need for retreatment of infants with recurrent skin lesions is undetermined and is also under study.

Infants with ocular involvement due to HSV infection should receive a topical ophthalmic drug (specifically, 1% to 2% trifluridine, 1% iododeoxyuridine, or 3% vidarabine), as well as parenteral antiviral therapy. Ophthalmologic consultation is strongly advised.

Genital Infection.

Primary. In adults, acyclovir diminishes the duration of symptoms and viral shedding in primary genital herpes. Oral acyclovir initiated within 6 days of onset of the disease has been demonstrated to shorten by approximately 3 to 5 days the median duration of the signs and symptoms and viral shedding from primary lesions. Intravenous acyclovir should be used only for primary genital herpes in patients with a severe or complicated course that requires hospitalization. Topical acyclovir (5%) ointment applied to primary genital herpes minimally reduces viral shedding and symptoms. Systemic or topical treatment of primary herpetic lesions does not affect the subsequent risk or severity of recurrences.

Recurrent. Antiviral therapy has minimal effect on recurrent genital herpes. Oral acyclovir initiated within 2 days of onset of symptoms shortens the mean clinical course by 1 day. Topical acyclovir is not beneficial in immunocompetent hosts.

Oral acyclovir administered daily to adults for suppressive therapy has been effective in decreasing the frequency of recurrences of active disease in persons with frequent recurrences (six or more episodes per year) of genital HSV infection. After 1 year of continuous daily therapy, acyclovir should be discontinued and the patient's recurrence rate should be assessed. Usually, however, the disease recurs at the same frequency as before the course of suppressive therapy. Acyclovir appears to be safe in adults receiving the drug for 3 years, but the long-term effects are unknown.

Acyclovir is not recommended for pregnant women.

Other Mucocutaneous HSV Infections.

Immunocompromised Hosts. Intravenous acyclovir and vidarabine have been effective in the treatment and prevention of dissemination of mucocutaneous HSV infections. Topical acyclovir can also accelerate the healing of recurrent lesions in immunocompromised patients. Both oral and intravenous acyclovir have been beneficial in reducing the rate of recurrences during, but not after, the course of therapy.

In the immunocompromised patient who has received prolonged or recurrent treatment with acyclovir for HSV infection, acyclovir-resistant HSV may be isolated from unresponsive lesions or lesions that occur or expand while the patient is receiving acyclovir. In this circumstance, foscarnet is the drug of choice.

Immunocompetent Hosts. Insufficient information is available to determine if the effects of acyclovir on primary or recurrent nongenital mucocutaneous herpetic disease are similar to those observed for genital HSV infections. In adults, minimal therapeutic benefit has been demonstrated from use of oral acyclovir in individuals with recurrent herpes labialis ("cold sores"). Children with primary gingivostomatitis have been treated with acyclovir but definitive data on efficacy are lacking.

In a small, controlled study in adults with recurrent herpes labialis (6 or more episodes per year), prophylactic acyclovir given in a dose of 400 mg twice daily was effective in reducing the frequency of recurrent episodes.

Ocular. Treatment of eye lesions usually should be undertaken with the help of an ophthalmologist. A variety of DNA inhibitors, such as 1% to 2% trifluridine, 1% iododeoxyuridine, and 3% vidarabine, have been successful for topical therapy of superficial keratitis. Many ophthalmologists also treat with oral acyclovir. Topical steroids are contraindicated in suspected HSV conjunctivitis. However, ophthalmologists may choose to use steroids in conjunction with antiviral drugs to treat more locally invasive infections.

Encephalitis. Acyclovir given intravenously is the drug of choice for the treatment of patients with HSV encephalitis; it is more likely to be beneficial if treatment is initiated early in the illness. Therapy is less effective in adults than in children, and less effective in comatose and semicomatose patients than in those who are not. Duration of therapy is for 14 to 21 days.

Isolation of the Hospitalized Patient:

Neonates With HSV Infection. Neonates with HSV infection, or with positive cultures in the absence of disease, should be hospitalized in a private room, if possible, and managed with contact isolation precautions for the duration of the illness.

Neonates Exposed to HSV During Delivery. Neonates with documented perinatal exposure to HSV may be in the incubation phase of infection and should be carefully observed. One method of infection control is to have the infant room in continuously with the mother in a private room. Infants born vaginally, or by cesarean delivery if membranes have been ruptured for more than 4 to 6 hours, to a mother with active HSV lesions should be physically separated from other infants and placed in contact isolation if they are hospitalized in the nursery during the incubation period. Some experts recommend separation of infants born by cesarean delivery irrespective of the duration of ruptured membranes before delivery. The risk of HSV infection in possibly exposed infants (eg, those born to a mother with a history of recurrent genital herpes) is low. Although expert opinion varies, special isolation precautions for these infants are not needed in most instances.

Women in Labor and Postpartum Women With HSV Infection. Women in labor who have active HSV lesions, or whose viral cultures or Papanicolaou smear are positive, should be managed during labor, delivery, and the postpartum period with contact isolation or drainage/secretion precautions, depending on the extent of the mucocutaneous disease. These mothers should be instructed on the importance of careful hand washing before and after caring for their infant. A clean covering gown may be used to help avoid contact of the infant with the lesions or infectious secretions. A mother with herpes labialis ("cold sores") or stomatitis should wear a disposable surgical mask when touching her newborn until the lesions have crusted and dried. She should not kiss or nuzzle her newborn until the lesions have cleared. Herpetic lesions on other skin sites should be covered.

Breast-feeding is acceptable if no lesions are present on the breast and if active lesions elsewhere on the mother are covered (see Human Milk, p 73).

Children With Mucocutaneous HSV Infection. For patients with severe mucocutaneous HSV infection, contact isolation is advised. Patients with localized recurrent lesions should be managed with drainage/secretion precautions for the duration of the illness or until the virus no longer can be recovered from the lesions.

Patients With Central Nervous System HSV Infection. Patients with infection limited to the CNS do not require special isolation precautions.

Control Measures:

Prevention of Neonatal Infection. Expert opinion on the appropriate management of pregnant women to minimize the risk of neonatal HSV infection has changed considerably in the past decade. Weekly HSV cultures during pregnancy are no longer recommended, and women with history of genital HSV infection and signs or symptoms of infection during pregnancy, or those whose sexual partners have genital HSV infection, are recognized to be at low (albeit somewhat increased) risk of transmitting HSV to their infants (see Epidemiology, p 243). In addition, intrapartum cultures have not had sufficient predictive value to be useful.

Experts differ about the recommendations for the prevention of neonatal infection in the many different circumstances that occur. Management of the infant exposed to HSV during delivery, in particular, will differ according to the status of the mother's infection, mode of delivery, and expert opinion (see Care of Newborns Whose Mothers Have Active Genital Lesions, p 249). Current recommendations for management of pregnant women for the prevention of HSV infection include the following:

- *During pregnancy.* All pregnant women should be questioned during a prenatal visit about history of HSV infection in themselves or in their sexual partners, and signs and symptoms of current infection should be sought as part of prenatal care.
- *Women in labor.* During labor, all women should be questioned about recent and current HSV symptoms and carefully examined for evidence of genital HSV infection. Cesarean delivery of women in labor who have clinically apparent HSV infection (particularly primary infection) may reduce the risk of neonatal HSV infection unless the membranes have been ruptured for more than 4 to 6 hours. The risk when the membranes have been ruptured for longer periods is uncertain. Most experts suggest that infants should be delivered by cesarean section whenever the birth canal is infected, even if the membranes have been ruptured for 6 or more hours. A history of genital HSV for a woman in labor is not an indication for cesarean section. Scalp monitors should be avoided when possible in infants of women suspected of having HSV infection.

A cesarean section should be performed immediately on a woman who presents with ruptured membranes and active genital lesions at term, or at a time when the fetal lung is known to be mature. In a woman who presents with ruptured membranes and active genital lesions at a time when the fetal lung is immature, the appropriate course of action is not clear. The options include (1) expectant management (ie, labor is allowed to follow its natural course), with or without administration of intravenous acyclovir (15 mg/kg in three divided doses) to the mother; (2) delay of delivery until betamethasone can be given to enhance the maturity of the fetal lungs; and, (3) cesarean delivery with administration of topical surfactant to the infant. The value and risks of acyclovir in this situation of expectant management is unknown. Use of acyclovir in this circumstance is not approved by the Food and Drug Administration, and it cannot be recommended for routine use. Since acyclovir given to the mother might decrease her duration of viral shedding and does result in appreciable drug concentrations in the fetus, the risk of HSV disease in the infant might be reduced.

Care of Newborns Whose Mothers Have Active Genital Lesions. [*]

- *By vaginal delivery.* Since the risk to infants exposed to HSV lesions during delivery varies in different circumstances from less than 5% to 50% or more, the decision to treat the asymptomatic, exposed infant empirically with intravenous acyclovir is controversial and difficult. The infection rate of infants born to mothers with active recurrent genital herpes infections is 5% or less. Most experts would not empirically treat these infants with acyclovir. However, for those infants born of mothers with a first-episode, primary genital infection, the risk of infection is high (at least 33% to 50%). Risk is also increased for exposed infants born prematurely or those who have a history of instrumentation or lacerations during delivery. Some experts, therefore, recommend empiric acyclovir treatment at birth after HSV cultures have been obtained (see Recommendations, p 250) in the case of infants who are exposed during delivery to maternal HSV infection and who have one or more of the aforementioned risk factors. Other experts would obtain HSV cultures 24 to 48 hours after delivery, assuming that the infant is asymptomatic, and they would initiate acyclovir if the result of cultures is positive. However, if the infant develops manifestations suggestive of HSV infection, such as skin or scalp rashes (especially vesicular lesions) and/or unexplored clinical manifestations (such as those of sepsis), then cultures should be obtained, irrespective of age, and acyclovir should be initiated immediately.

    In assessing the risk of HSV infection for the exposed infant, differentiation of primary, first-episode genital infection from recurrent HSV infection in the mother is helpful, but this differentiation is often difficult or impossible. In addition, primary infection and first-episode infection are not necessarily the same, as some primary infections are asymptomatic, in which case the first symptomatic episode is a secondary (recurrent) infection. In selected instances, serologic testing can be useful. For example, a woman with lesions who is seronegative for HSV antibody has primary infection, and her infant has a high risk of infection if born vaginally. Assessment of seropositive women, however, necessitates differentiation of HSV-1 antibodies from HSV-2 antibodies. In the future, reliable type-specific antibody

---

*For further information and the recommendations of the Infectious Disease Society of America, see Prober CG, Corey L, Brown ZA, et al. The management of pregnancies complicated by genital infections with herpes simplex virus. *Clin Infect Dis.* 1992;15:1031-1038

assays may allow the determination of the presence or absence of HSV-2 antibodies to assist in the categorizing of maternal infection.

Recommendations. In the management of exposed, asymptomatic infants, those who were delivered vaginally of mothers with active genital lesions can be categorized according to the type of maternal infection as follows:

- Mother with primary, first-episode infection.
- Mother with known, recurrent lesions.
- Mother whose status (primary vs recurrent) is not known.

Infants in each category should be cultured for HSV at 24 to 48 hours after birth (and sooner if symptoms develop), including swabs or specimens for the eyes, CSF, urine, stool or rectum, and nasopharynx (see Diagnostic Tests, p 244). For infants whose mothers have primary, first-episode infection, experts differ on the indications for acyclovir, as previously described (see p 245).

The infant whose mother has known, recurrent genital lesions should be observed carefully for skin or scalp rashes, especially vesicular lesions and unexplained clinical manifestations including respiratory distress, seizures, and signs of sepsis. If an infant has any of these manifestations, he or she should be evaluated for possible HSV as well as for bacterial infection. Skin lesions, conjunctiva, nasopharynx, mouth, CSF, and urine should be cultured for HSV. Acyclovir should be initiated if culture(s) from the infant become positive, if the CSF findings are abnormal, or if HSV infection is otherwise strongly suspected while awaiting culture results (assuming bacterial culture results are negative or pending, and no other causes of the infant's clinical manifestations are found).

Infants born to mothers in whom the differentiation between primary and recurrent infection cannot be made should be managed as recommended for those born to mothers with recurrent infection.

- *By cesarean delivery.* The infant born to a mother with herpetic lesions at delivery (primary, secondary, or unknown in status) should be observed carefully, and cultures should be obtained, as recommended for the potentially exposed infant born by vaginal delivery. Similarly, antiviral therapy should be initiated if culture(s) from the infant are positive, or if HSV is strongly suspected while awaiting culture results (assuming other causes of the infant's manifestations are not identified).

   Data confirming the benefit or need for antiviral therapy in these circumstances of the exposed infant born by vaginal or cesarean delivery are not yet available.

- *Infants born to mothers with history of genital HSV but no active lesions at delivery.* These infants should be carefully evaluated, as previously described. The value of the intrapartum cultures from these women is unclear. One or more positive cultures indicates only exposure and does not necessarily indicate infection. Cerebrospinal fluid examination of asymptomatic neonates is not necessary.

Other Recommendations:

- The length of in-hospital observation for infants at increased risk for neonatal HSV is empiric and based on factors specific to the infant and local resources, such as the family's ability to observe the infant at home, availability of follow-up care, and clinical assessment.

- Delay of elective or ritual circumcision for about a month for infants at highest risk of disease is prudent.
- Since neonatal HSV infection can occur as late as 6 weeks after delivery, physicians must be vigilant and not ignore a new rash or symptoms that might be caused by HSV.

Care of Persons With Dermatitis. Patients with dermatitis are at risk of developing eczema herpeticum. If these patients are hospitalized, special care should be taken to avoid exposure to HSV. They should not be kissed by persons with "cold sores" or handled by people with herpetic whitlow.

Care of Children With Mucocutaneous Infections Who Are in Child Care or School. Oral HSV infections are common in children who are in child care or school. Most of these infections are asymptomatic. In addition, recurrent shedding of virus in saliva in the absence of clinical disease is common. Only those children with HSV gingivostomatitis (ie, primary infection) who do not have control of oral secretions should be excluded from child care. Exclusion of children with "cold sores" (ie, recurrent infection) from child care or school is not indicated (see Children in Out-of-Home Child Care, p 81).

Children with uncovered lesions on exposed surfaces and who were infected with HSV as newborn infants or as a result of sexual abuse pose a small potential risk to contacts. If children are certified by a physician to have recurrent HSV infection, covering the active lesions with clothing, a bandage, or an appropriate dressing when they attend child care or school is prudent.

HSV Infections in Wrestlers and Rugby Players. Herpes simplex virus type 1 infection has been transmitted during athletic competition involving close physical contact and frequent skin abrasions, such as wrestling (herpes gladiatorum) and rugby (herpes rugbiaforum or scrum pox). Young competitors often do not recognize or may deny possible infection. Transmission of these infections can be limited or prevented by the following: (1) examination of wrestlers and rugby players dressed in underwear or competition outfits for vesicular or ulcerative lesions on exposed areas of their bodies and around their mouths or eyes before practice or competition by a person familiar with the appearance of different mucocutaneous infections (including HSV, herpes zoster, and impetigo); (2) exclusion of athletes with these conditions from competition or practice until healing occurs or a physicians' note declaring their condition noninfectious is obtained; and (3) wiping of wrestling mats with a freshly prepared solution of 1/64 household bleach (1/4 cup diluted to 1 gallon of water) at least daily, and preferably between matches. However, HSV spread during wrestling and other sports involving close, personal contact can still occur through contact with saliva of asymptomatic excreters.

Infected Hospital Personnel. Transmission of HSV in newborn nurseries from infected personnel to newborn infants has been documented rarely. The risk of transmission to infants by personnel who have labial HSV infection ("cold sores") or who are asymptomatic oral shedders of the virus is not known, but is probably low. Compromising patient care by excluding personnel with "cold sores" who are essential for the operation of the nursery must be weighed against the potential risk of infecting newborn infants. Personnel with cold sores who have contact with infants (1) should cover and not touch their lesions, (2) should carefully observe hand washing policies, and (3) must not kiss or nuzzle newborn infants or children with dermatitis. Transmission of HSV infection from personnel with genital lesions is not likely as long as hand washing policies are carefully observed. Personnel with active herpetic whitlow should not have responsibility for direct care of neonates, immunocompromised patients, or patients in an intensive care unit.

Histoplasmosis

Clinical Manifestations: Histoplasmosis encompasses a spectrum of clinical diseases. Acute pulmonary histoplasmosis is an influenza-like illness with pulmonary infiltrates and hilar adenopathy. Chronic pulmonary histoplasmosis resembles chronic tuberculosis in adults. Acute disseminated histoplasmosis is most frequent in infants younger than 2 years of age. Symptoms include fever, cough, hepatosplenomegaly, adenopathy, pneumonitis, skin lesions, diarrhea, and pancytopenia resembling acute lymphatic leukemia. Chronic histoplasmosis ranges from a single pulmonary lesion to disseminated disease. It is rare in children. Patients with AIDS are at increased risk for disseminated histoplasmosis.

Etiology: *Histoplasma capsulatum* is a dimorphic fungus. In soil, it exists in the mycelial form, but it converts to a yeast form at the body temperature (37°C) of mammals.

Epidemiology: *Histoplasma capsulatum* is encountered in many parts of the world and is endemic in the eastern and central United States. Infection is acquired through inhalation of airborne spores (conidia). Asymptomatic infection is common. The source of the organism is soil or dust in barnyards and other locations harboring bat and bird droppings. Histoplasmosis is not transmitted from person to person.

The **incubation period** is variable but is usually a few weeks from the time of exposure.

Diagnostic Tests: A positive reaction to the histoplasmin skin test* indicates either current or previous *Histoplasma* infection. Detection of *H capsulatum* polysaccharide antigen in urine or serum is a sensitive and rapid method for the diagnosis of disseminated histoplasmosis in HIV-infected patients.

Direct demonstration of intracellular yeast cells in smears of bone marrow or biopsy material from infected tissues is helpful in disseminated or chronic histoplasmosis. Wright and Giemsa stains are usually adequate, but the Gomori silver methenamine stain is more likely to detect sparse organisms.

---

*Available from Parke-Davis, Morris Plains, NJ.

A chemiluminescent DNA probe has recently become available for identification of cultures of *H capsulatum*.* The procedure can be applied to nonsporulating cultures, thereby reducing the risk of exposure of laboratory personnel to infectious forms of the fungi.

Bone marrow, blood, sputum, and material from lesions may be cultured on brain-heart infusion and modified Sabouraud's medium at room temperature. The lysis-centrifugation method is preferred for blood cultures. Laboratory workers should be aware of the hazards of conidia-bearing mycelia and resulting potential for infection.

Both mycelial-phase (histoplasmin) and yeast-phase antigens are used in serologic testing for complement-fixing antibodies to *H capsulatum*. Low titers are often present in healthy persons living in endemic areas. A fourfold rise in yeast-phase titers or a single high titer of 1:32 or greater is presumptive evidence of active infection. Serum titers of mycelial but not the yeast-phase antibodies can increase slightly after skin testing with mycelium-derived histoplasmin. In the immunodiffusion precipitin test, H bands, although rarely encountered, are highly suggestive of active infection. Cross-reacting antibodies can result from *Blastomyces dermatiditis* and *Coccidioides immitis* infections.

Treatment: Uncomplicated, primary pulmonary histoplasmosis requires no specific therapy. Amphotericin B is effective in progressive, disseminated disease, and is the drug of choice in such cases and in immunocompromised patients (eg, those with AIDS) with histoplasmosis (see Systemic Treatment With Amphotericin B, p 562).

Both itraconazole and ketoconazole are useful in the treatment of histoplasmosis. A recent multicenter trial in adults demonstrated that itraconazole is at least as effective as ketoconazole and is better tolerated with lower or negligible toxicity.

Duration of treatment is determined from clinical and laboratory evidence that active fungal infection has subsided. The minimum duration of treatment with amphotericin B is 6 weeks. Patients with HIV infection require longer courses, including suppressive therapy. Doses of amphotericin B given every other day, weekly, or biweekly have been used successfully. Itraconazole is the drug of choice for suppressive therapy.

Isolation of the Hospitalized Patient: No special precautions are recommended.

Control Measures: Investigation for the common source of infection in outbreaks is indicated.

---

*Accuprobe, Gene-Probe Inc, San Diego, CA.

HIV Infection and AIDS

Clinical Manifestations: Human immunodeficiency virus (HIV) infection in children causes a broad spectrum of disease and a varied clinical course. Acquired immunodeficiency syndrome (AIDS) represents the most severe end of the clinical spectrum. The current Centers for Disease Control and Prevention (CDC) surveillance definition for AIDS is given in Table 3.18 (p 255). Patients meeting these criteria for AIDS (see Table 3.18) must be reported to the appropriate public health department. In many states, HIV infection must be reported. The CDC has established a pediatric classification system for children younger than 13 years who are born to HIV-infected mothers or are known to be infected with HIV (see Table 3.19, p 256). This classification is currently being revised (as of December 1993).

The manifestations of HIV infection include generalized lymphadenopathy, hepatomegaly, splenomegaly, failure to thrive, oral candidiasis, recurrent diarrhea, parotitis, cardiomyopathy, hepatitis, nephropathy, central nervous system (CNS) disease (including developmental delay, which can be progressive), lymphoid interstitial pneumonia, recurrent invasive bacterial infections, opportunistic infections, and specified malignancies (Table 3.18, p 255).

Pneumocystis carinii pneumonia (PCP) is the most common, serious opportunistic infection in children with HIV infection, and it is associated with high mortality (see *Pneumocystis carinii Infections*, p 376). Most frequently, PCP occurs in infants between 3 and 12 months of age who acquired infection before or at birth, but it can occur in infants younger than 3 months of age. Other common opportunistic infections in children include *Candida* esophagitis, disseminated cytomegalovirus infection, chronic or disseminated herpes simplex virus infection, *Mycobacterium avium* complex (MAC) infection, chronic enteritis caused by *Cryptosporidium* or other agents, and, less commonly, disseminated or CNS cryptococcal or *Toxoplasma* infection.

Malignancies in pediatric HIV infection have been relatively uncommon to date, but certain lymphomas, including those of the CNS and non-Hodgkin's B-cell lymphomas of the Burkitt type, occur much more frequently in children with HIV infection than in nonimmunocompromised children. Kaposi's sarcoma is very rare in children.

The development of opportunistic infections, particularly PCP, progressive neurologic disease, and severe wasting is associated with a poor prognosis. The prognosis for survival is also poor in children infected perinatally who become symptomatic in the first year of life. With earlier and more effective treatment, survival is likely to improve.

Laboratory findings. The most notable finding, particularly as the disease progresses, is an increasing loss of T-lymphocyte immunity. Initially, the peripheral blood lymphocyte count can be normal, but, eventually, lymphopenia develops because of a decrease in the total number of circulating T-lymphocytes. The cells most affected are the T-helper (CD4) lymphocytes. The T-suppressor (CD8) lymphocytes usually increase in number initially and are not depleted until late in the course of the infection. These changes in cell populations result in a decrease of the normal CD4-to-CD8 cell ratio. This nonspecific finding, although characteristic of HIV infec-

TABLE 3.13—Centers for Disease Control and Prevention
Surveillance Case Definition for AIDS—Diagnoses Indicative of
AIDS in Children, Adolescents, and Adults[a]

1. All ages:
Candidiasis of the esophagus[b,c]
Candidiasis of the trachea, bronchi, or lungs[b]
Coccidioidomycosis, disseminated or extrapulmonary[d]
Cryptococcosis, extrapulmonary[b]
Cryptosporidiosis, chronic intestinal[b]
Cytomegalovirus disease (other than liver, spleen, nodes) onset at >1 month
   of age[b]
Cytomegalovirus retinitis (with loss of vision)[b,c]
Herpes simplex ulcer, chronic (>1 month duration) or pneumonitis
   or esophagitis onset at >1 month of age[b]
HIV encephalopathy[d]
Histoplasmosis, disseminated or extrapulmonary[d]
Isosporiasis, chronic intestinal (>1 month duration)[d]
Kaposi's sarcoma[b,c]
Lymphoma, primary brain[b]
Lymphoma (Burkitt's, or immunoblastic sarcoma)[d]
Mycobacterium avium complex or *M kansasii*, disseminated, or
   extrapulmonary[b]
M tuberculosis disseminated, or extrapulmonary[d]
Mycobacterium, other species or unidentified species, disseminated or
   extrapulmonary[c]
Pneumocystis carinii pneumonia[b,c]
Progressive multifocal leukoencephalopathy[b]
Toxoplasmosis of brain, onset at 1 month of age[b,c]
Wasting syndrome due to HIV[d]

2. Additional diagnoses applicable for children <13 years of age:
Lymphoid interstitial pneumonitis[b,c]
Multiple or recurrent serious bacterial infections[d]

3. Additional diagnoses for adolescents (≥13 years of age) and for adults:
Cervical cancer, invasive[d]
M tuberculosis, pulmonary[d]
Pneumonia, recurrent[d]
Salmonella septicemia, recurrent[d]
CD4 T-lymphocyte count of <200 cells/mm^3 or a CD4 percentage of <14[d]

---

[a]Adapted from Centers for Disease Control and Prevention. 1993 revised classification
system for HIV infection and expanded surveillance case definition for AIDS among adolescents and adults. *MMWR*. 1992;41(RR-17):1-19.
[b]If indicator disease is diagnosed definitively (eg, by biopsy or culture) and no other cause
of immunodeficiency is present, laboratory documentation of HIV infection is not required.
[c]Presumptive diagnosis of indicator disease is accepted if laboratory evidence of HIV infection is present.
[d]Laboratory evidence of HIV infection is required.

TABLE 3.19—Classification System for HIV Infection in Children Younger Than 13 Years*

Class P–O.	Indeterminate Infection. Includes perinatally exposed infants and children younger than 15 months who cannot be classified as definitely infected according to the above definition but who have antibody to HIV, indicating exposure to a mother who is infected.
Class P–1.	Asymptomatic Infection.
	Subclass A. Normal immune function
	Subclass B. Abnormal immune function
	Subclass C. Immune function not tested
Class P–2.	Symptomatic Infection.
	Subclass A. Nonspecific findings
	Subclass B. Progressive neurologic disease
	Subclass C. Lymphoid interstitial pneumonitis
	Subclass D. Secondary infectious disease
	Category D–1. Specified secondary infectious diseases listed in the CDC surveillance definition for AIDS
	Category D–2. Recurrent serious bacterial infections
	Category D–3. Other specified secondary infectious diseases
	Subclass E. Secondary cancers
	Category E–1. Specified secondary cancers listed in the CDC surveillance definition for AIDS
	Category E–2. Other cancers possibly secondary to HIV infection
	Subclass F. Other diseases possibly due to HIV infection. Includes children with other conditions possibly due to HIV infection not listed in the above subclasses, such as hepatitis, cardiopathy, nephropathy, hematologic disorders (anemia, thrombocytopenia), and dermatologic diseases.

*From Centers for Disease Control: Classification for human immunodeficiency virus (HIV) infection in children under 13 years of age. *MMWR.* 1987;36:225-230,235-236.

tion, also occurs with other acute viral infections, such as those caused by cytomegalovirus or Epstein-Barr virus. The normal values for peripheral CD4 lymphocyte counts and percentages are age related (see Treatment, p 261, including Table 3.20, p 262). Response of T-lymphocytes to plant lectin mitogens (phytohemagglutinin, concanavalin A, and particularly pokeweed) are decreased or absent, and patients may be anergic to skin test antigens such as mumps, *Candida*, *Trichophyton*, tetanus, and tuberculin (Purified Protein Derivative [PPD]).

B-lymphocytes remain normal or are increased in number. Serum immunoglobulin (IG) concentrations, particularly IgG and IgA, are frequently elevated. A few patients will develop panhypogammaglobulinemia. Specific antibody responses to antigens to which the patient has not previously been exposed can be abnormal. Measuring the serum antibody response to measles vaccine administered to children 12 months or older, or to tetanus after three doses of DTP can be useful for assessing humoral responsiveness.

Etiology: AIDS is caused by RNA cytopathic human retroviruses, specifically, human immunodeficiency virus type 1 (HIV-1) and, less commonly, HIV-2, a related virus that is extremely uncommon in the United States but is more common in West Africa. Human immunodeficiency virus is particularly tropic for T-helper (CD4) lymphocytes and other cells such as macrophages that have CD4 receptors. The role of cofactors, such as simultaneous infection with other infectious agents or malnutrition, in the natural history of HIV infection is not known.

Epidemiology: Humans are the only known reservoir of HIV, although related viruses have been identified in monkeys. Since retroviruses integrate into the target cell genome as proviruses and the viral genome is copied during cell replication, the virus persists in infected individuals for life. Human immunodeficiency virus has been isolated from blood (including lymphocytes, macrophages, and plasma), other body fluids such as cerebrospinal fluid, pleural fluids, human milk, semen, cervical secretions, saliva, urine, and tears. However, only blood, semen, cervical secretions, and human milk have been implicated epidemiologically in the transmission of infection.

Currently, the predominant modes of HIV transmission in the United States are via (1) sexual contact (both homosexual and heterosexual); (2) percutaneous or mucous membrane exposure to contaminated needles or other sharp instruments; and (3) mother-to-infant transmission before or around the time of birth. Transfusion of blood, blood components, or clotting factor concentrates is now rarely a mode of HIV transmission because of exclusion of infected donors, heat treatment of clotting factor concentrates, and the availability of recombinant clotting factors. In the absence of documented parenteral, mucous membrane, or skin contact with blood, transmission of HIV, as of December 1993, has rarely been demonstrated to occur in families or households, in schools or child care settings, or with routine care in hospitals or clinics.

Accidental exposure of health care personnel to HIV, such as from needlestick injuries, has rarely resulted in HIV infection. The risk of infection after a needlestick exposure to HIV-infected blood is approximately 0.3%. Many of the cases that have occurred might have been prevented by careful adherence to infection control measures, especially during emergencies.

AIDS in children and adolescents has accounted for 2% of all reported cases of AIDS in the United States. However, the total number of reported cases in these age groups continues to increase. Acquisition of HIV during adolescence contributes to the large number of AIDS cases in young adults. Adolescent risk factors for HIV infection are similar to those for adults.

Most infected children in the United States have been born to families in which one or both parents have HIV infection. The remainder, including patients with hemophilia or other coagulation disorders, received contaminated blood, its components, or clotting factor concentrates. A few cases of HIV infection in children have resulted from sexual abuse by an HIV-seropositive individual. Less than 5% of cases have been reported to have no identifiable risk factor, and after careful investigation, most are reclassified into one of the established risk factor groups. In some cases, available information is inadequate to determine reclassification.

The risk of infection for an infant born to an HIV-seropositive mother is estimated to be between 13% and 39%. The exact timing of transmission from an infected mother to her infant is uncertain, but evidence suggests that transmission may occur in utero, around the time of delivery, or postpartum through breast-feeding. The available evidence suggests that the majority of infections occur in the perinatal period. Some studies suggest higher rates of perinatal transmission in women with advanced disease, low peripheral CD4 lymphocyte counts, and high viral concentrations as evidenced by HIV p24 antigenemia. Prevention of transmission by cesarean section has not been clearly demonstrated.

Human immunodeficiency virus DNA has been detected in both the cellular and cell-free fractions of human breast milk, and breast-feeding has been implicated in the transmission of HIV infection, especially in mothers who acquired HIV in the postpartum period. These women may have a higher rate of transmission because they, as a result of recent HIV acquisition, have high concentrations of virus. The additional risk of HIV transmission to infants through breast-feeding for women who were infected before pregnancy or early in gestation is uncertain. Data from different populations are inconsistent and analyses are confounded by the different epidemiologic circumstances and study methods in these populations.

The **incubation period** of symptomatic HIV infection (ie, disease) is variable, ranging from months to years. The median age of onset of symptoms is estimated to be 3 years for infants infected perinatally. However, some children exhibit manifestations of infection during the first year of life, whereas others are asymptomatic until they are 5 years or older. In transfusion-associated cases in young children, the median incubation period for onset of clinical disease has been estimated to be 3.5 years, but with considerable individual variability. Other than infants born of infected mothers, persons infected with HIV usually develop serum antibody to HIV within 6 to 12 weeks after infection.

Diagnostic Tests: Diagnosis of HIV infection is usually made by serum antibody tests except in children younger than 18 months of age in whom passively acquired maternal antibody may be present.

Enzyme immunoassays (EIA) are most widely used to screen for HIV antibody. These tests are highly sensitive and specific, but false-positive results occur in a small percentage of cases. Repeat EIA testing of initially reactive specimens is required to reduce the likelihood of laboratory error; repeatedly reactive tests are highly reliable. Western blot or immunofluorescent antibody tests should be used for confirmation. A positive HIV antibody test in a child 18 months of age or older is usually indicative of infection.

Serum antibodies to HIV are present in almost all infected persons, although some patients with AIDS become seronegative late in disease. Some children with HIV infection may test negative for HIV antibody because they have hypogammaglobulinemia, or late in disease may be unable to produce antibody. Rarely, an HIV-infected child is antibody negative by EIA testing but positive on Western blot or positive by other virologic tests, such as culture or polymerase chain reaction (PCR).

Infants born to HIV-seropositive women pose a special diagnostic challenge since these infants are almost always seropositive at birth as the result of transplacental acquisition of maternal antibody, whether or not they are infected, and these serum antibodies can be detectable in the infant for as long as 18 months after birth. Thus, IgG antibody tests for HIV are not useful for diagnosis in the child younger than 18 months of age. However, the diagnosis can be made in infants in the first few months of life by other tests, specifically, positive HIV culture, detection of HIV DNA sequences using the PCR, detection of IgA-specific anti-HIV antibodies (after 3 months of age), and positive HIV-p24 antigen assay after acid dissociation. One or more of these tests are generally available at referral centers caring for HIV-infected children.

Using these assays, most infected infants can be diagnosed by 3 to 6 months of age. For an infant born to an HIV-seropositive mother, an initial diagnostic assay should be performed by approximately 1 month of age or as soon as possible thereafter. If the assay is negative, repeat testing between 3 and 6 months of age is indicated. A positive HIV culture, PCR and/or p24 antigen detection assay constitutes presumptive evidence of HIV infection, and a second diagnostic test should be subsequently performed, using either the same assay or one of the other two assays, to confirm the diagnosis. If an infant younger than 18 months of age who has a positive serologic test for HIV develops an AIDS-defining illness (see Table 3.18, p 255), the diagnosis of HIV infection is established even if virologic tests are negative.

The child who has negative virologic tests at 6 months of age requires continued serologic follow-up to document disappearance of maternal HIV antibody. An infant born to a seropositive mother who is HIV antibody negative at two consecutive times by 18 months of age, has normal immune function studies, and never has had a positive virologic test (culture, PCR, or p24 antigen) for HIV is a seroreverter and should be considered not to be infected. Despite two or more negative serologic tests, the National Pediatric HIV Resource Center recommends a final test at 24 months of age to decrease the possibility of misdiagnosing an infected, but antibody-negative child.*

Since interpretation of the available diagnostic tests may be complex, the pediatrician should consult with an HIV specialist to assist in the interpretation of diagnostic assays.

---

*Working Group on Antiretroviral Therapy: National Pediatric HIV Resource Center. Antiretroviral therapy and medical management of the human immunodeficiency virus-infected child. *Pediatr Infect Dis J.* 1993;12:513-522

Perinatal HIV Serologic Testing. Recommendations of the AAP Task Force on Pediatric AIDS include the following*:

- HIV testing should be routinely offered to all pregnant women and women of childbearing age throughout the United States.
- HIV testing should be routinely recommended and encouraged for all pregnant women and women of childbearing age at increased risk of HIV infection because of high-risk behaviors or because they live in areas (eg, state, metropolitan area, or city) with an HIV seroprevalence rate among pregnant women and newborns of 1:1,000 or more.
- Newborn testing should be routinely recommended and encouraged in mothers with known high-risk behaviors or from high-seroprevalence areas who have not been tested.
- HIV testing should be recommended and encouraged for abandoned infants and for infants otherwise in need of foster or adoptive care, as needed to facilitate placement and care. Courts should adopt methods for rapid processing of court orders to allow HIV testing of abandoned infants or those in foster care when follow-up adoption or initial placement may be facilitated by such testing.
- Testing in the perinatal period should be determined by specified policies that ensure retesting, education, informed consent, counseling, and follow-up criteria.
- Anonymous seroprevalence surveys should be continued and expanded to provide ongoing information on HIV seroprevalence in specific metropolitan areas and states. These surveys are not a substitute for individual counseling and testing, but they provide important public health information.
- Pediatricians or other primary pediatric caregivers should be informed whenever an infant is born to a known HIV-seropositive mother so that appropriate care and follow-up testing can be undertaken.
- Development of testing programs without addressing access to care is inappropriate. However, testing programs that may benefit the mother, fetus, and newborn cannot be delayed until access problems have been resolved completely.
- The Academy opposes mandatory (involuntary) maternal and/or newborn testing at this time.

Informed Consent for HIV Serologic Testing. Testing for HIV infection is unlike most routine blood testing in that substantial psychosocial risks can be incurred. When testing an infant or child, parents or other primary caretakers, and patients, if old enough to comprehend, should be counseled about the possible risks and benefits of testing and the consequences of HIV infection. Oral consent should be obtained from the parent or legal guardian and recorded in the patient's chart. Special written consent procedures for HIV testing should be discouraged as they can inhibit the performance of testing without adding significant benefit. Nevertheless, state and local laws and hospital regulations should be considered in deciding whether written consent is required. The necessity for counseling and consent should not deter efforts to

---

*For further information, see Task Force on Pediatric AIDS. Perinatal human immunodeficiency virus (HIV) testing. *Pediatrics*. 1992;89:791-794

undertake appropriate diagnostic testing for HIV infection. Refusal to give consent does not relieve the physician of the professional and legal responsibilities to their patients. If the physician believes that testing is essential to the child's health, authorization for testing will need to be obtained by other means. The results of serologic tests should be discussed in person with the family, primary caretaker, and, if appropriate according to age, the patient; if positive, appropriate counseling and subsequent follow-up care must be provided. Maintaining confidentiality in all cases is essential to preserving patient and parent trust and consent.

Treatment: Primary care physicians are encouraged to actively participate in the care of HIV-infected patients.

Antiretroviral therapy has become a standard of care for all children with symptomatic HIV infection. Guidelines for the institution of antiretroviral therapy in infants and children with HIV infection have been formulated by the Working Group on Antiretroviral Therapy convened by the National Pediatric HIV Resource Center.[*] The clinical and immunologic criteria for initiating therapy are listed in Table 3.20 (p 262). Current data are insufficient to recommend therapy in asymptomatic children with normal age-adjusted CD4 lymphocyte counts, including those with normal physical examinations as well as those with only lymphadenopathy, hepatomegaly, or hypergammaglobulinemia.

Oral zidovudine has been approved for use in children as well as in adolescents and adults. It is recommended for HIV-infected adults and adolescents with symptomatic HIV infection and often for those with CD4 lymphocyte counts of less than 500/mm³. For children 4 weeks of age or older with symptomatic HIV infection or immunosuppression (see Table 3.20, p 262), zidovudine is also recommended as initial therapy and is generally well tolerated. For dosage recomme ndations, see Antiviral Drugs, p 567. The most common side effect is hematologic toxicity (anemia and/or neutropenia). Hence, complete blood and platelet counts should be monitored monthly during therapy.

Changes in antiretroviral therapy should be made in consultation with a specialist experienced in the management of HIV infection, especially since therapeutic alternatives are limited. Disease progression in children is usually defined as deterioration of CNS function or growth failure. Other evidence of disease progression can include development of a new AIDS-defining opportunistic infection (Table 3.18, p 255), symptomatic HIV-associated cardiomyopathy, nephrotic syndrome, or significant, otherwise unexplained serum transaminase elevations (more than five times normal). Laboratory criteria for disease progression mandating a change in drug therapy are not clearly defined in children, particularly in the absence of clinical progression.

Didanosine (DDI), formerly termed dideoxyinosine, is an alternative therapy for children who cannot tolerate zidovudine or whose disease has progressed while receiving zidovudine therapy. For dosage recommendations,

---

[*]For detailed, further information, see Working Group on Antiretroviral Therapy: National Pediatric HIV Resource Center. Antiretroviral therapy and medical management of the human immunodeficiency virus-infected child. *Pediatr Infect Dis J.* 1993;12:513-522

TABLE 3.20—Recommendations for Use of Antiretroviral Therapy in Infants and Children With Proven HIV Infection*

- The presence of any of the HIV-associated clinical conditions listed below warrants initiation of antiretroviral therapy, independent of CD4 lymphocyte count:

    a. AIDS-defining opportunistic infection
    b. Wasting disease (crossing two percentiles over time)
    c. Failure to thrive (below the 5th percentile for age and falling from the growth curve)
    d. Progressive encephalopathy
    e. Malignancy
    f. Recurrent septicemia/meningitis
    g. Thrombocytopenia <75,000 platelets/mm^3
    h. Hypogammaglobulinemia (total IgG/IgM/IgA <250 mg/mL)

- If CD4 lymphocyte counts are less than the following age-adjusted concentrations, therapy should be initiated independent of clinical findings:

    CD4 absolute count

    <1,750 cells/mm^3 for children younger than 1 y
    <1,000 cells/mm^3 for children 1-2 y
    <750 cells/mm^3 for children 2-6 y
    <500 cells/mm^3 for children older than 6 y

    CD4 percentage (of the total peripheral lymphocyte count)

    <30% for children younger than 1 y
    <25% for children 1-2 y
    <20% for children older than 2 y

- Therapy should also be considered in children with the following clinical conditions, even if occurring as an isolated finding, independent of the CD4 lymphocyte count:

    Lymphoid interstitial pneumonitis
    Parotitis
    Splenomegaly
    Persistent oral candidiasis
    Recurrent and/or chronic diarrhea
    Cardiomyopathy
    Nephropathy
    Hepatitis
    Endocrinopathy
    Recurrent and/or chronic bacterial infections, such as sinusitis/pneumonia
    Recurrent herpes simplex and/or varicella-zoster infections
    Neutropenia (<750 neutrophils/mm^3)
    Anemia
    Neurodevelopmental abnormalities

*For further information, see Working Group on Antiretroviral Therapy: National Pediatric HIV Resource Center. Antiretroviral therapy and medical management of the human immunodeficiency virus-infected child. *Pediatr Infect Dis J.* 1993;12:513-522

see Antiviral Drugs (p 567). For optimal absorption of DDI, adequate buffering of stomach acid is necessary, and no food or drink should be taken for at least 30 minutes before and after drug administration. Side effects include pancreatitis and peripheral retinal depigmentation without associated visual impairment. Peripheral neuropathy has been reported in adults but not in children receiving the commonly used doses. Monthly monitoring of complete blood counts and of the serum amylase, or whenever abdominal symptoms occur, is essential.

Zalcitabine (DDC) has recently been approved for use in adults, but it is not yet approved for use in children. It is indicated for use in combination with zidovudine for adults with symptomatic HIV infection or CD4 lymphocyte counts equal to or less than 300/mm^3. Multicenter clinical trials are evaluating drug combinations, including zidovudine with DDI, and zidovudine with DDC, in children.

Other new antiretroviral drugs, immunomodulators, and vaccines for therapeutic use are under evaluation. Further information on therapeutic trials in HIV-infected children can be obtained from the Pediatric Clinical Trials Group, Pediatric Branch, National Cancer Institute (see Directory of Telephone Numbers, p 601).

The value of intravenous immune globulin (IGIV) in children with HIV infection has been evaluated in several trials. The Working Group on Antiretroviral Therapy has recommended routine IGIV therapy in combination with an antiviral agent for children with humoral immunodeficiency including (1) hypogammaglobulinemia (IgG less than 250 mg/mL); (2) recurrent, serious bacterial infections (defined as two or more serious bacterial infections such as bacteremia, meningitis, or pneumonia in a 1-year period; (3) children who fail to form antibodies to common antigens; and (4) children living in areas where measles is highly prevalent who have not developed an antibody response after two doses (1 month or more apart) of MMR.* The dose of IGIV is 400 mg/kg per dose given every 4 weeks. Intravenous immune globulin may also be useful in the treatment of HIV-associated thrombocytopenia at a dose of 500 to 1,000 mg/kg/d for 3 to 5 days. In addition, children with bronchiectasis despite treatment with the standard medical regimen of cyclic antibiotics and aggressive respiratory therapy might benefit from adjunctive IGIV therapy at 600 mg/kg per dose, given monthly.

Early diagnosis and aggressive treatment of opportunistic infections may prolong survival. Since PCP can be an early complication of perinatally acquired HIV infection and mortality is high, chemoprophylaxis should be given to HIV-infected children at risk for PCP. For further information, see *Pneumocystis carinii* Infections, p 377.

Chemoprophylaxis may also be warranted for MAC infections (see Diseases Caused by Nontuberculous Mycobacteria, p 503).

Immunization Recommendations (see also Table 3.21, p 264).

Children With Symptomatic HIV Infection. In general, live-virus (eg, oral poliovirus) vaccines and live-bacterial (eg, bacillus Calmette-Guerin) vac-

---

*Working Group on Antiretroviral Therapy: National Pediatric HIV Resource Center. Antiretroviral therapy and medical management of the human immunodeficiency virus-infected child. *Pediatr Infect Dis J.* 1993;12:513-522.

TABLE 3.21—Recommendations for Routine Immunization of HIV-Infected Children in the United States*

Vaccine†	Known Asymptomatic HIV Infection	Symptomatic HIV Infection
Hepatitis B	Yes	Yes
DTP	Yes	Yes
OPV	No	No
IPV	Yes	Yes
MMR	Yes	Yes
Hib	Yes	Yes
Pneumococcal	Yes	Yes
Influenza	Should be considered	Yes

*See Table 1.3 (p 23) for age at which specific vaccines are indicated.
†DTP = diphtheria and tetanus toxoids and pertussis vaccine; OPV = oral poliovirus vaccine; IPV = inactivated poliovirus vaccine; MMR = live-virus measles, mumps, and rubella; Hib = *Haemophilus influenzae* type b conjugate.

cines should not be given to patients with AIDS or other clinical manifestations of HIV infection who are immunosuppressed. Measles, mumps, and rubella (MMR) vaccine combined is an exception. For routine immunizations, DTP, hepatitis B, *Haemophilus influenzae* type b conjugate, inactivated poliovirus (IPV), and MMR vaccines should be given according to the usual immunization schedule (see Tables 1.3 and 1.4, pp 23 and 24). Pneumococcal vaccine at 2 years of age and yearly influenza vaccination beginning at age 6 months are also recommended.

The occurrence of severe measles in symptomatic HIV-infected children and the lack of reported serious or unusual reactions to immunization with MMR vaccine have led to the recommendation for measles immunization of HIV-infected children, regardless of symptoms, with MMR vaccine. Although MMR is usually given at 12 to 15 months, if the risk of exposure to measles is increased, such as during an outbreak, these children should receive vaccine at a younger age (see Measles, p 312).

In general, children with symptomatic HIV infection have poor immunologic responses to vaccines. Hence, such children, when exposed to a vaccine-preventable disease such as measles or tetanus, should be considered susceptible regardless of the history of vaccination, and should receive, if indicated, passive immunoprophylaxis (see Passive Immunization of Children With HIV Infection, p 265).

Children With Asymptomatic HIV Infection. Children with asymptomatic HIV infection should receive DTP, IPV, *Haemophilus influenzae* type b conjugate, hepatitis B, IPV, and MMR vaccines, according to the usual immunization schedules (see Tables 1.3 and 1.4, pp 23 and 24). Although oral poliovirus vaccine (OPV) has been given to these patients without adverse effect, IPV is recommended because both the child and family members may be immunosuppressed as the result of HIV infection and, therefore, may be at risk for vaccine-associated paralytic poliomyelitis caused by vaccine virus infection.

Pneumococcal vaccination is indicated for HIV-infected children 2 years and older in view of their high incidence of invasive pneumococcal infection. Yearly influenza vaccination should be considered for children 6 months or older.

In areas of low tuberculosis prevalence, BCG vaccine is not recommended. However, in areas where the prevalence of tuberculosis is high, the World Health Organization recommends that BCG should be given to all infants at birth, regardless of maternal HIV infection, if the infants are asymptomatic.

Seronegative Children Residing in the Household of a Patient With Symptomatic HIV Infection. In a household with an adult or child immunocompromised as the result of HIV infection, seronegative as well as seropositive children should receive IPV vaccine because the live polioviruses in OPV can be excreted and transmitted to immunosuppressed contacts. MMR vaccine may be given because MMR vaccine viruses are not transmitted. To reduce the risk of transmission of influenza to patients with symptomatic HIV infection, yearly influenza vaccination is indicated for their household contacts (see Influenza, p 280).

Passive Immunization of Children With HIV Infection.

1. *Measles* (see Measles, p 311).
   * Symptomatic HIV-infected children who are exposed to measles should receive immune globulin (IG) prophylaxis (0.5 mL/kg, maximum 15 mL), regardless of vaccination status.
   * Exposed, asymptomatic HIV-infected patients who are susceptible should also receive IG; the recommended dose is 0.25 mL/kg.
   * Children who have received IGIV within 3 weeks of exposure do not require additional passive immunization.
2. *Tetanus.* In the management of wounds classified as tetanus prone (see Tetanus, p 460 and Table 3.45, p 461), children with HIV infection should receive Tetanus Immune Globulin (Human) (TIG) regardless of vaccination status.
3. *Varicella.* Children infected with HIV who are exposed to varicella or zoster and who are susceptible should receive Varicella-Zoster Immune Globulin (VZIG) (see Varicella-Zoster Infections, p 516). Children who have received IGIV or VZIG within 3 weeks of exposure do not require additional passive immunization.

Isolation of the Hospitalized Patient: Universal blood and body fluid precautions should be scrupulously followed by all hospital personnel (see Isolation Precautions, p 92). The risk to health care personnel of acquiring HIV infection from a patient is minimal, even after accidental exposure from a needlestick injury. Nevertheless, every effort should be made to avoid exposures to blood and other body fluids that could contain HIV (see Table 2.4, p 94).

Control Measures:

Adolescent Education.* Adolescents at risk for HIV infection should have access to HIV testing and knowledge of their serostatus. Attention to the need for

---

*For further information, see Task Force on Pediatric AIDS. Adolescents and human immunodeficiency virus infection: the role of the pediatrician in prevention and intervention. *Pediatrics.* 1993;92:626-630.

informed consent for either testing or the release of information regarding serostatus is crucial. Decisions regarding the disclosure of HIV status to a sexual partner without the consent of the patient should be based on several factors, including whether the partner has a reasonable cause to suspect the risk and take precautions without specific warning; the likelihood the partner is in fact at risk; relevant law that might prohibit or require such disclosure; and the possible effects of such disclosure upon future patients.

Specific recommendations of the AAP Task Force on Pediatric AIDS for pediatricians caring for adolescents are as follows:

- Information regarding HIV infection and AIDS should be regarded as an important component of the anticipatory guidance provided by pediatricians to their adolescent patients. This guidance should include information about transmission, implications of infection, and strategies for prevention including abstinence from behaviors that place adolescents at risk and safer sex practices for those who opt to be sexually active.
- Young persons at risk for HIV infection should be offered diagnostic testing in addition to other educational and counseling services.
- Parental involvement in adolescent health care is a desirable goal. However, the consent of the adolescent alone should be sufficient to provide evaluation and treatment for suspected or confirmed HIV infection.
- The maintenance of confidentiality regarding HIV status is of great importance. Respecting this confidentiality, the pediatrician should use all reasonable means to persuade an infected adolescent to inform his or her sexual partner on a voluntary basis. Involuntary disclosure is a complex question that should be decided on the basis of local law, the relationship between the physician and the patient, the relationship of the physician to the partner, and the degree of perceived risk to the unsuspecting sexual partner.

If adolescents are sexually active, they should be counseled about the correct and consistent use of condoms to reduce the risk of infection (see Sexually Transmitted Diseases, p 103).

School Attendance and Education of Children With HIV Infection. In the absence of blood exposure, HIV infection is not acquired through the types of contact that usually occur in a school setting, including contact with saliva or tears. Hence, children with HIV infection should not be excluded from school for the protection of other children or personnel. Specific recommendations concerning school attendance of children and adolescents with HIV infection are the following:

- Most school-aged children and adolescents infected with HIV should be allowed to attend school without restrictions, provided the child's physician gives approval.
- The need for a more restricted school environment for some infected children should be evaluated on a case-by-case basis considering conditions that may pose an increased risk to others, such as aggressive biting behavior or the presence of exudative, weeping skin lesions that cannot be covered.
- No one besides the child's parents, other guardians, and physician has an absolute need to know that the child is HIV-infected. The number of personnel aware of the child's condition should be kept to the minimum

needed to ensure proper care of the child. The family has the right to inform the school. Persons involved in the care and education of an infected student must respect the student's right to privacy.

- All schools should adopt routine procedures for handling blood or blood-contaminated fluids, including the disposal of sanitary napkins, regardless of whether students with HIV infection are known to be in attendance. School health care workers, teachers, administrators, and other employees should be educated about procedures (see Housekeeping Procedures for Blood and Body Fluids, p 268).
- Children infected with HIV develop progressive immunodeficiency, which increases their risk of experiencing severe complications from infections such as varicella, tuberculosis, measles, cytomegalovirus, and herpes simplex virus. The child's physician should regularly assess the risk of an unrestricted environment on the health of the HIV-infected student, including evaluation of possible contagious diseases in the school (eg, measles, varicella, tuberculosis).
- Routine screening of schoolchildren for HIV infection is not recommended.

As the incidence of HIV infection in children increases, the school population of children with this disease will increase. With the advent of new drug therapy, these children will likely have longer survival, resulting in an increasing number of HIV-infected children entering school. An understanding of the effect of chronic illness and the recognition of neurodevelopmental problems in these children is essential to provide appropriate educational programs. The AAP Task Force on Pediatric AIDS has made the following recommendations regarding the education of children with HIV infection[*]:

- All children with HIV infection should receive an appropriate education that is adapted to their evolving special needs. The spectrum of needs differs with the stage of the disease.
- HIV infection should be treated like other chronic illnesses that require special education and other related services.
- Continuity of education must be assured whether at school or at home.
- Because of the stigmatization that still exists with this disease, maintaining confidentiality is essential. Disclosures of information should be only with the informed consent of the parents or legal guardians and age-appropriate assent of the student.

Child Care[†] and Foster Care. Current AAP recommendations are as follows[‡]:

- No reason exists to restrict foster care or adoptive placement of children who have HIV infection to protect the health of other family members. The risk of transmission of HIV infection in family environments is negligible.
- No need exists to restrict the placement of HIV-infected children in child care settings to protect personnel or other children because the risk of transmission of HIV in these settings is negligible.

---

[*]For further information, see Task Force on Pediatric AIDS. Education of children with human immunodeficiency virus infection. *Pediatrics.* 1991;88:645-648.
[†]For additional discussion of recommendations for child care, see Children in Out-of-Home Child Care, p 89.
[‡]Adapted from American Academy of Pediatrics Task Force on Pediatric AIDS. Guidelines for human immunodeficiency virus (HIV)-infected children and their families. *Pediatrics.* 1992;89: 681-683.

- Child care personnel need not be informed of the HIV status of a child to protect the health of caregivers or other children in the child care environment. In some jurisdictions the child's diagnosis cannot be divulged without the written consent of the parent or legal guardian. Parents may choose to inform the child care provider of the child's diagnosis to support a request that the caregiver observe the child closely for signs of illness that might require medical attention and assist the parents with the child's special emotional and social needs.
- Recommended universal precautions should be followed in all child care settings when blood or bloody fluids are being handled, to minimize the possibility of transmission of any blood-borne disease (see Housekeeping Procedures for Blood and Body Fluids, below).
- All preschool child care programs should routinely inform all families whenever a highly infectious illness, such as measles or chickenpox, occurs in any child in that setting. This process will help families protect their immunodeficient children.
- To facilitate foster care or adoptive placement, courts should adopt methods for rapid processing of court orders to allow HIV testing of infants and young children whenever such testing would promote placement. Placement would be promoted most clearly when such court-ordered testing is pursued in areas of high seroprevalence or when the child comes from a high-risk setting.

Adults With HIV Infection Working in Child Care or Schools. Asymptomatic HIV-infected adults may care for children in school or child care settings provided that they do not have exudative skin lesions or other conditions that would allow contact with their body fluids. No data indicate that HIV-infected adults have transmitted HIV in the course of normal child care or school responsibilities.

Adults with symptomatic HIV infection are immunocompromised and at increased risk from infectious diseases of young children. They should consult their physicians regarding the safety of their continuing work.

Housekeeping Procedures for Blood and Body Fluids. In general, routine housekeeping procedures using a commercially available cleaner (detergents, disinfectant-detergents, or chemical germicides) compatible with most surfaces are satisfactory for cleaning spills of vomitus, urine, and feces. Nasal secretions can be removed with tissues and discarded in routine waste containers. For spills involving blood or other body fluids: organic material should be removed, then the surface disinfected with diluted bleach (ie, 1:10 to 1:100). A 1:64 dilution is 1/4 cup bleach diluted in 1 gallon of water. Reusable rubber gloves may be useful for cleaning large spills to avoid contamination of the hands of the person cleaning the spill, but gloves are not essential for cleaning small amounts of blood that can be contained easily by the material used for cleaning. Persons involved in cleaning contaminated surfaces should avoid exposure of open skin lesions or mucous membranes to blood or bloody fluids. Whenever possible, disposable towels or tissues should be used and properly discarded, and mops should be rinsed in the disinfectant.

Management and Counseling of Families. Infection acquired by children before or during birth is a disease of the family. Serologic screening of siblings and parents is recommended. In each case, the physician needs to provide education and ongoing counseling regarding HIV and its transmission, and to outline precautions to be taken within the household and the community to prevent spread of this virus.

Infected women need to be made aware of the risk of having an infected child if they become pregnant, and they should be referred for family planning counseling. Infected individuals should not donate blood, plasma, sperm, organs, corneas, bone, other tissues, or breast milk.

The infected child should be taught good hygiene and behavior. How much he or she is told about the illness will depend on age and maturity. Older children and adolescents should be made aware that the disease can be transmitted sexually, and they should be provided with appropriate counseling. Most families are not willing to share the diagnosis with others, since it can create social isolation. Feelings of guilt are common. Family members, including children, can become clinically depressed and require psychiatric counseling.

Breast-feeding (see also Human Milk, p 73). The risk of HIV transmission by breast-feeding, especially from mothers who acquire HIV infection during the postpartum period, has been reported in some studies to be increased. In the United States, where safe, alternative, effective sources of feeding are readily available and affordable, an HIV-infected woman should be counseled not to breast-feed her infant or donate to milk banks. The World Health Organization has recommended that mothers residing in areas where infectious disease and malnutrition are an important cause of mortality early in life should be advised to breast-feed their infants regardless of the mother's HIV serologic status.

Sexual Abuse. After sexual abuse by a person with or at risk for HIV infection, the child should be tested at the time of abuse and at 3 and 6 months after sexual contact for antibodies to HIV (see Sexual Abuse, p 110). If feasible, serologic evaluation of the abuser for HIV infection should be obtained. Counseling of the child and family needs to be provided.

Blood, Blood Components, and Clotting Factors. Screening blood and plasma for HIV antibody has dramatically reduced the risk of infection through transfusion. Nevertheless, careful scrutiny of the requirements of each patient for blood, its components, or clotting factors is important.

Transmission of HIV through contaminated clotting-factor concentrates has been virtually eliminated in the United States. All plasma-derived factor VIII and factor IX concentrates available in the United States are now manufactured from plasma screened for HIV antibody. Additionally, the concentrates are treated with heat, solvents, or detergents for inactivation of HIV (as well as other agents including hepatitis B and hepatitis C viruses). Some concentrates also undergo monoclonal antibody purification. Cryoprecipitate from single or pooled donor plasma is screened for anti-HIV antibody but does not undergo any process to inactivate HIV or other viruses. Patients with hemophilia should be managed in consultation with specialists familiar with current aspects of treatment, such as desmopressin for the treatment of individuals with mild or moderate factor VIII deficiency. Recombinant factor replacement is now available.

*Exposed Health Care Workers.** Management of the health care worker who has had a percutaneous or mucous membrane exposure to blood or bloody secretions from an HIV-positive patient should include the following:

1. Confirmation that the patient is HIV positive.
2. Evaluation of the health care worker clinically and serologically for evidence of HIV infection as soon as possible after the exposure. If the health care worker is seronegative, he or she should be retested at 6 weeks, 3 months, and 6 months after exposure to determine whether transmission has occurred. Most exposed individuals who have been infected will seroconvert during the first 12 weeks after exposure.
3. Immediately informing the exposed health care worker of the availability of zidovudine for chemoprophylaxis. The data on the use of zidovudine for postexposure prophylaxis, however, are inadequate to establish its efficacy or safety. In the absence of conclusive data, many medical centers have adopted a protocol for offering zidovudine chemoprophylaxis after occupational exposures. If given, zidovudine should be started as soon as possible after exposure at a dose (for adults) of 200 mg every 4 hours for 4 to 6 weeks.
4. Counseling about the risks from the exposure and possible benefits of zidovudine.

Hookworm Infections (*Ancylostoma duodenale* and *Necator americanus*)

Clinical Manifestations: After contact with contaminated soil, initial skin penetration of larvae, usually involving the feet, causes stinging or burning followed by pruritus and a papulovesicular rash persisting for 1 to 2 weeks. Pneumonitis associated with migrating larvae in this phase is uncommon and usually mild except in severe infections. Disease following oral ingestion of infectious *Ancylostoma duodenale* larvae can present with pharyngeal itching, hoarseness, nausea, and vomiting shortly after ingestion. Colicky abdominal pain with diarrhea and marked eosinophilia can develop 29 to 38 days after exposure. Chronic infection is a common cause of hypochromic, microcytic anemia in tropical, developing countries, and severe infection can cause hypoproteinemia and edema secondary to blood loss. Cardiac decompensation occasionally develops in children with hemoglobin concentrations of less than 6 g/dL.

Etiology: Infection is caused by *A duodenale* and *Necator americanus*, two worms with similar life cycles.

---

*For additional information, see Centers for Disease Control. Guidelines for prevention of transmission of human immunodeficiency virus and hepatitis B virus to health-care and public-safety workers. *MMWR.* 1989;38(5-6):9-10.

TABLE 3.22—Intensity of Infection (Beaver Technique)

Egg Count per mg of Stool	Clinical Significance
≥50 eggs	Massive Infection
≥20 eggs	Anemia in well-nourished patients
≥5 eggs	Anemia in malnourished patients
<5 eggs	Minimal clinical significance

Epidemiology: Humans are the major reservoir. Well-nourished, lightly infected individuals are often asymptomatic. Hookworms are prominent in rural, tropical, and subtropical areas where human fecal soil contamination is common. Larvae and eggs survive in loose, sandy, moist, shady, well-aerated, warm soil (optimal temperature 23° to 33°C). Although both worms are equally prevalent in many areas, *A duodenale* is the predominant species in Europe, the Mediterranean region, northern Asia, and the west coast of South America, and *N americanus* is predominant in the Western hemisphere, subsaharan Africa, southeast Asia, and a number of Pacific islands. Percutaneous infection occurs after exposure to infectious larvae. Peroral and possibly transmammary infection can occur with *A duodenale*. Infectious larvae are found in contaminated soil within 5 to 7 days, and can persist for weeks to months. Untreated infected patients who do not become reinfected can harbor worms for 5 to 15 years but a reduction in worm burden of at least 70% generally occurs within 1 to 2 years.

The **incubation period**, the time from exposure to eggs in the stool (prepatent period), is 4 to 6 weeks.

Diagnostic Tests: The microscopic demonstration of hookworm eggs in the feces is diagnostic. Adult worms or larvae are rarely seen. During the acute infection, eggs will not be present in the stool. A direct stool smear with potassium iodide saturated with iodine is adequate for the diagnosis of significant hookworm infection; light infections require concentration techniques. To determine the clinical significance of infection, quantification techniques are necessary (see Table 3.22, above).

Treatment: Mebendazole or pyrantel pamoate is the drug of choice (see Drugs for Parasitic Infections, p 574). In children younger than 2 years of age, in whom experience with both drugs is limited, the risks and benefits of therapy should be considered before administering either drug. In pregnancy, mebendazole is not recommended and pyrantel pamoate has not been adequately studied. Therefore, adequate protein and iron nutrition should be maintained throughout pregnancy, and treatment is delayed until after delivery. A repeat stool examination, using a concentration technique, should be performed 2 weeks posttreatment, and, if positive, retreatment is indicated. Nutritional supplementation, including iron, is important when anemia is present. Severely affected children may require blood transfusion.

Isolation of the Hospitalized Patient: No special precautions are recommended.

Control Measures: Sanitary disposal of feces to prevent contamination of the soil, particularly in endemic areas, is necessary but rarely accomplished. Treatment of all known infected patients and screening of high-risk groups (ie, children and agriculture workers) in endemic areas can help reduce environmental contamination. Wearing shoes is also helpful.

Human Herpesvirus 6
(Formerly Roseola)

Clinical Manifestations: Major clinical manifestations of primary infection include roseola (exanthem subitum, sixth disease), undifferentiated febrile illness without rash or localizing signs, and other acute febrile illnesses, possibly accompanied by respiratory or gastrointestinal signs. Fever is characteristically high, lasting 3 to 7 days. In roseola, fever is followed by an erythematous maculopapular rash lasting hours to days. Seizures occur during the febrile period in approximately 10% of primary human herpesvirus 6 (HHV-6) infections. Encephalitis is a rare complication. The full spectrum of primary infection has yet to be determined.

The virus may persist and subsequently reactivate. The clinical circumstances and manifestations of reactivation in healthy persons are currently unclear. Reactivation has been described primarily in immunosuppressed hosts in whom clinical signs, such as fever, hepatitis, bone marrow suppression, and pneumonia have occasionally been described.

Etiology: Human herpesvirus 6 is a newly identified member of the family *Herpesviridae*, which contains a large, double-stranded DNA genome. Strain variation occurs, the import and extent of which are yet to be defined.

Epidemiology: Humans are the only known natural hosts. Transmission to the infant most likely occurs via the respiratory secretions of an asymptomatic family member or caretaker. Human herpesvirus 6 has been identified in the saliva of some healthy adults. During primary infection, HHV-6 can be isolated from peripheral blood lymphocytes in which it may subsequently persist. The attack rate is highest in children between the ages of 6 and 24 months of age. Infection is rare before 3 months or after 4 years of age. Virus-specific maternal antibody is uniformly present in infants at birth and is protective. As antibody declines with increasing age, infection is increasingly common. By the age of 4 years, almost all individuals are seropositive. Human herpesvirus 6 infections occur throughout the year without a distinct seasonal pattern. Secondary cases are rarely identified, although occasional outbreaks of roseola have been reported. Communicability is most likely greatest during the febrile and viremic phase of the illness. Virus is infrequently isolated from healthy children after defervescence.

The mean **incubation period**, based on experimental infection, is estimated to be approximately 9 days.

Diagnostic Tests: The diagnosis of primary HHV-6 infection currently necessitates primarily viral isolation from peripheral blood, which is available only in research laboratories. Commercial assays for antibody and antigen detection are being developed but are problematic in that they are unlikely to differentiate between primary infection and persistence or reactivation of the virus.

Treatment: Supportive.

Isolation of the Hospitalized Patient: No special precautions are recommended.

Control Measures: None.

Infectious Mononucleosis Due to Epstein-Barr Virus

Clinical Manifestations: Infectious mononucleosis is typically manifested by fever, exudative pharyngitis, lymphadenopathy, hepatosplenomegaly, and atypical lymphocytosis. However, the spectrum of disease is extremely variable, ranging from asymptomatic to fatal infection. Infections are frequently unrecognized in infants and young children. Rash, which is more frequent in patients treated with ampicillin, can occur. Central nervous system complications include aseptic meningitis, encephalitis, and the Guillain-Barré syndrome. Rare complications include splenic rupture, thrombocytopenia, agranulocytosis, hemolytic anemia, orchitis, and myocarditis. Usually, the replication of Epstein-Barr virus (EBV) in B-lymphocyte and the resulting lymphoproliferation is inhibited by natural killer and T-cell responses, but in patients who have congenital or acquired cellular immune deficiencies, fatal disseminated infection or B-cell lymphomas can occur. The chronic fatigue syndrome, formerly called "chronic" infectious mononucleosis, is not specifically related to EBV infection. However, a small group of patients with recurrent symptoms have markedly abnormal serologic tests for EBV and other viruses as well.

Two other syndromes caused by EBV assume much greater importance than infectious mononucleosis outside the United States. Burkitt B-cell lymphoma, found in Central Africa, and nasopharyngeal carcinoma, found in Southeast Asia, appear to be caused by persistent EBV infection.

Etiology: Epstein-Barr virus, a DNA virus, is a herpesvirus.

Epidemiology: Humans are the only source of EBV. Close personal contact is usually required for transmission. Epstein-Barr virus is also occasionally transmitted by blood transfusion. Infection is frequently contracted early in life, particularly among lower socioeconomic groups, in which intrafamilial spread is common. Endemic infectious mononucleosis is common in group settings of adolescents, such as in educational institutions. No seasonal pattern has been documented. Respiratory tract viral excretion can occur for many months after infection, and asymptomatic carriage is common. The period of communicability is indeterminate.

The **incubation period** is estimated to be 30 to 50 days.

Diagnostic Tests: Epstein-Barr virus isolation from oropharyngeal secretions is possible, but techniques for performing this procedure are usually not available in routine diagnostic laboratories, and viral isolation does not necessarily indicate acute infection. Hence, diagnosis depends on serologic testing. Nonspecific tests for heterophile antibody, including the Paul-Bunnell test and slide agglutination reaction, are most commonly available. These tests are often negative in infants and children younger than 4 years with EBV infection, but they identify approximately 90% of cases (proven by EBV-specific serology) in older children and adults.

Multiple specific serologic antibody tests for EBV are available in diagnostic virology laboratories (see Table 3.23, p 275). The most commonly performed test is for antibody against the viral capsid antigen (VCA). Since IgG antibody against VCA is found in high titers early after onset of infection, testing of paired sera for anti-VCA may not be useful in establishing infection. Testing for IgM anti-VCA antibody and for antibodies against early antigen (EA) are useful in identifying recent infections. Serum antibody against EBV nuclear antigens (EBNA) is present only several weeks to months after onset of the infection. The demonstration of anti-EBNA antibody excludes recent infection.

Epstein-Barr virus serologic tests are particularly valuable for studying patients who have heterophile-negative infectious mononucleosis. Testing for other viral agents, especially cytomegalovirus, is indicated in these patients. In research studies, culture of saliva or peripheral blood mononuclear cells for EBV, in situ DNA hybridization, or the polymerase chain reaction can determine the presence of EBV or EBV DNA, and may link a syndrome, such as lymphoproliferation, with the virus.

Treatment: Steroids have been useful for control of tonsillar swelling and other lymphadenopathy but are only considered in cases with complications. Although acyclovir has in vitro antiviral activity against EBV, the clinical benefits of treatment have not been demonstrated, with the possible exception of HIV-infected patients with the hairy leukoplakia. Reduced immunosuppressive therapy is beneficial in patients with EBV-induced lymphoproliferation.

Isolation of the Hospitalized Patient: No special precautions are recommended.

TABLE 3.23—Serum EBV Antibodies in EBV Infection

Infection	Anti-VCA-IgG*	Anti-VCA-IgM†	Anti-EA (D)‡	Anti-EBNA§
No previous infection	0	0	0	0
Acute infection	+	+	+/0	0
Recent infection	+	+/0	+/0	+/0
Past infection	+	0	0	+

*Anti-VCA-IgG: IgG class antibody to viral capsid antigen.
†Anti-VCA-IgM: IgM class antibody to viral capsid antigen.
‡EA(D): early antigen diffuse staining.
§EBNA: Epstein-Barr nuclear antigen.
0 = <1:10 or < 1:2 for EBNA.
+ = ≥1:10 or ≥ 1:2 for EBNA.

Control Measures: Patients with a recent history of EBV infection or an illness similar to infectious mononucleosis should not donate blood

Influenza

Clinical Manifestations: Influenza is characterized by the sudden onset of fever, frequently with chills or rigors, headache, malaise, diffuse myalgia, and a dry cough. Subsequently, the respiratory signs of sore throat, nasal congestion, and cough become more prominent. Conjunctival infection, abdominal pain, nausea, and vomiting can be present. In some children, influenza can appear as a simple upper respiratory tract infection or as a febrile illness with few respiratory signs. In young infants, influenza can produce a sepsis-like picture and occasionally cause croup or pneumonia. Acute myositis characterized by calf tenderness and refusal to walk may develop after several days of influenza, especially type B infection. Reye syndrome has been associated primarily with influenza B, but also with influenza A infection. Influenza can alter the metabolism of certain medications, especially theophylline, possibly resulting in the development of toxicity from high serum concentrations.

Etiology: Influenza viruses are orthomyxoviruses of three antigenic types (A, B, and C). Epidemic disease is caused by types A and B. Influenza A strains are subclassified by two antigens, hemagglutinin (H) and neuraminidase (N). Three immunologically distinct hemagglutinin subtypes (H1, H2, and H3) and two neuraminidases (N1 and N2) have been recognized as causing human infection. Specific antibodies to these various antigens are important determinants of immunity. Major changes in either of these antigens, such as H1 to H2, are called antigenic shifts. Minor variations within the same subtypes are called antigenic drifts. Antigenic shift has occurred only with influenza A, usually at intervals of 10 or more years. Antigenic drift, which occurs almost annually in both influenza A and B viruses, can result during a period of several years in susceptibility to infection with a type of influenza with which persons were previously infected or immunized.

Epidemiology: Influenza is spread from person to person by direct contact, large droplet infection, or articles recently contaminated by nasopharyngeal secretions. In some explosive outbreaks, airborne spread by small-particle aerosols has appeared to be an important mode of transmission. During an outbreak of influenza, the highest attack rates occur in school-aged children. Secondary spread to adults and other children within the family is common. The attack rates depend in part on the immunity developed by previous experience (either by natural disease or immunization) with the circulating strain or a related strain. Antigenic shift or major drift in the circulating strain is most likely to produce widespread epidemics. In temperate climates, epidemics almost always occur during the winter months and last 4 to 8 weeks within a community; the peak usually occurs within 2 weeks of the onset. In recent years, activity of two or three types of influenza virus in a community has been common and has been associated with a prolongation of the influenza season to 3 months or more. Influenza is highly contagious, especially among institutionalized populations. Patients are most infectious in the 24 hours before onset of symptoms and during the period of peak symptoms. Viral shedding in the nasal secretions usually ceases within 7 days of the onset of illness, but it can last longer in young children.

The impact of influenza on children is appreciable during interepidemic as well as epidemic years in both healthy children and those with underlying high-risk conditions. Attack rates in healthy children have recently been estimated at 10% to 40% each year, and approximately 1% of these infections can result in hospitalization. The risk of lower respiratory tract disease complicating influenza infection, primarily pneumonia and bronchiolitis, has ranged from 0.2% to 25%. A wide variety of complications, such as Reye syndrome, myositis, and central nervous system (CNS) manifestations can occur. The risk of subsequent Reye syndrome, which occurs primarily in school-aged children, has decreased in recent years. In contrast to patterns of respiratory disease in adults, other respiratory viruses (eg, respiratory syncytial virus and the parainfluenza viruses) cause yearly outbreaks of infection that can produce life-threatening illness in young children. As a result, morbidity and mortality rates in children for influenza are more difficult to determine and the effect of control measures for influenza can be more difficult to measure in children.

Excess rates of hospitalization have been documented for children with influenza who are neonates or who have sickle-cell disease, bronchopulmonary dysplasia, severe asthma, cystic fibrosis, malignancies, diabetes, or chronic renal disease. Pulmonary complications such as bronchitis and pneumonia appear to be more common in these children. Influenza in neonates has been associated with considerable morbidity, including a sepsis-like syndrome, apnea, and lower respiratory tract disease.

The **incubation period** is usually 1 to 3 days.

Diagnostic Tests: Cultures, when performed, should be obtained during the first 72 hours of illness because the quantity of virus shed subsequently decreases rapidly. Nasopharyngeal secretions obtained by swab or aspirate should be placed in appropriate transport media for culture. After inoculation into eggs or tissue culture, virus can usually be isolated within 2 to 6 days. The sensitivity of rapid diagnostic tests such as immunofluorescence for identification of influenza antigen in nasopharyngeal specimens has been variable. Serologic diagnosis can be made retrospectively by a significant change in antibody titer between acute and convalescent sera, as determined by complement fixation, hemagglutination inhibition, neutralization, or enzyme immunoassay tests.

Treatment: Both amantadine and its closely related analogue rimantadine are approved by the Food and Drug Administration (FDA) for use in children and adults for prophylaxis against influenza A infection, but in children only amantadine is currently approved for treatment. Studies evaluating either amantadine or rimantadine are limited in children, but they indicate that treatment with either drug diminished the severity of the signs and symptoms of influenza A infection when administered within 48 hours of the onset of illness. Amantadine and rimantadine are not effective in influenza B infections, and they are not FDA approved for use in infants (ie, children younger than 1 year).

Influenza A therapy with rimantadine or amantadine should be considered for (1) patients in whom the amelioration of clinical symptoms may be particularly beneficial, such as those with underlying conditions rendering them at high risk for severe or complicated influenza infection; (2) normal children with more severe illness; and (3) those with special environmental, family, or social situations, such as examinations and athletic competitions. Influenza A viral isolates may become resistant to amantadine and rimantadine after several days of treatment. Although this resistance has not been demonstrated to affect the clinical benefit of treatment, the epidemiologic implications of routinely using amantadine or rimantadine for treatment of influenza are unclear.

For children aged 9 years or younger, the recommended dosage for amantadine and rimantadine is 5 mg/kg/d, in one or two divided doses, given orally, not to exceed 150 mg/d. For older children weighing 40 kg or more, the dosage is 200 mg/d in one or two divided doses. For children older than 9 years but weighing less than 40 kg, the dosage is 5 mg/kg/d in one or two divided doses (see Table 3.24, p 278). Little information is available on the use of amantadine or rimantadine in children younger than 1 year. Therapy should be started as soon as possible after the onset of symptoms and continued for 2 to 7 days, depending on clinical improvement. Dosage should be reduced in patients with severe renal insufficiency. Either drug may cause mild CNS symptoms, which resolve with discontinuation of the drug. The incidence of these side effects appears to be higher in amantadine recipients than in those receiving rimantadine. An increased incidence of convulsions has been reported in children with epilepsy who receive amantadine. Seizures or seizure-like activity has also been observed in a small number of patients

TABLE 3.24—Dosage Recommendations for Amantadine and Rimantadine*,†,‡

	Age		
	1–9 y	Children ≥10 y	
		Weight <40 kg	Weight ≥40 kg
Treatment	5 mg/kg/d, maximum 150 mg/d, in 1 or 2 divided doses	5 mg/kg/d in 1 or 2 divided doses	200 mg/d in 1 or 2 divided doses
Prophylaxis	Dosages may be the same as those for treatment. An alternative and equally acceptable dosage for children >20 kg and adults is 100 mg/d. For either regimen, the total daily dosage may be given in 1 or 2 divided doses.		

*Amantadine and rimantadine are not FDA approved for use in children younger than 1 y of age.
†Rimantadine is FDA approved for prophylaxis in children but not for treatment of children.
‡Patients, including elderly persons, with any degree of renal insufficiency should be monitored for adverse effects, and the dosage reduced or the drug discontinued as necessary (see package insert for further information).

with a history of convulsions while taking rimantadine, although the incidence has not been adequately evaluated.

Both influenza A and B viruses are sensitive in vitro to ribavirin. In clinical trials of normal, young adults with natural influenza A and B infections, therapy with aerosolized ribavirin has been associated with a modest shortening of clinical symptoms. Ribavirin, however, is not approved for the treatment of influenza infections at this time.

Control of fever with acetaminophen or ibuprofen may be important in young children because the fever of influenza can precipitate febrile convulsions. **Children with influenza should not receive salicylates because of the resulting increased risk of developing Reye syndrome.**

Isolation of the Hospitalized Patient: For children hospitalized with influenza or an influenza-like illness, contact isolation precautions are recommended for the duration of the illness. Respiratory secretions should be considered infectious, and strict hand washing procedures should be used.

Control Measures:

Influenza Vaccine. The current influenza vaccines produced in embryonated eggs are immunogenic, safe, and associated with minimal side effects. The vaccines are multivalent and contain different viral subtypes; the composition is periodically changed in anticipation of the expected prevalent influenza strains. The preparations currently in use are the inactivated whole-virus vaccine prepared from the intact, purified virus particles; the subvirion vaccine prepared by the additional step of disrupting the lipid-containing membrane of the virus; and purified surface-antigen vaccine. Only the subvirion or purified surface-antigen vaccines, ie, those termed "split"-virus vaccines, should be used for children younger than 13 years of age.

Immunogenicity in Children. In children with little previous experience with influenza, two doses of vaccine administered 1 month apart are necessary to produce a satisfactory antibody response (see Table 3.25, page 280). Children previously primed with a related strain of influenza by infection or vaccination almost uniformly exhibit a brisk antibody response to one dose of the vaccine.

Vaccine Efficacy. The impact of influenza immunization on acute respiratory illness is less likely to be evident in pediatric than adult populations because of the frequency of colds, upper respiratory tract infections, and influenza-like illness caused by other viral agents in young children. The efficacy of the currently available killed vaccines has also been difficult to assess because of yearly variation in the strains of the circulating viruses and their resulting variation in similarity to the antigens contained in the available vaccines. The protection in healthy subjects from either the whole-virus or split-virus vaccines against homologous viral-type challenge is usually 70% to 80%, with a range of 50% to 95%. Efficacy has not been evaluated in infants in the first 6 months of life.

Special Considerations:

- In immunosuppressed children receiving chemotherapy, influenza immunization with a new vaccine antigen results in a sufficient immune response in only a minority of children. The optimal time to immunize children with malignancies who still must undergo chemotherapy is 3 to 4 weeks after chemotherapy has been discontinued and the peripheral granulocyte and lymphocyte counts are greater than 1,000/mm^3. Children who are no longer receiving chemotherapy generally have high rates of seroconversion.
- The immune response and safety of influenza vaccine in children with hemodynamically unstable cardiac disease (another large group of children potentially at high risk for complications of influenza) are comparable to those in healthy children.
- The effect of steroid therapy on influenza vaccine immunogenicity is unknown. Since a high dose of steroids (ie, a dose equivalent to either 2 mg/kg or a total of 20 mg/d of prednisone) may impair antibody responses, particularly in unvaccinated or previously uninfected persons, vaccination could be deferred temporarily during the time of receipt of high doses, provided deferral does not compromise the likelihood of immunization before the recommended time of administration, ie, before the start of the influenza season (see Vaccine Administration, p 281). Steroid therapy should not unnecessarily delay the administration of influenza vaccine, particularly in children with asthma who require intermittent or maintenance steroid therapy.
- Infants younger than 6 months with high-risk conditions, especially those with cardiopulmonary compromise, may have the same risk as, or a greater risk than, older children. However, no information is available about the reactivity, immunogenicity, or efficacy of the influenza vaccines in infants during the first 6 months of life. In addition, the effect of influenza antigens in an inactivated vaccine on the infant's future immune response to influenza is not known. Thus, alternative methods of protection for young infants should be considered (see Chemoprophylaxis: Alternative Method of Protecting Children Against Influenza, p 282).

TABLE 3.25—Schedule for Influenza Immunization*

Age	Recommended Vaccine†	Dose‡	Number of Doses
6–35 mo	Split virus only	0.25 mL	1-2§
3–8 y	Split virus only	0.5 mL	1-2§
9–12 y	Split virus only	0.5 mL	1
>12 y	Whole or split virus	0.5 mL	1

*Vaccine is administered intramuscularly.
†Split-virus vaccine may be termed "split," "subvirion," or "purified surface-antigen" vaccine.
‡Dosages are those recommended in recent years. Since they could change in future years, physicians should refer to the product circular for dosage for each vaccine.
§Two doses are recommended if the child is receiving influenza vaccine for the first time. If the hemagglutinin and neuraminidase of vaccine strains have not changed, subsequent immunization may be achieved with one dose yearly.

Recommendations for Influenza Immunization:
Targeted High-Risk Children. Yearly immunization is recommended for children 6 months of age and older with one or more specific risk factor. Data are insufficient on the severity of influenza in several of these groups of children; however, based on available data and knowledge of the pathophysiology of these disorders, children with the following risk factors warrant immunization:
• Those with asthma and other chronic pulmonary diseases.
• Those with hemodynamically significant cardiac disease.
• Those undergoing immunosuppressive therapy (for the optimal time of administration, see Special Considerations, p 279).
• Those with sickle-cell anemia and other hemoglobinopathies.
Other High-Risk Children. Children who should be considered potentially at increased risk for complicated influenza illness and who may benefit from influenza immunization are those with one or more of the following conditions:
• HIV infection (see HIV Infection and AIDS, p 263)
• Diabetes mellitus
• Chronic renal disease
• Chronic metabolic diseases
• Recipients of long-term aspirin therapy such as children with rheumatoid arthritis or Kawasaki disease who, thus, may be at increased risk for developing Reye syndrome. Influenza vaccination may also be considered for children who are marginally compromised from any underlying condition, since even uncomplicated influenza can produce adverse effects on the course of an underlying disease.
Close Contacts of High-Risk Patients. Immunization and chemoprophylaxis of adults who are in close contact with high-risk children may be an important means of protection for these children, especially for infants younger than 6 months for whom vaccination is not recommended. The immunization of pregnant women may be beneficial to their soon-to-be-born

infants, since transplacentally acquired antibody appears to protect them from infection with influenza A virus. The following is recommended:

- Immunization of hospital personnel in contact with pediatric patients should be encouraged.
- Household contacts, including siblings and primary caretakers of high-risk children, should be immunized.
- Children who are members of households with high-risk adults, including those with symptomatic human immunodeficiency virus (HIV) infection, should be immunized.

Other Children. Vaccination should be considered for groups of individuals whose close contact facilitates rapid transmission and resulting disruption of routine activities. Examples are students in colleges, schools, and other institutions of learning, particularly those who reside in dormitories or who are members of athletic teams, and those living in residential institutions.

Physicians should administer influenza vaccine to any child or adolescent whose parents or guardian wishes to reduce the child's or adolescent's chance of developing illness due to influenza infection. The morbidity from influenza in normal children can be appreciable, but routine immunization of all normal children at this time is not feasible.

Foreign Travel. Persons traveling to foreign areas in which influenza outbreaks are or may be occurring should be considered candidates for vaccination, since the likelihood of exposure to influenza during travel is increased and the resulting illness can spoil the trip. The decision to give influenza vaccine will depend on the destination, duration of travel, and risk of acquiring influenza (because of the season of the year and other factors) and the possible consequences.

Vaccine Administration. Influenza vaccine should be administered in the autumn before the start of the influenza season, which is usually December or later but in some years has occurred earlier. The recommended vaccine, dose, and schedule for different age groups are given in Table 3.25 (p 280). Annual vaccination is recommended because of declining immunity in the year after vaccination, and in most years at least one of the antigens is changed to increase the antigenic similarity between vaccine and circulating strains.

Influenza vaccine may be administered simultaneously (but at a separate site and with a different syringe) with other routine vaccinations in children, including pertussis vaccine (DTP or DTaP). Since influenza vaccine in young children can cause fever, DTaP may be preferable in those children 15 months and older who are receiving the fourth (or fifth) dose of pertussis vaccine.

Reactions, Adverse Effects, and Contraindications. Febrile reactions in children younger than 13 years are infrequent, especially after split-virus vaccine administration, and occur primarily 6 to 24 hours after vaccination in children younger than 24 months of age. For children older than 12 years and for adults the side effects and immunogenicity of the whole-virus and split-virus vaccines are similar when used at the recommended doses (see Table 3.25, p 280). Local reactions are infrequent in children younger than 13 years. In children 13 years or older, they occur in approximately 10% after immunization with either whole- or split-virus vaccine.

Unlike the 1976-77 swine influenza vaccine, subsequent vaccines prepared from other virus strains have not been clearly associated with an increased frequency of Guillain-Barré syndrome (GBS). However, estimating the precise risk for a rare condition such as GBS is difficult. In 1990-91, although no overall increase in frequency of GBS among vaccine recipients was observed, a small increase in GBS cases in vaccinated persons 18 to 64 years of age, but not those aged 65 years or older or those younger than 18 years, may have occurred. In contrast to the swine influenza vaccine, the epidemiologic features of the possible association of the 1990-91 vaccine with GBS were not as convincing. Even if GBS were a true side effect, the very low estimated risk of GBS is less than that of severe influenza that could be prevented by immunization. In addition, GBS has **not** been associated with influenza immunization of children.

Immunization of children who have asthma with the currently available influenza vaccines is not associated with a detectable increase in adverse reactions, including bronchial reactivity and leukocyte histamine release.

Children demonstrating severe, anaphylactic reaction to chickens or eggs can experience, on rare occasion, a similar type of reaction to killed influenza vaccines. Although influenza vaccine has been safely administered to such children after skin testing and even desensitization, these children generally should not receive influenza vaccine in view of the risk of reactions, the likely need for yearly vaccination, and the availability of chemoprophylaxis against influenza A infection.

Chemoprophylaxis: Alternative Method of Protecting Children Against Influenza.

Most studies demonstrating the efficacy of amantadine or rimantadine as a chemoprophylactic agent against influenza A infection have been performed in adults. Several studies in children have indicated a similar beneficial effect in diminishing the spread of influenza among institutionalized children and family members and on pediatric wards. Both drugs are FDA approved for prophylaxis in children and adults. The usual recommended doses of rimantadine and amantadine for prophylaxis are the same as those for treatment. However, studies have demonstrated that a dose of 100 mg/d for prophylaxis in adults and in children weighing more than 20 kg is as effective as the recommended dose of 200 mg/d for treatment and may be associated with fewer side effects. This dosage of 100 mg/d, given in one or two divided doses, thus, is also acceptable for these persons. The prophylactic dosage for children weighing 20 kg or less remains the same as the therapeutic dosage and may be given in one or two divided doses. These recommendations are summarized in Table 3.24 (p 278).

Indications. Persons for whom chemoprophylaxis is or may be indicated are as follows:

• Children* and adolescents at high risk who were vaccinated after influenza A activity in the community has begun. Chemoprophylaxis during the interval before a vaccine response (2 weeks after the recommended vaccine schedule of one or two doses has been completed) can be beneficial.

---

*Use of amantadine and rimantadine in infants (ie, children younger than 1 year of age) has not been adequately evaluated and neither drug is FDA approved for use in infants.

- Unimmunized persons providing care to high-risk individuals.
- Immunodeficient persons whose antibody response to vaccine is likely to be poor.
- Persons at high risk for whom vaccine is contraindicated, specifically those with anaphylactic hypersensitivity to egg protein who do not receive desensitization (see Reactions, Adverse Effects, and Contraindications, p 281).

Isosporiasis
(Isospora belli)

Clinical Manifestations: Protracted watery diarrhea is the most common presenting symptom. Clinical manifestations are similar to those caused by *Cryptosporidium* and include abdominal pain, anorexia, and weight loss. Infection can be life threatening in immunocompromised patients, particularly those with AIDS. Fever, malaise, abdominal pain, and headache have all been reported.

Etiology: *Isospora belli* is a coccidian protozoan.

Epidemiology: Humans are the only known host for *I belli*. Frequency of this parasite, especially in asymptomatic persons, is unknown. Infection is more common in tropical and subtropical than in temperate climates and in areas of poor sanitary conditions. Human infection probably occurs by the oral-fecal route. Oocysts are resistant to most disinfectants and may remain viable for months in a cool, moist environment.

The **incubation period** is estimated to be 8 to 14 days, based on a small number of persons who had laboratory exposure to the organism.

Diagnostic Tests: Demonstration of oocysts in feces or in duodenal aspirates or finding developmental stages of the parasite in biopsy specimens of the small intestine is diagnostic. Oocysts in stool can be distinguished by their size, which is ten times larger than *Cryptosporidium*, and by their oval shape. Oocysts can be detected by a modified Kinyoun acid-fast stain and by auramine-rhodamine stains. Concentration techniques may be needed since organisms are often present in small numbers.

Treatment: Trimethoprim-sulfamethoxazole or pyrimethamine-sulfadoxine (Fansidar) are effective. In HIV-infected patients who are allergic to sulfonamides, treatment of adults with pyrimethamine (75 mg/d), followed by daily prophylactic administration of pyrimethamine (25 mg/d) has been effective.

Isolation of the Hospitalized Patient: Enteric precautions are recommended, but risk of nosocomial infection is unknown.

Control Measures: None.

Kawasaki Disease

Clinical Manifestations: Kawasaki disease is a febrile, exanthematous, multisystem illness in which the acute phase is self-limited. It occurs predominantly in children younger than 5 years of age. Within 3 days of the abrupt onset of fever, the other characteristic features of the illness usually appear, including (1) discrete bulbar conjunctival injection without exudate; (2) erythematous mouth and pharynx, strawberry tongue, and red, cracked lips; (3) a polymorphous generalized erythematous rash that can be morbilliform, maculopapular, or scarlatiniform, or may resemble erythema multiforme; (4) changes in the peripheral extremities consisting of induration of the hands and feet with erythematous palms and soles; and (5) a usually solitary, frequently unilateral cervical lymph node enlarged to more than 1.5 cm in diameter. These early manifestations progress with drying, cracking, and fissuring of the lips, usually apparent by the sixth day of illness. Periungual desquamation and peeling of the palms and, to a lesser extent, soles, occur during the second to third week. For the diagnosis to be made, patients should have fever and at least four of these five features. Patients with fever and fewer than four of these manifestations can be diagnosed as having atypical Kawasaki disease when coronary artery disease is detected. Associated features include anterior uveitis (80%) in the first week of illness, sterile pyuria (70%), arthritis or arthralgias (35%), aseptic meningitis (5%), carditis with congestive heart failure (less than 5%), pericardial effusion or arrhythmias (20%), and gallbladder hydrops with or without obstructive jaundice (less than 10%).

Without aspirin or intravenous immunoglobulin therapy, the mean duration of fever is 12 days. After the fever resolves, patients can remain anorectic or irritable for 2 to 3 weeks. During this subacute phase, the characteristic peripheral desquamation can occur, usually between days 10 and 20 of the illness.

Carditis and arthritis can develop at any time during the acute and subacute phases (the first 3 weeks of illness) and generally resolve by 6 to 8 weeks after the onset of the manifestation. Routine two-dimensional echocardiography or angiography demonstrates coronary aneurysm(s) in approximately 20% of untreated patients. Patients at increased risk for development of coronary aneurysms include males, infants (ie, younger than 12 months of age), those whose fever persists for more than 10 days, and those who manifest signs or symptoms of cardiac involvement (such as arrhythmias or pericardial effusion). Coronary aneurysms have been detected within 3 days after the onset of symptoms. The peak prevalence of coronary aneurysms and coronary dilation is approximately 2 to 4 weeks after onset of disease. In some children with mild coronary dilation, the coronary artery size returns to baseline by 8 weeks after onset of disease. Prospective studies indicate that coronary aneurysms frequently regress to normal lumen size within 1 year. However, coronary stenosis may accompany aneurysm regression, and aneurysm regression does not always result in a normal blood vessel. Other arterial aneurysms (eg, iliac, femoral, and axillary vessels) can occur. In addition to coronary artery disease, carditis can involve the pericardium, myocardium, or endocardium, and mitral and aortic regurgitation can occur.

The current mortality rate in the United States is less than 0.5%. Death results from coronary occlusion with myocardial infarction due to thrombosis or progressive stenosis. Seventy-five percent of fatalities occur within 6 weeks of the onset of symptoms, but myocardial infarction and sudden death can occur months to years after the acute episode. Long-term prognosis is unknown.

Etiology: The etiology is not known. However, the epidemiology and clinical presentation suggest an infectious etiology.

Epidemiology: Peak age of occurrence in the United States is between 6 months and 5 years. Fifty percent of patients are younger than 2 years and 80% are younger than 5 years; children older than 8 years seldom have the disease. The male to female ratio is 1.6:1. The incidence is highest in Asians. Two thousand to 4,000 cases are estimated to occur annually in the United States.

Kawasaki disease was first described in Japan where a pattern of endemic occurrence with superimposed epidemic outbreaks has emerged. A similar pattern of steady or increasing endemic disease with sharply defined community-wide epidemics has been recognized in diverse locations in North America and Hawaii. Epidemics generally occur during the winter and spring at 2- to 3-year intervals. No evidence indicates person-to-person or common-source spread, although the incidence is higher in siblings of children with Kawasaki disease.

Diagnostic Tests*: No specific tests are available. The diagnosis is established by fulfillment of the clinical criteria (see Clinical Manifestations) and exclusion of other possible illnesses, including measles, streptococcal infections (ie, scarlet fever), viral and rickettsial exanthems, drug reactions (eg, Stevens-Johnson syndrome), staphylococcal scalded skin syndrome, toxic shock syndrome, juvenile rheumatoid arthritis, leptospirosis, and mercury poisoning. An elevated sedimentation rate and C-reactive protein during the first 2 weeks and an elevated platelet count (above 450,000/mm^3) after the 10th day of illness are common laboratory features. These values usually return to normal within 6 to 8 weeks.

Treatment*: Management consists of supportive care, detection of coronary artery disease, and anti-inflammatory therapy. **Specific therapy should be initiated when the diagnosis is established.** Specific recommendations are as follows:

Immune Globulin Intravenous (IGIV). High-dose IGIV therapy initiated within 10 days of the onset of fever in conjunction with aspirin decreases the prevalence of coronary artery dilation and aneurysms detected 2 and 7 weeks later in comparison to treatment with aspirin alone. The mechanism of action

---

*For further information on the diagnosis of Kawasaki disease, see the statement prepared by the Committee on Rheumatic Fever, Endocarditis, and Kawasaki Disease of the American Heart Association: Dajani AS, Taubert KA, Gerber MA, et al. Diagnosis and therapy of Kawasaki disease in children. *Circulation.* 1993;87:1776-1780

of IGIV has not been identified. Significant and rapid resolution of fever and other indicators of acute inflammation have also been demonstrated. Hence, IGIV in conjunction with aspirin is recommended to treat patients who meet the criteria for Kawasaki disease (see Clinical Manifestations, p 284). Therapy with IGIV should be initiated as soon as possible and within 10 days of the onset of illness. The efficacy of such therapy if initiated later than 10 days after onset of illness or after aneurysms have been detected has not been evaluated. Therapy with IGIV should be considered for those patients diagnosed after day 10 who have signs of ongoing inflammation (eg, fever and increased sedimentation rate) or of evolving coronary artery disease.

Dosage. The optimal therapeutic dose of IGIV is not known. In the initial studies demonstrating the therapeutic benefit of IGIV, the dosage schedule was 400 mg/kg/d in a 2-hour infusion for 4 consecutive days. In a later well-controlled study, a dosage schedule of 2 g/kg as a single dose, given during a 10- to 12-hour period, was at least as effective in decreasing the prevalence of subsequent coronary artery disease and ameliorating the resolution of fever and other acute inflammatory indices. Complications from this regimen were few and no more than those associated with the 4-day schedule. Advantages of the single-dose regimen (2 g/kg) are (1) shorter duration of intravenous therapy, (2) earlier defervescence, and (3) possible earlier hospital discharge of the child. Therefore, the single infusion of 2 g/kg is preferred. Other studies have used single doses of 1 g/kg IGIV, but no trials comparing the efficacies of single doses of 1 g/kg and 2 g/kg have been reported.

Retreatment. Approximately 10% of children with Kawasaki disease treated with IGIV may not respond to the initial dose and may experience persistent or recrudescent fever. Other clinical indications of inflammation, such as conjunctivitis and rash, may also persist or recur. If the diagnosis remains likely when the patient is reevaluated, retreatment with a second infusion of 1 to 2 g/kg, given in a 10- to 12-hour period, should be considered.

Aspirin. Aspirin is given initially in high dosage for its anti-inflammatory effect, and, subsequently, in low dosage for its antiplatelet aggregation action. An anti-inflammatory dose of 80 to 100 mg/kg/d in four divided doses can reduce the duration of fever if started during the first week. Serum salicylate concentrations should be followed during high-dose therapy because gastrointestinal absorption is highly variable. After fever is controlled, aspirin should be decreased. A suggested dose is 3 to 5 mg/kg (maximum, 80 mg/d) given in one daily dose; this regimen should be maintained for at least 2 months or until both the platelet count and sedimentation rate are normal to reduce the likelihood of spontaneous coronary thrombosis. Because the risk of Reye syndrome associated with treatment of influenza or varicella with aspirin may outweigh the benefit of aspirin therapy, parents of children receiving aspirin should be instructed to contact their child's physician promptly if their child develops symptoms of varicella or influenza.

Cardiac Care. An echocardiogram should be obtained early in the acute phase of the illness, 3 weeks after onset and 8 weeks after onset. The care of patients with carditis should involve a cardiologist experienced in the management of patients with Kawasaki disease and in echocardiographic studies of coronary arteries in children. Children must be examined repeatedly during the first 2 months to detect arrhythmias, congestive heart failure, valvular insufficiency, and myocarditis. In addition to prolonged low-dose aspirin therapy to suppress platelet aggregation in patients with persistent coronary artery abnormalities, some experts recommend dipyridamole in a dose of 4 mg/kg/d, given in three divided doses.

Corticosteroids. These drugs are contraindicated except in very unusual circumstances. Corticosteroid use has resulted in increased frequency of coronary aneurysms, according to several studies.

Subsequent Immunization. Measles vaccination in children who have received high-dose IGIV for treatment of Kawasaki disease should be deferred for 11 months, after receipt of IGIV (see Measles, p 318). An exception is if the child's risk of exposure to measles is high, in which case he or she should be vaccinated and then revaccinated at or after 11 months following the receipt of IGIV, unless serologic testing indicates that the child was successfully immunized by the earlier dose. Subsequent administration of other childhood immunizations should not be interrupted. Yearly influenza vaccination is indicated in patients requiring long-term aspirin therapy because of the possible increased risk of developing Reye syndrome (see Influenza, p 280).

Isolation of the Hospitalized Patient: No special precautions are indicated.

Control Measures: None.

Legionella pneumophila Infections

Clinical Manifestations: Infection results in at least the following two distinct syndromes:
- Pneumonia (Legionnaires' disease), which varies in severity from a mild respiratory tract illness to severe multisystem disease with gastrointestinal tract, central nervous system, renal, and progressive pulmonary manifestations. Respiratory failure and death can occur.
- Pontiac fever, which is an abrupt-onset, self-limited, influenza-like illness without pneumonia.

Etiology: *Legionella* are fastidious, weakly staining, Gram-negative bacilli. Eighteen different species have been implicated in human disease, but the majority of *Legionella* infections in the United States are caused by *L pneumophila* serogroup 1.

Epidemiology: Legionnaires' disease is acquired through inhalation of aerosolized water contaminated with *Legionella*. Person-to-person transmission has not been demonstrated. More than 80% of cases appear to be sporadic in occurrence and unrelated to outbreaks; the sources of infection for these cases have not been well characterized. Outbreaks have been ascribed to common-source exposure to contaminated air-conditioning cooling towers, evaporative condensers, and potable water systems. Outbreaks have occurred in hospitals, hotels, and other large buildings. The disease occurs most commonly in elderly and immunocompromised persons. Infection in children is uncommon and is usually asymptomatic or mild, and unrecognized. Severe disease has occurred in children with leukemia, severe immunodeficiency, and chronic granulomatous disease.

The **incubation period** for Legionnaires' disease (pneumonia) is 2 to 10 days; for Pontiac fever it is 1 to 2 days.

Diagnostic Tests: The recovery of *Legionella* from respiratory tract secretions by culture using special media is definitive evidence of infection. The bacterium can be demonstrated in these specimens by direct immunofluorescence and by DNA probes, but these tests are less sensitive than culture. For serologic diagnosis, a fourfold or greater rise in titer of antibody to *L pneumophila* serogroup 1 to 1:128 or greater, measured by an indirect immunofluorescence antibody assay (IFA), also indicates acute infection. Newer serologic assays, such as enzyme immunoassay or tests using *Legionella* antigens other than serogroup 1, are commercially available but have not been adequately standardized. A single titer of 1:256 or more in a patient with compatible clinical manifestations is considered presumptive evidence of infection, but approximately 5% of healthy adults will have a titer of this magnitude. Antibodies to *Mycoplasma pneumoniae*, several Gram-negative organisms, *Mycobacterium tuberculosis*, and *Campylobacter jejuni* may cause false-positive IFA tests. Detection of *L pneumophila* serogroup 1 antigen in urine by radioimmunoassay allows rapid diagnosis of infection with this subtype. Antibody titers usually rise within 1 to 6 weeks after onset of symptoms but can be delayed for as many as 12 weeks. Titer rises from cross-reacting antibodies can also occur.

Treatment: Erythromycin (30 to 60 mg/kg/d, maximum 2 to 4 g/d in four divided doses) is the drug of choice. Intravenous high-dose therapy is generally given initially. Once the patient is improving, oral therapy can be substituted. The addition of rifampin (15 mg/kg/d, maximum 600 mg/d) is recommended for patients with confirmed disease who do not respond promptly to intravenous erythromycin. Newer antimicrobial agents such as ciprofloxacin, ofloxacin, azithromycin, and clarithromycin may also be effective. The quinolones are not approved by the Food and Drug Administration for persons younger than 18 years of age. Duration of therapy is usually 3 weeks.

Isolation of the Hospitalized Patient: No special precautions are recommended.

Control Measures: Methods for decontaminating water supplies in common-source outbreaks have included hyperchloridation (or other chemical decontaminants) and/or superheating (to 70°C, 158°F) in conjunction with appropriate mechanical cleaning.

Leishmaniasis

Clinical Manifestations: The three major clinical syndromes are as follows:

1. *Cutaneous leishmaniasis.* After inoculation of parasites by the bite of an infected sand fly, local proliferation results in an erythematous macule or nodule that ultimately forms a shallow ulcer with raised borders. Lesions are typically located on exposed areas of the face and extremities and may be accompanied by satellite lesions and regional adenopathy. The clinical manifestations of Old World and New World cutaneous leishmaniasis are similar. Spontaneous resolution of lesions may take from weeks to years and usually results in residual scarring.

2. *Mucosal leishmaniasis (espundia).* After the initial cutaneous infection by species of the New World *Leishmania braziliensis* complex, parasites may disseminate over months to years to midline facial structures, including the oral and nasopharyngeal mucosa. In some patients, granulomatous ulceration follows, leading to facial disfigurement, infection, and mucosal perforation.

3. *Visceral leishmaniasis (kala-azar).* After cutaneous inoculation of parasites, organisms spread throughout the mononuclear macrophage system and are concentrated in the spleen, liver, and bone marrow. The resulting clinical illness is marked by fever, anorexia, weight loss, splenomegaly, hepatomegaly, lymphadenopathy, anemia, leukopenia, thrombocytopenia with hemorrhage, and hypergammaglobulinemia. Secondary pyogenic, enteric, and mycobacterial infections are common. Active, untreated visceral disease is often fatal. Reactivation of latent visceral leishmaniasis has been reported in patients with concurrent human immunodeficiency virus infection.

Etiology: Cutaneous leishmaniasis is caused by multiple species of the protozoan genus *Leishmania*, including *Leishmania tropica*, *Leishmania aethiopica*, and *Leishmania major* (Old World species); and *Leishmania mexicana*, *Leishmania peruviana*, and *L braziliensis* (New World species). Mucosal leishmaniasis is caused by subspecies of the *L braziliensis* complex, and visceral infection is caused by *Leishmania donovani*, *Leishmania infantum*, *Leishmania chagasi*, and *Leishmania tropica*. *Leishmania* species are obligate intracellular parasites in the human host.

Epidemiology: Leishmaniasis is a zoonosis with a variety of mammalian reservoir hosts, including canines and rodents. The vector is the phlebotomine sand fly. The distribution of Old World cutaneous leishmaniasis includes the Middle East, some Asian and African countries, countries of the former Soviet Union, and, sporadically, southern Europe. New World cutaneous leishmaniasis is found from the Yucatan region of Mexico to northern Argentina, although a few cases have been reported as far north as Texas. Mucosal leishmaniasis occurs primarily in the Amazon basin and the central plains of Brazil but also has been reported in other countries in South and Central America. The distribution of visceral leishmaniasis includes the Old World from China to India, the Middle East, southern Europe, the Mediterranean basin, and East Africa. Small endemic foci have also occurred in both South and Central America, particularly in Brazil.

The **incubation period** of the different forms of leishmaniasis range from several days to months. In cutaneous leishmaniasis, primary skin lesions typically appear several weeks after parasite inoculation. In visceral infection, the incubation period can vary from 6 weeks to 6 months. However, incubation periods from 10 days to 10 years have been reported, and reactivation of previously asymptomatic latent infection can occur in immunosuppressed patients.

Diagnostic Tests: Definitive diagnosis is usually established by microscopic identification of intracellular leishmanial organisms on Giemsa-stained smears or histologic sections of infected tissues. In cutaneous disease, tissue can be obtained by a 3-mm punch biopsy, lesion scrapings, or a needle aspiration of the raised nonnecrotic edge of the lesion. In visceral leishmaniasis, the organisms are usually present in the spleen and may be present in bone marrow, liver, and lymph nodes. Whenever possible, isolation of parasites by culture of appropriate tissue specimens in specialized media should be attempted. Culture media and further information can be provided by the Centers for Disease Control and Prevention (CDC).

The diagnosis of visceral leishmaniasis and some cases of cutaneous infection can also be aided by serologic testing available at the CDC. However, a negative serologic test should never be interpreted as excluding the possibility of a leishmanial infection. In addition, occasional false-positive results occur in patients with other infectious diseases, especially American trypanosomiasis (Chagas' disease).

Treatment: Because cutaneous lesions may heal without specific therapy, treatment is not always necessary. Treatment is indicated when the ulcers are disabling or disfiguring, when healing is delayed, or when the patient may be infected with a subspecies of the *L braziliensis* complex. Drug therapy is always indicated when mucosal or visceral infection is present.

In the United States, the standard drug of choice for leishmaniasis is stibogluconate sodium, a parenteral pentavalent antimonial that is usually given daily for a minimum of 20 days. It is available from the Drug Service of the CDC (see Directory of Telephone Numbers, p 601). It is generally well tolerated in young, otherwise healthy patients, but cardiac and hepatic toxicity can occur. Meglumine antimoniate is a similar antimonial compound that can be administered as an alternative to stibogluconate (see Drugs for Parasitic Infections, p 574). For patients with disease that is refractory to antimonial therapy, amphotericin B, or pentamidine, may also be considered. In selected cases of American cutaneous leishmaniasis, ketoconazole and allopurinol, as well as local heat, have been used successfully.

Isolation of the Hospitalized Patient: No special precautions are necessary.

Control Measures: Since elimination of infected animal reservoirs and/or sand fly populations is unlikely in most regions that are endemic for leishmaniasis, travelers should be advised to minimize their exposure to sand fly bites by the use of screened accommodations, fine-mesh bed netting, protective clothing, and insect repellents, and by minimizing outdoor exposures from dusk to dawn. Patients with visceral leishmaniasis should not donate blood.

Leprosy

Clinical Manifestations: Leprosy is a chronic disease involving mainly skin, peripheral nerves, and the mucosa of the upper airway. The clinical syndromes of leprosy represent a spectrum that reflects the cellular immune response to *Mycobacterium leprae*. Characteristic features are the following:
- Tuberculoid: one or few well-demarcated, hypopigmented or erythematous, hypoesthetic or anesthetic skin lesions, frequently with raised, active, spreading edges and central clearing. Cell-mediated immune responses are intact.
- Lepromatous: initial numerous, ill-defined, hypopigmented or erythematous macules that progress to papules, nodules, or plaques; and late-occurring hypesthesia. Dermal infiltration of the face, hands, and feet in a bilateral and symmetric distribution can occur without preceding maculopapular lesions. *Mycobacterium leprae*-specific, cell-mediated immunity is greatly diminished. However, antibody responses to *M leprae*-derived antigens may occur, or nonspecific antibodies (such as rheumatoid factor or nontreponemal tests for syphilis) may be elevated.
- Borderline (dimorphous): single or multiple well-defined skin lesions similar to tuberculoid but with a raised central area; and delayed development of dysesthesia. Borderline disease is often subdivided into borderline lepromatous, borderline, and borderline tuberculoid.
- Indeterminate: an early form of leprosy that may develop into any of the other forms; typified by hypopigmented macules with indistinct edges and no associated dysesthesia.
  Serious consequences of leprosy occur from nerve involvement with resulting anesthesia, which can lead to repeated, unrecognized trauma, ulcerations, fractures, and bone resorption.

Etiology: Leprosy is caused by the bacteria *M leprae*.

Epidemiology: The major mode of transmission is contact with humans who have untreated or drug-resistant multibacillary disease (lepromatous or borderline types). A long duration of exposure, such as to a household contact, is common. However, 70% to 80% of cases in endemic areas do not have a history of household exposure or other contact with a known or suspected case of leprosy, suggesting the possibility of other sources of infection. The major source of infectious material is probably nasal secretions from patients with untreated multibacillary forms from whom organisms are found in large numbers. Little shedding of *M leprae* from patients' intact skin occurs. In the United States, 90% of reported cases are imported, occurring in immigrants and refugees from areas endemic for leprosy, particularly Mexico and Southeast Asia. Indigenous cases continue to occur in Texas, California, Louisiana, and Hawaii. The infectivity of lepromatous patients probably ceases soon after treatment is instituted, frequently within a few days or weeks of initiating rifampin therapy or about 3 months after initiating therapy with dapsone or clofazimine.

The **incubation period** ranges from 1 to many years; usually, it is 3 to 5 years. The incubation period of tuberculoid cases tends to be shorter than that for lepromatous cases.

Diagnostic Tests: Histopathologic examination by an experienced pathologist is the best method for establishing the diagnosis and is the basis for the classification of leprosy. Acid-fast bacilli may be found in slit-smears or biopsies from skin lesions, but rarely from patients with the tuberculoid and indeterminate forms of disease. Organisms have not been successfully cultured in vitro. Drug resistance is tested by the mouse footpad inoculation test. However, this test is only performed in specialized laboratories and results are not available for at least 6 months. Therefore, changes in medication are usually based on clinical findings. The demonstration of morphologically normal bacilli, ie, organisms with solid-staining of the capsule on AFB stains, despite usually effective therapy, should suggest possible drug resistance (or poor compliance with therapy), indicating the possible need for a change in therapy.

High titers of predominantly IgM serum antibodies against phenolic glycolipid-1 of *M leprae* have been detected in untreated patients with lepromatous or borderline disease. Because elevated antibody titers frequently occur in persons without disease, this test is not diagnostic for leprosy. Titers of these antibodies slowly decrease after years of therapy. This test is experimental and available only in a few reference laboratories.

Treatment: Therapy of patients with leprosy should be undertaken in consultation with an expert in leprosy. The Gillis W. Long Hansen's Disease Center (GWLHDC), Carville, Louisiana (800/642-2477), provides consultation on clinical and pathologic issues and can provide information about local Hansen's disease clinics and/or clinicians who have experience with the disease.

Dapsone is one of the primary drugs used in the treatment of leprosy. It is usually administered in a dose of 100 mg/d for adults and 1 mg/kg/d for children. Individuals in high-risk groups for glucose-6-phosphodehydrogenase deficiency should be tested for this condition before administration. Because primary dapsone resistance of *M leprae* has been reported, dapsone should not be used as monotherapy. To reduce the risk of drug resistance and possibly to shorten the duration of therapy, multidrug therapy is necessary in all patients. Rifampin (600 mg/d for adults or 10 mg/kg/d for children) should be given with dapsone for 6 months for paucibacillary (indeterminate, tuberculoid, and borderline tuberculoid) disease, with close follow-up to detect relapses. Clofazimine (50 mg/d for adults or 1 mg/kg/d for children) should be added for multibacillary (borderline, borderline lepromatous, and lepromatous) disease and continued for at least 2 years and until skin smears are negative. Corticosteroids are used to treat erythema nodosum leprosum (ENL), which commonly occurs in patients with multibacillary forms after drug therapy is initiated. Occasionally, ENL occurs in untreated patients as well. Short-term, high-dose steroids, followed by maintenance thalidomide, are often useful for managing severe or recurrent ENL reactions. Thalidomide is available from the GWLHCD as an experimental drug for selected patients and should never be given to a woman of childbearing age unless she is following a reliable means of contraception. Other agents including clofazimine can also be used to treat ENL.

Another type of reaction seen primarily in patients with borderline disease is the reversal reaction, which is characterized by delayed type hypersensitivity reactions at the site of current or former leprosy lesions and/or acute neuropathies. Reversal reactions, especially those with neuropathies, should be treated aggressively with corticosteroids to avoid permanent neurologic sequelae.

Most patients can be treated as outpatients. Rehabilitative measures, including surgery and physical therapy, may be necessary in some patients.

Isolation of the Hospitalized Patient: No special precautions are necessary. A private room should be sufficient for a newly diagnosed patient.

Control Measures: Hand washing is recommended for all persons in contact with a lepromatous patient. Disinfection of nasal secretions, handkerchiefs, and other fomites should be considered until treatment is established. Household contacts, particularly those with multibacillary disease, should be examined initially and then annually for at least 5 years. Household contacts of patients with borderline or lepromatous leprosy who are younger than 25 years should be treated prophylactically with dapsone for 3 years at the same doses used for treatment. Local public health department regulations for leprosy vary and should be consulted.

Newly diagnosed cases of leprosy should be reported to public health authorities.

Leptospirosis

Clinical Manifestations: The onset of leptospirosis is usually abrupt, with nonspecific, influenza-like, constitutional symptoms of fever, chills, headache, severe myalgia, and malaise. Gastrointestinal tract symptoms can also occur. The clinical course is frequently biphasic and protean, and can result in hepatic (abnormal function tests, hepatomegaly, jaundice, and failure), renal (abnormal urinalysis, azotemia, and failure), and central nervous system (aseptic meningitis and altered sensorium) involvement. Myositis is common. Weil's syndrome refers to severe leptospirosis with jaundice. Conjunctival suffusion, the most characteristic physical finding, occurs in less than half the patients. The duration of the illness varies from less than 1 week to 3 weeks.

Etiology: The etiologic agent is the spirochete *Leptospira interrogans*. Approximately 250 serotypes (serovars) comprising 19 serogroups have been recognized. Disease in the United States has been caused by more than ten serovars, the most common of which are *icterohaemorrhagiae* and *canicola*.

Epidemiology: The sources for human infection include many species of wild and domestic mammals, particularly dogs, rats, and livestock, that excrete *Leptospira* organisms in the urine. Most cases in the United States result from recreational exposure. Disease occurs most commonly in the summer among teenagers and adults, especially in the tropics. Those predisposed by occupation include abattoir and sewer workers, veterinarians, farmers, and field workers. Transmission is zoonotic, either by direct or indirect contact with urine or carcasses of infected animals. Indirect contact occurs from swimming, wading, or splashing in pools, streams, or puddles contaminated by leptospiruric animals; occasionally, indirect exposure causes common-source outbreaks. Asymptomatic and symptomatic human infections occur. Communicability in infected animals exists during the 1-month to more than 3-month phase of prolonged leptospiruria. Humans with leptospirosis usually excrete the organism in urine for 4 to 6 weeks and occasionally for as long as 18 weeks. Person-to-person transmission is rare.

The **incubation period** is usually 7 to 13 days, with a range of 2 to 26 days.

Diagnostic Tests: Blood and cerebrospinal fluid in the first 7 to 10 days of illness, and urine after the first week and during convalescence should be cultured on special media. Because such media are not available routinely, laboratory personnel should be consulted in cases of suspected leptospirosis. The organism can also be recovered by inoculation of body fluids into guinea pigs. Serum antibody measured by enzyme immunoassay or agglutination reactions develop in the second week of illness, but titer rises can be delayed or absent in some patients. Microscopic agglutination is the confirmatory serologic test and is performed in reference laboratories. Direct darkfield examination of blood and other body fluids has pitfalls that obviate its usefulness, and it is not recommended.

Treatment: Penicillin is the drug of choice for severely ill patients. Intravenous, high-dose penicillin (1.5 million units given every 6 hours to adults) for 7 days appears to be effective even in patients in whom therapy is not started until after the fourth day of the illness. Oral doxycycline therapy in persons with mild illness also appears to shorten the course of illness and reduces the incidence of convalescent leptospiruria. Tetracycline drugs should not be given to children younger than 9 years of age unless the benefits of therapy justify the risk of dental staining.

Isolation of the Hospitalized Patient: Universal precautions should be scrupulously followed for the duration of hospitalization. These precautions also include urine, which in patients with leptospirosis, is potentially infectious.

Control Measures:
- Vaccination of dogs and livestock prevents disease but not infection and leptospiruria in animals. Its effect on human disease is unproven.
- Protective clothing, boots, and gloves should be worn to reduce occupational exposure.
- Rodent control is indicated.
- Doxycycline, 200 mg, given orally once weekly to adults, is effective prophylaxis and should be considered for high-risk occupational groups with short-term exposure. However, indications for doxycycline use in children have not been established. Tetracycline drugs generally should not be given to children younger than 9 years of age.

Listeria monocytogenes Infections (Listeriosis)

Clinical Manifestations: Puerperal and neonatal *Listeria* infections are relatively uncommon. Neonatal illness has early-onset and late-onset syndromes similar to those of group B streptococcal infections. Pneumonia, septicemia, and maternal symptoms are common in early-onset disease. Late-onset infection occurs after the first week of life and often results in meningitis. Maternal infection can be associated with an influenza-like illness, fever, malaise, headache, gastrointestinal tract symptoms, and back pain. Approximately 65% of women experience a symptomatic prodromal illness before diagnosis of listeriosis in their fetus or newborn infant. Amnionitis during labor or asymptomatic infection can occur. Infection occurs most commonly in the perinatal period and in patients with decreased cell-mediated immunity resulting from cancer chemotherapy, steroid therapy, congenital immunodeficiency, hepatic or renal disease, or HIV infection.

Etiology: *Listeria monocytogenes* is a small, aerobic, non-spore-forming, Gram-positive bacillus that is beta-hemolytic on blood agar.

Epidemiology: *Listeria monocytogenes* is distributed widely in the environment, especially in the food chain. Food-borne transmission is a major cause of epidemics and sporadic infections. Incriminated foods include unpasteurized milk, cheese and other dairy products, undercooked poultry, and prepared meats such as paté. Asymptomatic fecal and vaginal carriage can result in sporadic neonatal disease, which can cause early-onset neonatal infections from transplacental or ascending intrauterine infection or from exposure during delivery. Maternal infection has been associated with preterm delivery and other obstetric complications. Late-onset neonatal infection can result from acquisition of the organism during passage through the birth canal or possibly from environmental sources. Nosocomial nursery outbreaks have also occurred. Infection is possibly acquired by inhalation or genital contact.

The median **incubation period** for food-borne transmission is 21 days.

Diagnostic Tests: The organism can be recovered from cultures of blood, cerebrospinal fluid (CSF), meconium, gastric washings, placenta, and other infected tissues on blood agar plates. Special techniques (eg, enrichment and selective media) may be needed to recover *Listeria* from sites with mixed flora. Gram stain of gastric aspirate or CSF from an infected newborn infant may demonstrate the organism. As the result of morphologic similarity to diphtheroids, a culture isolate of *Listeria* can mistakenly be considered a contaminant or saprophyte. The value of serologic tests is not established.

Treatment:
- Initial therapy with intravenous ampicillin and an aminoglycoside, usually gentamicin, is recommended for severe infections. This combination is more effective than ampicillin alone in animal models of *Listeria* infection. After clinical response occurs, or for less severe infections in normal hosts, ampicillin alone may be given. The optimal therapeutic regimen, however, has not been established. For the penicillin-allergic patient, the alternative regimen is intravenous trimethoprim-sulfamethoxazole. Cephalosporins, including the newer derivatives, are not active against *Listeria*.
- In invasive infections caused by *Listeria*, including uncomplicated meningitis, 14 days of treatment is usually satisfactory.
- The usefulness of culturing the cervix and stool of the mother of an infected infant and treatment of the mother, if either culture is positive, has not been established. Similarly, no data suggest that reculturing during a subsequent pregnancy has any value.

Isolation of the Hospitalized Patient: No special precautions are indicated.

Control Measures:
- Antimicrobial therapy of infection diagnosed during pregnancy may prevent fetal or perinatal infection and its consequences.
- The existence of listeriosis in herds of sheep or cattle should preclude the use of untreated manure on crops destined for human consumption, although the role of raw vegetables as a source of infection needs further study.
- Pregnant women and immunosuppressed patients should avoid unpasteurized dairy products, soft cheeses, and undercooked meats.
- Cases of listeriosis should be reported to the state or local health department to facilitate early recognition and control of common-source outbreaks of listeriosis.

Lyme Disease
(Borrelia burgdorferi)

Clinical Manifestations: Early disease usually begins with a distinctive rash, referred to as erythema migrans, at the site of a recent tick bite. The lesion begins as a red macule or papule, is 5 cm or more in diameter (median, 15 cm), and typically expands to form large annular erythema, with partial central clearing. The presentation of erythema migrans can vary greatly in size and shape. Multiple secondary annular lesions, evanescent red blotches or circles, malar rash or urticaria, conjunctivitis, periorbital edema, or diffuse erythema can develop. Fever, malaise, headache, mild neck stiffness, and arthralgia can occur. These symptoms are typically intermittent and variable during a period of several weeks in untreated patients.

Weeks to months later, manifestations involving joints, eyes, and the cardiac and nervous systems can occur. Nervous system findings include seventh cranial nerve (facial) palsies, aseptic meningitis, and peripheral radiculoneuropathy. Brief, recurrent attacks of nonsymmetric arthritis in large joints are characteristic. Chronic arthritis is uncommon in children. Late manifestations can be present without the typical history of early Lyme disease or erythema migrans.

Adverse pregnancy outcomes, including congenital heart disease, syndactyly, cortical blindness, intrauterine fetal death, prematurity, and rash in the newborn, have been associated with infection in pregnant women. However, although transplacental transmission can occur, resulting prematurity and fetal deaths or malformations have not been proven.

Etiology: The cause is the spirochete *Borrelia burgdorferi*.

Epidemiology: Lyme disease is clustered primarily in three distinct geographic regions of the United States. Most cases are reported in the Northeast from Massachusetts to Maryland, in the Midwest in Wisconsin and Minnesota, and in California. The occurrence of cases in the United States correlates with the known distribution and frequency of infection of known tick vectors (*Ixodes scapularis* [previously known as *Ixodes dammini*] in the East and Midwest; *Ixodes pacificus* in the West). However, cases of Lyme disease have been reported from 48 states, many of which are outside the usual range of these ticks, and in which the existence of infected vectors has not been established. Although *B burgdorferi* transmission may be documented in some of these states in the future, false-positive serologic tests may have resulted in misdiagnosis in some of these reported cases. Lyme disease has also been reported from Canada, Europe, Scandinavia, the Soviet Union, China, and Japan. Onset of illness generally occurs between May 1 and November 30; most cases occur before August. Patients of all ages and both sexes may be affected.

The **incubation period** for erythema migrans is 3 to 31 days. It is typically 7 to 10 days.

Diagnostic Tests: Diagnosis is made clinically in the early stages of the disease if erythema migrans is present. A biopsy of the perimeter of this lesion frequently yields *B burgdorferi*, but cultures require special medium, are commercially available, and growth is not rapid. In patients without a rash or who manifest a later disease stage, diagnosis should also be based on clinical findings, using the presently available serologic tests as an adjunct.

Both an indirect fluorescent antibody (IFA) test and an enzyme immunoassay (EIA) are available. The EIA is more widely used and is more sensitive and specific. However, these tests are not yet standardized and results from nonreference laboratories often vary. Western blot analysis is available as a confirmatory test, but criteria for positivity are not standardized and interpretation of results will vary. Both false-negative and false-positive IFA and EIA test results occur. The IgM antibody titer usually reaches a peak between the third and sixth weeks after onset of the disease; specific IgG antibody titers usually rise slowly and generally are highest months later. Patients with Lyme disease may not have elevated titers during the first several weeks of illness, particularly if they received antimicrobial therapy, but thereafter most patients with untreated Lyme disease will have a positive serologic test. Titers to *Borrelia burgdorferi* are particularly useful in differentiating Lyme disease from other rheumatic syndromes. *B burgdorferi* antibody cross-reacts with other spirochetes, including *Treponema pallidum*, but patients with Lyme disease do not have positive nontreponemal syphilis tests (eg, VDRL or RPR).

Definitive diagnosis can be made by isolation of *B burgdorferi* on culture from an erythema migrans lesion, blood, or other body fluid, but cultures are usually not necessary for diagnosis, and positive cultures from blood and body fluids are rare. Spirochetes are visualized rarely by microscopic examination of blood, skin transudate, or tissue specimens.

Treatment (see Table 3.26, p 299):

Early-Stage Disease. At the time of the appearance of erythema migrans or shortly thereafter, oral doxycycline or amoxicillin is the drug of choice for children 9 years and older. For children younger than 9 years of age, amoxicillin or penicillin V is recommended. On the basis of antibiotic susceptibility testing, amoxicillin is probably the preferred choice in this age group. Alternative drugs are cefuroxime axetil and erythromycin for the penicillin-allergic patient, although erythromycin may be less effective. Clarithromycin and azithromycin are active in vitro against *B burgdorferi*. Length of therapy is dependent on clinical response and manifestations.

A patient with early disease should be seen after 10 to 14 days of antibiotic therapy. If all symptoms have resolved, no further therapy is indicated. If symptoms persist, continued therapy for 7 additional days, or, occasionally, 14 days, may be warranted. Maximum total duration is 30 days. Relapses are unusual but can occur, and they require retreatment with the same or another antibiotic.

Early treatment of erythema migrans should prevent development of later manifestations.

TABLE 3.26—Recommended Treatment for Lyme Disease in Children

Disease Category	Drug(s) and Dose*	
Early Disease		
≥9 y	Doxycycline	100 mg twice daily
<9 y	Amoxicillin†,‡	25-50 mg/kg/d, divided into 3 daily doses (maximum 1-2 g/d)
	Penicillin V‡	25-50 mg/kg/d, divided into 3 daily doses (maximum 1-2 g/d)
Other Manifestations, Including Late-Stage Disease		
Isolated facial palsy	Same as for early disease (oral regimen)	
Arthritis	Same as for early disease (oral regimen)	
Mild carditis	Same as for early disease (oral regimen)	
Persistent arthritis	Ceftriaxone, 75-100 mg/kg, IV or IM, once daily (maximum 2 g/d); or penicillin, 300,000 U/kg/d, IV, given in divided doses every 4 h (maximum, 20 million U/d)	
Severe carditis	Ceftriaxone, 75-100 mg/kg, IV or IM, once daily (maximum 2 g/d); or penicillin, 300,000 U/kg/d, IV, given in divided doses every 4 h (maximum, 20 million U/d)	
Meningitis or encephalitis	Ceftriaxone, 75-100 mg/kg, IV or IM, once daily (maximum 2 g/d); or penicillin, 300,000 U/kg/d, IV, given in divided doses every 4 h (maximum, 20 million U/d)	

*Duration of therapy for oral regimens is 10 to 30 d; for parenteral therapy it is 14 to 21 d. Duration of therapy is usually based on severity of disease and rapidity of response.
†Amoxicillin may be preferred.
‡For penicillin-allergic patients, cefuroxime axetil and erythromycin are alternative drugs.

Other Manifestations, Including Late-Stage Disease. Isolated seventh nerve palsy with normal cerebrospinal fluid findings, mild carditis, or arthritis should be treated with one of the oral regimens recommended for early-stage disease, and treatment may need to be extended beyond 14 days. Severe carditis, persistent arthritis, or neurologic involvement should be treated with parenteral antibiotics. Ceftriaxone or parenteral penicillin G is indicated for persistent arthritis, severe carditis, and central nervous system disease. The optimal duration of therapy is not well established for these different indications. Duration, thus, is usually based on severity of disease and rapidity of response. Oral regimens are generally given for 14 to 30 days, and parenteral therapy is given for 14 to 21 days. A total of more than 4 weeks is not indicated.

The Jarisch-Herxheimer reaction, with fever, chills, and malaise, can occur when therapy is initiated.

Pregnancy. The most appropriate therapy for Lyme disease during pregnancy has not been determined. Tetracyclines are contraindicated. Otherwise, most experts recommend the same therapy as for nonpregnant persons.

Isolation of the Hospitalized Patient: No special precautions are recommended other than the routinely recommended universal precautions.

Control Measures:
Ticks. Avoidance of tick-infested areas is the best preventive measure. If a tick-infested area is entered, clothing should cover as much of the arms and legs as possible. Permethrin can be sprayed on clothing to prevent tick attachment. Tick repellents, used on exposed skin, require repeated applications every 1 to 2 hours to be effective. If DEET* is used, it should be applied sparingly because seizures have been reported coincident with its application in young children. Daily self-inspection, inspection of family members, and prompt removal of any ticks are recommended (see Control Measures for Prevention of Tick-Borne Infections, p 114).

Antimicrobial prophylaxis after a tick bite in an endemic area is not routinely warranted. Animal studies indicate that transmission requires a prolonged (more than 24 hours) time of tick attachment. In published studies of prophylaxis, the risk of infection with *B burgdorferi* after a recognized deer tick bite is so low that prophylactic antimicrobial treatment is not routinely indicated. However, factors such as a long duration of feeding by a tick (eg, as indicated by removal of an engorged tick) or pregnancy may alter the decision not to administer prophylactic antimicrobial therapy.

Blood Donation. Patients with active disease should not donate blood because spirochetemia occurs early in Lyme disease. Patients who were previously treated for Lyme disease can be considered for blood donation.

Lymphocytic Choriomeningitis

Clinical Manifestations: Infection may result in a mild to severe nonspecific illness, including fever, malaise, myalgia, retro-orbital headache, photophobia, anorexia, and nausea. Fever usually lasts 1 to 3 weeks. A biphasic febrile course is frequent. Neurologic manifestations varying from aseptic meningitis to severe encephalitis can occur. Arthralgia or arthritis, respiratory symptoms, orchitis, and leukopenia occasionally develop. Infection during pregnancy has been associated with abortion and with hydrocephalus and chorioretinitis in the fetus.

Etiology: Lymphocytic choriomeningitis (LCM) virus is an arenavirus.

Epidemiology: Lymphocytic choriomeningitis is a chronic infection of the common house mouse. These mice are often asymptomatically infected in

---

*N, N-diethyl-m-toluamide.

nature. In addition, laboratory mice and colonized golden hamsters can be infected with significant virus shedding. Humans are infected incidentally by inhalation or ingestion of dust or food contaminated with the virus from the urine, feces, blood, or nasopharyngeal secretions of infected rodents. Pet hamsters have been found to be a source of infection. The disease is most prevalent in young adults. Human-to-human spread of the virus has not been reported.

The **incubation period** is usually 6 to 13 days; occasionally it is as long as 3 weeks.

Diagnostic Tests: The spinal fluid may contain hundreds to thousands of white blood cells, predominantly lymphocytes, and hypoglycorrhachia can occur. The LCM virus can be isolated from blood, cerebrospinal fluid (CSF), urine, or, occasionally, nasopharyngeal secretions. Acute and convalescent sera can be tested for increases in antibody titers; demonstration of IgM antibodies in serum and CSF is useful. Infection of mice trapped in or around houses may be identified by demonstrating serum antibody or viral antigen in liver impression smears.

Treatment: Supportive.

Isolation of the Hospitalized Patient: No special precautions are recommended.

Control Measures: Infection can be controlled by preventing rodent infection in animal and food storage areas of wholesalers and others dealing in the sale of hamsters or other rodents. Because the virus is excreted by rodent hosts for long periods of time, attempts should be made to monitor colonies for infection. Pet or wild rodents in the patient's home should be considered likely sources of infection.

Malaria

Clinical Manifestations: The classic symptoms are high fever with chills, rigor, sweats, and headache. These symptoms occur in paroxysms. As the infection becomes synchronized, the fever and paroxysms generally occur in a cyclic pattern. Depending on the infecting species, fever may appear every other or every third day. Other symptoms can include nausea, vomiting, arthralgia, and abdominal and back pain. Pallor and jaundice caused by hemolysis can be present. Hepatosplenomegaly may be present and is more prominent in chronic infections. Infection by *Plasmodium falciparum* is potentially fatal and may present with one of the following clinical syndromes:

- *Cerebral malaria*, which may have variable neurologic manifestations including seizures, signs of increased intracranial pressure, confusion, and progression to stupor, coma, and death.

- *Pulmonary edema*, which is difficult to manage and may be fatal.
- *Renal failure*, caused by acute tubular necrosis.
- *Vascular collapse and shock*, associated with hypothermia and adrenal insufficiency.
- *Dysentery.*
- *Black water fever*, which describes the hemoglobinuria after massive hemolysis and acute renal failure. It occurs in nonimmune persons traveling in endemic areas.

Syndromes associated with *Plasmodium malariae* infection are as follows:

- *Tropical splenomegaly*, with significant enlargement of the spleen, hemolytic anemia, and lymphocytic infiltration of the portal triads of the liver.
- *Nephrotic syndrome*, from the deposition of immune complexes in the kidney.
- *Congenital malaria*, which can resemble neonatal sepsis, including nonspecific symptoms of poor appetite, restlessness, fever, and lethargy.

Etiology: The *Plasmodium* species infecting humans are *Plasmodium vivax, P malariae, Plasmodium ovale,* and *P falciparum.*

Epidemiology: Malaria is endemic throughout the tropical areas of the world. Half of the world's population live in areas where transmission occurs. Areas of highest prevalence include subsaharan Africa, parts of Central and South America, and many parts of Oceania but not Polynesia. However, transmission is possible in more temperate climates, including areas in the United States where *Anopheles* mosquitos are present. Infections are usually acquired from bite of female *Anopheles* mosquitos. Transmission can also be congenital, through transfusions, or via the use of contaminated needles.

Plasmodium vivax and P falciparum are the most common species. *Plasmodium vivax* malaria occurs worldwide, including in some temperate regions. *Plasmodium falciparum* infection is found only in the tropics and subtropics. *Plasmodium malariae* is transmitted less commonly in temperate and tropical areas. *Plasmodium ovale* occurs most often in West Africa, although cases have been reported from other areas. Relapses may occur in *P vivax* and *P ovale* malaria because of a persistent hepatic stage of the infection. Recrudescence of *P falciparum* and *P malariae* infection occurs when a persistent low-concentration parasitemia causes a recurrence of the disease. Of increasing importance is the spread of strains of chloroquine-resistant *Plasmodia* species throughout the world.

Diagnostic Tests: Definitive diagnosis relies on identification of the parasite on stained blood films. Both thick and thin blood films should be made. The thick film allows for concentration of the blood to find the parasite that may be present in small numbers. Species identification is easier on thin films. A rapid screening test for malarial parasites, the Quantitative Buffy Coat Analysis (QBC), is available, but blood smears should always be performed when malaria is a possible diagnosis since the data available are insufficient to justify using QBC only. Confirmation and speciation of malaria parasites on blood smear is important in guiding therapy. Serology is generally not helpful except in epidemiologic surveys. New diagnostic tests using polymerase chain reaction, DNA probes, and malarial ribosomal RNA are under development and may be valuable diagnostic methods in the future.

Treatment: Chemotherapy is based upon the infecting species (see Table 3.27, p 304). In patients with *P falciparum* malaria, sequential blood smears are indicated to monitor the treatment.

Isolation of the Hospitalized Patient: Universal precautions should be scrupulously followed.

Control Measures: Control measures are directed to control of the *Anopheles* mosquito population, chemotherapy of infected persons, and chemoprophylaxis of travelers in endemic areas. Decreased contact with mosquitos is also effective through use of bed nets impregnated with insecticide while sleeping, mosquito repellents, and protective clothing. The most current information on risks, drug resistance, and resulting recommendations for travelers can be obtained by contacting the Centers for Disease Control and Prevention (see Directory of Telephone Numbers, p 601).

Chemoprophylaxis for Travelers to Endemic Areas.* The appropriate chemoprophylactic regimen is determined by the traveler's risk of acquiring malaria in the area(s) to be visited and by the risk of exposure to chloroquine-resistant *P falciparum*. Chemoprophylaxis should begin 1 week before arrival in the endemic area, allowing time for development of adequate blood concentration and evaluation of any adverse reactions.

Chloroquine-resistant *P falciparum* has not yet been reported in Haiti, the Dominican Republic, Central America west of the Panama Canal, and the Middle East, including Egypt. Travelers to areas where chloroquine-resistant malaria species have not been reported should take chloroquine, once weekly, for the duration of exposure and for 4 weeks after departure from the endemic area.

Travelers to areas where chloroquine-resistant *P falciparum* exists should take mefloquine, once weekly, starting 1 week before travel, continuing weekly during travel, and for 4 weeks after travel has concluded (see Table 3.28, p 306). Mefloquine, however, is not recommended for use in children weighing less than 15 kg, pregnant women during the first trimester, patients taking beta blockers or other drugs that can prolong or alter cardiac conduction, patients with history of epilepsy or severe psychiatric disorders (eg, psychosis), and travelers involved in tasks requiring fine coordination and spatial discrimination (such as airline crews). Because of the frequency of side effects, mefloquine should not be used for presumptive self-treatment.

---

*For further information on prevention of malaria in travelers, see the following: Centers for Disease Control and Prevention. Recommendations for the prevention of malaria among travelers. *MMWR.* 1990;39(RR-3):1-10; and the US Public Health Service's annual publication, *Health Information for International Travel,* Superintendent of Documents, US Government Printing Office, Washington, DC

TABLE 3.27—Treatment of Malaria

Drug	Adult Dosage	Pediatric Dosage

All *Plasmodium* species except chloroquine-resistant *P falciparum*

Oral drug of choice:

| Chloroquine phosphate | 600 mg base (1 g), then 300 mg base (500 mg) 6 h later, and 300 mg base (500 mg/d) at 24 and 48 h | 10 mg base/kg (max 600 mg base), then 5 mg base/kg 6 h later (max 300 mg), and 5 mg base/kg/d at 24 and 48 h (maximum 300 mg) |

Parenteral drug of choice:

Quinidine gluconate[a]	10 mg/kg loading dose, IV (maximum 600 mg), over 1-2 h, then 0.02 mg/kg/min continuous infusion until oral therapy can be started	Same as adult
OR		
Quinine dihydro-chloride[a]	600 mg in 300-mL normal saline, IV, over 2 to 4 h; repeat every 8 h until oral therapy can be started (maximum 1,800 mg/d)	25 mg/kg/d; give 1/3 of daily dose over 2-4 h; repeat every 8 h until oral therapy can be started (maximum 1,800 mg/d)

P falciparum acquired in areas of known chloroquine resistance

Oral drug of choice:

Quinine sulfate[b]	650 mg 3 times daily for 3 to 7 d	25 mg/kg/d in 3 doses for 3 d
PLUS		
Tetracycline[c]	250 mg 4 times daily for 7 d	5 mg/kg 4 times daily for 7 d (maximum 250 mg 4 times daily)
or		
Clindamycin	900 mg 3 times daily for 3 d	20-40 mg/kg/d in 3 doses for 3 d
or		
Pyrimethamine-sulfadoxine[d] (Fansidar)	Single dose of 3 tablets	<1 y: single dose of 1/4 tablet 1-3 y: single dose of 1/2 tablet 4-8 y: single dose of 1 tablet 9-14 y: single dose of 2 tablets >14 y: single dose of 3 tablets

TABLE 3.27—Treatment of Malaria *(continued)*

Drug	Adult Dosage	Pediatric Dosage
Alternative drug:		
Mefloquine hydrochloride[e]	Single dose of 1,250 mg	25 mg/kg in single dose (maximum 1,250 mg)
Parenteral drug of choice:		
Quinidine gluconate[a]	Same as above	Same as above
Prevention of Relapses: *P vivax* and *P ovale* only		
Drug of choice:		
Primaquine phosphate[f]	15 mg base (26.3 mg)/d for 14 d or 45 mg base (79 mg)/wk for 8 wk	0.3 mg/kg/d for 14 d (maximum 26.3 mg/d)

[a]Electrocardiogram monitoring is recommended to detect arrhythmias, widening QRS complex, or prolonged QT interval. Patients should also be monitored for hypotension.

[b]For treatment of *P falciparum* infections acquired in Thailand, quinine should be given for 7 d.

[c]Physicians must weigh the benefits of tetracycline therapy against the possibility of dental staining in children younger than 9 y.

[d]Use of Fansidar, which contains 25 mg pyrimethamine and 500 mg sulfadoxine per tablet, is contraindicated in patients with history of sulfonamide or pyrimethamine intolerance, in pregnant women at term, and in infants younger than 2 mo. Pregnant women should take chloroquine.

[e]Mefloquine should not be used in children lighter than 15 kg, pregnant women in the first trimester, patients using beta blockers (or other cardiac drugs that may prolong or alter cardiac conduction), or patients with history of epilepsy or psychiatric disorder. Quinidine or quinine may exacerbate the known side effects of mefloquine; patients not responding to mefloquine therapy or failing mefloquine prophylaxis should be closely monitored if they are treated with quinidine/quinine.

[f]Primaquine phosphate can cause hemolytic anemia in patients with glucose-6-phosphate dehydrogenase erythrocyte deficiency. A G6PD screen should be done before initiating treatment. Primaquine should not be used during pregnancy.

For short-term travelers unable to take mefloquine, doxycycline alone is the preferred alternative regimen (see Table 3.28, p 306). Travelers taking doxycycline should be advised of the possible side effects, including diarrhea, photosensitivity, and increased risk of monilial vaginitis. Use of doxycycline is contraindicated in pregnant women and usually in children younger than 9 years because of the risk of dental staining.

In other travelers for whom mefloquine is contraindicated and doxycycline is inappropriate (eg, for reasons of age or length of stay), chloroquine alone or chloroquine plus proguanil may be effective alternatives (see Table 3.28, p 306). In addition, these travelers should carry pyrimethamine-sulfadoxine for use as presumptive self-treatment if a febrile illness develops while taking chloroquine and professional medical care is not readily available. Self-treatment should not be considered a replacement for seeking prompt medical

TABLE 3.28—Prevention of Malaria[a]

Drug[b]	Adult Dosage	Pediatric Dosage
Chloroquine phosphate	300 mg base (500 mg salt), orally, once per wk beginning 1 wk before exposure, and continuing for 4 wk after last exposure.	5 mg/kg base (8.3 mg/kg salt) once per wk, maximum dose is 300 mg base (adult dose)
	CHLOROQUINE-RESISTANT AREAS	
Mefloquine[c]	250 mg, orally, once per wk, beginning 1 wk before travel, and continuing for 4 wk after last exposure	15-19 kg: 1/4 tablet per wk 20-30 kg: 1/2 tablet per wk 31-45 kg: 3/4 tablet per wk >45 kg: 1 tablet per wk
Alternatives:		
Doxycycline[d] OR	100 mg/d, starting 1-2 d before exposure, and continuing for 4 wk after last exposure	>8 y: 2 mg/kg/d of body weight, orally, up to adult dose of 100 mg/d
Chloroquine phosphate **with or without**	Same as above	
Proguanil[e] plus	200 mg/d during exposure, and for 4 wk after last exposure	<2 y: 50 mg/d 2-6 y: 100 mg/d 7-10 y: 150 mg/d >10 y: 200 mg/d
Pyrimethamine-sulfadoxine (Fansidar)[f] for presumptive treatment	Carry a single dose (3 tablets) for self-treatment of febrile disease when medical care is not immediately available	Used as for adults in the following doses: <1 y: 1/4 tablet 1-3 y: 1/2 tablet 4-8 y: 1 tablet 9-14 y: 2 tablets >14 y: 3 tablets

[a]At present, no drug regimen guarantees protection against malaria. Travelers to countries with risk of malaria should be advised to avoid mosquito bites by using personal protective measures (see text for a discussion of these measures).

[b]All drugs should be continued for 4 wk after last exposure.

[c]Mefloquine should not be used by children lighter than 15 kg, pregnant women in the first trimester, people using beta blockers (or other cardiac drugs that may prolong cardiac conduction), travelers involved in tasks requiring fine coordination and spatial discrimination (eg, airline crews), or persons with history of epilepsy or psychiatric disorder. Due to the frequency of side effects, especially dizziness, mefloquine should not be used for presumptive self-treatment.

[d]Physicians who prescribe doxycycline as malaria chemoprophylaxis should advise patients to limit exposure to direct sunlight to minimize the possibility of photosensitivity reaction. Use of doxycycline is contraindicated in pregnant women and in children younger than 9 y.

[e]Proguanil is not available in the United States but is widely available overseas. It is recommended primarily for use in Africa south of the Sahara. Failures in prophylaxis with chloroquine and proguanil have been reported in travelers to Kenya, however.

[f] Use of Fansidar, which contains 25 mg pyrimethamine and 500 mg sulfadoxine per tablet, is contraindicated in patients with history of sulfonamide or pyrimethamine intolerance, in pregnant women at term, and in infants younger than 2 mo.

help. Pyrimethamine-sulfadoxine should not be taken by patients with known intolerance to either drug, pregnant women at term, infants younger than 2 months of age, or for routine prophylaxis.

Prevention of relapses. To prevent relapses of *P vivax* or *P ovale* infection after departure from areas where these species are endemic, use of primaquine phosphate can be considered. Primaquine can cause hemolysis in patients with glucose-6-phosphate dehydrogenase deficiency; thus, all patients should be screened for this condition before primaquine therapy.

Protective Measures. All travelers to areas where malaria is endemic should be advised to use personal protective measures, including (1) using insecticide-impregnated mosquito nets while sleeping, (2) remaining in well-screened areas, (3) wearing protective clothing, and (4) using mosquito repellents containing DEET.* To be effective, these repellents require reapplication every 1 to 2 hours. Adverse reactions associated with DEET include skin rashes, toxic encephalopathy, and seizures. Hence, it should be used sparingly on exposed skin and, where possible, it should be used on clothing to limit skin exposure. Travelers, particularly children, should be advised against using products containing high concentrations of DEET directly on skin.

Malassezia furfur Invasive Infections

Clinical Manifestations: Invasive disease is rare but includes dacryocystitis, folliculitis, and mastitis. More serious invasive disease, including fungemia, chronic sinusitis, peritonitis, life-threatening pulmonary infections, and pulmonary infarct, is associated with continuous peritoneal dialysis, central venous catheters, central nervous system catheters, and immunosuppression. Neonates with fungemia have fever, pneumonitis, apnea, leukocytosis, thrombocytopenia, and bradycardia.

Etiology: *Malassezia furfur* is a lipid-dependent fungus (that also causes superficial skin infection [see Tinea Versicolor, p 468]).

Epidemiology: Fungemia occurs primarily in premature infants and other neonates who are receiving parenteral nutrition that includes fat emulsions. In one study, 64% of neonates in an intensive care unit had skin colonization with *M furfur*, whereas only 3% of healthy infants did. Nosocomial colonization provides the likely source of invading strains that colonize the catheter and result in hematogenous dissemination of the fungus.

The **incubation period** is unknown.

Diagnostic Tests: The diagnosis can be made from scale scrapings or smears of skin lesions. In potassium hydroxide preparations or methylene blue stained smears, short septate hyphae of variable length plus clusters of oval or budding (phialiolic) yeasts 4 to 8 micrometers in size are diagnostic.

---

*N, N-diethyl-m-toluamide.

Routine media may not support growth of this organism since medium- and long-chain fatty acids are required. However, Sabouraud medium overlaid with sterile olive oil provides an effective culture system.

Treatment: Removal of catheters and temporary cessation of lipid infusions are usually adequate therapy. Although the organism is frequently sensitive to antifungal drugs, treatment with these drugs without catheter removal is usually not successful. The need for antifungal therapy in addition to catheter removal in patients with positive cultures from sites other than blood has not been determined.

Isolation of the Hospitalized Patient: No special precautions are recommended.

Control Measures: Strict adherence to routine infection control measures, such as hand washing, is essential. In addition, aseptic technique when managing intravascular, central nervous system, and intraperitoneal catheters and devices, particularly when administering hyperalimentation fluids, is indicated in neonatal nursery outbreaks.

Measles

Clinical Manifestations: Measles is an acute disease characterized by fever, cough, coryza, conjunctivitis, an erythematous maculopapular rash, and a pathognomonic enanthem (Koplik spots). Complications such as otitis media, bronchopneumonia, laryngotracheobronchitis (croup), and diarrhea occur more commonly in young children. Encephalitis, which frequently results in permanent brain damage, occurs in approximately 1 of every 1,000 cases. Since 1989, death, predominantly from respiratory and neurologic complications, has occurred in 3 of every 1,000 cases reported in the United States. Case-fatality rates are increased in immunocompromised children; these patients sometimes do not develop the characteristic rash.

Subacute sclerosing panencephalitis (SSPE), a rare degenerative central nervous system disease characterized by behavioral and intellectual deterioration and convulsions, is a result of a persistent measles virus infection. With widespread measles vaccination, this complication has virtually disappeared.

Etiology: Measles virus is an RNA virus with one antigenic type, classified as a morbillivirus in the *Paramyxovirus* family.

Epidemiology: Measles is transmitted by direct contact with infectious droplets or, less commonly, by airborne spread. In temperate areas, the peak incidence of infection in unvaccinated populations occurs during the winter and spring. In the prevaccine era, measles was an epidemic disease with biennial cycles in urban areas. Most cases occurred in preschool-aged and young school-aged children, and few persons were still susceptible by age 20 years. The childhood immunization program in the United States has resulted in a greater than 95% reduction in the reported incidence of measles. Since 1963 when measles vaccine was first licensed, the incidence of measles has decreased dramatically in all age groups. The decline has been greatest in children 5 to 14 years of age.

From 1989 to 1991 the incidence of measles in the United States increased, especially in preschool-aged children (younger than 5 years) in large, urban settings. The greatest increase occurred among children too young (less than 15 months) to be immunized according to routine recommendations. The majority of cases in children 15 months to 4 years occurred in unvaccinated children who should have been vaccinated. Outbreaks involving children and young adults 5 to 24 years of age became less prominent in the early 1990s than they were in the 1980s, during which time outbreaks initially occurred primarily among vaccinated adolescents in junior and senior high schools and on college campuses.

The major factor contributing to the most recent recrudescence of measles is low immunization rates in preschool-aged children, especially in urban areas. Vaccine failure occurs in as many as 5% of individuals appropriately vaccinated at 15 months or older. Although some evidence indicates possible waning immunity after vaccination as a factor, most measles vaccine failures appear to occur in children who did not respond to the vaccine, ie, primary vaccine failure.

Patients are contagious from 1 to 2 days before the onset of symptoms (3 to 5 days before the rash) to 4 days after the appearance of the rash. Immuno-compromised patients who may have prolonged excretion of the virus in respiratory secretions can be contagious for the duration of the illness. Patients with SSPE are not contagious.

The **incubation period** is generally 8 to 12 days from exposure to onset of symptoms; the average interval from exposure to appearance of the rash is 14 days. In family studies, the average interval between appearance of rash in the source case and subsequent cases is 14 days, with a range of 7 to 18 days. In SSPE, the mean incubation period of 84 cases reported between 1976 and 1983 was 10.8 years.

Diagnostic Tests: Measles virus infection can be diagnosed by viral isolation in tissue culture from nasopharyngeal secretions, conjunctiva, blood, and urine during the febrile phase of the illness. However, virus isolation is technically difficult and usually not available. Many measles cases can be diagnosed by comparing the antibody concentrations in acute sera obtained shortly after appearance of the rash with that in convalescent sera collected as early as 1, but preferably 2 to 4, weeks later. Some patients will already have experienced a substantial rise in antibody titer if the initial serum is obtained 4 or more days after the onset of rash. Some laboratories, however, can use a single specimen to detect the presence of measles-specific IgM antibody. Correct interpretation of serologic data requires knowledge of the time at which specimens were obtained relative to the onset of the rash and the characteristics of the antibody assay. This point is especially important when interpreting negative serum IgM results, since IgM antibody may not be detectable on the first day or two after the onset of the rash and is usually undetectable 30 to 60 days after the onset of the rash.

Some IgM-specific measles antibody testing is not always positive even in confirmed cases.

In SSPE, high titers of measles antibody are found in serum and cerebrospinal fluid.

Treatment: No specific antiviral therapy is available. Measles virus is susceptible in vitro to ribavirin, which has been given by the intravenous and/or aerosol route to treat severely affected and immunocompromised children with measles. However, no controlled trials have been conducted, and ribavirin is not approved by the Food and Drug Administration for the treatment of measles.

Vitamin A. The World Health Organization (WHO) and the United Nations International Children's Emergency Fund (UNICEF) recommend that vitamin A be administered to all children diagnosed with measles in communities where vitamin A deficiency is a recognized problem and where mortality related to measles is 1% or greater. Several recent investigations indicate that vitamin A treatment of children with measles in developing countries has been associated with reduction in morbidity and mortality.

Although vitamin A deficiency is not recognized as a major problem in the United States, low serum concentrations of vitamin A have been found in children with more severe measles. Hence, although the available data are incomplete and insufficient to determine the appropriate use of vitamin A for all children with measles, the Academy recommends that vitamin A supplementation should be considered in the following circumstances:

1. Patients 6 months to 2 years of age hospitalized with measles and its complications (eg, croup, pneumonia, and diarrhea). Limited data are available regarding the safety and need for vitamin A supplementation for infants younger than 6 months of age.
2. Patients older than 6 months of age with measles who have any of the following risk factors and who are not already receiving vitamin A:
   - Immunodeficiency (eg, acquired immunodeficiency syndrome, congenital immunodeficiencies, and immunosuppressive therapy).
   - Ophthalmologic evidence of vitamin A deficiency including night blindness, Bitot's spots (grayish white deposits on the bulbar conjunctiva adjacent to the cornea) or xerophthalmia.
   - Impaired intestinal absorption (eg, biliary obstruction, short bowel syndrome, and cystic fibrosis).
   - Moderate to severe malnutrition, including that associated with eating disorders.
   - Recent immigration from areas where high mortality rates from measles have been observed.

The available vitamin A formulation in the United States is a solution, 50,000 IU/mL, for oral administration. The recommended dosage should be similar to that recommended by the WHO and UNICEF, and is as follows:

- Single dose of 200,000 IU, orally, for children 1 year and older (100,000 IU for children 6 months to 1 year of age). The higher dose may be associated with vomiting and headache for a few hours.
- The dose should be repeated the next day and at 4 weeks for children with ophthalmologic evidence of vitamin A deficiency.

Isolation of the Hospitalized Patient: Respiratory isolation is indicated for 4 days after the onset of rash. In immunocompromised patients, isolation should be maintained for the duration of the illness.

Control Measures:

Care of Exposed Persons.

Use of Vaccine. Exposure to measles is not a contraindication to vaccination. Available data suggest that live-virus measles vaccine, if given within 72 hours of measles exposure, will provide protection in some cases. If the exposure does not result in infection, the vaccine should induce protection against subsequent measles infection. Vaccine should be the intervention of choice for control of school-based measles outbreaks.

Use of Immune Globulin (IG). Immune globulin can be given to prevent or modify measles in a susceptible person within 6 days of exposure. The usual recommended dose is 0.25 mL/kg of body weight given intramuscularly; immunocompromised children should receive 0.5 mL/kg (maximum dose in either instance is 15 mL). Immune globulin is indicated for susceptible household contacts of measles patients, particularly contacts younger than 1 year, immunocompromised persons, and pregnant women for whom the risk of complications is highest. Infants younger than 5 months of åge usually have partial or complete protection from passively acquired measles antibodies. However, when measles is diagnosed in mothers, unimmunized children of all ages in the household should receive IG, since the mothers will not have transmitted protective antibodies to the children before birth.

Intravenous immune globulin (IGIV) preparations generally contain measles antibodies at approximately the same concentration as IG although the concentration may vary by lot and manufacturer. For patients who regularly receive IGIV, the usual dose of 100 to 400 mg/kg should be more than sufficient for measles prophylaxis after exposures occurring up to 3 weeks or more, after receiving IGIV.

For children who receive IG for modification or prevention of measles after exposure, measles vaccine (if not contraindicated) should be given 5 months (if the dose was 0.25 mL/kg) or 6 months (if the dose was 0.5 mL/kg) after IG administration, provided that the child is at least 12 months old. Longer intervals are required after larger doses of IGIV (see Precautions and Contraindications, p 318).

HIV Infection. Children and adolescents with symptomatic HIV infection who are exposed to measles should receive IG prophylaxis (0.5 mL/kg), regardless of vaccination status (see HIV Infection and AIDS, p 265). An exception is the patient receiving IGIV at regular intervals whose last dose was received within 3 weeks of exposure. Immune globulin is also indicated for measles-susceptible household contacts with asymptomatic HIV infection, particularly those younger than 1 year of age.

Children Younger Than 1 Year. The risk of complications resulting from measles is high among infants younger than 1 year of age. Therefore, considering the benefits and risks for postexposure immunoprophylaxis, infants as young as 6 months may be vaccinated if the vaccine is given within 72 hours of exposure. If exposure occurred within the previous 6 days, IG may be given to prevent or modify the disease.

Hospital Personnel. To decrease nosocomial infection, vaccination programs should be established to ensure that health care personnel who will be in contact with patients with measles are immune to the disease (see Health Care Personnel, p 65).

Measles Virus Vaccine. The only measles vaccine currently licensed in the United States is a live further-attenuated strain prepared in chick embryo cell culture. Measles vaccines provided through the Expanded Programme on Immunization (EPI) in developing countries meet World Health Organization standards and are usually comparable to the vaccine available in the United States. Measles vaccine is available in monovalent (measles only) formulation and in combination formulations, ie, measles-rubella (MR) and measles-mumps-rubella (MMR) vaccines. MMR is the vaccine of choice for use in routine vaccination programs for children. In all situations where measles vaccine is to be used, a combination vaccine should be given if the recipients are also likely to be susceptible to rubella and/or mumps.

After administration of a single dose of live-virus vaccine at 15 months or older, approximately 95% or more of vaccine recipients develop serum measles antibody. The protection conferred by a single dose is durable in most persons. However, a small percentage of vaccinated individuals may lose protection after several years. Measles vaccination of seronegative persons causes a mild or inapparent, noncommunicable infection. Vaccination is not deleterious for individuals who are already immune.

Improperly stored vaccine may fail to protect against measles. Since 1979, an improved stabilizer has been added to the vaccine that makes it more resistant to heat inactivation. However, during storage before reconstitution, measles vaccine should be kept at 2° to 8°C (35.6° to 46.4°F) or colder. Freezing is not harmful to the lyophilized vaccine. Measles vaccine must also be protected from ultraviolet light (especially after reconstitution), which can inactivate the virus. Vaccine should be shipped at 10°C (50°F) or colder and may be shipped on dry ice. The vaccine diluent (sterile water) vials may break if frozen. Therefore, the diluent should not be frozen. Reconstituted vaccine should be stored in a refrigerator and discarded if not used within 8 hours.

Vaccine Recommendations (see Table 3.29, p 313, for summary).

General. Measles vaccine is indicated for persons susceptible to measles, unless otherwise contraindicated. Persons can be considered immune to measles only if they have had a documented episode of physician-diagnosed measles, have laboratory evidence of measles immunity, were born before 1957, or have had documented immunization.

Effective measles control necessitates identification and immunization of all susceptible persons, especially preschool-aged children. Because of the continuing occurrence of cases in older children and young adults, emphasis must be placed on identifying and appropriately immunizing adolescents and young adults in high school, college, and health care settings. Special emphasis should be placed on the administration of the first dose of vaccine at 12 to 15 months of age. Delays in administering the first dose contributed to large outbreaks from 1989 to 1991.

TABLE 3.29—Recommendations for Measles Vaccination*

Group	Remarks
Unvaccinated, no history of measles (12-15 mo)	A 2-dose schedule (with MMR) is recommended if born after 1956. The first dose is recommended at 12-15 mo; the second is recommended at 11-12 y (by entry to middle school or junior high school). In localities where revaccination at school entry is mandated by law, no additional, subsequent doses are indicated.
Children 12 mo in areas of recurrent measles transmission	Vaccinate; a second dose is indicated during the school years
Children 6-12 mo in epidemic situations†	Vaccinate; if vaccinated before the first birthday, revaccination (with MMR) at 12-15 mo of age is necessary and another dose is indicated during the school years
Children 11-12 y who have received one dose of measles vaccine at ≥12 mo	Revaccinate
Students in college and other post-high-school institutions who have received one dose of measles vaccine at ≥12 mo	Revaccinate
History of vaccination before the first birthday	Consider susceptible and vaccinate
Unknown vaccine, 1963-1967	Consider susceptible and vaccinate
Further attenuated or unknown vaccine given with IG	Consider susceptible and vaccinate
Egg allergy, nonanaphylactic	Vaccinate; no reactions likely
Neomycin allergy, nonanaphylactic	Vaccinate; no reactions likely
Tuberculosis	Vaccinate; vaccine does not exacerbate infection
Measles exposure within 72 h	Vaccination may protect (alternatively, IG should be given if household exposure)
HIV-seropositive	Vaccinate
Immunoglobulin or blood product received	Vaccinate at the appropriate interval (see Table 3.30, p 319)

*See text for details.
†See Outbreak Control (p 321).

By 12 years of age, persons should have received two doses of live-virus measles vaccine, the first of which should be given on or after the first birthday. The interval between doses should be 1 month or more. The Academy recommends that the second dose be given at entry to junior high school or middle school, ie, at age 11 to 12 years. Some public health jurisdictions mandate the second dose at school entry, and physicians should comply with local requirements. A third dose is not indicated under these circumstances unless the first dose was given before the child's first birthday. Current recommendations for routine reimmunization allow for flexibility in the age of administration of the second dose.

Adolescents and adults should be considered susceptible unless they have documentation of physician-diagnosed measles, have laboratory evidence of immunity to measles, have documentation of two doses of measles vaccine (as previously described), or were born before 1957. Since the two-dose schedule is not yet completely implemented in the United States, the number of doses required will depend on the age of the child and the year that the two-dose requirement was instituted in the area. In future years, an increasing number of students will have received a second dose, and eventually adequate vaccination for all adolescents and young adults will be defined by receipt of two doses.

A parental report of immunization is not considered adequate documentation. A physician should provide an immunization record for a patient only if he or she has administered the vaccine or has seen a record documenting vaccination.

Dose and Vaccine. Measles vaccine (as a monovalent or combination product) in a dose of 0.5 mL is given subcutaneously.

Measles and measles-containing vaccines can be given simultaneously with other vaccines (see Simultaneous Administration of Multiple Vaccines, p 25). Immune globulin should not be given with measles vaccine.

MMR is given for the initial dose when administered at 12 months of age or older. For reimmunization, MMR is also preferred in order to provide additional immunization against mumps and rubella. Recently, the number of cases of mumps in previously vaccinated persons has increased, and revaccination may be particularly important for control of mumps. Monovalent measles vaccine may be substituted for the second dose of MMR if cost is a factor. The anticipated side effects after MMR vaccination are expected to be infrequent after a second dose because most vaccinees will be immune.

Age of Routine Vaccination (see Tables 1.3 and 1.4, pp 23 and 24). The first dose should be given at age 12 to 15 months. It has been given usually at 15 months of age, but it should be administered at 12 months in high-risk areas, such as those with recurrent measles transmission. The second dose is recommended by the Academy to be given to children 11 or 12 years of age (the age of usual entry to middle school or junior high school). Revaccination at this age (or before) is recommended because the risk of measles increases substantially soon after entrance to middle school or junior high school. Thus, revaccination increases rates of immunity in the population soon before the high-risk period, and in individual patients it reinforces possible waning immunity. Vaccination at this age can easily be accomplished within the existing recommendations for health maintenance visits.* Alternatively, because of feasibility or local public health regulations, the second dose may be given at school entry (age 4 to 6 years). In jurisdictions where no law stipulates the age of revaccination, parents should be informed of the reasons for the recommendation for revaccination at 11 or 12 years of age.

Colleges and Other Institutions for Education Beyond High School. Colleges and other institutions should require that all entering students have documentation of physician-diagnosed measles, serologic evidence of immunity, birth before 1957, or receipt of two doses of measles-containing vaccines. Students without documentation of any measles vaccination or immunity should receive a dose on entry, followed by a repeat dose 1 or more months later.

Vaccination of Preschool-aged Children in Areas of Recurrent Measles Transmission. Initial vaccination at 12 months of age is recommended for preschool-aged children in high-risk areas. Guidelines for defining such areas are as follows: (1) a county with more than 5 cases among preschool-aged children during each of the last 5 years; (2) a county with a recent outbreak among unvaccinated preschool-aged children; and (3) a county with a large inner-city population.

During an outbreak, monovalent measles vaccine may be given to infants as young as 6 months (see Outbreak Control, p 321). If monovalent vaccine is not available, MMR is not contraindicated and may be given. However, seroconversion rates for measles, mumps, and rubella antigens are significantly lower in children vaccinated before the first birthday than seroconversion rates in children vaccinated after the first birthday. Therefore, children vaccinated before their first birthday should be vaccinated with MMR at 12 to 15 months and again at age 11 or 12 (or at school entry if locally required).

International Travel. Persons traveling to foreign countries should be immune to measles. From 1985 to 1991, 993 reported cases of measles in the United States were attributable to exposure in foreign countries and an additional 943 cases occurred in contacts of these imported cases. Therefore, vaccination against measles is particularly important for international travelers. A second dose should be given to persons born after 1956 who travel internationally, have not previously received two doses of measles vaccine, and otherwise do not have documented evidence of measles immunity.

For young children traveling to areas where measles is endemic or epidemic, the age for initial measles vaccination may need to be lowered. Children 12 to 14 months should be given their first dose of MMR before departure. Infants 6 to 11 months should receive a dose of monovalent measles vaccine (or MMR) before departure; at 12 to 15 months they should be revaccinated with MMR (at least 1 month after the initial measles vaccination), ie, children 16 months or older should have received two doses of measles-containing vaccine to assure immunity. A subsequent dose at or before 11 or 12 years of age is also recommended in accordance with the requirements for routine measles vaccination.

*See American Academy of Pediatrics, Committee on Psychosocial Aspects of Child and Family Health. *Guidelines for Health Supervision II.* Elk Grove Village, IL: American Academy of Pediatrics; 1988

Since most infants younger than 6 months are protected by maternally derived antibodies, immunization is not needed for infants in countries with ongoing measles transmission until they are 6 to 9 months of age.

Medical Facilities. Evidence of having had measles, measles immunity, or receipt of two measles vaccinations is desirable before beginning employment for nurses, nursing and medical students, residents, and other staff born after 1956 (see Health Care Personnel, p 65). For recommendations during an outbreak, see Outbreak Control (p 321).

Revaccination of Persons Vaccinated According to Pre-1989 Recommendations.

- *Persons vaccinated before 12 months of age.* These children should be considered susceptible and receive a dose at 12 to 15 months of age and again at age 11 or 12 years (or earlier if required by local immunization requirements for school entry).

- *Persons vaccinated at 12 to 14 months of age.* These children should be considered to have received an acceptable first vaccination, and they should receive a second dose, according to previously described recommendations.

- *Recipients of inactivated (killed) vaccine.* Two doses of live-measles vaccine separated by no less than 1 month are recommended for individuals vaccinated at any age with inactivated vaccine, and for those vaccinated with inactivated vaccine followed by live vaccine within 3 months. When recipients of inactivated-measles vaccine are exposed to natural virus, they are at risk for developing the atypical measles syndrome, which can be severe and can result in serious complications. Inactivated, as well as live-virus measles vaccine was available in the United States from 1963 to 1967. In Canada, inactivated vaccine was not distributed after 1970.

  As many as 50% of recipients of inactivated measles vaccine have reactions after revaccination with live measles vaccine. Most of these reactions are mild and consist of local swelling and erythema, with or without low-grade fever lasting 1 to 2 days. Rarely, more severe reactions, including prolonged high fever, lymphadenopathy, and extensive local reactions, occur and may necessitate hospitalization of the patient. However, recipients of inactivated measles vaccine are more likely to have serious illness when exposed to natural measles than when given live measles virus vaccine.

- *Persons with documented vaccination after 1967.* Because inactivated measles vaccine was not distributed in the United States after 1967 (and in Canada after 1970), persons with documentation of vaccination after 1967 on or after their first birthday with a vaccine of unknown type need not be revaccinated.

- *Persons who received IG with vaccine.* Edmonston B measles vaccine was effective when administered with IG, but the response to further attenuated strains (ie, Schwarz or Attenuvax) may be impeded by simultaneous or previous receipt of IG. A person who received further attenuated vaccine or a vaccine of an unknown type with IG after 1965 should be considered susceptible and should be given two additional doses of vaccine, as previously described (see also Precautions and Contraindications, p 318).

Adverse Reactions. About 5% to 15% of susceptible vaccinees develop a fever of 39.4°C (103°F) or higher, usually beginning 7 to 12 days after vaccination; the fever generally lasts 1 to 2 days (and as many as 5 days). Most persons with fever are otherwise asymptomatic. Transient rashes have been reported in approximately 5% of vaccinees. Transient thrombocytopenia has occurred after administration of measles-containing vaccines, specifically MMR. Central nervous system conditions, including encephalitis and encephalopathy, have been reported in an approximate frequency of less than one per million doses administered in the United States. Because the incidence of encephalitis or encephalopathy after measles vaccination in the United States is lower than the observed incidence of encephalitis of unknown etiology, some or most of the reported severe neurologic disorders may be only temporally, rather than causally, related to measles vaccination. After revaccination, reactions are expected to be clinically similar but much less frequent in occurrence since most vaccine recipients are already immune.

Allergic reactions occur rarely and are attributable in most cases to egg or egg-related antigens in the vaccine formulation (see Precautions and Contraindications, p 318). Anaphylaxis is extremely rare in these cases. Hypersensitivity reactions to the trace amounts of neomycin in the vaccine also have been reported.

Very-high-titer vaccines have been associated in several developing countries with increased mortality several months to years after vaccination. These high-titer vaccines were never licensed in the United States and are no longer in use in foreign countries.

Convulsions. As with any condition that induces fever during the second year of life, children predisposed to febrile seizures can experience seizures after measles immunization. Most of these seizures are simple febrile seizures. These seizures do not increase the risk of subsequent epilepsy or other neurologic disorders. Studies have suggested an increased risk of convulsions after administration of measles-containing vaccines to children who have history of previous seizures or whose first-degree family members have history of seizures. Although the exact risk cannot be determined, it appears to be low. Children with personal histories of convulsions or those whose first-degree relatives have histories of convulsions should be immunized because the benefits greatly outweigh the risks. This recommendation is based on the risks from measles disease, the large number of children with personal or family history of seizures (5% to 7%), the low incidence of seizures after measles vaccination, and the lack of association of these seizures with permanent brain damage.

Subacute Sclerosing Pancephalitis (SSPE). Measles vaccine, by protecting against measles, significantly reduces the possibility of developing SSPE. The marked decline in the number of SSPE cases after the introduction of measles vaccine is additional strong evidence of a protective effect of measles vaccination. Subacute sclerosing pancephalitis has been rarely reported in children with no history of natural measles but with history of receiving measles vaccine. Other children have developed SSPE without a history of having had measles or measles vaccine. Some of these children have had unrecognized measles and some children with a history of measles vaccine have only been exposed to measles or have had measles-like illnesses before vaccination. However, the risk of SSPE is not enhanced from live measles vaccine given to individuals who previously received live measles vaccine or had natural measles infection.

Precautions and Contraindications (see also Tables 3.30 and 3.31, pp 319 and 320).

- *Pregnancy.* Live measles vaccine, when given as a component of MR or MMR, should not be given to women known to be pregnant or who are considering becoming pregnant within 3 months of vaccination. Women who are given monovalent measles vaccine should not become pregnant for at least 30 days. This precaution is based on the theoretical risk of fetal infection, which applies to the administration of any live-virus vaccine to women who might be pregnant or who might become pregnant shortly after vaccination. No evidence, however, substantiates this theoretical risk.

  In the immunization of adolescents and young adults against measles, asking women if they are pregnant, excluding those who are, and explaining the theoretical risks to the others are recommended precautions.

- *Allergies.* Live measles vaccine is produced in chick embryo cell culture. Hypersensitivity reactions rarely follow the administration of live measles vaccine and are attributable in most cases to egg or egg-related antigens in the vaccine formulation. Most of these reactions are considered minor and consist of wheal-and-flare reactions or urticaria at the injection site. After distribution of more than 190 million doses of measles vaccine in the United States, less than 10 cases of immediate severe allergic reactions in children with history of anaphylactic reactions to egg ingestion have been reported. These anaphylactic reactions could have been life threatening, as some children experienced difficulty breathing and one had hypotension. Persons with histories of anaphylactic reactions (hives, swelling of the mouth and throat, difficulty breathing, hypotension, and shock) after egg ingestion should be vaccinated only with extreme caution (see Hypersensitivity Reactions to Vaccine Constituents, p 36). Persons are not at increased risk if they have egg allergies that are not anaphylactic in type, and they should be vaccinated in the usual manner. Persons with allergies to chickens or feathers are also not at increased risk of reaction to the vaccine.

  Because measles vaccine contains trace amounts of neomycin (25 µg), persons who have experienced anaphylactic reactions to topically or systemically administered neomycin should not receive measles vaccine. Most often, neomycin allergy manifests as a contact dermatitis, which is a delayed-type (cell-mediated) immune response rather than anaphylaxis. In such persons, an adverse reaction to neomycin in the vaccine would be an erythematous, pruritic nodule or papule 48 to 96 hours after vaccination. A history of contact dermatitis to neomycin is not a contraindication to receiving measles vaccine. Measles vaccine does not contain penicillin.

- *Recent administration of immune globulin.* Immune globulin preparations interfere with the serologic response to measles vaccine for variable time periods depending upon the dose administered. For example, vaccination should be deferred for 3 months after a person has received IG for postexposure prophylaxis against hepatitis A or B, but substantially longer intervals are indicated after larger doses of IG, IGIV, or other IG-containing products, such as in the case of patients with

TABLE 3.30—Suggested Intervals Between Immune Globulin Administration and Measles Vaccination (MMR or Monovalent Measles Vaccine)

Indication for Immune Globulin (IG)	Route	Dose U or mL	mg IgG/kg	Interval (mo)[a]
Tetanus (as TIG)	IM	250 U	~10	3
Hepatitis A prophylaxis (as IG)				
Contact prophylaxis	IM	0.02 mL/kg	3.3	
International travel	IM	0.06 mL/kg	10	3
Hepatitis B prophylaxis (as HBIG[b])	IM	0.06 mL/kg	10	
Rabies prophylaxis (as RIG[c])	IM	20 IU/kg	22	4
Measles prophylaxis (as IG)				
Standard	IM	0.25 mL/kg	40	5
Immunocompromised host	IM	0.50 mL/kg	80	6
Varicella prophylaxis (as VZIG[d])	IM	125 U/10 kg (maximum 625 U)	20–39	5
Blood transfusion:				
Washed red blood cells (RBCs)	IV	10 mL/kg	Negligible	0
RBCs, adenine-saline added	IV	10 mL/kg	10	3
Packed RBCs	IV	10 mL/kg	20–60	5
Whole blood	IV	10 mL/kg	80–100	6
Plasma/platelet products	IV	10 mL/kg	160	7
Replacement (or therapy) of immune deficiencies (as IGIV)	IV		300–400	8
ITP[e] (as IGIV)	IV		400	8
ITP	IV		1000	10
ITP or Kawasaki disease	IV		1600	11
Kawasaki disease	IV		2000	11

[a]These intervals should provide sufficient time for decreases in passive antibodies in all children to allow for an adequate response to measles vaccine. Physicians should not assume that children are fully protected against measles during these intervals. Additional doses of IG or measles vaccine may be indicated after exposure to measles (see text).
[b]Hepatitis B Immune Globulin.
[c]Rabies Immune Globulin.
[d]Varicella-Zoster Immune Globulin.
[e]Immune (formerly termed "idiopathic") thrombocytopenic purpura.

TABLE 3.31—Contraindications for Measles Vaccination

Underlying Condition	Rationale
Known pregnancy	Theoretical risk of fetal damage
Anaphylaxis to egg ingestion	Vaccinate with caution after skin testing*
Anaphylactic allergy to neomycin	Vaccine contains neomycin
Compromised immunity (except HIV infection)	Possibility of severe infection with vaccine virus

*See Hypersensitivity Reactions to Vaccine Constituents (p 36).

immune (formerly termed "idiopathic") thrombocytopenia (ITP) or Kawasaki disease. Suggested intervals between IG administration and measles vaccination are given in Table 3.30 (p 319). If vaccine is given at less than the indicated intervals, as may be warranted if the risk of exposure to measles is imminent, the child should be revaccinated at or after the appropriate interval for immunization, unless serologic testing indicates that measles-specific antibodies were produced (ie, the child was successfully immunized by the earlier dose of vaccine).

If IG is to be administered in preparation for international travel, administration of vaccine should precede receipt of IG by at least 2 weeks to preclude interference with replication of the vaccine virus.

- *Tuberculosis.* Tuberculin skin testing is not a prerequisite for measles vaccination. Although tuberculosis may be exacerbated by natural measles infection, live-virus measles vaccine is not known to have a deleterious effect and the value of protection against natural measles far outweighs the theoretical hazard of possible exacerbation of unsuspected tuberculosis. If tuberculin skin testing is otherwise indicated, it can be done on the day of vaccination. Otherwise, it should be postponed for 4 to 6 weeks since measles vaccination may temporarily suppress tuberculin skin test reactivity.
- *Altered immunity.* Significantly immunocompromised patients, with the exception of those with HIV infection, should not be given live-virus measles vaccine (see Immunodeficient and Immunosuppressed Children, p 53). Replication of the measles vaccine virus can be potentiated in patients with immunodeficiency diseases and by the suppressed immune responses associated with leukemia, lymphoma, or generalized malignancy, or resulting from therapy with alkylating drugs, antimetabolites, radiation, or large systemic doses of corticosteroids. Patients with such conditions should not be vaccinated with live-virus measles vaccine. Their risk of exposure to measles can be reduced by vaccinating their close susceptible contacts. Vaccinated persons do not transmit vaccine virus. Management of immunodeficient patients exposed to measles can be facilitated by prior knowledge of their immune status. Susceptible patients with immunodeficiencies should receive IG after exposure (see Care of Exposed Persons, p 311).

After cessation of immunosuppressive therapy, live measles virus vaccine is generally withheld for an interval of not less than 3 months. This interval is based on the assumption that immunologic responsiveness will have been restored in 3 months and the underlying disease for which immunosuppressive therapy was given is in remission or under control. However, because the interval can vary with the intensity and type of immunosuppressive therapy, radiation therapy, underlying disease, and other factors, a definitive recommendation for an interval after cessation of immunosuppressive therapy when measles vaccine can be safely and effectively administered is often not possible.

- *HIV infection.* Measles vaccination (given as MMR) is recommended for patients with symptomatic or asymptomatic HIV infection at the usually recommended ages. These recommendations are based on reports of severe and often fatal measles in these patients and the lack of complications from live-virus vaccine in children with HIV infection (see HIV Infection and AIDS, p 263). Regardless of vaccination status, symptomatic HIV-infected patients who are exposed to measles should receive IG prophylaxis because the children may not be protected from the vaccine (see Care of Exposed Persons, p 311). An exception may be the patient receiving IGIV at regular intervals whose last dose was received within 3 weeks of exposure.

- *Personal and/or family history of convulsions.* Children with this history should be vaccinated after discussion of the risks and benefits of immunization with parent or guardian (see Adverse Reactions, p 317). The parents or guardians of children who have either a personal or immediate family history of seizures should be advised that such children have a slightly increased risk of seizures after measles vaccination.

  Since fever induced by measles vaccine usually occurs between 7 and 12 days after immunization, prevention of vaccine-related febrile seizures is difficult. Parents should be alert to the occurrence of fever after vaccination and should treat their children appropriately.

  Children who are receiving anticonvulsants should continue to take such therapy after measles vaccination. However, prophylactic use of anticonvulsants may not be feasible, as therapeutic concentrations of many of the currently prescribed anticonvulsants (eg, phenobarbital) are not achieved for some time after the initiation of therapy.

- *Febrile illness.* Children with minor illnesses, with or without fever, such as upper respiratory tract infections, may be vaccinated (see Vaccine Safety and Contraindications, p 29). Fever per se is not a contraindication to immunization. However, if other manifestations suggest a more serious illness, the child should not be vaccinated until recovery. Most studies have demonstrated that children with afebrile upper respiratory infections had serologic responses similar to those in well children after measles vaccination.

Outbreak Control (see Table 3.32, p 322, for summary). All reports of suspected measles cases should be investigated promptly. A measles outbreak exists in a community whenever one case of measles is confirmed. Once this occurs, preventing the spread of measles depends on the prompt vaccination of susceptible persons. Persons who cannot readily provide documentation of measles immunity should be vaccinated or excluded from the setting (eg, school). Documentation of vaccination is adequate only if the date of vaccination is

TABLE 3.32—Recommendations for Measles Outbreak Control*

Setting	Control Measures
Outbreaks in preschool-aged children	Age for vaccination should be lowered to 6 mo in outbreak area if cases are occurring in children <1 y.†
Outbreaks in institutions: child care centers, K-12th grades, colleges, and other institutions	All students, their siblings, and school personnel born in or after 1957 who do not have documentation of immunity to measles‡ should have received 2 doses of measles vaccine.
Outbreaks in medical facilities	Revaccination of all medical workers born after 1956 who have direct patient contact and who do not have proof of immunity to measles.‡ Vaccination may also be considered for workers born before 1957.
	Susceptible personnel who have been exposed should be relieved from direct patient contact from the 5th to the 21st day after exposure (regardless of whether they received measles vaccine or IG) or, if they become ill, for 4 d after they develop rash.

*Revaccination should be limited to populations at risk, such as students attending institutions where cases occur. Mass revaccination of entire populations is not necessary.
†Children initially vaccinated before the first birthday should be revaccinated at 12-15 mo of age. A second dose should be administered during the school years.
‡Proof consists of documentation of physician-diagnosed measles disease, serologic evidence of immunity to measles, or documentation of receipt of 2 doses of measles vaccine on or after the first birthday.

provided. Almost all persons who are excluded from an outbreak area because they lack documentation of immunity quickly comply with vaccination requirements. Persons who have been exempted from measles vaccination for medical, religious, or other reasons should be excluded from the setting until at least 2 weeks after the onset of rash in the last case of measles.

Schools and Child Care Centers. A program of revaccination with MMR vaccine is recommended during outbreaks in child care centers; elementary, middle, junior, and senior high schools; and colleges and other institutions of higher education. Consideration should be given to revaccination in unaffected schools that may be at risk of measles transmission. Revaccination should include all students and their siblings and personnel born after 1956 who cannot provide documentation that they received two doses of measles-containing vaccine on or after their first birthday or other evidence of measles immunity. Persons revaccinated, as well as unvaccinated persons receiving their first dose as part of the outbreak control program, may be immediately readmitted to school. Mass revaccination of entire communities is not necessary.

Imposing quarantine measures for outbreak control is both difficult and disruptive to schools and other organizations. Under special circumstances, restriction of an event might be warranted; however, such action is not recommended as a routine measure for outbreak control.

Children Under 1 Year of Age. The risk of complications from measles is high among infants younger than 1 year. Therefore, considering the benefits and risks, vaccination with monovalent measles vaccine (or MMR if monovalent vaccine is not available) is recommended for infants as young as 6 months when exposure to natural measles is considered likely. Children vaccinated before the first birthday should be revaccinated with MMR when they are 12 to 15 months and again during their school years (see Vaccine Recommendations, p 312).

Medical Settings. If an outbreak occurs in an area served by a hospital or within a hospital, all employees with direct patient contact who were born after 1956 who cannot provide documentation that they have received two doses of measles vaccine on or after their first birthday or other evidence of immunity to measles should receive a dose of measles vaccine. Since some medical personnel who have acquired measles in medical facilities were born before 1957, vaccination of older employees who may have occupational exposure to measles should also be considered. Susceptible personnel who have been exposed should be relieved from direct patient contact from the 5th to the 21st day after exposure regardless of whether they received vaccine or IG after the exposure. Personnel who become ill should be relieved from patient contact for 4 days after they develop rash.

Meningococcal Infections

Clinical Manifestations: Invasive infection usually results in meningococcemia and/or meningitis. Onset is abrupt in meningococcemia with fever, chills, malaise, prostration, and a rash that initially may be urticarial, maculopapular, or petechial. In fulminant cases, purpura, disseminated intravascular coagulation, shock, coma, and death (Waterhouse-Friderichsen syndrome) can ensue within several hours despite appropriate therapy. The signs of meningococcal meningitis are indistinguishable from those of acute meningitis caused by *Haemophilus influenzae* and *Streptococcus pneumoniae*. Invasive meningococcal infections can be complicated by arthritis, myocarditis, pericarditis, endophthalmitis, or pneumonia. Other less common diseases include primary pneumonia, occult febrile bacteremia, conjunctivitis, and chronic meningococcemia.

Etiology: *Neisseria meningitidis* is a Gram-negative diplococcus with multiple serogroups known to cause invasive disease (A, B, C, X, Y, Z, 29-E, and W-135). Serogroups B and C are currently the most prevalent in the United States, each accounting for approximately 45% of reported cases. Group A has been frequently associated with epidemics elsewhere in the world.

Epidemiology: Asymptomatic colonization of the upper respiratory tract is frequent and provides the focus from which the organism is spread. Transmission is from person to person through droplets of respiratory tract secretions. Disease occurs most often in children younger than 5 years of age; the peak attack rate occurs in the 3- to 5-month age group. Close contacts of patients with meningococcal disease are at an increased risk for developing infection; outbreaks have occurred in semiclosed communities, including child care centers, nursery schools, colleges, and military recruit camps. Patients with deficiency of a terminal complement component (C5-9) are at particular risk for invasive and recurrent meningococcal disease. Patients are considered capable of transmitting infection for approximately 24 hours after initiation of effective treatment.

The **incubation period** is from 1 to 10 days, most commonly less than 4 days.

Diagnostic Tests: Cultures of blood and cerebrospinal fluid (CSF) are indicated in all patients with suspected invasive meningococcal disease. Cultures of petechial scraping, synovial fluid, sputum, and other body fluids are positive in some patients. Gram stain of a petechial scraping, CSF, and buffy coat of blood can be helpful on occasion. Antigen detection tests of CSF, serum, and urine with group-specific meningococcal antisera can allow rapid diagnosis and can be particularly useful if antibiotics were administered before collection of specimens for culture. In some cases, the value of the test is limited by lack of adequate sensitivity and specificity of the reagents, especially that of group B meningococcal antisera (which also reacts with K1 *Escherichia coli*). A polymerase chain reaction test has been used to detect and type meningococci directly from clinical specimens.

Treatment:
- Penicillin G should be administered intravenously in a high dose every 4 to 6 hours for patients with invasive disease. Cefotaxime and ceftriaxone are acceptable alternatives. In the patient with penicillin allergy of the anaphylactoid type, chloramphenicol is indicated. Five to 7 days of antibiotic therapy is usually adequate for most cases of invasive meningococcal disease. In the few areas (Spain and parts of Africa) where penicillin in vitro resistance has been reported, cefotaxime, ceftriaxone, or chloramphenicol is recommended.
- Dexamethasone therapy should be considered in infants and children 2 months or older with bacterial meningitis after consideration of the benefits and possible risks (see Dexamethasone Therapy for Bacterial Meningitis in Infants and Children, p 558).

Isolation of the Hospitalized Patient: Respiratory isolation is indicated for 24 hours after initiation of effective therapy.

Control Measures:
Care of Exposed Persons.
   Careful Observation. Exposed household, school, or child care contacts must be carefully observed. Exposed individuals who develop a

febrile illness should receive prompt medical evaluation. If indicated, antimicrobial therapy appropriate for invasive meningococcal infections should be administered.

Household, Child Care Center, and Nursery School Contacts. Antibiotic prophylaxis should be given as soon as possible, preferably within 24 hours of the diagnosis of the primary case. Prophylaxis is also warranted for persons who have had contact with the patient's oral secretions through kissing or sharing of food or beverages. Prophylaxis is not recommended routinely for medical personnel except those who have had intimate exposure (such as occurs with mouth-to-mouth resuscitation, intubation, or suctioning) before antibiotic therapy was begun. Respiratory tract cultures are not of value in deciding who should receive prophylaxis.

Chemoprophylaxis. The drug of choice in most instances is rifampin. The recommended regimen for rifampin prophylaxis is 10 mg/kg (maximum dose, 600 mg) every 12 hours, for a total of four doses in 2 days. Some experts recommend reducing the dose to 5 mg/kg for infants younger than 1 month of age. A liquid preparation can be formulated, or the powder can be mixed with other vehicles such as applesauce. For adults, each dose is 600 mg. The 4-day rifampin regimen, given for prophylaxis of *Haemophilus influenzae* type b disease, of 20 mg/kg (600 mg maximum) once daily for 4 days, is also effective for meningococcal prophylaxis.

Ceftriaxone given in a single intramuscular dose (125 mg for children younger than 12 years; 250 mg for children older than 12 years and for adults) has been demonstrated to be more effective than oral rifampin in eradicating pharyngeal carriage of group A meningococci. Although ceftriaxone is not recommended routinely for prophylaxis because its efficacy has been confirmed only for group A strains, its effect is likely to be similar for other strains. It has the advantages of possible greater efficacy than rifampin, easier dosage administration, and safety in pregnancy.

Sulfisoxazole is recommended when an isolate is known to be sulfasusceptible. For sulfisoxazole chemoprophylaxis, the dose is 500 mg/d for infants younger than 1 year, 500 mg every 12 hours for children 1 to 12 years, and 1 g every 12 hours for children older than 12 years and for adults. The duration of therapy is 2 days.

Ciprofloxacin given as a single, oral dose of 500 mg to adults is also effective in eradicating meningococcal carriage. At present, ciprofloxacin is not recommended for use in persons younger than 18 years of age.

Immunoprophylaxis. Because secondary cases can occur several weeks or more after onset of disease in the index case, meningococcal vaccine is a possible adjunct to chemoprophylaxis when the outbreak is caused by a serogroup contained in the vaccine. The results of one study demonstrated efficacy of the vaccine in lowering the occurrence of secondary cases.

Meningococcal Vaccine. A serogroup-specific quadrivalent meningococcal vaccine* against groups A, C, Y, and W-135 *N meningitidis* is available in the United States. The vaccine consists of 50 µg each of the respective purified bacterial capsular polysaccharides. The vaccine is administered subcutaneously as a single 0.5-mL dose.

---

*Meningococcal Polysaccharide Vaccine, Groups A, C, Y, W-135 Combined (Menomune) is available from Connaught Laboratories, Inc, Swiftwater, PA.

The group A component is immunogenic in children 3 months and older. For children younger than 18 months, two doses 3 months apart have been given in epidemic control. If the quadrivalent vaccine is used in infants, response to the other meningococcal group polysaccharides is usually poor. Group C component is effective in children 2 years and older. The duration of protection is not established but is likely to be less than 3 years against group A infections in children immunized when younger than 4 years of age.

Indications. Routine vaccination of children with meningococcal vaccine is not recommended. However, vaccination should be considered in children 2 years and older in high-risk groups, including those with functional or anatomic asplenia (see Asplenic Children, p 57), or those with terminal complement component deficiencies. The vaccine can be considered as an adjunct to chemoprophylaxis (see Care of Exposed Persons, p 324). It should be used to control outbreaks of disease caused by serogroups represented in the vaccine and may be of benefit to travelers to countries recognized to have hyperendemic or epidemic disease.

The vaccine is currently given to all American military recruits.

Revaccination. For persons at high risk of infection, particularly children who were first immunized when younger than 4 years of age, revaccination may be indicated. Such children should be considered for revaccination after 2 or 3 years if they remain at high risk. The need for revaccination in older children and adults is unknown.

Adverse Reactions and Precautions. Infrequent and mild adverse reactions occur, the most common of which is localized erythema for 1 to 2 days. The safety of the vaccine in pregnant women has not been established. Hence, pregnant women should be immunized only if they have a substantial risk of infection.

Microsporidia Infections (Microsporidiosis)

Clinical Manifestations: Patients with intestinal infection have watery, nonbloody diarrhea. Fever is uncommon. Intestinal infection has been recognized only in immunocompromised individuals, especially those who are infected with HIV. The clinical course is complicated by malnutrition and progressive weight loss.

Etiology: *Microsporidia* are intracellular protozoa. At least four genera — *Encephalitozoon*, *Nosema*, *Pleistophora*, and *Enterocytozoon* — infect humans.

Epidemiology: *Enterocytozoon bieneusi* is an important cause of chronic diarrhea in patients with HIV infection. Other clinical syndromes associated with other *Microsporidia* genera in HIV-infected patients include keratoconjunctivitis, nephritis, hepatitis, and peritonitis, but they have occurred infrequently. Information about the epidemiology and mode of transmission is limited. In animals, transmission occurs by ingestion of *Microsporidia* spores in food or contact with spores shed into the environment through stools or urine. In humans, fecal-oral contact may play a role in transmission.

The **incubation period** is not known.

Diagnostic Tests: Infection with *E bieneusi* can be documented by identification of organisms in biopsy specimens from the small intestine. *Microsporidia* spores can be detected in formalin-fixed stool specimens or duodenal aspirates stained with a chromotrope-based stain, which is a modification of the trichrome stain, and viewed by light microscopy. Gram, acid-fast, periodic acid-Schiff, and Giemsa stains can also be used to detect organisms in tissue sections. The organisms are often not noticed because they are small, stain poorly, and evoke minimal inflammatory response. Use of one of the stool concentration techniques does not appear to improve the ability to detect *E bieneusi* spores. Identification for classification purposes and diagnostic confirmation of species requires the use of transmission electron microscopy.

Treatment: No effective therapy for patients with microsporidiosis is known. In a limited number of patients, albendazole has been reported to produce remission.

Isolation of the Hospitalized Patient: Enteric precautions are recommended.

Control Measures: None.

Molluscum Contagiosum

Clinical Manifestations: Molluscum contagiosum is a benign, usually asymptomatic viral disease of the skin. It is characterized by a relatively small number (usually 2 to 20) of discrete, papular, waxy lesions, some with central umbilication in a generalized distribution. An eczematous reaction may encircle the lesions in about 10% of patients. It has no systemic manifestations.

Etiology: The cause is a poxvirus.

Epidemiology: Humans are the only known source of the virus. It is spread by direct contact, including sexual contact, or by fomites. The infectivity is generally low, but occasional outbreaks have been reported. The period of communicability is unknown.

The **incubation period** appears to vary between 2 and 7 weeks but may extend to 6 months.

Diagnostic Tests: The diagnosis can usually be made from the characteristic clinical appearance of the lesions. However, staining of the material expressed from the central core of the lesions reveals characteristic intracytoplasmic inclusions. Electron microscopic examination will identify the typical poxvirus particles.

Treatment: Mechanical removal of the central core of each lesion usually results in resolution. Alternatively, topical application of cantharidin, peeling agents such as salicylic and lactic acid preparations, or liquid nitrogen may be successful. Although lesions can regress spontaneously, removal is advisable, when possible, to prevent autoinoculation and spread to other individuals.

Isolation of the Hospitalized Patient: Drainage/secretion precautions are recommended.

Control Measures: No control measures are known for isolated cases. For outbreaks, such as are commonly found in the tropics, restricting direct body contact between affected and unaffected children can reduce the spread.

Moraxella catarrhalis Infections

Clinical Manifestations: Infections include otitis media and paranasal sinusitis in children. Bronchopulmonary infection in patients with chronic lung disease can occur. Rare manifestations are bacteremia in children (healthy or immunocompromised) and conjunctivitis in neonates.

Etiology: *Moraxella catarrhalis* (formerly called *Branhamella catarrhalis*) is a Gram-negative diplococcus. Beta-lactamase production mediating resistance to penicillins has been identified in more than 75% of strains.

Epidemiology: *Moraxella catarrhalis* is part of the normal flora in the upper respiratory tract of humans. Carriage may be more frequent during the fall and winter than during the spring and summer. The mode of transmission is presumed to be direct contact with contaminated respiratory tract secretions and/or droplet spread. Infection is most frequent in infants but occurs at all ages. Transmission in families, schools, and day care centers has not been studied. The duration of carriage by infected and colonized children, and the period of communicability are unknown.

The **incubation period** is unknown.

Diagnostic Tests: The organism can be isolated readily on common culture media (blood or chocolate agar) after incubation in air or with increased CO_2 (candle jar). Culture of middle ear or sinus fluid is indicated in patients with unusually severe infection, in some who are treatment failures, and in neonates or other highly susceptible children. Recovery of *M catarrhalis* with other pathogens (*Streptococcus pneumoniae* or *Haemophilus influenzae*) can occur, indicating a mixed infection.

Treatment: Since most strains of *M catarrhalis* produce beta-lactamase and are ampicillin resistant, appropriate antimicrobial choices include amoxicillin-clavulanate, cefixime, cefaclor, cefuroxime, erythromycin-sulfisoxazole, and trimethoprim-sulfamethoxazole. If parenteral drugs are needed to treat *M catarrhalis* infection or other concurrent bacteria in a mixed infection, in vitro data indicate that the following drugs will be effective: cefuroxime, cefotaxime, ceftriaxone, ceftazidime, chloramphenicol, and trimethoprim-sulfamethoxazole.

Isolation of the Hospitalized Patient: No special precautions are recommended.

Control Measures: None.

Mumps

Clinical Manifestations: Mumps is a systemic disease, characterized by swelling of the salivary glands. Approximately one third of infections, however, do not cause clinically apparent salivary gland swelling. Meningeal signs are reported in 10% to 30% of cases. Encephalitis occurs in approximately 1 in 6,000 cases and has an average case fatality rate of 1.4%; permanent sequelae are rare. Orchitis is a common complication after puberty but sterility rarely occurs. Other rare complications include arthritis, renal involvement, thyroiditis, mastitis, pancreatitis, and hearing impairment.

Etiology: Mumps is caused by a paramyxovirus.

Epidemiology: Humans are the only known natural hosts. The virus is spread by direct contact via the respiratory route. Infection occurs throughout childhood. Mumps during adulthood is more likely to produce severe disease, including orchitis. Death from mumps is rare; more than half the fatalities occur in persons older than 19 years. Mumps infection during the first trimester of pregnancy can increase the rate of spontaneous abortion, which has been reported to be as high as 27%. Although mumps virus can cross the placenta, no evidence indicates that mumps infection in pregnancy causes congenital malformations. The infection is more common during the late winter and spring. The incidence has declined markedly since the introduction of the mumps vaccine. The United States experienced a minor resurgence of mumps in 1986 to 1987, peaking at 12,848 reported cases in 1987. Reported cases in 1988 to 1992 have been slightly higher than those in 1981 to 1985. The peak incidence continues to be between the ages of 10 and 14; incidences in 5- to 9-year-olds and 15- to 19-year-olds are not substantially lower. Outbreaks can occur in highly vaccinated populations, indicating that mumps transmission can be sustained among the few persons not protected by vaccination. The period of communicability is usually 1 to 2 days but has been reported to be as many as 7 days before the onset of parotid swelling, and is usually 5 (although occasionally as many as 9 days) after onset.

The **incubation period** is usually from 16 to 18 days, but cases may occur from 12 to 25 days after exposure.

Diagnostic Tests: Mumps virus can be isolated in tissue culture inoculated with throat washings, urine, and spinal fluid. The complement fixation (CF), neutralization, or hemagglutination inhibition (HAI) test or an enzyme immunoassay (EIA) can be used to serologically confirm infection or vaccination. Although paired sera are desirable, a single serum specimen containing complement-fixing antibody against the soluble component of mumps virus suggests recent infection. An EIA or neutralization test, although the latter is not always readily available, should be used for assessing immunity; CF or HAI tests are unreliable for this purpose. Skin tests are unreliable and should not be used to test immune status.

Treatment: Supportive.

Isolation of the Hospitalized Patient: Respiratory isolation is indicated. Patients should be isolated until 9 days after the onset of parotid swelling.

Control Measures:

School and Child Care. Children should be excluded until 9 days after the onset of parotid gland swelling. For control measures during an outbreak, see Outbreak Control, p 332.

Care of Exposed Persons. Mumps vaccine has not been demonstrated to be effective in preventing infection after exposure. However, mumps vaccine can be given after exposure, as immunization will provide protection against subsequent exposures. No increased risk of reactions or contraindications exist after vaccination of a person during the incubation period of mumps or from vaccination of a person who is already immune. Because approximately 90% of adults who have no knowledge of past infection are immune on serologic testing, mumps vaccine is not routinely advised for those born before 1957 unless they are proven to be susceptible (ie, seronegative). Mumps immune globulin is of no value and is no longer manufactured.

Mumps Virus Vaccine. Live mumps virus vaccine is prepared in chick embryo cell cultures. Vaccine is administered by subcutaneous injection of 0.5 mL, either alone or as a combined vaccine containing measles and rubella vaccines (MMR). More than 95% of all persons susceptible to mumps develop antibody after a single dose. Serologic and epidemiologic evidence extending through 25 years indicates that vaccine-induced immunity is long lasting.

Vaccine Recommendations.
  • Mumps vaccine should be given routinely to children at 12 months of age or older. It is usually administered in combination with measles and rubella vaccine (MMR) and is usually given at 15 months of age (see Tables 1.3 and 1.4, pp 23 and 24). A second dose of mumps vaccine administered as MMR is advised; the recommended age is determined by the measles vac-

cination schedule (see Measles, p 312). Mumps revaccination is particularly important because mumps can occur in highly vaccinated populations and substantial numbers of cases have occurred in persons with history of mumps vaccination. Administration of MMR is not harmful if given to an individual already immune to one or more of the viruses (from either infection or vaccination).

- Mumps vaccination is of particular value for susceptible children approaching puberty and for susceptible adolescents and adults. At office visits of prepubertal children and adolescents, the status of immunity to mumps should be assessed. Persons should be considered susceptible unless they have documentation of physician-diagnosed mumps, adequate immunization for age, or serologic evidence of immunity.

- *International travel*. Mumps is still endemic throughout most of the world. Although vaccination against mumps is not a requirement for entry into any country, susceptible children, adolescents, and adults born after 1956 should be offered mumps vaccination (usually as MMR) before beginning travel. Because of concern about inadequate seroconversion due to persisting maternal antibodies and because the risk of serious disease from mumps infection is relatively low, persons younger than 12 months need not be given mumps vaccine before travel.

- Mumps vaccine is not routinely advised for those born before 1957 unless they are considered susceptible, as defined by seronegativity. However, vaccination is not contraindicated in these persons if their serologic status is unknown.

- Mumps vaccine can be given simultaneously with other vaccines (see Simultaneous Administration of Multiple Vaccine, p 25).

Adverse Reactions. Adverse reactions attributed to live mumps vaccine are extremely rare. Temporally related reactions, including febrile seizures, nerve deafness, parotitis, meningitis, encephalitis, rash, pruritus, and purpura, may not be related etiologically. In the United States, the frequency of central nervous system complications after mumps vaccination has been lower than the observed background incidence in the normal population. Orchitis and parotitis have been reported rarely. Allergic reactions attributable to egg or egg-related antigens in the vaccine formulation are very rare (see Precautions and Contraindications, below).

Reimmunization with mumps vaccine (monovalent or MMR) is not associated with an increased incidence of reactions. Reactions would be expected only among those not protected by the first dose.

Precautions and Contraindications:

- *Pregnancy.* Susceptible postpubertal females should not be vaccinated if known to be pregnant, and they should be counseled before vaccination about the potential hazard of fetal infection with vaccine virus. Live-virus mumps vaccine can infect the placenta, but virus has not been isolated from fetal tissues of susceptible females who received vaccine and underwent elective abortions. In view of the theoretical risk, however, conception should be avoided for 3 months after vaccination.

- *Allergies.* Mumps vaccine is virtually devoid of allergenic substances derived from the chick embryo cell cultures used for growth of the live vaccine viruses. However, a remote, potential risk of hypersensitivity reactions in patients allergic to eggs does exist. The large-scale use of the vaccine since 1967 has resulted in only rare, isolated reports of allergic reactions. Persons with anaphylactic reactions to eggs should receive mumps-containing vaccines only with extreme caution (see Hypersensitivity Reactions to Vaccine Constituents, p 36). Mumps vaccine does not contain penicillin.

- *Recent administration of immune globulin (IG).* Live mumps vaccine should be given at least 2 weeks before or at least 3 months after administration of IG or blood transfusion because of the possibility that antibody will neutralize vaccine virus and prevent a successful immunization. Since mumps vaccine is usually given as MMR, and high doses of immunoglobulin (such as those given for the treatment of Kawasaki disease) can inhibit the response to measles vaccine for longer intervals, mumps vaccination with MMR necessitates deferral for longer periods in such circumstances (see Measles, p 318). Large doses of immune globulin administered for replacement therapy of individuals with immunodeficiency disorders or for treatment of Kawasaki disease could also inhibit the response to mumps vaccine for longer intervals.
- *Altered immunity.* The following persons should not receive live mumps virus vaccine: (1) patients with immunodeficiency diseases; (2) those receiving immunosuppressive therapy (eg, patients with leukemia, lymphoma, or generalized malignancy); (3) those receiving large systemic doses of corticosteroids, alkylating agents, antimetabolites, or radiation; and (4) patients who are otherwise immunocompromised. The exceptions are patients with symptomatic HIV infection who are to be immunized against measles with MMR (see HIV Infection and AIDS, p 263). The risk of mumps exposure for patients with altered immunity can be reduced by vaccinating their close susceptible contacts. Vaccinated persons do not transmit mumps vaccine virus.

  After cessation of immunosuppressive therapy, live-virus mumps vaccine is generally withheld for an interval of not less than 3 months. This interval is based on the assumption that immunologic responsiveness will have been restored in 3 months and the underlying disease for which immunosuppressive therapy was given is in remission or under control. However, because the interval can vary with the intensity and type of immunosuppressive therapy, radiation therapy, underlying disease, and other factors, a definitive recommendation for an interval after cessation of immunosuppressive therapy when mumps vaccine can be safely and effectively administered is often not possible.
- *Febrile illness.* Children with minor illnesses with or without fever, such as upper respiratory tract infections, may be vaccinated (see Vaccine Safety and Contraindications, p 29). Fever per se is not a contraindication to immunization. However, if other manifestations suggest a more serious illness, the child should not be vaccinated until recovery.

Outbreak Control. In determining means to control outbreaks, exclusion of susceptible students from affected schools and schools judged by local public health authorities to be at risk for transmission should be considered. Such exclusion should be an effective means of terminating school outbreaks and rapidly increasing rates of immunization. Excluded students can be readmitted immediately after vaccination. Pupils who have been exempted from mumps vaccination because of medical, religious, or other reasons should be excluded until at least 26 days after the onset of parotitis in the last person with mumps in the affected school. Experience with outbreak control for other vaccine-preventable diseases indicates that almost all students who are excluded from the outbreak area because they lack evidence of immunity quickly comply with requirements and can be readmitted to school.

Mycoplasma pneumoniae Infections

Clinical Manifestations: Initial symptoms in patients who develop pneumonia, the most prominent infection, are malaise, fever, and, in some cases, headache. Nonproductive cough develops within several days, can become productive (in older children, adolescents, and adults), and persists for 3 to 4 weeks. Roentgenographic abnormalities vary, but bilateral, diffuse infiltrates are common. The most common clinical syndromes are upper respiratory tract infections, including tracheobronchitis, pharyngitis, and, occasionally, otitis media or myringitis, which may be bullous. Coryza (ie, the common cold) is infrequent. Much less frequent manifestations are aseptic meningitis, encephalitis, cerebellar ataxia, peripheral neuropathy, myocarditis, pericarditis, polymorphous mucocutaneous eruptions (including Stevens-Johnson syndrome), hemolytic anemia, and arthritis. Patients with sickle-cell disease, immunodeficiencies, and chronic cardiorespiratory disease can develop severe pneumonia.

Etiology: *Mycoplasma pneumoniae* is the cause. Mycoplasmas, the smallest free-living organisms, lack cell walls.

Epidemiology: Infected humans are the only source of infection. Acquisition is most likely from symptomatic patients and is presumed to be by droplet spread. Individuals at any age can be infected, but specific disease syndromes are age related. *Mycoplasma pneumoniae* is an uncommon cause of infection in children younger than 5 years of age but is the leading cause of pneumonia in school-aged children and young adults. Military and college populations have a high incidence of the disease. Infections occur throughout the world, in any season, and in all geographic settings. Epidemics may occur every 4 to 8 years. Familial spread over many months frequently occurs, resulting in cumulative household attack rates that approach 100%. Clinical illness within a group, particularly a family, can range from tracheobronchitis to pneumonia. Asymptomatic carriage after infection can occur for prolonged intervals, commonly for weeks. Immunity after infection is not long lasting.

The **incubation period** is 2 to 3 weeks.

Diagnostic Tests: Recovery of *M pneumoniae* in cultures requires special media, takes 7 to 21 days, and is not widely available. Isolation of *M pneumoniae* in a compatible clinical situation suggests causation. Because this organism can be excreted from the respiratory tract for several weeks after an acute infection despite appropriate therapy, isolation of the organism may not indicate recent infection.

Of the different antibody tests used to demonstrate a fourfold or greater increase in titer between acute and convalescent sera, the complement fixation antibody test is most widely available. Since *M pneumoniae* antibody cross-reacts with some other antigens, particularly with those of other mycoplasmas, results of this test should be interpreted cautiously in evaluating febrile illnesses of unknown origin. However, no cross-reactivity with other respiratory pathogens causing diseases clinically similar to those caused by *M pneumoniae* exists. False-negative results can occur, as the sensitivity of this serologic test is 50% to 80%. Serum cold hemagglutinin titers of 1:64 or more are present in 50% of infected patients; fourfold increases in titer between acute and convalescent sera occur more often in patients with severe *Mycoplasma* pneumonia than in those with less severe disease. Other etiologic agents, including adenoviruses, Epstein-Barr virus, and measles, can cause illnesses in infants or children associated with a rise in titer of cold hemagglutinins. A negative test for cold agglutinins does not exclude the diagnosis of mycoplasmal infection.

Two rapid diagnostic tests are commercially available. One is a radiolabeled DNA probe that detects *M pneumoniae* ribosomal RNA in respiratory secretions. Positive tests correlate well with positive cultures; however, cultures are more sensitive, and the test does not detect many infections indicated by antibody conversions. The second test is a slide agglutination reaction to detect *M pneumoniae* antibodies. Since infections are common and resulting antibodies persist for months or years, measurement of antibody in a single serum sample is of little diagnostic value. Recently, a polymerase chain reaction test for *M pneumonia* has been demonstrated to be effective.

Treatment: Erythromycin is the preferred antimicrobial agent in children younger than 9 years. Other new macrolides, such as clarithromycin and azithromycin, are also likely to be effective and may be better tolerated, but, as of 1993, have not been approved by the Food and Drug Administration for use in preadolescent children. Tetracycline is equally effective and may be used in children 9 years and older. Most studies with these antimicrobial agents have been conducted in adults, and definitive evidence for their efficacy in children with *M pneumoniae* infection is lacking.

Isolation of the Hospitalized Patient: Respiratory isolation is recommended.

Control Measures: Diagnosis of an infected patient should lead to an increased index of suspicion for *Mycoplasma* infection in household members and close contacts. Case finding should be instituted if *Mycoplasma* organisms have affected many individuals in a group. Appropriate therapy for each contact should be given if a compatible clinical illness occurs. Because therapy does not affect the rate of transmission to exposed persons, antibiotic prophylaxis for contacts is not indicated.

Nocardiosis

Clinical Manifestations: A common presentation in nonimmunocompromised children is cutaneous or lymphocutaneous disease after contamination of an abrasion. Usually in these cases the lesions remain localized. Invasive disease occurs most commonly in immunocompromised patients, particularly those with chronic granulomatous disease or HIV infection. Infection characteristically begins in the lung, with hematogenous spread to the liver, brain, kidneys, and other organs. Pulmonary disease resembles that of tuberculosis and systemic fungal infection.

Etiology: *Nocardia* species are fungus-like bacteria. Disease is caused most commonly by *Nocardia asteroides*, less frequently by *Nocardia braziliensis*, and occasionally by other *Nocardia* species.

Epidemiology: *Nocardia* species are free living in nature, in soil, and in compost, and are found worldwide. Infectious particles are airborne, and the lung is the probable portal of entry. Direct skin inoculation occurs, often as the result of minor trauma and/or soil contamination. Person-to-person transmission does not occur.

The **incubation period** is unknown.

Diagnosis: Stained smears of sputum, cerebrospinal fluid, or pus can demonstrate beaded, branched, weakly-Gram-positive rods that are variably acid fast. The Brown and Brenn and the methenamine silver stains are recommended for demonstrating microorganisms in tissue. Growth of typical colonies occurs on Sabouraud's dextrose agar without added antibiotics. Blood specimens should be cultured on brain-heart infusion media. These organisms are slow growing; therefore, cultures should be maintained for 7 to 10 days.

Treatment: Trimethoprim-sulfamethoxazole or a sulfonamide (eg, sulfadiazine,* sulfisoxazole, or triple sulfonamide combinations) is the drug of choice. Blood concentrations of the sulfonamide should be maintained at 15 to 20 mg/dL. Immunocompetent patients with lymphocutaneous disease usually respond after 6 to 12 weeks of therapy. Immunocompromised patients and those with invasive disease should be treated for 6 to 12 months. The disease can recur months or years after therapy. Patients with AIDS may need long-term therapy. Patients with meningitis or brain abscess should be monitored with serial brain scans. If response to sulfa drugs does not occur, streptomycin, amikacin, minocycline, or tetracycline may be added. Tetracycline drugs should not be given to children younger than 9 years unless the benefits of therapy outweigh the risks. Incision and drainage of abscesses is beneficial.

Isolation of the Hospitalized Patient: No special precautions are recommended.

Control Measures: None.

---

*As of 1993, sulfadiazine is no longer marketed in the United States. Until a domestic source of the drug is reestablished, the drug may be obtained from the Division of Parasitic Diseases at the Centers for Disease Control and Prevention (see Directory of Telephone Numbers, p 601).

Onchocerciasis
(River Blindness)

Clinical Manifestations: The disease involves the skin, subcutaneous tissues, lymphatics, and eyes. Subcutaneous nodules of varying sizes, containing adult worms, develop 6 to 12 months after the initial infection. In patients in Central America, the nodules are usually on the head or upper torso. In patients in Africa, the nodules are usually on the lower torso, pelvis, and lower extremities. After the worms mature, microfilariae are produced and migrate in the tissues, where they may cause a chronic, generalized, pruritic dermatitis. After a period of years, the skin can become lichenified and hypo- or hyperpigmented. The presence of microfilariae, living or dead, in the ocular structures, leads to photophobia and inflammation of the cornea, iris, ciliary body, retina, choroid, and optic nerve. Blindness can result if the disease is untreated.

Etiology: *Onchocerca volvulus* is a filarial nematode.

Epidemiology: The larvae are transmitted by the bites of an infected *Simulium* black fly that breeds in fast-flowing streams and rivers (hence the colloquial name of the disease, "river blindness"). Disease occurs primarily in equatorial Africa, but small foci are found in southern Mexico, Guatemala, northern South America, and Yemen. Prevalence is greatest among those who live near vector-breeding areas. The adult worms continue to produce microfilariae capable of infecting flies for as long as a decade. The infection is not transmissible by person-to-person contact or blood transfusion.

The **incubation period** from larval inoculation to microfilariae in the skin is approximately 6 to 12 months.

Diagnostic Tests: Direct examination of a shave biopsy of the epidermis (taken from scapular or posterior hip area) usually will reveal microfilariae. Specimens should be incubated in saline solution overnight and examined unstained under a microscope. A slit-lamp examination of the anterior chamber of the eye may reveal motile microfilariae or corneal lesions typical of onchocerciasis. Eosinophilia is common, but microfilariae are rarely found in blood. Specific serologic tests are available only at selected research laboratories.

Treatment: Ivermectin, a microfilaricidal agent, is the drug of choice for treatment of onchocerciasis. Ivermectin is available from the Drug Service of the Centers for Disease Control and Prevention (see Directory of Telephone Numbers, p 601). Treatment reduces dermatitis and the risk of developing ocular disease, but it does not kill the adult worms and, thus, is not curative. A single oral dose (150 µg/kg) should be given each year for 5 to 10 years. Adverse reactions are caused by the death of the microfilariae and include rash, edema, fever, exacerbation of astnma, and hypotension (which is rarely severe). Contraindications to treatment include pregnancy, central nervous system disorders, and body weight of less than 15 kg.

Isolation of the Hospitalized Patient: No special precautions are recommended.

Control Measures: Repellents and protective clothing (long sleeves and pants) can reduce exposure to black fly bites. Treatment of vector breeding sites with larvicides has been effective for controlling black fly populations, particularly in West Africa. A major effort to distribute ivermectin in hyperendemic communities has been undertaken.

Papillomaviruses

Clinical Manifestations: Human papillomavirus (HPV) produces epithelial tumors (warts) of the skin and mucous membranes. Cutaneous nongenital warts include common skin warts, plantar warts, flat warts, and thread-like filiform warts on the neck and face. Those affecting membranes include anogenital warts, epidermodysplasia verruciformis, and respiratory papillomatosis.

Common skin warts are dome shaped with conical projections that give the surface a rough appearance. They are usually asymptomatic and multiple, occurring on the hands and around or under the nails. When small dermal vessels thrombose, black dots appear in the warts. Plantar warts on the foot can be painful and are characterized by marked hyperkeratosis, sometimes with black dots. Flat warts, commonly found on the face and extremities, are usually small, multiple, and flat topped; they seldom exhibit papillomatosis and rarely cause pain. Thread-like filiform warts occur on the face and neck. Cutaneous warts are benign.

The manifestations of anogenital HPV infection range from asymptomatic infection to condylomata acuminata, skin-colored growths with a cauliflower-like surface that vary in size from a few millimeters to several centimeters in diameter. In males, such warts may be found on the shaft of the penis, penile meatus, scrotum, and perianal areas. In females, usual sites of HPV infection are the cervix, introitus, labia, perineum vagina, and perianal areas. Most anogenital warts are asymptomatic but occasionally cause itching, burning, local pain, or bleeding. Some HPV types are associated with genital carcinoma, including carcinoma of the cervix.

Laryngeal papillomas, which appear to be comparable to genital warts, are rare. They occur mostly in children younger than 10 years of age, and are manifested by a voice change or abnormal cry.

Epidermodysplasia verruciformis is a rare, lifelong, severe papillomavirus infection, believed to be a consequence of an inherited immunodeficiency. The lesions can resemble flat warts but are often similar to tinea versicolor covering the torso and upper extremities. Most appear in the first decade of life but do not undergo malignant transformation until adulthood.

Etiology: Human papillomaviruses (HPV) are members of the *Papovaviridae* family and are DNA viruses. More than 60 types have been identified, but a small number of HPV types account for most warts. Those causing nongenital warts are distinct from those causing anogenital infections. Of the latter, only a small number have been associated with malignancies.

Epidemiology: Papillomaviruses are widely distributed among mammals but are species specific. Cutaneous warts occur frequently among school-aged children; prevalence rates are as high as 50%. Human papillomavirus infections are thought to be transmitted from person to person by close contact. Nongenital warts are acquired through minor trauma to the skin. An increase in the incidence of plantar warts has been associated with swimming in public pools.

Anogenital warts are primarily transmitted by sexual contact but can be acquired at the time of delivery. Particularly when found in a child beyond infancy, sexual abuse must be considered. Evidence of genital human papillomavirus infection has been detected in as many as 38% of sexually active adolescent females.

Laryngeal papillomas are believed to be transmitted through aspiration of infectious secretions during passage through the infected birth canal.

The **incubation period** is unknown but is estimated to range from 3 months to several years. Papillomavirus acquired by a neonate at the time of delivery may not cause clinical manifestations for several years.

Diagnostic Tests: Most warts are diagnosed by clinical inspection. Clinical detection of anogenital warts can be enhanced by soaking the area in 3% to 5% acetic acid (vinegar), which causes the lesion to turn white. When the diagnosis is questionable, histologic examination of a biopsy or cytology specimen is diagnostic. No culture for HPV is available.

Treatment: Most nongenital warts eventually regress spontaneously, but they may persist for months or years. The optimal treatment for warts that do not resolve spontaneously has not been identified. Most methods of treatment rely on chemical or physical destruction of the infected epithelium, such as the application of salicylic acid products or cryotherapy with liquid nitrogen. Care must be taken to avoid a deleterious cosmetic result of therapy.

The optimal treatment for anogenital warts has not been identified. The application of podophyllin is often the initial therapy of choice. It has not been tested for safety and efficacy in children. Other treatment modalities are intravaginal fluorouracil, trichloracetic acid, electrocautery, laser surgery, and surgical excision. Two newer therapies, intralesional interferon and patient-applied podofilox (the major cytotoxic ingredient of podophyllin), have not been evaluated in children. Since treatment does not eradicate infection, relapses can occur.

Laryngeal papillomas are very difficult to treat. Local recurrence is common, and repeated surgical procedures for removal are usually necessary. Extension or seeding of laryngeal papillomas into the trachea, bronchi, or lung parenchyma results in increased morbidity and mortality. Interferon has been used as an investigational treatment and may be of benefit for patients with frequent recurrences.

Isolation of the Hospitalized Patient: No special precautions are recommended.

Control Measures: Suspected child abuse should be reported to the appropriate local agency. Sexual transmission of anogenital warts can be decreased by using condoms. Other measures are those for other sexually transmitted diseases (see Sexually Transmitted Diseases, p 103), such as refraining from intercourse until therapy is completed and lesions have healed.

Paracoccidioidomycosis (South American Blastomycosis)

Clinical Manifestations: Typical features are chronic granulomatous lesions of the mucous membranes, especially the mouth and rectum, and the skin adjacent to the mouth, lymph nodes, and viscera.

Etiology: *Paracoccidioides brasiliensis* is a dimorphic fungus with a yeast and a mycelial (mold) form.

Epidemiology: The infection occurs primarily in South America, where it is the predominant systemic fungal disease. A few cases have been found in Central America and Mexico. The habitat is not known, but soil is suspected. The mode of transmission is not known.

The **incubation period** is highly variable, ranging from 1 month to many years.

Diagnostic Tests: Round, multiple-budding cells may be seen in 10% potassium hydroxide preparations of sputum or material from lesions. The organism can be cultured easily on most enriched media, including blood agar at 37°C and Sabouraud agar (preferably with added cycloheximide) at room temperature. Complement fixation and immunodiffusion serologic antibody tests are useful diagnostic aids. Skin hypersensitivity can develop but is nonspecific, as false-positive tests in patients with histoplasmosis can occur as the result of immunologic cross-reactivity.

Treatment: The treatment of choice for paracoccidioidomycosis in children is usually ketoconazole. Limited experience indicates that ketoconazole is safe in children younger than 2 years of age. Miconazole has also been used. Newer azoles, such as itraconazole and fluconazole, which have fewer adverse effects, are promising. For acute and severe paracoccidioidomycosis, amphotericin B is usually recommended (see Systemic Treatment with Amphotericin B, p 562). Prolonged therapy is necessary.

Isolation of the Hospitalized Patient: No special precautions are recommended.

Control Measures: None.

Paragonimiasis

Clinical Manifestations: The disease has an insidious onset and a chronic course. The initial symptom is cough, which eventually becomes productive of blood-tinged sputum. Pleural pain and dyspnea follow. Bacterial pneumonitis and lung abscesses can complicate the course. Pleural effusion and pneumothorax have also been reported. Because of pulmonary fibrosis and bronchiectasis, clubbing of the fingers and toes can develop. Abdominal disease, occurring when the worms invade the intestinal wall, is associated with dull pain, nausea, vomiting, and diarrhea. Involvement of the lymph nodes can lead to suppuration and abscesses. Symptoms tend to subside after approximately 5 years, but can persist for as many as 20 years. Invasion of the brain occurs rarely; acutely, it may resemble meningoencephalitis and cause seizures.

Etiology: The adult *Paragonimus westermani* is a fluke, 10 to 12 mm long and 5 to 7 mm wide. The pathologic lesions are caused by the eggs, not the worms (except for those in the brain); the eggs elicit an eosinophilic inflammatory response.

Epidemiology: Transmission occurs when raw or uncooked freshwater crabs or crayfish containing larvae (metacercariae) are ingested. They excyst in the small intestine and penetrate the abdominal cavity, where they undergo further development. After several days, most of the larvae travel to the lungs through the diaphragm, but some remain in the abdomen and others reach aberrant sites. They burrow into the tissues, become encapsulated, and begin laying eggs after approximately 4 to 6 weeks. When sputum that contain eggs is swallowed, the eggs are passed in the stool. Eggs in fresh water embryonate, hatch within 3 weeks, and yield miracidia that penetrate snails. Cercariae emerge several weeks later, and they encyst on and within the muscles and viscera of freshwater crustaceans and mature into infective metacercariae.

Areas of the highest prevalence are limited to the Far East, especially Japan, Korea, Taiwan, and the Philippines. The disease is also endemic in some parts of Australia and in West Africa. The Western hemisphere has endemic foci in Colombia, Venezuela, Ecuador, Peru, Costa Rica, and Mexico. Foxes, civets, tigers, leopards, panthers, mongooses, wolves, pigs, dogs, and cats serve as animal reservoirs. No person-to-person transmission occurs.

The **incubation period** is not known.

Diagnostic Tests: Microscopic examination of stools, sputum, pleural effusion, cerebrospinal fluid, and other tissue aspirates can reveal the eggs. Serologic antibody tests are available at the Centers for Disease Control and Prevention (CDC), but these tests do not distinguish active from past infection. Charcot-Leyden crystals and eosinophils in sputum are characteristic.

Treatment: Praziquantel is the drug of choice. An alternative drug, bithionol, is effective but is associated with side effects including gastrointestinal disturbances and allergic rashes. It is available from the Drug Service of the CDC (see Directory of Telephone Numbers, p 601).

Isolation of the Hospitalized Patient: No special precautions are recommended.

Control Measures: Complete control is impossible because of the animal reservoirs. Boiling of crabs for several minutes until the meat has congealed and turned opaque kills the metacercariae.

Parainfluenza Virus Infections

Clinical Manifestations: Parainfluenza viral infections are the major cause of laryngotracheobronchitis (croup), but they also frequently result in upper respiratory tract infection, pneumonia, or bronchiolitis. Parainfluenza viral infections can be particularly severe and persistent in immunodeficient children.

Etiology: Parainfluenza viruses are large, enveloped RNA viruses classified as paramyxoviruses. Four antigenically distinct types—1, 2, 3, and 4 (with two subtypes, 4A and 4B)—have been identified.

Epidemiology: Parainfluenza viruses are believed to be transmitted from person to person by direct contact and exposure to contaminated nasopharyngeal secretions through respiratory droplets and/or fomites. Parainfluenza viral infections are ubiquitous and are both epidemic and sporadic. Type 1 viruses tend to produce outbreaks of respiratory illness in the fall of every other year. A major increase in the number of cases of croup in the autumn is indicative of a parainfluenza type 1 outbreak. Type 2 virus can also cause outbreaks of respiratory illness in the fall, often in conjunction with type 1 outbreaks, but type 2 outbreaks tend to be less severe, irregular, and less frequent. Parainfluenza type 3 virus usually produces infections during a somewhat longer period, occurring predominantly during the spring and summer in temperate climates. Infections with types 4A and 4B are less commonly recognized, sporadic, and generally clinically mild. Infection with type 3 virus is usually first acquired during infancy and is a major cause of lower respiratory tract disease in children in the first year of life. Illness from primary infection with types 1 and 2 occurs predominantly in 2- to 6-year-old children. Reinfections can occur at any age, but they are usually milder, causing primarily upper respiratory tract illness. Immunodeficient individuals can develop severe lower respiratory tract disease, with prolonged shedding of the virus. Healthy children with primary infection from type 1 shed the virus for an average of 4 to 7 days, but this shedding can last as long as 2 weeks.

The average period of shedding for type 3 infections is 8 to 9 days, but can last as long as 3 weeks.

The **incubation period** is from 2 to 6 days.

Diagnostic Tests: Virus may be isolated from nasopharyngeal secretions in tissue culture, usually within 4 to 7 days. More rapid identification of viral antigen in the nasopharyngeal secretions can be accomplished by immunofluorescent and enzyme immunoassay methods, but the sensitivity of the tests can be variable. Serologic diagnosis, made retrospectively by a significant rise in antibody titer between acute and convalescent sera, is generally less helpful and can be confusing, as heterotypic antibody rises are common with infections caused by other serotypes of parainfluenza and mumps viruses. Furthermore, infection may not always be accompanied by a significant homotypic antibody response.

Treatment: Racemic epinephrine aerosol is frequently given to severely affected, hospitalized patients with laryngotracheobronchitis to reduce airway obstruction. Dexamethasone in high doses (more than 0.3 mg/kg) results in diminished severity and duration of symptoms in patients with severe laryngotracheobronchitis. Management is otherwise supportive.

Isolation of the Hospitalized Patient: Contact isolation is recommended for hospitalized infants and young children with parainfluenza viral infections. Strict adherence to infection control procedures, including prevention of contamination by respiratory secretions and careful hand washing, will help control nosocomial spread.

Control Measures: Efforts should be aimed at reducing nosocomial infection. Hand washing should be emphasized.

Parasitic Diseases

Parasitic diseases have traditionally been considered exotic and, therefore, are frequently not included in differential diagnoses in the United States and Europe. Nevertheless, they are among the most common causes of morbidity and mortality worldwide. Many of these infections can be encountered anywhere in the world. Tourists returning to their own countries, immigrants from endemic areas (eg, refugees from Indochina, Central America, and the Caribbean), and immunosuppressed patients are potential victims of infections in nonendemic areas. In the United States, a noticeable increase in the number of reports of several parasitic infections has occurred in recent years, and many physicians and clinical laboratories are seeing patients with these infections and their diagnostic specimens for the first time.

Consultation and assistance in the diagnosis and management of parasitic diseases are available from government agencies (eg, Centers for Disease Control and Prevention [CDC] and state health departments) and from uni-

TABLE 3.33—Additional Parasitic Diseases*

Disease and/or Agent	Where Infection May Be Acquired	Definitive Host	Intermediate Host	Modes of Human Infection	Directly Communicable (Person to Person)	Diagnostic Laboratory Test in Humans	Causative Form of Parasite	Manifestation
							Diseases in Man	
Angiostrongylus cantonensis	Pacific islands, Eastern Asia, Puerto Rico, Cuba, Africa	Rat	Snails and slugs	Eating uncooked, infected mollusks	No	Eosinophils in CSF. Identification of larvae in CSF	Larval worms	Meningo-encephalitis
Angiostrongylus costaricensis	Central and South America	Rodents	Snails and slugs	Eating uncooked, infected mollusks	No	Gel diffusion	Larval worms	Abdominal pains
Anisakiasis	Cosmopolitan, mainly Japan	Marine mammals	Certain saltwater fish	Eating uncooked, infected fish	No	Identification of recovered larvae in granulomas or vomitus	Larval worms	Acute GI disease
Clonorchis sinensis	Far East	Humans, cats, dogs, other animals	Certain freshwater snails	Eating uncooked, infected fish	No	Eggs in stool or duodenal fluid	Larvae and mature flukes	Abdominal pain; hepatobiliary disease

TABLE 3.33—Additional Parasitic Diseases* *(continued)*

Disease and/or Agent	Where Infection May Be Acquired	Definitive Host	Intermediate Host	Modes of Human Infection	Directly Communicable (Person to Person)	Diagnostic Laboratory Test in Humans	Diseases in Man	
							Causative Form of Parasite	Manifestation
Dracontiasis, *Dracunculus medinensis*	Foci in India, Africa, Middle East	Humans	Cyclops crustacea	Drinking infected water	No	Adult worm in skin, subcutaneous tissues	Adult female worm	Inflammatory response; systemic and local in skin and subcutaneos tissue
Fascioliasis, *Fasciola hepatica*	Foci throughout tropics and temperate areas	Humans and many animals	Certain freshwater snails and vegetation	Eating uncooked, infected plants such as watercress	No	Eggs in feces, duodenal fluid or bile	Larvae and mature worms	Disease of liver and biliary tree; acute GI disease
Fasciolopsiasis, *Fasciolopsis buski*	Far East	Humans, pigs, dogs	Certain freshwater snails, plants	Eating uncooked, infected plants	No	Eggs or worm in feces or duodenal fluid	Larvae and mature worms	Gastroenteritis
Intestinal capillariasis, *Capillaria philippinensis*	Philippines	Humans	Fish	Ingestion of uncooked, infected fish	Uncertain	Eggs and parasite in feces	Larvae and mature worms	Protein-losing enteropathy

*For recommended drug treatment, see Drugs for Parasitic Infections (p 574).

versity departments of geographic medicine, tropical medicine, infectious disease, international health, and public health.

The CDC distributes a number of drugs for the treatment of parasitic diseases that are not available commercially in the United States. These drugs are indicated by footnotes in the tables on Drugs for Parasitic Infections (p 574), and in the chapters on specific parasitic infections. To request these drugs, a physician must contact the CDC Drug Service (see Directory of Telephone Numbers, p 601), and provide the following information: (1) the physician's name, address, and telephone number; (2) the type of infection to be treated and the method by which it was diagnosed; and (3) the patient's name, age, weight, sex, and, if the patient is a woman, whether she is pregnant. Prior consultation with a medical officer from the CDC may be required.

Important human parasitic infections are discussed in individual chapters in this book. The diseases are arranged alphabetically and the discussions include recommendations for drug treatment. Table 5.7, reproduced from *The Medical Letter* (see Drugs for Parasitic Infections, p 574), gives specific antiparasitic drug and dosage recommendations. Although the recommendations for administration of these drugs given in the discussion of the diseases and in the table are similar, they may not be identical in all instances because of differences of opinion among authorities. Both sources should be consulted.

Table 3.33 (p 343) gives details on some less commonly encountered parasitic diseases.

Parvovirus B19
(Erythema Infectiosum, Fifth Disease)

Clinical Manifestations: Parvovirus B19 infection is most often manifested as erythema infectiosum (EI), which is characterized by mild systemic symptoms, fever in 15% to 30% of patients, and, frequently, a distinctive rash. On the face, this rash is intensely red with a "slapped cheek" appearance and circumoral pallor. A symmetric maculopapular, lace-like rash can also be noted on the arms, moving caudally to involve the trunk, buttocks, and thighs. The rash can recur and fluctuate in intensity with environmental changes, such as temperature and exposure to sunlight for weeks and sometimes months. Arthralgia and arthritis occur infrequently in children but commonly in adults, especially women.

Infection with the etiologic agent of EI, human parvovirus B19, can also cause asymptomatic infection, a mild respiratory illness with no rash, a rash atypical for EI that may be rubelliform, arthritis in adults (in the absence of manifestations of EI), chronic anemia in immunodeficient patients, and aplastic crisis lasting 7 to 10 days in patients with chronic hemolytic anemias (eg, sickle-cell disease). Patients with aplastic crisis may have a prodromal illness with fever, malaise, and myalgia, but rash is usually absent. The red blood cell aplasia is related to the replication of the agent in erythrocyte precursors.

Parvovirus B19 infection that occurs during pregnancy can cause fetal hydrops and death. The risk of fetal death is less than 10% after proven maternal infection in the first half of pregnancy and may be negligible in the second half. Congenital anomalies among newborn infants associated with B19 infection have not been reported.

Etiology: Human parvovirus B19, a small DNA-containing virus, is the cause of EI and associated syndromes.

Epidemiology: Humans are the only known hosts. The mode of spread probably involves respiratory secretions and blood. Early in the illness, respiratory secretions have been demonstrated to contain viral DNA, and blood has been found to have viral particles. Parvovirus B19 infections are ubiquitous, and cases of EI can occur sporadically or as part of community outbreaks. The outbreaks frequently occur in elementary or junior high schools in spring months. Secondary spread among susceptible household members—adults or children—is common, occurring in about 50% of contacts. Rates of infection in schools are less, but infection can be an occupational risk for school and child care personnel, affecting 19% of susceptible persons in one outbreak. However, 50% or more of adults have serologic evidence of past infection and are probably not susceptible to reinfection. In young children, only 5% to 10% are immune. The timing of the presence of B19 DNA in serum and respiratory secretions indicates that persons with EI are most infectious before onset of illness and are unlikely to be infectious after onset of the rash and other associated symptoms. In contrast, patients with aplastic crises are highly contagious from before the onset of clinical symptoms through the week after onset or even longer. Transmission to hospital personnel has been infrequently reported but in one institution occurred in 38% of susceptible contacts.

Household studies of secondary cases suggest that the **incubation period** is usually between 4 and 14 days but can be as long as 20 days. Data from human volunteer studies suggest that rash and joint symptoms occur 2 to 3 weeks after acquisition.

Diagnostic Tests: The most feasible method for detecting infection in the healthy host is assaying for serum B19-specific IgM antibody, the presence of which confirms infection within the past several months. Serum IgG antibody indicates previous infection and immunity. These assays are available in commercial laboratories and some state health and research laboratories. Their sensitivity and specificity, especially for IgM antibody, may vary, however. The best method for detecting chronic infection in the immunocompromised patient is to demonstrate virus by nucleic acid hybridization assay or the polymerase chain reaction assay, but these tests are investigational. Virus can sometimes be detected in serum by electron microscopy but this method is probably too insensitive to be of value in most cases. Viral B19 antigens can be detected by radioimmunoassay or enzyme immunoassay. Parvovirus B19 has not been grown in standard tissue-culture systems but can be isolated in selected cell lines.

Treatment: For most patients, supportive care only is indicated. In treating chronic infection in the immunodeficient patient, intravenous immunoglobulin therapy appears to be effective and should be considered.

Isolation of the Hospitalized Patient: For patients hospitalized with EI, no special precautions are indicated.

Contact isolation, including use of gowns and gloves, is indicated for hospitalized children with aplastic crises or immunosuppressed patients with chronic aplastic anemia for the duration of the illness. Masks should also be worn during close contact. Pregnant health care workers should know about the potential risks to the fetus from B19 infections and about preventive measures that may reduce these risks, including the possibility of not caring for patients with aplastic crises who are highly contagious.

Control Measures:

- Women who are exposed to children either at home or at work (eg, teachers or child care workers) are at increased risk of infection with parvovirus B19. However, because of widespread inapparent infection in both adults and children, all women are at some degree of risk of exposure, particularly those with school-aged children. In view of the high prevalence of B19, the low incidence of ill effects on the fetus, and the fact that avoidance of child care or teaching can only reduce but not eliminate the risk of exposure, routine exclusion of pregnant women from the workplace where EI is occurring is not recommended. When IgG testing for parvovirus B19 antibody becomes more widely available, women at increased risk may be able to have their susceptibility determined.
- Pregnant women who find that they have been in contact with children who were in the incubation period of EI or who were in aplastic crisis should have the relatively low potential risk explained to them, and the option of serologic testing should be offered, if possible. Fetal ultrasound may be useful when assessing damage to the fetus.
- Children with EI may attend child care or school, as they are not contagious.
- Transmission of infection is likely to be lessened by routine hygienic practices for control of respiratory infections, which include hand washing and the disposal of facial tissues containing respiratory secretions.
- Pediatricians, as school medical advisors, should act as consultants in providing greater access to testing facilities, assistance in interpreting test results, and reassurance to pregnant women.

Pasteurella multocida Infections

Clinical Manifestations: The most common manifestation is cellulitis at the site of a scratch or bite of a cat, dog, or other animal. This finding usually occurs within 24 to 48 hours of the bite or scratch and includes swelling, erythema, tenderness, and serous or sanguinopurulent discharge. Regional lymphadenopathy, chills, and fever can occur. Local complications such as septic arthritis, osteomyelitis, and tenosynovitis are common. Less common complications include meningitis, respiratory infections (eg, chronic bronchitis, chronic sinusitis, chronic otitis media, pulmonary abscesses, empyema, and pneumonia), appendicitis, hepatic abscess, spontaneous peritonitis, urinary tract infection, and ocular infections, including conjunctivitis, corneal ulcer, and endophthalmitis.

Etiology: *Pasteurella multocida* organisms are bipolar staining, Gram-negative coccobacilli.

Epidemiology: The organism is found in the oral flora of 70% to 90% of cats, 25% to 50% of dogs, and the mouths of many other animals. Transmission occurs from the bite or scratch of an infected animal, usually a cat. Respiratory spread from animals to humans also occurs. Human-to-human spread via drainage from a lesion or respiratory discharge has not been documented.

The **incubation period** is usually less than 24 hours.

Diagnostic Tests: *Pasteurella multocida* can be isolated from skin lesion drainage or other sites of infection (eg, joint fluid, cerebrospinal fluid, sputum, pleural fluid, or suppurative lymph nodes). The organism resembles several other organisms morphologically (such as *Haemophilus influenzae*, *Neisseria* species, and some enteric organisms), but laboratory differentiation is not difficult.

Treatment: The drug of choice is penicillin or ampicillin. In patients allergic to penicillin, either chloramphenicol or tetracycline are effective. Tetracycline drugs should not be given to children younger than 9 years unless the benefits of therapy are considered greater than the risks of dental staining. For polymicrobial infection, which may occur with *Staphylococcus aureus*, oral amoxicillin-clavulanate can be given. Parenterally administered cephalosporins, such as cefotaxime or cefoxitin, are active against *P multocida* in vitro, but therapeutic experience with these drugs in *P multocida* infections is limited. New oral cephalosporins (such as cefixime, cefpodoxime, and ceftibuten) have not been studied but may prove effective. The duration of therapy is usually 7 to 10 days for local infections and 10 to 14 days for invasive infections. Wound drainage or debridement may be necessary.

Isolation of the Hospitalized Patient: Drainage/secretion precautions are recommended for cutaneous disease.

Control Measures: Limiting contact with wild and domestic animals can prevent *Pasteurella* infections. Animal bites and scratches should be promptly irrigated, cleansed, and debrided; whenever possible, surgical closure of the wounds should be avoided. Antimicrobial prophylaxis with penicillin or the combination drug of amoxicillin and clavulanic acid may be given, but efficacy of prophylactic regimens has not been proven.

Pediculosis

Clinical Manifestations:

Pediculosis capitis: Itching is the most common symptom of head lice infestation, although some children with light infestations (1 to 5 lice) do not complain. Adult lice or eggs (nits) are found in the hair usually behind the ears and near the nape of the neck. Excoriations and crusting are common and can be associated with secondary bacterial infection and regional lymphadenopathy. In temperate climates, head lice deposit their eggs on the hair shaft 3 to 4 mm from the scalp. The duration of infestation can be estimated by the distance of the nit from the scalp.

Pediculosis pubis: Pruritus of the anogenital area is a common symptom in pubic lice infestations. Many hairy areas of the body can be infested with the pubic louse including the eyelashes, eyebrows, beard, scalp, axilla, and perianal area. A characteristic sign of heavy pubic lice infestation is the presence of bluish or slate-colored macules on the chest, abdomen, or thighs.

Pediculosis corporis: Intense itching, particularly at night, is common with body lice infestations. Body lice and their eggs live on the seams of clothing. Infrequently, a louse can be seen feeding on the skin.

Etiology: Three species or subspecies of lice infest humans: *Pediculus humanus capitis*, the head louse; *Pediculus humanus corporis*, the body louse; and *Pthirus pubis*, the pubic or crab louse. Ova hatch in 6 days. Both nymphs and adult lice feed on human blood.

Epidemiology:

Pediculosis capitis: Head lice infestation in child care and school-aged children is common in the United States. All socioeconomic groups are affected. Infestations are less common in blacks than in people of other races. Hair length does not influence infestation. Head lice infestation is not a sign of uncleanliness. Head lice are not a major health hazard. Transmission occurs by direct contact with infested individuals or indirectly by contact with their personal belongings such as combs, brushes, and hats. Lice can survive only 1 to 2 days away from the scalp.

Pediculosis pubis: Pubic lice infestations are common in adolescents and young adults and are transmitted through sexual contact. Infested individuals should be investigated for other sexually transmitted diseases. The pubic louse can also be transferred by contaminated items such as towels. Pubic lice can be found on the eyelashes of younger children and, while other modes of transmission are possible, may be evidence of sexual abuse.

Pediculosis corporis: Body lice are generally found on persons with poor hygiene. Fomites play a role in their transmission. Body lice cannot survive away from a blood source for longer than 10 days. Body lice are well recognized vectors of disease (eg, epidemic typhus, trench fever, and relapsing fever).

The **incubation period** of louse eggs is 6 to 10 days.

Diagnostic Tests: Identification of eggs, nymphs, and lice with the naked eye is possible; the diagnosis can be confirmed by using a hand lens or microscope.

Treatment:

Pediculosis capitis: Although the following agents are effective in treating pediculosis of the scalp (see Table 3.34, p 351, for trade names), permethrin has distinct advantages over the other pediculicides.

1. *Permethrin.* A synthetic pyrethroid in a 10-minute hair rinse is available without a prescription, has low potential for toxicity, and has a very high cure rate. Because permethrin has high ovicidal activity, a single treatment is usually adequate; nonetheless, some experts advise a second treatment 7 to 10 days after the first.

2. *Natural pyrethrin-based products.* These 10-minute shampoos are available without prescription. Ovicidal activity is low and repeat application 7 to 10 days later is advised to kill newly hatched lice. Resistance to these synergized natural pyrethrins has not been reported.

3. *Lindane (1%).* This 4-minute shampoo has the highest potential toxicity of all pediculicides, but serious adverse effects have not been reported when used according to package instructions. Toxicity with lindane has been reported only with misuse, such as ingestion or prolonged administration. Ovicidal activity is low and repeat application 7 to 10 days later is often recommended. Lindane resistance has been reported from England, Egypt, the Netherlands, and Panama.

4. *Malathion (0.5%).* This 8- to 12-hour lotion is less toxic than lindane and has better ovicidal activity than lindane or pyrethrin products. Its alcohol base is flammable until it dries.

After treatment with an appropriate pediculicide, removal of nits is not necessary to prevent spread. If the removal of nits is attempted for aesthetic reasons, it may be facilitated by (1) combing with a fine-toothed nit comb designed for this purpose and by applying a damp towel to the scalp for 30 to 60 minutes, or by (2) soaking the hair with white vinegar (3% to 5% acetic acid) and then applying a damp towel soaked in the same solution for 30 to 60 minutes.

Pediculosis pubis: Any of the pediculicides for pediculosis capitis is effective in the treatment of pubic lice. Retreatment is recommended 7 to 10 days later. For infestation of eyelashes by pubic lice, petrolatum ointment applied 3 to 4 times daily for 8 to 10 days is effective. Nits should be removed mechanically from the eyelashes.

Pediculosis corporis: Treatment consists of improving hygiene and cleaning clothes. Infested clothing can be washed and dried at hot temperatures to kill the lice. Pediculicides are not necessary.

Isolation of the Hospitalized Patient: Contact isolation without masks is recommended until the patient has been treated with an appropriate pediculicide.

TABLE 3.34—Medications for Treatment of Pediculosis*

Drug	Trade Names (examples)	Manufacturer
Lindane, 1%	Kwell	Reed & Carnick
Malathion, 0.5%	Ovide	GenDerm
Natural pyrethrin-based products	A-200 RID R & C	Beecham Lieming Reed & Carnick
Permethrin (synthetic pyrethroid)	Nix	Burroughs Wellcome

*Compiled from the *Physicians Desk Reference*. Oradel, NJ: Medical Economics Company, Inc; 1993

Control Measures:

Pediculosis capitis: Contacts should be examined and treated if infested. Differentiation of nits from benign hair casts (a layer of follicular cells that easily slide off the hair shaft) from plugs of desquamated epithelial cells or external debris can be difficult. Bedmates should be treated prophylactically. Children should be allowed to return to school or child care after their first treatment or to their classroom if they are treated at school by a nurse since the risk of transmission is promptly reduced by treatment. Reinfestation of children from an untreated, infested contact is more common than treatment failure after proper application of an effective pesticide.

"No nit" policies requiring that children be free of nits before return to child care or school have not been demonstrated to be effective in controlling head lice. Combing out of nits after treatment with an appropriate pediculicide is, nonetheless, required by some school officials.

Clothing, bedding, or cloth toys can be disinfected by machine washing or drying (using hot cycles), since temperatures exceeding 53.5°C (128.3°F) for 5 minutes are lethal to lice and eggs. Dry cleaning or simply storing clothing in plastic bags for about 10 days is also effective. For disinfecting combs and brushes, soaking in hot water for 10 minutes or washing with a pediculicide shampoo is recommended. No evidence indicates that the use of environmental insecticides is a useful adjunctive measure in the control of head lice.

Pediculosis pubis: All sexual contacts should be treated.

Pediculosis corporis: The most important factor in the control of body lice infestation is the ability to change and wash clothing. Close contacts should be examined and treated appropriately.

Pelvic Inflammatory Disease

Clinical Manifestations: Pelvic inflammatory disease (PID) denotes a spectrum of inflammatory disorders of the female upper genital tract including salpingitis, endometritis, and pelvic peritonitis, but it may be asymptomatic ("silent PID"). In symptomatic patients, frequent presenting complaints are abdominal or pelvic pain that may be vague, abnormal vaginal bleeding, dyspareunia, or unexplained vaginal discharge.

Common findings include lower abdominal or adnexal tenderness (which may be unilateral), tenderness on motion of the cervix, fever and palpation of an inflammatory mass on bimanual pelvic examination, or its demonstration by ultrasonography. The onset of symptoms often follows menses. Most cases have only mild symptoms and few clinical findings. Many patients are afebrile, do not have an abnormal vaginal discharge, and have normal leukocyte counts. No single historical, physical, or laboratory finding is both sensitive and specific for the diagnosis of acute PID. Combinations of findings that improve sensitivity (ie, detection of more women who have PID) or specificity (ie, exclusion of more women who do not have PID) do so only at the expense of the other.

Complications of acute PID include perihepatitis (Fitz-Hugh-Curtis syndrome) and tubo-ovarian abscess. Important long-term sequelae are tubal infertility (in 10% to 30% of patients after a single episode, depending on the severity; in 50% to 75% after three or more episodes) and ectopic pregnancy.

Etiology: Sexually transmitted organisms, especially *Neisseria gonorrhoeae* and *Chlamydia trachomatis,* are implicated in most PID cases, but the etiology in many cases is polymicrobial. Other organisms isolated from the upper genital tract of PID patients include mixed anaerobic organisms (*Bacteroides* species and *Peptostreptococcus* species), facultative bacteria (*Gardnerella vaginalis, Streptococcus* species, coliform bacteria), and genital tract mycoplasmas (*Mycoplasma hominis, Ureaplasma urealyticum,* and *Mycoplasma genitalium*). The organisms causing upper tract infection are not reliably predicted by cervical culture or known infection in a partner.

Epidemiology: The incidence of PID is highest among sexually active adolescents. Other risk factors include multiple sexual partners, use of an intrauterine device, douching, and a previous episode of PID. Pelvic inflammatory disease is a frequent complication of common sexually transmitted diseases. Approximately 10% to 20% of females with endocervical *N gonorrhoeae* and 10% to 30% of those with endocervical *C trachomatis* develop overt PID. Asymptomatic upper genital tract infection is common in apparently uncomplicated chlamydial infection. In prepubertal females, ascending infection resulting in PID is uncommon.

The **incubation period** varies with the etiology (see Gonococcal Infections, p 196, and *Chlamydia trachomatis*, p 155).

Diagnostic Tests: The diagnosis is usually based on clinical findings and is supported by evidence of *N gonorrhoeae* or *Chlamydia* in the cervical secretions, increased leukocytes in the cervical smear, leukocytosis, and/or an elevated C-reactive protein or erythrocyte sedimentation rate. Endocervical and rectal cultures for *N gonorrhoeae* and an endocervical test for *C trachomatis* should be obtained before treatment. Laparoscopy definitively diagnoses salpingitis and can be used to obtain a more complete bacteriologic diagnosis, but this procedure will not detect endometritis and is not usually indicated or practical. If the patient's menses is late or she is not using reliable contraception, a pregnancy test should be done.

Treatment: Treatment is empiric and is directed against the common etiologic agents because microbiologic testing cannot determine which organisms are important in an individual patient. Antibiotic treatment should be instituted promptly, based on clinical diagnosis without awaiting culture results, to minimize the risk of progression of the infection and the risk of transmission of the organisms to other sexual partners. No substantial evidence indicates that any one of the current antibiotic regimens decreases the incidence of infertility or ectopic pregnancy more than any other.

Many experts recommend hospitalization for all PID patients, particularly adolescents, in whom the risk of sequelae is high and whose ability to follow a therapeutic regimen may be unpredictable. If the diagnosis is uncertain and ectopic pregnancy or appendicitis cannot be excluded, or if follow-up within 72 hours cannot be assured, hospitalization is indicated if the patient (1) has a pelvic or tubo-ovarian abscess, (2) has overt peritonitis, (3) is pregnant, (4) has an intrauterine device (IUD) in place, (5) is unable to follow or tolerate an outpatient regimen, and/or (6) has failed to respond to 48 hours of outpatient management.

No single therapeutic regimen of choice exists for all persons with PID. Antimicrobial regimens recommended by the Centers for Disease Control and Prevention are summarized in Table 3.35 (p 354). These empiric regimens provide broad coverage against the etiologic agents of PID. The specific antibiotics listed are examples only. If the patient has an IUD in place, it should be promptly removed.

Ambulatory patients should be monitored closely and re-evaluated within 3 days of initiating treatment. Pregnant or HIV-infected women who develop PID should ordinarily be hospitalized and managed aggressively.

Isolation of the Hospitalized Patient: No special precautions are indicated.

Control Measures:
- Male sexual partners of PID patients must be examined, cultured, and treated empirically for presumptive gonorrhea and chlamydial infection because they are likely to have asymptomatic urethral infection and reinfect the index case or other partners.
- Patients should be advised to abstain from intercourse until all symptoms have resolved and both the patient and her partner(s) have completed treatment.
- Patients should be offered a serologic test for syphilis and HIV counseling and screening.
- Patients and their partners with positive cultures for *N gonorrhoeae* and *C trachomatis* should be recultured 7 to 10 days after completing therapy.
- Because of the high risk of reinfection, some experts recommend that patients with PID should be cultured for *N gonorrhoeae* and *C trachomatis* 4 to 6 weeks after completing treatment.

TABLE 3.35—Recommended Treatment of Pelvic Inflammatory Disease (PID)

Inpatient Treatment	Ambulatory Treatment[a]
Regimen A[b] • Cefoxitin 2 g, IV, every 6 h (or Cefotetan[c] 2 g every 12 h) **PLUS** • Doxycycline[d] 100 mg, IV or PO, every 12 h, continued for at least 48 h after clinical improvement, and followed by doxycycline[d] 100 mg, orally, 2 times a day to complete a 14-d total course **OR** Regimen B[b] • Clindamycin 900 mg, IV, every 8 h (15 to 40 mg/kg/d) **PLUS** • Gentamicin[e]: loading dose 2.0 mg/kg, IV, followed by maintenance 1.5 mg/kg, IV, every 8 h **PLUS** • This regimen is continued for at least 48 h after the patient demonstrates significant clinical improvement and is followed by doxycycline[d] 100 mg, orally, 2 times a day, to complete a 14-d total course, or clindamycin 450 mg, PO, every 6 h, to complete a 14-d total course.	• Cefoxitin 2 g, IM, with concurrent administration of probenecid 1 g, PO **OR** • Equivalent cephalosporin[c] **PLUS** • Doxycycline[d] 100 mg, orally, 2 times a day for 14 d **OR** • For patients older than 18 y, oxfloxacin[f] 400 mg, PO, 2 times a day for 14 d **PLUS** • Clindamycin 450 mg, PO, 4 times a day, or metronidazole 500 mg, PO, 2 times a day for a total course of 14 d

[a]Patients who do not respond to outpatient therapy within 48 h should be hospitalized for parenteral therapy.

[b]When tubo-ovarian abscess is present, many clinicians use clindamycin since it provides more effective anaerobic coverage than doxycycline. Clindamycin administered intravenously appears to be effective against *C trachomatis* infection; the effectiveness of oral clindamycin against *C trachomatis*, however, has not been determined.

[c]The experience with cefotetan is less than that with cefoxitin, although cefotetan provides similar antimicrobial coverage and requires less frequent dosing. Clinical data are limited on other second- and third-generation cephalosporins (ceftizoxime, cefotaxime, and ceftriaxone) to replace cefoxitin or cefotetan, although many authorities believe they are also effective therapy for PID.

[d]Doxycycline administered orally has bioavailability similar to the IV formulation. Patients who do not tolerate doxycycline should receive erythromycin 500 mg, orally, 4 times a day (40 mg/kg/d) for 10 to 14 d, although this recommendation is based on limited clinical data. Use of doxycycline is ordinarily limited to patients 9 y or older because of the potential for dental staining. Doxycycline is preferred to tetracycline because of its greater bioavailability and better patient compliance.

[e]Although short courses of aminoglycosides (≤3 d) in healthy adolescents with normal renal function do not usually necessitate monitoring of serum concentrations, some practitioners may elect to do so.

[f]Quinolones are contraindicated for children and for adolescents younger than 18 y and for pregnant or nursing mothers.

Pertussis

Clinical Manifestations: Pertussis begins with mild upper respiratory symptoms (catarrhal stage) and can progress to severe paroxysms of cough (paroxysmal stage), often with a characteristic inspiratory whoop, followed by vomiting. Fever is absent or minimal. Symptoms wane gradually (convalescent stage). In infants younger than 6 months, apnea is a common manifestation and whoop can be absent. Similarly, older children and adults can have atypical manifestations, with persistent cough and no whoop. Duration of the illness in uncomplicated cases is 6 to 10 weeks. Complications include seizures, pneumonia, encephalopathy, and death. Pertussis is a particularly severe disease in the first year of life. According to surveillance data from 1980 to 1989 in the United States, pneumonia, seizures, and encephalopathy occurred in 21.7%, 3.0%, and 0.9%, respectively, of infants with pertussis. The case-fatality rate was 1.3% in children younger than 1 month and 0.3% in those 2 to 5 months and those 6 to 11 months of age. Infection in vaccinated children and older individuals is often mild.

Etiology: *Bordetella pertussis* is a fastidious, Gram-negative, pleomorphic bacillus. A whooping cough syndrome may also be caused by *Bordetella parapertussis*, *Chlamydia trachomatis*, and certain adenoviruses.

Epidemiology: Humans are the only known hosts of *B pertussis*. Transmission occurs by close contact via respiratory secretions. As many as 90% of nonimmune household contacts acquire the disease. Infants and young children are frequently infected by older siblings or adults who have a mild or atypical illness. In the United States, adolescents and adults have recently been recognized as major sources of pertussis. Asymptomatic infection has been demonstrated; its relative importance in transmission is uncertain. Pertussis occurs endemically with periodic outbreaks. Widespread active immunization with pertussis vaccine since the 1940s is primarily responsible for the current low morbidity and mortality rates of pertussis in the United States. Pertussis can occur at any age but is most often diagnosed in young children. Currently, approximately one third of pertussis hospitalizations and deaths in the United States are reported to the Centers for Disease Control and Prevention (CDC). Thirty-eight percent of cases reported to the CDC occurred in infants younger than 6 months, including a substantial proportion in those younger than 3 months; 71% occur in children younger than 5 years. Mortality and the hospitalization rate are highest in the first month of life and progressively decrease as children become older.

Patients are most contagious during the catarrhal stage before the onset of paroxysms; communicability then diminishes rapidly but may persist for as long as 3 weeks. Erythromycin therapy decreases infectivity and may limit secondary spread. Nasopharyngeal cultures usually become negative for *B pertussis* within 5 days after initiating erythromycin therapy.

The **incubation period** is 6 to 20 days, usually 7 to 10 days.

Diagnostic Tests: Culture of *B pertussis* requires inoculation of nasopharyngeal mucus, obtained by dacron or calcium alginate swab, on special media (such as Regan-Lowe or fresh Bordet-Gengou), with incubation for 7 days. Because these media may not be routinely available, the laboratory should be informed when *B pertussis* is suspected. The organism is most frequently recovered in the catarrhal or early paroxysmal stage and is rarely found after the fourth week of illness. A positive culture is diagnostic. False-negative cultures are common, particularly late in the course of the disease or from patients receiving antibiotics. The direct immunofluorescent assay (DFA) of nasopharyngeal secretions has variable sensitivity and specificity, and it requires experienced personnel for interpretation. Since false-positive and false-negative DFA results occur, culture confirmation of all suspected pertussis cases should be attempted. Although absolute lymphocytosis is often present in patients with classical pertussis, it is a nonspecific finding, especially in infants who often develop lymphocytosis from other infections. The degree of lymphocytosis usually parallels the severity of the patient's cough. No single serologic test is highly specific and sensitive. *Bordetella pertussis* infections stimulate a heterogenous antibody response that differs among individuals depending on age and previous exposure to the organism or to its antigens by immunization. New serologic tests, such as enzyme immunoassays for IgG antibody to pertussis toxin and IgA antibody to *B pertussis* filamentous hemagglutinin, are promising diagnostic methods but are currently available only in research laboratories.

Treatment:
- Infants younger than 6 months and other patients with potentially severe disease often require hospitalization for supportive care to manage coughing paroxysms, apnea, cyanosis, feeding difficulties, or other complications. Intensive care facilities may be required for severe cases.
- Antimicrobials given during the catarrhal stage may ameliorate the disease. After paroxysms are established, however, antimicrobials usually have no discernible effect on the course of illness and are recommended primarily to limit the spread of the organisms to others. The drug of choice is erythromycin (40 to 50 mg/kg/d, orally, in four divided doses; maximum, 2 g/d); some experts prefer the estolate preparation. The recommended duration of therapy to prevent bacteriologic relapse is 14 days. Trimethoprim-sulfamethoxazole (8 mg/kg/d – 40 mg/kg/d, orally, in two divided doses) is a possible alternative for patients who do not tolerate erythromycin, but its efficacy is unproven.
- Corticosteroids and albuterol, a beta-2-adrenergic stimulant, have shown promise in reducing paroxysms of coughing but require further evaluation before they can be recommended.

Isolation of the Hospitalized Patient: The patient should be placed in respiratory isolation for 5 days after initiation of erythromycin, or until 3 weeks after the onset of paroxysms if appropriate antimicrobial therapy is not given.

Control Measures:

Care of Exposed Persons.

Child Care. Exposed children, especially those incompletely immunized, should be observed for respiratory symptoms for 14 days after contact has been terminated. Pertussis immunization and chemoprophylaxis should be given as recommended for household and other close contacts. Symptomatic children with cough should be excluded from day care, pending physician evaluation. Children with pertussis, if their medical condition allows, may return or enter a child care facility 5 days after initiation of erythromycin therapy.

Household and Other Close Contacts.

- *Immunization.* Close contacts younger than 7 years who are unimmunized or who have received fewer than four doses of pertussis vaccine (DTP or DTaP) should have pertussis immunization initiated or continued, according to the recommended schedule. Children who received their third dose 6 months or more before exposure should be given a fourth dose at this time. Those who have had at least four doses of pertussis vaccine should receive a booster dose of DTaP or DTP unless a dose has been given within the last 3 years or they are more than 6 years old.

- *Chemoprophylaxis.* Erythromycin (40 to 50 mg/kg/d, orally, in four divided doses; maximum, 2 g/d) for 14 days, as tolerated, is recommended for all household contacts and other close contacts, such as those in child care, **irrespective of vaccination status**. Some experts recommend the estolate preparation. Prompt use of erythromycin chemoprophylaxis in household contacts is effective in limiting secondary transmission. The rationale for administering chemoprophylaxis to all household and other close contacts irrespective of age or immunization status is that pertussis immunity is not absolute and may not prevent infection. Persons with mild illness that may not be recognized as pertussis can transmit the infection.

  For those patients who cannot tolerate erythromycin, trimethoprim-sulfamethoxazole is an alternative. However, its efficacy has not been established.

- Persons who have been in contact with an infected individual should be monitored closely for respiratory symptoms for 14 days after last contact with the infected individual.

Immunization. Universal immunization with pertussis vaccine of children younger than 7 years is critical for the control of pertussis. The pertussis vaccines currently available in the United States include whole-cell and acellular vaccines in combination with diphtheria and tetanus toxoids. Diphtheria-tetanus-pertussis vaccine is a suspension of inactivated *B pertussis* cells and contains multiple antigens. Acellular vaccines contain immunogens derived from *B pertussis* organisms. These antigens include an inactive form of pertussis toxin (PT) also known as lymphocytosis-promoting factor (LPF), filamentous hemagglutinin (FHA), agglutinogens, a 69-kd outer membrane protein (periactin), and others. As of December 1993, two acellular pertussis-containing vaccines (DTaP) are licensed in the United States (see Table 3.36, p 358). Although these two vaccines differ in their formulation of pertussis antigens, their efficacy in the prevention of disease and safety are similar.

TABLE 3.36—Licensed Acellular Pertussis Vaccines (DTaP) in the United States (as of December 1993)

Manufacturer	Pertussis Antigens	Trade Name	Date of FDA Licensing
Lederle Laboratories	Filamentous hemagglutinin Pertussis toxoid* Agglutinogens 69-kd protein	ACEL-IMUNE	December 1991
Connaught Laboratories, Inc	Filamentous hemagglutinin Pertussis toxoid*	Tripedia	August 1992

*Pertussis toxin inactivated by formaldehyde.

Both whole-cell and acellular pertussis vaccines are combined with diphtheria and tetanus toxoids and adsorbed onto an aluminum salt, and, thus, are administered intramuscularly. Whole-cell DTP should be used for the first three doses in infants and children. Acellular pertussis vaccines are currently licensed in the United States for use only for the fourth and fifth doses for children aged 15 months or older.

Based on household studies of young children exposed to pertussis, the efficacy of whole-cell pertussis vaccine for children who have received at least three doses is estimated to be approximately 80%. Observed protection varies according to the definition used for pertussis cases and is greatest for culture-confirmed, more severe cases. Vaccine-induced immunity persists for at least 3 years and diminishes thereafter with time. Disease in those previously immunized is usually mild.

Comparable efficacy of some acellular pertussis vaccines has been demonstrated in Japan in children 2 years of age and older but not in infants. Studies are now in progress to compare the efficacy in infants of acellular and whole-cell pertussis vaccines.

When acellular pertussis vaccines are used for the fourth and fifth doses in infants previously vaccinated with whole-cell pertussis vaccine, the immunogenicity of the antigens in the acellular vaccine is similar to that of whole-cell DTP vaccine. However, antibody responses do not correlate with protection against disease and, thus, cannot be used to predict efficacy. The rates of local reactions (erythema and induration at the injection site), fever, and other common systemic symptoms (drowsiness, fretfulness, and anorexia) are lower after acellular pertussis vaccination than those after whole-cell DTP. Whether the rare, more serious adverse events associated with DTP will occur less frequently after acellular pertussis vaccine is not known (see Adverse Events After Pertussis Vaccination, p 361).

Schedule for Routine Childhood Immunization (see Tables 1.3 and 1.4, pp 23 and 24). Five doses of pertussis vaccine, given intramuscularly, are recommended unless contraindicated or unless the fourth dose was given after the fourth birthday. The first dose is usually given at about 2 months, followed by two additional doses at intervals of approximately 2 months. A fourth dose is recommended 6 to 12 months after the third dose, usually at 15 to 18 months of age, to complete the initial series; it may be given as early as 12 months of age, provided that the interval after the third dose is at least 6 months and DTP is given. A fifth dose is given before school entry (kindergarten or elementary school) at 4 to 6 years of age to protect these children from pertussis in ensuing years and to decrease transmission of the disease to younger children. Pertussis vaccines may be given concurrently with other vaccines, including *Haemophilus influenzae* type b conjugate vaccines (see Simultaneous Administration of Multiple Vaccines, p 25, and *Haemophilus influenzae* Infections, p 207).

If pertussis is prevalent in the community, immunization can be started as early as 4 weeks of age, and doses can be given as frequently as 4 weeks apart.

Pertussis immunization is not routinely indicated at present in individuals 7 years or older.

As of 1993, whole-cell pertussis vaccine is the only product recommended for the first three doses, even for children who are only partially immunized at 15 months or older. Acellular pertussis vaccines (DTaP) may be used only for the fourth and fifth doses for children 15 months and older. For DTaP immunization, the two currently licensed products (see Table 3.36, p 358) are considered interchangeable. If additional acellular pertussis vaccines are licensed in the United States for the fourth and fifth doses, they are likely to be similarly interchangeable unless otherwise noted in the Food and Drug Administration approval.

Either acellular or whole-cell vaccines may be used for the fourth and fifth doses. However, since the occurrence of fever and local reactions is appreciably less with acellular pertussis vaccines (see Table 3.37, p 360), acellular pertussis vaccine is advantageous for the fourth and fifth doses for children who have a personal or family history of seizures and are at increased risk for seizures after whole-cell DTP (presumably because of the fever it induces).

Dose and Route. The DTP and DTaP dose is 0.5 mL, given intramuscularly. The use of reduced volume of individual doses of pertussis vaccines or multiple doses of reduced volume (fractional doses) is not recommended. The effect of such practices on the frequency of serious adverse events and on protection against disease has not been determined.

Antipyretic Prophylaxis. Administration of acetaminophen (15 mg/kg per dose) or other appropriate antipyretic at the time of immunization and at 4 and 8 hours after immunization decreases the incidence of febrile and local reactions. Since convulsions after pertussis vaccine are almost always associated with fever, antipyretic prophylaxis may benefit children at increased risk of seizures (see Adverse Events After Pertussis Vaccination, p 361). For such children, administration of an antipyretic every 4 to 6 hours for as long as 24 hours after vaccination should be considered. Caretakers should be aware that antipyretic therapy could also obscure fever caused by concomitant, unrelated infection.

Recommendations for Scheduling Pertussis Vaccine in Special Circumstances.
• For the child whose pertussis immunization is resumed after deferral or interruption of the recommended schedule, the next dose in the sequence

TABLE 3.37—Comparison of Frequency (%) of Adverse Events Occurring Within 72 Hours of Vaccination With DTaP[a] or Whole-Cell DTP in Children Given the Fourth DTP Dose at 15 to 20 Months of Age and the Fifth DTP Dose at 4 to 6 Years of Age[b]

Events	Vaccination at 15 to 20 Months of Age		Vaccination at 4 to 6 Years of Age	
	DTaP[a] (N=372)	Whole-Cell DTP (N=189)	DTaP[a] (N=240)	Whole-Cell DTP (N=76)
Local				
Any erythema	18[c]	29	31[d]	61
Erythema >2.5 cm	3[d]	13	18[d]	47
An induration	11[d]	40	28[d]	59
Induration >2.5 cm	2[d]	14	NA[e]	NA[e]
Pain/tenderness	14[d]	77	46[d]	93
Systemic				
Fever ≥38°C (100.4°F)[f]	20[d]	44	7[d]	22
Fever ≥39°C (102.2°F)[f]	1[g]	6	1	1
Drowsiness	12[d]	33	15[c]	33
Fretfulness	21[d]	68	16[d]	45
Vomiting	2	3	1.7	1.3

Adapted from Centers for Disease Control. Pertussis vaccination: acellular pertussis vaccine for the fourth and fifth doses of the DTP series; update to supplementary ACIP statement. Recommendations of the Advisory Committee on Immunization Practices (ACIP). *MMWR*. 1992;41(RR-15):4

[a]BIKEN Acellular DTP Vaccine (Tripedia, available from Connaught Laboratories, Inc, Swiftwater, PA).

[b]All children had been previously vaccinated with 3 or 4 doses of whole-cell DTP. Whole-cell DTP, available from Connaught, was used in the whole-cell comparison group.

[c]$p<0.05$

[d]$p<0.001$

[e]NA - not available

[f] Sample sizes for fever were 361, 186, 209, and 67, respectively.

[g]$p<0.01$

should be given, irrespective of the interval since the last dose; ie, the schedule is not reinitiated (see Lapsed Immunizations, p 26).

- If the fourth dose of pertussis vaccine is not given until after the fourth birthday, no further doses of pertussis vaccine are necessary.
- For children who have received fewer than the recommended number of doses of pertussis vaccine but who have received the recommended number of DT doses for their age (ie, those started on DT, then given DTP or DTaP), dose(s) of DTP or DTaP should be given to complete the recommended pertussis immunization schedule. However, the total number of doses of diphtheria and tetanus toxoids (as either DT, DTP, or DTaP)

should not exceed six before the fourth birthday. A monovalent pertussis vaccine preparation* may be used instead.

- Children who have recovered from culture-proven pertussis need not receive further pertussis immunization.
- During pertussis outbreaks, such as in a hospital, pertussis immunization is not usually recommended for adult contacts. Some experts advise a booster dose of 0.25 mL of monovalent pertussis vaccine for health care and child care center personnel and for close contacts who have chronic pulmonary disease in addition to antibiotic prophylaxis. However, the efficacy of immunoprophylaxis and chemophrophylaxis in these circumstances is unproven. Evaluation of acellular pertussis vaccines for use in adults at increased risk for pertussis is in progress.

Medical Records. Charts of those children for whom DTP vaccination has been deferred should be flagged, and the immunization status of these children should be periodically assessed to ensure that they are appropriately immunized.

Adverse Events After Pertussis Vaccination.

- *Local and febrile reactions.* Redness, edema, induration, and tenderness at the injection site; drowsiness; fretfulness; anorexia; vomiting; crying; and slight-to-moderate fever are common reactions to DTP vaccination (see Table 3.38, p 362). These manifestations occur within several hours of immunization and subside spontaneously without sequelae. Children with such reactions should receive subsequent doses of pertussis vaccine as scheduled. They are more likely to have the same reactions after subsequent DTP immunization than those who have not reacted previously. The incidence of local and febrile reactions tends to increase with age and with the number of doses of DTP vaccine. In general, the frequency of local and common systemic events after acellular pertussis vaccine (DTaP) is one-fifth to one-half the frequency of these events after whole-cell pertussis vaccine (DTP) (see Table 3.37, p 360).

  Bacterial or sterile abscesses at the site of the injection are infrequent (six to ten per million injections of DTP). Bacterial abscesses indicate contamination of the product or nonsterile technique and should be reported (see Reporting of Adverse Reactions, p 30). The causes of sterile abscesses are unknown. Their occurrence usually does not contraindicate further doses of DTP or DTaP. .

- *Allergic reactions.* The rate of anaphylaxis is estimated to be approximately two cases per 100,000 injections of DTP. Severe anaphylactic reactions and resulting deaths, if any, are extremely rare. The transient urticarial rashes that occasionally occur after DTP immunization, unless appearing immediately (ie, within minutes), are unlikely to be anaphylactic (IgE-mediated) in origin. These rashes probably represent a serum sickness-type reaction due to circulating antigen-antibody complexes resulting from one of the antigens in DTP or DTaP and corresponding antibody acquired either from an earlier dose or transplacentally. Because formation of such complexes is dependent on a precise balance between

*Distributed by the Division of Biologic Products, Michigan Department of Public Health (see Directory of Telephone Numbers, p 601).

TABLE 3.38—Adverse Events Occurring Within 48 Hours of DTP Immunization*

Categories	Rate (%) per Dose
Redness at site	37.4
Redness >2.4 cm in diameter	7.2
Swelling at site	40.4
Swelling >2.4 cm in diameter	8.9
Pain at site	51
Fever ≥38°C (100.4°F)	47
Fever ≥40.5°C (104.9°F)	0.3
Drowsiness	32
Fretfulness	53
Anorexia	21
Vomiting	6
Persistent crying, for 3 to 21 h	1
High-pitched, unusual cry	0.1
Convulsions	0.06
Collapse with shock-like state	0.06

*These data are derived from 15,752 DTP immunizations (modified from Cody CL, Baraff LJ, Cherry JD, Marcy SM, Manclark CR. Nature and rates of adverse reactions associated with DTP and DT immunizations in infants and children. *Pediatrics*. 1981;68:650-660).

concentrations of circulating antigen and antibody, such reactions are unlikely to recur after a subsequent dose and are not contraindications to further doses.

- *Seizures*. The incidence of seizures occurring within 48 hours of adminis-tration of pertussis vaccine is 1:1,750 doses administered, based on a large prospective study.* Most seizures occurring after DTP immuniza-tion are brief, self-limited, and generalized, and they occur in febrile chil-dren. These characteristics suggest that seizures associated with pertussis vaccine are usually febrile convulsions. These seizures have not been demonstrated to result in the subsequent development of recurrent afeb-rile seizures (ie, epilepsy) or other neurologic sequelae. Predisposing factors to seizures occurring within 48 hours include underlying con-vulsive disorder, personal history of convulsions, and family history of convulsions (see Infants and Children With Underlying Neurologic Disor-ders, p 365; and Children With Personal or Family History of Seizures, p 59.)
- *Unusual crying*. Persistent, severe, inconsolable screaming or crying for 3 or more hours (1:100 doses administered*) is sometimes observed within 48 hours of pertussis vaccination. Distinguishing between these features and crying from pain can be difficult and requires close questioning of the

---

*Cody CL, Baraff LJ, Cherry JD, Marcy SM, Manclark CR. Nature and rates of adverse reactions associated with DTP and DT immunizations in infants and children. *Pediatrics*. 1981;68:650-660.

patient's caretaker. The significance of persistent crying is unknown. It has been noted after receipt of immunizations other than pertussis vaccine and is not known to be associated with sequelae.

- *Collapse.* Collapse or shock-like state (hypotonic-hyporesponsive episode) has been observed after pertussis vaccination (1:1,750*). However, reported incidence rates vary widely, from 3.5 to 291 cases per 100,000 immunizations.[†] A recent follow-up study of a group of children who had experienced such episodes demonstrated no evidence of serious neurologic damage or intellectual impairment as a result of these episodes.

Moderate to severe systemic events, including fever of 40.5°C (104.9°F) or higher; persistent, inconsolable crying lasting 3 hours or more; and collapse (hypotonic-hyporesponsive episode) rarely have been reported after vaccination with DTaP. Each of these events appears to occur less often than with whole-cell DTP. When these events occur after the administration of whole-cell DTP, they appear to be without sequelae; the limited experience with DTaP suggests a similar outcome. Because DTaP causes fever less frequently than whole-cell DTP, events such as convulsions are anticipated to be less common after receipt of DTaP.

Alleged Reactions. The temporal relation of immunization and severe adverse events, such as death, encephalopathy, onset of a seizure disorder, developmental delay, or learning or behavioral problems, does not establish causation by a vaccine. Many of the manifestations of alleged vaccine reactions have other causes, such as viral encephalitis, other concurrent infections, pre-existing neurologic disorders, and metabolic and other congenital abnormalities. For example, whereas infantile spasms frequently have their onset in the first 6 months of life and, in some cases, have been temporally related to the administration of pertussis vaccine, epidemiologic data demonstrate that the vaccine does not cause infantile spasms. Sudden infant death syndrome (SIDS) has occurred after DTP immunization, but several studies provide evidence that DTP immunization is not associated with SIDS. A large case-control study of SIDS in the United States demonstrated that SIDS victims were no more likely to have recently received DTP vaccination than control children who did not have SIDS. Since SIDS occurs most commonly at the age when DTP immunization is recommended, coincidental, temporal associations between the death and immunization by chance alone are expected.

Evaluation. Appropriate diagnostic studies should be undertaken to establish an etiology of serious adverse events occurring temporally with immunization rather than assuming that they are caused by the vaccine. However, the cause of events temporally related to immunization cannot always be established even after diagnostic studies.

Severe Acute Neurologic Illness and Permanent Brain Damage. Permanent neurologic disability (brain damage) and even death have previously been considered uncommon sequelae of rare, severe, adverse neurologic events

---

*Cody CL, Baraff LJ, Cherry JD, Marcy SM, Manclark CR. Nature and rates of adverse reactions associated with DTP and DT immunizations in infants and children. *Pediatrics.* 1981;68:650-660.
†Howson CP, Fineberg HV. Adverse events following pertussis and rubella vaccines. Summary of a report of the Institute of Medicine. *JAMA.* 1992; 267:392-396.

temporally related to pertussis vaccine. Because no specific clinical syndromes or neuropathologic findings have been recognized in these cases, determination of whether pertussis vaccine is the cause of a specific child's deficit is not possible. Such adverse events can occur in both vaccinated and unvaccinated children, particularly in the first year of life. Hence, epidemiologic studies have been necessary to determine the risk of severe sequelae after acute events temporally related to pertussis immunization.

The only case-control study that addresses the issue of whether acute neurologic illness associated with DTP immunization results in permanent brain damage is the National Childhood Encephalopathy Study (NCES) in England, conducted from 1976 to 1979. This study examined the causes and natural history of serious acute neurologic illness in 1,182 children aged 2 to 36 months admitted to a hospital. More than 95% of cases of encephalopathy were unrelated temporally to DTP vaccination. Only 35 of these children had received pertussis vaccine within 7 days, and in many of these the temporal relation between acute neurologic illness and vaccination may have occurred by chance. Six of these children had infantile spasms, which was shown in a separate analysis not to be attributable to DTP vaccine. Analysis of the results indicated that very rarely (1:140,000 DTP doses) pertussis vaccine may be associated with the development of severe acute neurologic illness in children who were previously normal. Whereas later neurologic assessment of these children appeared to indicate that permanent neurologic sequelae could occur in some cases, the conclusion of an expert group that subsequently reviewed the NCES was that because of the small number of cases and limitations of the design and methods, the study could not provide valid information regarding whether acute neurologic illness associated with DTP vaccine results in permanent neurologic sequelae. Additional studies have not provided evidence to support a causal relationship between DTP vaccination and serious acute neurologic illness that results in permanent neurologic injury. Although each of these studies individually is of insufficient size to provide definitive answers, taken together the results are consistent with that of the reanalysis of the NCES findings.

The Committee concludes, based on currently available data, that pertussis vaccine has not been proven to be a cause of brain damage. Although the data do not prove that pertussis vaccine can never cause brain damage, they do indicate that if it does so, such occurrences must be exceedingly rare. Furthermore, in individual cases, the role of pertussis vaccine is impossible to determine on the basis of clinical or laboratory findings. Limited experience with acellular pertussis vaccine does not allow conclusions to be drawn as to the frequency of rare, serious, adverse effects temporally associated with its administration.

Contraindications and Precautions to Pertussis Immunization. Adverse events after pertussis immunization that contraindicate further administration of either DTP or DTaP are as follows:
- An immediate anaphylactic reaction.
- Encephalopathy within 7 days, defined as severe, acute, central nervous system disorder unexplained by another cause, which may be manifested by major alterations of consciousness or by generalized or focal seizures that persist for more than a few hours without recovery within 24 hours.

Studies indicate that such events associated with DTP are evident within 72 hours of immunization; prudence, however, usually justifies considering such an illness occurring within 7 days of DTP as a possible contraindication to further doses of pertussis vaccine.

If the following adverse events occur in temporal relation to DTP or DTaP, the decision to administer additional doses of pertussis vaccine should be carefully considered. Although these events were once regarded as contraindications to DTP, they are now considered precautions because of circumstances such as a pertussis outbreak in which the potential benefits of pertussis immunization outweigh the possible risks, particularly since the following events have not been proven to cause permanent sequelae:

- A convulsion, with or without fever, occurring within 3 days of DTP or DTaP vaccination.
- Persistent, severe, inconsolable screaming or crying for 3 or more hours within 48 hours.
- Collapse or shock-like state (hypotonic-hyporesponsive episode) within 48 hours.
- Temperature of 40.5°C (104.°9F) or higher, unexplained by another cause, within 48 hours.

Before administration of each dose of DTP or DTaP, the child's parent or guardian should be questioned about possible adverse events after the previous dose.

Although the risks of giving subsequent doses of pertussis vaccine to a child who has had one of these events are not known, the possibility of another reaction of similar or greater severity may justify discontinuing pertussis immunization. In each case, the decision to give or withhold immunization should be based on the clinical assessment of the earlier reaction, the likelihood of pertussis exposure in the child's community, and the potential benefits and risks of pertussis vaccine.

Infants and Children With Underlying Neurologic Disorders. The decision to give pertussis vaccine to infants and children with underlying neurologic disorders can be difficult and must be made on an individual basis after careful and continuing consideration of the risks and benefits (see also Children With Personal or Family History of Seizures, p 59). In some cases, these disorders may constitute a cause for deferring DTP or DTaP immunization and, based on the medical history of the child, subsequent administration of pertussis vaccine. The different circumstances and recommendations are categorized as follows:

- *A progressive neurologic disorder characterized by developmental delay or neurologic findings.* These conditions are reason for deferral of pertussis immunization. Administration of DTP may coincide with or hasten the recognition of inevitable manifestations of the disorder, with resulting confusion about causation. Examples include infantile spasms, uncontrolled epilepsy, and progressive encephalopathy. Such disorders should be differentiated from those that are nonprogressive and in which the symptoms may change as the child matures.
- *Infants and children with personal history of convulsions.* These patients have an increased risk of convulsions after receipt of pertussis-containing

vaccines. A retrospective review of adverse events after the receipt of DTP vaccine indicated that children with a personal history of seizure were seven times more likely to have a seizure after DTP vaccination than children who had local or other nonneurologic, post-DTP adverse events. No evidence indicates that these vaccine-associated seizures induce permanent brain damage, cause epilepsy, aggravate neurologic disorders, or affect the prognosis in children with underlying disorders. However, because the risk of a postvaccination convulsion is increased, pertussis immunization of children with recent seizures should be deferred until a progressive neurologic disorder is excluded or the child's diagnosis has been established. Because outbreaks of pertussis continue to occur in the United States, the decision to defer immunization should be reassessed at each subsequent medical visit; the decision to give pertussis vaccine should be based on the adjudged risks and consequences of seizure after DTP or DTaP vaccination in comparison to the risk of pertussis and its complications. Infants and children with well-controlled seizures or those in whom a seizure is unlikely to recur may be vaccinated. Children with associated neurologic deficits may be at increased risk of complications if they develop pertussis. Children traveling to or residing in areas of endemic or epidemic pertussis are at increased risk of developing pertussis. Efforts should be undertaken to ensure pertussis immunization of children attending child care centers, special clinics, or residential care institutions.

Because fever may lower the threshold for seizures in such patients, acetaminophen (15 mg/kg per dose) should be considered at the time of pertussis vaccination and every 4 hours for the ensuing 24 hours. DTaP is recommended for the fourth and fifth doses since it is less frequently associated with moderate to high fever than is whole-cell DTP.

- *Infants and children known to have, or suspected of having, neurologic conditions that predispose either to seizures or neurologic deterioration.* Such conditions include tuberous sclerosis and certain inherited metabolic or degenerative diseases. Deferral of pertussis immunization should be considered for these patients. Convulsions or encephalopathy can occur in the normal course of these disorders and, thus, may occur after any immunization. DTP, DTaP, or DT vaccination may be associated with the occurrence of overt manifestations of the disorders with resulting confusion about causation. Hence, children with unstable or evolving neurologic disorders that may predispose to seizures or neurologic deterioration should be observed for a period of time to ascertain the diagnosis and prognosis of the primary neurologic disorder before immunization. Pertussis immunization should be reconsidered at each visit. Children whose condition is resolved, corrected, or controlled can be vaccinated. No evidence indicates that prematurity in the absence of other factors increases the risk of seizures after immunization and is not a reason to defer vaccination (see Preterm Infants, p 51). Similarly, stable neurologic conditions, such as developmental delay or cerebral palsy, are not contraindications to pertussis immunization.

Temporary Deferment. Children in the first year of life with neurologic disorders that necessitate temporary deferment of pertussis immunization should not receive either DT or DTP because the risk of acquiring diphtheria or tetanus in children younger than 1 year in this country is remote. At or before the first birthday, however, the decision to give either DTP or DT should be made to ensure that the child is immunized at least against diphtheria and tetanus because as children become ambulatory, their risk of tetanus-prone wounds increases.

Children in whom DTP or DT immunization is deferred may not respond optimally to *Haemophilus influenzae* type b conjugate vaccines that use carrier proteins related to tetanus or diphtheria toxoids, such as HbOC or PRP-T. For such children, vaccination with PRP-OMP may be advantageous.

Children with neurologic disorders that are recognized after the first birthday frequently will have received one or more doses of DTP. The physician may temporarily defer additional doses of DTP or DTaP in anticipation of stabilization of the child's neurologic status. If the physician determines that the child probably should not receive further pertussis immunizations, DT immunization should be completed according to the recommended schedule. (See Diphtheria, p 180, and/or Tetanus, p 461). If pertussis immunization is continued, DTaP is preferred for the fourth and fifth doses.

Children With Family History of Convulsions (see also Children with Personal or Family History of Seizures, p 59). A history of seizure disorders or adverse events after receipt of a pertussis-containing vaccine in a family member is not a contraindication to pertussis immunization. Although the risk of seizures after DTP in children with family history of seizures is increased, these seizures are usually febrile in origin and have a generally benign outcome. In addition, this risk is outweighed by the continuing risk of pertussis in the United States and the substantial number of children with family history of seizures who, if not vaccinated, would remain susceptible to pertussis. DTaP is preferred for the fourth and fifth doses for children with a family history of seizures because it causes fever less frequently.

Advice to Parents of Children at Increased Risk of Seizures. Parents of children who may be at increased risk of a seizure after pertussis immunization, such as from personal or family history of convulsions, should be informed of the risks and benefits of pertussis immunization in these circumstances. Advice should be provided about fever, its control (see Antipyretic Prophylaxis, p 359), and appropriate medical care in the unlikely event of a seizure.

Pinworm Infection
(*Enterobius vermicularis*)

Clinical Manifestations: Pinworm infection (enterobiasis) causes pruritus ani and, rarely, pruritus vulvae. Although pinworms have been found in the lumen of the appendix, most evidence indicates that they are not causally related to acute appendicitis. Many symptoms, such as grinding of the teeth at night and enuresis, have been attributed to pinworm infections, but proof of a relationship has not been established. Vaginitis, salpingitis, and pelvic peritonitis can occur because of aberrant migration of the adult worm from the perineum.

Etiology: *Enterobius vermicularis* is a nematode.

Epidemiology: Enterobiasis is distributed worldwide and commonly occurs in family clusters, but it has no sex preference or seasonal variation in incidence. In the past, 5% to 15% of the population in the United States was estimated to be infected, but reports suggest that the incidence has declined. Prevalence rates are higher in preschool-aged and school-aged children, in mothers of infected children, and in the institutionalized, where 50% of the population may be infected. Adult gravid female nematodes usually die after depositing eggs on the perianal skin. Thus, reinfection by autoinfection or infection acquired from others is necessary to maintain enterobiasis in an individual. The period of communicability is as long as the gravid female nematodes are discharging eggs on perianal skin and the eggs remain infective in an indoor environment; this period is usually 2 to 3 weeks. Humans are the only hosts.

The **incubation period** is not known.

Diagnostic Tests: Diagnosis is made by application of transparent (not merely translucent) adhesive tape to the perianal skin to pick up any eggs; the tape is then applied to a glass slide and examined under a low-power microscopic lens. These specimens are best collected when the patient first awakens in the morning and before washing.

Treatment: The drug of choice is pyrantel pamoate or mebendazole; both are given in a single dose and repeated in 2 weeks (see Drugs for Parasitic Infections, p 574). In children younger than 2 years, in whom experience with both of these drugs is limited, the risks and benefits of the drugs should be considered before administration. Alternatives include piperazine and pyrvinium pamoate, but they are less effective and cumbersome to use. No unusual cleansing or hygienic measures should be undertaken. Excessive zeal in this regard can induce guilt and is counterproductive. Because of the high frequency of reinfection, families should be informed that recurrence is common. Repeated infections should be treated the same as the first one. Families may need to be treated as a group. Vaginitis is self-limited and does not require separate treatment.

Isolation of the Hospitalized Patient: No special precautions are indicated.

Control Measures: Control is difficult in child care centers and schools because the rate of reinfection is extremely high. In institutions, mass and simultaneous treatment, repeated in 2 weeks, can be effective.

Plague

Clinical Manifestations: Plague is usually accompanied by fever and painful lymphadenitis (bubonic plague). Pneumonic, septicemic, meningeal, and pharyngeal forms of plague are uncommon.

Etiology: Plague is caused by *Yersinia pestis*, a pleomorphic, bipolar staining, Gram-negative bacillus.

Epidemiology: Plague is an enzootic infection of rodents and their fleas in many parts of the world, including the western United States, parts of South America, Africa, and Asia. Most human cases in the United States occur singly or in small clusters and are associated with epizootic infection in wild rodents. Epidemics can occur when the domestic rodent populations become infected and their infected ectoparasites (fleas) spread the disease to humans. Bubonic plague is associated primarily with bites by infected fleas, particularly the oriental rat flea (*Xenopsylla cheopis*) outside the United States and by other rodent fleas in the United States. Direct contact with infected rodents, rabbits, and domestic animals, especially cats, can result in transmission. Bubonic plague is communicable by contact with purulent discharge from a bubo, and by bites of human fleas. Pneumonic and pharyngeal plague are transmitted by the droplet route during direct contact with an infected animal or person.

The **incubation period** is 2 to 6 days for bubonic plague and 2 to 4 days (occasionally shorter but rarely longer) for pneumonic plague.

Diagnostic Tests: *Yersinia pestis* can be isolated by culture of bubo aspirates, blood, or cerebrospinal fluid (CSF), and from sputum in pneumonic or pharyngeal plague. Identification of isolates as *Y pestis* can be confirmed by bacteriophage sensitivity, fluorescent antibody tests, animal pathogenicity tests, and agglutination tests. The characteristic bipolar staining of the organism is best seen with Wayson's stain. Giemsa stain, Gram stain, and fluorescent antibody studies of the bubo aspirate, CSF, occasionally peripheral blood, or sputum can provide presumptive evidence of *Y pestis*. Paired sera from the acute and convalescent phases of illness, 3 to 4 weeks apart, should be obtained to demonstrate seroconversion or a fourfold antibody titer rise by the passive hemagglutination test.

Treatment: Streptomycin* (30 mg/kg/d) is the drug of choice. Tetracycline (20 to 30 mg/kg/d, given intravenously, in four divided doses), chloramphenicol (75 to 100 mg/kg/d, given intravenously, in four divided doses) or sulfonamides are also effective. Tetracycline should not be given to children younger than 9 years unless the benefits of therapy are greater than the risks of dental staining. Chloramphenicol, with or without streptomycin, should be

---

*As of December 1993, available from Pfizer Streptomycin Program, Pfizer Pharmaceuticals, New York, NY (800/254-4445).

used for plague meningitis. The optimum duration of antibiotic therapy is not known. Five to 7 days of streptomycin, 10 to 14 days of tetracycline, or 10 days of chloramphenicol is usually sufficient.

Drainage of buboes and abscesses may be necessary, but should not be attempted until at least 24 hours after initiating antimicrobial therapy because of the potentially highly infectious nature of the drainage.

Isolation of the Hospitalized Patient: All patients should be in strict isolation until pneumonia is excluded and therapy has been initiated. Drainage/secretion precautions are recommended for patients with bubonic plague; strict isolation is mandatory for patients with pneumonic plague. Isolation should be continued for 3 days after the start of effective antimicrobial therapy.

Control Measures:

Care of Exposed Persons. A person with intimate exposure to a person with bubonic plague should be placed under surveillance for 7 to 10 days. If fleas are known to be present, disinfestation of clothing and residence of the exposed person with an insecticide effective against local fleas should be considered. The person exposed to pneumonic plague should (1) have clothing and quarters disinfested with an insecticide powder, if indicated; (2) be given chemoprophylaxis for 7 days with tetracycline (15 mg/kg/d), which is the preferred drug except for children younger than 9 years, or a sulfonamide (40 mg/kg/d); and (3) be closely observed (including twice daily recordings of temperature) for 7 to 10 days.

Vaccine. An inactivated whole-cell bacterial vaccine* is useful for persons whose occupation may regularly lead to contact with potentially infected rodents or their fleas (eg, biologists, geologists, or laboratory workers). Routine vaccination is not recommended for persons living in plague enzootic areas of the western United States. Vaccination is recommended for those traveling to or residing in areas where plague is occurring and where domestic rats are known to be infested. Primary immunization consists of three intramuscular injections of vaccine, the first two at 30-day intervals and the third 3 to 6 months after the second dose.

Booster doses are indicated at 6-month intervals until a total of five doses are given, then at 12- to 24-month intervals for as long as the danger of exposure exists. The package insert should be consulted for further information, including the dose.

Other Measures. Periodic surveys in enzootic areas to determine the prevalence of infested rats, other rodents, and fleas should be performed by public health workers. Health officials must be notified when a presumptive diagnosis of plague is made so that control measures can be instituted.

Suppression of the rodent population is important in epidemic control, but it must not be done without prior or concurrent ectoparasite (flea) control during an active plague epizootic. Ratproofing buildings, reducing breeding

---

*Available from Miles, Inc, West Haven, CT.

areas, and rat control on ships by ratproofing and periodic fumigation are important, as is flea control of domestic cats and dogs. If field surveys indicate a need, treatment of premises or other human contact areas with residual insecticides should be performed. In enzootic areas the public should be educated about the role of domestic animals and their fleas in zoonotic transmission of disease.

Pneumococcal Infections

Clinical Manifestations: Pneumococci are the most common cause of acute otitis media and a frequent cause of pneumonia, meningitis, and sinusitis in children. They are also the most common cause of bacteremia in infants and children 1 to 24 months of age, some of whom have no evidence of a primary focus of infection.

Etiology: *Streptococcus pneumoniae* (the pneumococci) are lancet-shaped, Gram-positive diplococci. Eighty-four pneumococcal serotypes have been identified. Certain serotypes are prevalent in adults; others are prevalent in children. Serotypes in groups 14, 6, 18, 19, 23, 4, 9, 7, 1, and 3 (in order of decreasing prevalence) cause most childhood pneumococcal infections. Serotypes 6, 14, 19, and 23 are the most frequent ones associated with resistance to penicillin.

Epidemiology: Pneumococci are ubiquitous; many persons carry organisms in the upper respiratory tract without symptoms. Transmission is from person to person, presumably by respiratory droplet contact. Disease is more likely to occur when predisposing conditions exist, including immunoglobulin deficiency, Hodgkin's disease, congenital or acquired immunodeficiency (including human immunodeficiency virus [HIV] infection), nephrotic syndrome, some viral upper respiratory tract infections, splenic dysfunction (including sickle-cell anemia), splenectomy, and organ transplantation. Invasive pneumococcal disease is often the first clinical manifestation of HIV infection, indicating significant humoral immunodeficiency early in the course of HIV infection in children. Pneumococcal infections are most prevalent when respiratory disease is most common, usually during the winter months. The period of communicability is unknown. It may be as long as the organism is present in respiratory seretions but is probably less than 24 hours after effective antimicrobial therapy is begun.

Mortality from pneumococcal disease is highest in patients who have bacteremia or meningitis. Patients with one of the aforementioned predisposing conditions are at increased risk for developing severe pneumococcal disease because of impaired immunologic response to *S pneumoniae*. Certain other patients may also be at increased risk for severe pneumococcal infections, such as those with diabetes mellitus, congestive heart failure, chronic pulmonary disease, or renal failure. Patients with cerebrospinal fluid (CSF) leakage, complicating skull fracture, or neurosurgical procedures can have recurrent pneumococcal meningitis.

The **incubation period** varies by type of infection and can be as short as 1 to 3 days. Illness usually occurs within 1 month after a new pneumococcal serotype is acquired in the upper respiratory tract. Illness is seldom associated with preceding prolonged carriage.

Diagnostic Tests: Material obtained from a suppurative focus should be Gram stained and cultured by appropriate microbiologic techniques. Blood cultures should be obtained in all patients suspected of having invasive pneumococcal disease; cultures of CSF and other body fluids (eg, pleural fluid) are also often indicated. The white blood cell (WBC) count may be of assistance in suspected bacteremic disease caused by *S pneumoniae*; young children with high temperatures and leukocytosis have an increased likelihood of bacteremia. Although the predictive value of an elevated WBC count for pneumococcal bacteremia is not high, a normal WBC count is highly predictive of the absence of bacteremia. Recovery of pneumococci from an upper respiratory tract culture is not proof of causation of otitis media, pneumonia, or sinusitis because of the frequent presence of these bacteria in uninfected persons. Rapid methods to detect pneumococcal capsular antigen in CSF, pleural fluid, serum, and concentrated urine can facilitate a rapid diagnosis in suspected bacteremia, pneumonia, and meningitis; a negative test result, however, does not exclude pneumococcal disease. These tests are particularly useful in patients who have received antibiotics before the collection of specimens for culture.

Treatment:
- Penicillin G is the drug of choice for the treatment of most pneumococcal infections. However, *S pneumoniae* strains with resistance to penicillin G have been identified from many regions of the United States and the world with increasing frequency in recent years. Most resistant strains have intermediate penicillin G resistance (in vitro minimal inhibitory concentration [MIC] of 0.1 to 1 µg/mL), although as many as 40% of strains in one community had high-concentration penicillin G resistance (MIC greater than 1 µg/mL). Therefore, oxacillin disk susceptibility testing should be performed on all isolates from blood, CSF, or other infected body fluids. Penicillin, cefotaxime, ceftriaxone, and vancomycin MICs of strains identified as resistant by oxacillin disk testing should be determined. In many instances, infections caused by strains with intermediate resistance to penicillin respond clinically to high-dose penicillin therapy. However, patients with meningitis caused by one of these intermediately resistant strains should not be treated with penicillin, and selection of an antibiotic should be based on in vitro susceptibility testing. If the strain is susceptible in vitro, cefotaxime, ceftriaxone, vancomycin, or chloramphenicol can be used. However, treatment failure has been reported with each of these drugs in patients with pneumococcal meningitis.
- Vancomycin or chloramphenicol are also appropriate alternative drugs for penicillin-allergic patients.

- Strains with high-level resistance to penicillin (MIC greater than 1 μg/mL) are frequently resistant to many other antimicrobial agents but are usually susceptible to vancomycin. In general, the MIC values for other beta-lactam antibiotics, such as cefotaxime, ceftriaxone, and imipenem-cilastatin, increase in parallel with the MIC to penicillin. Therefore, in cases of meningitis caused by strains highly resistant to penicillin, MICs must be determined before these agents are used. In addition, the use of imipenem-cilastatin is limited because it sometimes causes convulsions in infants and children with meningitis.
- For children with mild to moderately severe infections who are allergic to penicillins, erythromycin and trimethoprim-sulfamethoxazole are alternative drugs. Clindamycin, chloramphenicol, and cephalosporins are also effective therapeutic agents. For treatment of meningitis, CSF concentrations with the macrolides and older cephalosporins (such as cephalothin and cefazolin) are inadequate for these drugs to be used. The newer, extended-spectrum cephalosporins, such as cefotaxime and ceftriaxone, are effective in the treatment of meningitis. New beta-lactam-like antimicrobial agents may also be effective.
- The route and dosage of antimicrobial therapy depend on the severity of the illness (see Tables of Antibacterial Drug Dosages, p 541). For meningitis, a minimum of 10 days of therapy is generally required.
- In infants and children 2 months and older with bacterial meningitis, dexamethasone therapy should be considered after weighing the benefits and possible risks (see Dexamethasone Therapy for Bacterial Meningitis in Infants and Children, p 558).
- Treatment of carriers is not indicated.

Isolation of the Hospitalized Patient: No special precautions are recommended.

Control Measures:

Child Care. No isolation precautions are necessary for children in child care who have pneumococcal disease. Prophylactic antibiotic treatment of child care contacts of a person with pneumococcal disease is not recommended.

Active Immunization. The 23-valent pneumococcal vaccine is composed of purified, capsular polysaccharide antigens of 23 pneumococcal serotypes. It is given subcutaneously or intramuscularly. Each vaccine dose (0.5 mL) contains 25 μg of each polysaccharide antigen. These capsular antigens are those of serotypes causing 88% of cases of bacteremia and meningitis in adults, nearly 100% of cases of bacteremia and meningitis in children, and 85% of cases of acute otitis media. Like other polysaccharide antigens, some of the pneumococcal serotypes (eg, types 6 and 14) in the vaccine have limited immunogenicity in children younger than 2 years of age. The effectiveness of pneumococcal vaccines in preventing pneumonia has been demonstrated in healthy young adults and older children predisposed to a high incidence of pneumococcal disease. In one study, vaccinated children with sickle-cell disease or those who had undergone splenectomy experienced significantly less bacteremic pneumococcal disease than nonvaccinated patients.

Adverse Reactions. Mild side effects, such as erythema and pain at the injection site, are common. Fever, myalgia, and severe local reactions are very uncommon. Severe systemic reactions, such as anaphylaxis, have rarely been reported.

Recommendations for Vaccination:

- Children 2 years and older with increased risk of acquiring systemic pneumococcal infections or with increased risk of serious disease if they become infected should be vaccinated. Included in this high-risk category are children with (1) sickle-cell disease; (2) functional or anatomic asplenia; (3) nephrotic syndrome or chronic renal failure; (4) conditions associated with immunosuppression, such as organ transplantation or cytoreduction therapy; (5) CSF leaks; and (6) HIV infection (see HIV Infection and AIDS, p 263).

- In addition to administering pneumococcal vaccine to children with functional or anatomic asplenia, parents and patients should be informed that vaccination does not guarantee protection from fulminant pneumococcal disease and death (case fatality rates are 50% to 80%). Asplenic patients with unexplained fever or manifestations of sepsis should receive prompt medical attention including treatment for suspected bacteremia, the initial signs and symptoms of which may be subtle. Antimicrobials selected for initial empirical treatment should be effective against *S pneumoniae*, *Neisseria meningitidis*, and beta-lactamase-producing *Haemophilus influenzae* type b.

- When elective splenectomy is to be performed, pneumococcal vaccine should be given approximately 2 weeks or more before the operation, if possible, to increase the likelihood of eliciting a protective antibody response. Similarly, in planning cancer chemotherapy or immunosuppressive therapy for such patients as those with Hodgkin's disease or those who are to undergo bone marrow or solid-organ transplantation, vaccination should precede the initiation of chemotherapy or immunosuppression by approximately 2 weeks or more. Vaccination during chemotherapy or radiation therapy should be avoided because antibody responses are poor and vaccination is not likely to be effective in preventing pneumococcal infection. Patients who received vaccine during chemotherapy or radiation therapy should be immunized 3 months after discontinuation of the therapy.

- Vaccination with the current pneumococcal vaccine is not recommended for preventing otitis media during the first 2 years of life. Data are inadequate to evaluate the effectiveness of pneumococcal vaccine in preventing otitis media in children older than 2 years of age, although some experts recommend vaccination in older children with recurrent otitis media.

- Vaccination is not recommended for preventing upper or lower respiratory tract infection in healthy children living in the United States.

- Routine revaccination with the 23-valent vaccine of children who previously received the 14-valent vaccine is not recommended because the increased protection from more serotypes in the vaccine is modest and the duration of protection is not well defined. However, revaccination with the 23-valent vaccine should be strongly considered for persons who received the 14-valent vaccine if they are at high risk of fatal pneumococcal infection, such as asplenic patients.

- Revaccination of recipients of the 23-valent vaccine after 3 to 5 years should also be considered for children 10 years or younger who are at high risk of severe pneumococcal infection. These children include (1) those who are asplenic (functionally or anatomically); (2) those with asplenia from sickle-cell disease; and (3) those who have been demonstrated to have rapid antibody decline after initial vaccination, such as from nephrotic syndrome, renal failure, or transplantation. Revaccination should also be considered for high-risk, older children and adults who were vaccinated 6 years or more before.

- Vaccination generally should be deferred during pregnancy because the effect of the vaccine on the fetus is unknown. The risk of severe pneumococcal disease during pregnancy must be weighed against the potential hazards of the vaccine.

- Pneumococcal vaccine may be given concurrently with other vaccines (see Simultaneous Administration of Multiple Vaccines, p 25). No data indicate that administration of pneumococcal vaccine with DTP, poliovirus, influenza, or other vaccines increases the severity of reactions or diminishes antibody responses.

Passive Immunization. Intramuscular or intravenous immunoglobulin administration is recommended for preventing pneumococcal infection in patients with congenital or acquired immunodeficiency diseases, including those with HIV infection who have recurrent pneumococcal infections (see HIV Infection and AIDS, p 261).

Chemoprophylaxis (see also Asplenic Children, p 57). Many experts recommend that children with functional or anatomic asplenia receive daily antimicrobial prophylaxis. For prevention of pneumococcal disease, oral penicillin G or V (125 mg twice daily for children younger than 5 years; 250 mg twice daily for children 5 years and older) is recommended. The age at which to discontinue prophylaxis is decided empirically, since no studies of this question have been performed. Some experts continue prophylaxis throughout childhood and in particularly high-risk patients into adulthood.

The results of a multicenter study demonstrated that oral penicillin V (125 mg twice daily) given to infants and young children with sickle-cell disease reduces the incidence of severe bacterial infection by 84% compared with the placebo control group. Based on this study, a National Institutes of Health Consensus Development Panel recommended daily penicillin prophylaxis for children with sickle-cell hemoglobinopathy beginning before the age of 4 months.

Antimicrobial prophylaxis against pneumococcal infection may be particularly useful for asplenic children not likely to respond to vaccine, such as those younger than 2 years of age or those receiving intensive chemotherapy or cytoreduction therapy.

Pneumocystis carinii Infections

Clinical Manifestations: Infants characteristically develop a subacute, diffuse pneumonitis with dyspnea at rest, tachypnea, oxygen desaturation, cough, and fever. In immunocompromised children and adults, the onset can be more acute and fulminant. The chest roentgenogram often shows bilateral diffuse alveolar disease, but without a characteristic pattern. Occasionally, the chest roentgenogram at the time of diagnosis can even appear normal. Mortality in immunocompromised patients is high, ranging from 10% to 40% if treated, and close to 100% if untreated.

Etiology: Based on DNA sequencing, *Pneumocystis carinii* appears to be a fungus. Previously, it was presumed to be a sporozoan because of its morphology.

Epidemiology: *Pneumocystis carinii* is ubiquitous in mammals worldwide, particularly rodents. Whether *P carinii* in animals is infectious for humans has not been determined. Asymptomatic infection occurs early in life with more than 70% of healthy individuals acquiring antibody by 4 years of age. In developing countries and in times of famine in industrialized countries, *P carinii* pneumonia (PCP) has occurred in epidemics, primarily affecting malnourished infants and children. Epidemics have also been described in premature infants. In industrialized countries today, PCP occurs almost entirely in immunocompromised persons with deficient cell-mediated immunity, particularly those with HIV infection, including recipients of immunosuppressive therapy after organ transplantation or treatment for malignancy, and children with congenital immunodeficiency syndromes. *Pneumocystis carinii* pneumonia is the most common serious opportunistic infection in infants and young children with perinatally acquired HIV infection. Although onset of disease can occur at any age, including rare instances in the first month of life, PCP most frequently occurs between 3 and 12 months of age, and can be the initial HIV-related illness. The prognosis in infants and young children with HIV infection who develop PCP is poor, particularly when the diagnosis and resulting treatment are delayed. In patients with lymphoma or leukemia, the disease occurs during remission or relapse. The mode of transmission is unknown. Proposed hypotheses are (1) person-to-person transmission by the respiratory route, and (2) reactivation of latent infection resulting from immunosuppression. Circumstantial evidence suggests that person-to-person transmission can occur. Primary infection probably accounts for disease during infancy, whereas reactivation infection is presumably the mode of disease after the first 2 years of life. Recurrences in immunocompromised patients, especially those with AIDS, are common. The period of communicability is unknown.

The **incubation period** is unknown.

Diagnostic Tests: A definitive diagnosis of PCP is made by demonstration of organisms in lung tissue or lower respiratory tract secretions. The most sensitive and specific diagnostic procedures have been open-lung biopsy and transbronchial biopsy. However, bronchoscopy with broncho-alveolar lavage, induction of sputum in older children and adolescents, and intubation with deep endotracheal aspiration are less invasive, often diagnostic, and have been sufficiently sensitive in patients with HIV infection. Toluidine blue O and methenamine silver nitrate are the most useful stains for identifying the thick-walled cysts. Extracystic trophozoites are easier to identify with Giemsa, Wright, Gram-Weigert, or polychrome methylene blue stains. Serologic tests for detecting *P carinii* infection are still experimental and are not recommended for diagnosis. Many children and adults with HIV infection and PCP have elevated serum concentrations of lactate dehydrogenase, but this abnormality is not specific for PCP.

Treatment: The drug of choice is trimethoprim-sulfamethoxazole (TMP-SMX), usually given intravenously. Oral therapy should be reserved for patients with mild disease who do not have malabsorption or diarrhea. The rate of adverse reactions is higher in patients with AIDS than in other patients. The incidence in HIV-infected children treated with TMP-SMX has been estimated to be about 15%, but in adults with AIDS it may be as high as 60%. Of patients with AIDS who have an adverse reaction, 50%, nevertheless, have been subsequently treated successfully with TMP-SMX.

Parenterally administered pentamidine is an alternative drug for children and adults who cannot tolerate TMP-SMX or who have not responded to TMP-SMX after 5 to 7 days of therapy. The therapeutic efficacy of pentamidine in adults with PCP has been similar to that of TMP-SMX. However, pentamidine is associated with a high incidence of adverse reactions, including pancreatitis, renal dysfunction, hypoglycemia, hyperglycemia, hypotension, fever, and neutropenia. Pentamidine should not be used concomitantly with didanosine (DDI), since both drugs can cause pancreatitis. If a recipient of DDI develops PCP and requires pentamidine, DDI should be discontinued until 1 week after the pentamidine therapy has been completed.

Atovaquone (a hydroxynaphtho-quinone) is a new drug that has been approved for the oral treatment of mild to moderate PCP in adults who are intolerant of TMP-SMX. Experience with the use of atovaquone in children is limited. The initial pediatric formulation was inadequately absorbed and evaluation of a new formulation is in progress.

Other potentially useful drugs identified by in vitro studies, animal models, and clinical trials in adults include dapsone with TMP, trimetrexate with folinic acid, aerosolized pentamidine, pyrimethamine with sulfadoxine, and clindamycin and primaquine.

A minimum duration of 2 weeks of therapy is recommended. In patients with AIDS, 3 weeks is recommended because of the high incidence of recurrence.

Based on data in adults, corticosteroids appear to be beneficial in the treatment of HIV-infected patients with moderate to severe PCP. A panel of experts have recommended steroids as adjunctive therapy for persons older than 13 years with documented or suspected PCP who have moderate or severe hypoxia (as defined by an arterial oxygen pressure of less than 70 mm Hg, or an arterial-alveolar gradient of more than

35 mm Hg).* Oral prednisone 80 mg/d in two divided doses is recommended for days 1 through 5 of therapy, 40 mg/d on days 6 through 10, and 20 mg/d on days 11 through 21. Although no controlled studies of the use of steroids in young children have been performed, most experts would include steroids as part of the therapy for children with moderate to severe PCP. The optimal dose and duration of corticosteroid therapy for children have not been determined.

Prophylaxis. Chemoprophylaxis is strongly recommended by the United States Public Health Service for HIV-infected adults and adolescents who have already had an episode of PCP or other opportunistic infections, those with a peripheral blood T-helper (CD4) lymphocyte count of 200/mm^3 or less, and those patients with HIV-related symptoms such as thrush or unexplained fever higher than 100°F (37.8°C) for 2 weeks or more, regardless of their CD4 count.[†]

Because PCP can occur early in life, identification of infants as early as possible who have been perinatally exposed to HIV is essential. The initial evaluation of these children should include a CD4 lymphocyte count, and testing should be repeated at 3-month intervals during the first 24 months of life. Prophylaxis for PCP is recommended for any child who has had an episode of PCP, has a CD4 lymphocyte count lower than the age-adjusted threshold, or has a CD4 percentage of 20% or less of the total peripheral lymphocytes.[‡] In children, normal lymphocyte counts tend to be higher than in adults, and they vary with age. The age-adjusted CD4 lymphocyte counts at which PCP prophylaxis is recommended are as follows:

1 to 11 months: ≤1500/mm^3
12 to 23 months: ≤750/mm^3
2 through 5 years: ≤500/mm^3
6 years and older: ≤200/mm^3

Prophylaxis for PCP should be discontinued for children who are subsequently proven not to be infected with HIV.

The regimen that is recommended for all immunocompromised patients is trimethoprim-sulfamethoxazole (TMP-SMX) administered daily or for 3 days each week. TMP-SMX administered on 3 consecutive days each week is as effective as daily administration in immunosuppressed children with cancer. The dose, including those with HIV infection, is 150 mg/m^2/d (TMP) – 750 mg/m^2/d (SMX) (maximum, 160 mg – 800 mg) in two divided doses. For patients who cannot tolerate TMP-SMX, aerosolized pentamidine for those 5 years or older is an alternative. Intravenous pentamidine at a dose of 4 mg/kg monthly or biweekly has also been used, but it appears to be less effective than other prophylactic regimens.

---

*The National Institutes of Health-University of California Expert Panel for Corticosteroids as Adjunctive Therapy for Pneumocystis Pneumonia. Consensus statement on the use of corticosteroids as adjunctive therapy for pneumocystis pneumonia in the acquired immunodeficiency syndrome. *N Engl J Med.* 1990;323:1500-1504

†See the following for further information: Centers for Disease Control. Recommendations for prophylaxis against *Pneumocystis carinii* pneumonia for adults and adolescents infected with human immunodeficiency virus. *MMWR.* 1992;41(RR-4):1-11.

‡Centers for Disease Control. Guidelines for prophylaxis against *Pneumocystis carinii* pneumonia for children infected with human immunodeficiency virus. *MMWR.* 1991;40(RR-2):1-13.

Daily oral dapsone, 1 mg/kg/d, is another alternate drug for prophylaxis in children, especially those younger than 5 years of age. Clinical trials of its efficacy are in progress.

Other drugs for prophylaxis include oral pyrimethamine with dapsone and oral pyrimethamine-sulfadoxine. Evaluation of oral atovaquone is in progress. Experience with these drugs in children is limited. These agents should be considered for children only in unusual situations in which the recommended regimens are not tolerated or cannot be used.

Pneumocystis carinii pneumonia and extrapulmonary *P carinii* infections have occurred in adults and children receiving prophylaxis. The reason for these prophylaxis failures is not well understood but may be related to compliance with the drug regimen and absorption of the drug.

In certain immunosuppressed children with cancer, recipients of organ transplants, and congenital immunodeficiency syndrome, TMP-SMX prophylaxis to prevent *P carinii* has also been effective. The dosage recommendation is the same as for HIV-infected patients, and it can be given on 3 consecutive days of each week.

Isolation of the Hospitalized Patient: Patients with PCP should not have contact with immunocompromised patients.

Control Measures: Appropriate therapy of infected patients and prophylaxis in immunocompromised patients are the only available means of control.

Poliovirus Infections

Clinical Manifestations: Approximately 90% to 95% of poliovirus infections are asymptomatic. Nonspecific illness with low-grade fever and sore throat (minor illness) occurs in 4% to 8% of infections. Aseptic meningitis, sometimes with paresthesias, occurs in 1% to 5% of patients a few days after the minor illness has resolved. Rapid onset of asymmetric acute flaccid paralysis with areflexia of the involved limb occurs in 0.1% to 2% of infections, and residual paralytic disease involving the motor neurons (paralytic poliomyelitis) occurs in approximately 1 per 1,000 infections. Cranial nerve involvement (bulbar paralysis) and paralysis of respiratory muscles may occur. The cerebrospinal fluid (CSF) reveals a moderate lymphocytosis and elevated protein.

Etiology: Polioviruses are enteroviruses and consist of three types: 1, 2, and 3.

Epidemiology: Poliovirus infections occur only in humans. Spread is by the fecal-oral and possibly oral-oral (respiratory) routes. Perinatal transmission from mother to newborn infant occurs. Infection is more common in infants and young children, and occurs at an earlier age under conditions of poor hygiene. However, paralysis is more likely when infection occurs in older individuals. In temperate climates, poliovirus infections are most common in the summer and fall; in the tropics, the seasonal pattern is variable, with a less pronounced peak of activity.

Poliomyelitis is rare in the United States at the present time. The last epidemic occurred in 1979 in a group of persons who had refused immunization. As of December 1993, all endemic cases since 1979 (an average of nine cases per year) have been associated with oral poliovirus vaccine (OPV). The remainder of cases (an average of one case every 2 years) have been imported. Poliomyelitis is still prevalent in underdeveloped areas of the world and, therefore, is a potential threat for unimmunized travelers to these areas, as well as for importation into the United States.

Communicability is greatest shortly before and after onset of clinical illness when the virus is present in the throat and excreted in large amounts in the feces. The virus persists in the throat for about 1 week after onset of illness, and it is excreted in the feces for several weeks and occasionally for months. Patients are potentially contagious as long as fecal excretion persists. In recipients of OPV, the virus persists in the throat for 1 to 2 weeks; it is excreted in the feces for several weeks, although in rare cases it has been excreted for more than 2 months. Immunodeficient patients may excrete virus for prolonged periods.

The **incubation period** of abortive poliomyelitis is 3 to 6 days. For the onset of paralysis in paralytic poliomyelitis, the incubation period is usually 7 to 21 days, but occasionally it is as short as 4 days.

Diagnostic Tests: Poliovirus can be recovered from the feces, throat, urine, and, rarely, from CSF by isolation in tissue culture. Specimens for viral isolation should be obtained from all patients with paralytic disease suspected to be poliomyelitis. Fecal material is most likely to yield virus, but virus can also be recovered from rectal swabs. In children with aseptic meningitis caused by poliovirus, the rate of positive cultures from rectal swabs has been 50% to 60%, which is more than that for CSF (30%), throat (20%), or urine (20%) cultures.

If a poliovirus is isolated from a patient with paralysis, it should be sent to the Centers for Disease Control and Prevention through the state health department for testing to distinguish wild-type from vaccine strains. Since infants who are immunized with poliovirus vaccine can excrete virus in the feces for several weeks, proof that a disease is caused by the poliovirus necessitates viral isolation from a nongastrointestinal and nonpharyngeal source. The incidental isolation of poliovirus from enteric sites in healthy young infants should be assumed to be the result of administration of, or exposure to, vaccine virus, unless a reason to suspect otherwise exists. Serologic testing of acute and convalescent sera should be performed in patients suspected of having paralytic poliomyelitis. However, interpretation of serologic tests can be difficult. Hence, the diagnostic test of choice for confirming polio is stool cultures from at least two specimens collected in the first 15 days after onset of symptoms.

Treatment: Supportive.

Isolation of the Hospitalized Patient: For patients suspected of excreting wild poliovirus or who have poliomyelitis, enteric precautions are indicated for the duration of hospitalization.

Control Measures:

Immunization of Infants and Children. Two types of trivalent vaccine are available—live oral poliovirus vaccine (OPV) and inactivated poliovirus vaccine (IPV), given parenterally. Oral poliovirus vaccine contains poliovirus types 1, 2, and 3, which have been produced in monkey kidney cell cultures. Inactivated poliovirus vaccine is a mixture of the three types of poliovirus grown in human diploid cells or Vero cells and inactivated with formalin. The current IPV is of enhanced potency and is highly immunogenic; after only three doses it induces seroconversion rates equal to or greater than that of OPV. Both IPV and OPV are effective in preventing poliomyelitis.

Based on consideration of the risks and benefits, OPV is currently the vaccine of choice for routine immunization of most children in the United States because it (1) induces intestinal immunity, (2) is simple to administer, (3) is well accepted by patients, (4) results in immunization of some contacts of vaccinated persons, and (5) has eliminated disease caused by wild polioviruses in the United States. Multiple doses of OPV are given to ensure that infection and resulting immunity to all three types of poliovirus develops.

Oral poliovirus vaccine should not be given to infants and children living in households with an immunodeficient person, including persons known to be infected with human immunodeficiency virus (HIV), because OPV is excreted in the stool by healthy vaccinees and can infect an immunocompromised household member who may contract paralytic disease (see Adverse Vaccine Reactions, p 386). Inactivated poliovirus vaccine should be given to persons requiring poliovirus immunization in such households. For adults needing polio immunization, IPV is indicated in most cases (see Immunization Recommendations for Adults, p 383).

To ensure that vaccination is undertaken among fully informed persons, parents of prospective vaccinees should be made aware of the reasons and circumstances for specific vaccine recommendations at particular ages, and of the benefits and risks of poliovirus vaccines for both individuals and the community. Parents who refuse OPV for their children after being informed of the risks and benefits should be offered IPV for their children.

Recommendations for OPV. Ordinarily, the first dose of OPV is administered when the infant is approximately 6 to 8 weeks old and a second dose is given when the infant is 4 months old. Two doses produce an antibody response in excess of 90% to all three serotypes. A third dose of OPV is recommended when the child is 6 to 18 months of age to complete the primary series (see Table 1.3, p 23). Administration of the third dose at 6 months of age has the potential advantage of enhancing the likelihood of completion of the primary series and does not compromise seroconversion. An interval of 2 months between doses is recommended. The minimal interval in most circumstances is 6 weeks, but in children in whom accelerated poliomyelitis vaccination is warranted, this interval may be 4 weeks.

Oral poliovirus vaccine may be given concurrently with other vaccines (see Simultaneous Administration of Multiple Vaccines, p 25). A supplementary dose of OPV should be given before the child enters school, ie, at 4 to 6 years of age.

In geographic areas where polio is endemic, a dose may also be given when the newborn infant is discharged from the hospital, and supplemental doses are often administered during mass community-based programs.

Breast-feeding does not affect the overall success of immunization; hence, no interruption of the feeding schedule is necessary. No evidence for waning immunity exists.

For children who are not immunized in the first year of life (see Table 1.4, p 24), two doses of OPV should be given approximately 6 to 8 weeks apart, followed by a third dose 2 to 12 months later. If the risk of exposure to polio is substantial, such as for travelers to endemic areas, or for children whose receipt of vaccines has been delayed, the interval between doses may be 4 to 6 weeks. If the third dose is administered before the fourth birthday, a supplementary (fourth) dose should be given before the child enters school, ie, at 4 to 6 years of age.

Children at any age who are partially immunized should receive the number of doses necessary to complete the required series of three doses. If the schedule has been interrupted, the series does not need to be reinitiated.

Indications for OPV are summarized in Table 3.39 (p 383).

Recommendations for IPV. Persons who have refused OPV or in whom OPV is contraindicated (see Precautions and Contraindications to Immunization, p 385) should be immunized with IPV.

The primary series of IPV consists of three doses administered subcutaneously or intramuscularly, and it results in antibody responses to the three serotypes in more than 95% of vaccine recipients. The first two doses should be given at 4- to 8-week intervals beginning at 6 to 8 weeks of age, and the third dose should be given 6 to 12 months after the second dose. In infancy, the primary schedule of IPV is usually concomitant with the first two doses and the fourth dose of diphtheria-tetanus-pertussis (DTP) vaccine at 15 to 18 months of age (see Table 1.3, p 23).

Inactivated poliovirus vaccine may be given concurrently with other vaccines (see Simultaneous Administration of Multiple Vaccines, p 25). If OPV and DTP are given at the same time, they should be given in separate syringes because of possible interference. An investigational, special dual-chambered syringe that allows mixing of selective DTP and IPV preparations just before injection has been developed.

When entering school (ie, between the ages of 4 and 6 years), children should receive another dose of IPV. For IPV-immunized persons, booster doses of IPV every 5 years had previously been recommended; however, for recipients of enhanced-potency IPV (the vaccine currently in use in the United States), the need for 5-year boosters has not been established. Indications for IPV are summarized in Table 3.40 (p 384).

Incompletely Immunized Children and Vaccine Interchangeability. Children partially immunized with IPV or OPV should receive sufficient doses of either IPV or OPV to complete the primary immunization series (see Lapsed Immunizations, p 26). Incompletely immunized children who are at increased

TABLE 3.39—Persons for Whom OPV Immunization Is Indicated

Healthy infants and children receiving routine immunization.

Unimmunized or partially immunized children who are at imminent risk of exposure to poliovirus.

Adults at future risk of exposure to poliomyelitis who previously received one or more doses of OPV or IPV.

Adults at imminent (within 4 wk) risk of exposure to poliomyelitis who are unimmunized.

---

risk of exposure to poliovirus should be given the remaining recommended doses of IPV. If time does not permit completion of the routine schedule, the intervals between doses can be shortened, or OPV can be administered as long as the child is not immunocompromised or does not live in a household with an immunocompromised member. For children who received one or more doses of OPV and for whom OPV is subsequently contraindicated, the series can be completed with IPV. Schedules of an initial one or two doses of IPV followed by two or three doses of OPV are under investigation.

Immunization Recommendations for Adults.

- Routine primary poliovirus vaccination of previously unvaccinated adults (those 18 years or older) residing in the United States is **not** indicated unless they are at increased risk of exposure to wild-type virus or to OPV from household contact (see p 384).
- Immunization is recommended for certain adults who are at a greater risk of exposure to wild polioviruses than the general population, including the following:
  1. Travelers to areas or countries where poliomyelitis is or may be epidemic or endemic.
  2. Members of communities or specific population groups experiencing disease caused by wild polioviruses.
  3. Laboratory workers handling specimens that may contain polioviruses.
  4. Health care workers in close contact with patients who may be excreting polioviruses.

All persons should be fully informed of the two available poliovirus vaccines and of the benefits, risks, and reasons for immunization with one or the other vaccine. Recommendations for immunization of these individuals are as follows:

- *Unvaccinated adults.* Primary immunization with IPV is recommended whenever feasible. Inactivated poliovirus vaccine is preferred because the risk of vaccine-associated paralysis after OPV is slightly higher in adults than in children. Two doses of IPV should be given at intervals of 1 to 2 months; a third dose should be given 6 to 12 months after the second dose.

If time does not allow three doses of IPV to be given according to the recommended schedule before protection is required, the following alternatives are recommended:

TABLE 3.40—Persons for Whom IPV Immunization Is Indicated

Persons with compromised immunity who are unimmunized or partially immunized.

Symptomatic and asymptomatic persons known to be infected with the human immunodeficiency virus (HIV).

Household contacts of an immunodeficient individual, including those known to be HIV infected.

Partially immunized or unimmunized adults (or other close contacts) in households of children to be given OPV (see below).

Unimmunized adults at future risk of exposure to poliomyelitis.

Adults at future risk of exposure to poliomyelitis who have been partially immunized with IPV or OPV.*

Adults at future risk of exposure to poliomyelitis who have had a primary series of IPV.*

Individuals refusing OPV immunization.

*OPV is also acceptable.

1. If 2 months or more are available before protection is needed, three doses of IPV should be given at least 1 month apart.
2. If 1 to 2 months are available before protection is needed, two doses of IPV at least 1 month apart should be given.
3. If less than 1 month is available, a single dose of either OPV or IPV should be given.

In these instances, the remaining doses of vaccine to complete the primary immunization should be subsequently given at the recommended intervals if the person remains at an increased risk.

- *Incompletely immunized adults.* Those who previously received less than a full primary course of OPV or IPV should be given the remaining required doses of vaccine, either OPV or IPV, regardless of the interval since the last dose and the type of vaccine that was previously received.
- *Adults who are at an increased risk of exposure to poliomyelitis and who previously completed a primary course of OPV.* Such adults can be given another dose of OPV or IPV. The need for further supplementary doses has not been established. Adults who previously completed a primary course of IPV may be given a dose of either IPV or OPV. If IPV is used exclusively, additional doses may be given every 5 years, but their need in recipients of enhanced-potency IPV has not been established.

Management of Unimmunized or Inadequately Immunized Adults in Households in Which Children (or Close Contacts of Such Children) Are to Be Given Oral Poliovirus Vaccine.

Adults who have not been adequately immunized against poliomyelitis with OPV or IPV are at risk, albeit small, of developing OPV-associated paralytic poliomyelitis when children in the household or child care facility in which they work are given OPV (see Adverse Vaccine Reactions, p 386). The physician should avoid any unnecessary delay in infant immunization with OPV while minimizing the risk to adult contacts, which may include parents, older relatives, baby-sitters, child care center staff, and others with prolonged contact and opportunity for fecal-oral acquisition. Administering OPV to the infant is recommended regardless of the history of immunization in the adult contact after the responsible adult has been informed of the small risk involved and advised to take precautions concerning contact with feces. An acceptable alternative, provided complete immunization of the infant can be ensured, is to immunize the adult household contacts according to the following guidelines:

- For a susceptible adult who previously received a partial course of OPV or IPV, a dose of IPV is given, and the first dose of OPV is given to the infant.
- For a susceptible adult with no previous immunization or an unknown immunization status, two doses of IPV are given 1 month apart; at the time of the second dose of IPV, the first dose of OPV is administered to the infant. This process can be facilitated by giving the initial IPV dose to the mother and/or other adult contacts when the infant is discharged from the hospital. The remaining dose or doses can then be administered to the adult before or at the time OPV is given to the infant at 2 months of age.

No procedures should be adopted that decrease the likelihood of children being adequately immunized against poliomyelitis.

Precautions and Contraindications to Immunization.

- *Pregnancy.* Although no convincing evidence indicates that increased rates of adverse effects of either OPV or IPV occur in the pregnant woman or developing fetus, immunization during pregnancy should generally be avoided for reasons of theoretical risk. However, if exposure to poliomyelitis is likely, either vaccine can be administered. If immediate protection against poliomyelitis is needed, OPV is recommended.
- *Immunodeficiency disorders.* Patients with immunodeficiency disorders, including HIV infection, combined immunodeficiency, abnormalities of immunoglobulin synthesis, leukemia, lymphoma, or generalized malignancy, or those being given immunosuppressive therapy with pharmacologic agents (see Immunodeficient and Immunosuppressed Children, p 53) or radiation therapy should not receive OPV because of the theoretical or known risk of paralytic disease. Although a protective immune response to IPV in the immunodeficient patient cannot be ensured, IPV is safe and some protection may result from its administration.
- *Household contacts of persons with immunodeficiency disease, altered immune states, immunosuppression due to therapy for other disease, or known HIV infection.* Inactivated poliovirus vaccine is recommended for these individuals, and OPV should not be used. If OPV is inadvertently administered to a household contact of an immunodeficient or HIV-infected person, close contact between the patient and the OPV recipient should be minimized for approximately 2 months after vaccination (the period of maximum excretion of vaccine virus) to the extent that is feasible. Household members should be counseled on practices that will minimize the exposure of the immunodeficient or HIV-infected person to

excreted polio vaccine virus. Since virus is excreted in stool, the risk may be maximal with diaper changes, and persons who must change diapers should be instructed to scrupulously wash hands immediately after so doing.

- *Parents with one or more immunodeficient children.* Because of the possibility of immunodeficiency in other offspring, OPV should not be given to members of a household with this history until the immune status of the recipient and other family members is documented and immunodeficiency has been excluded.

Diarrhea and breast-feeding are not contraindications to either OPV or IPV administration.

Adverse Vaccine Reactions.[*] Oral poliovirus vaccine has been associated with paralysis in vaccinees and their contacts. The approximate risk in the United States is one case of paralytic disease in immunologically healthy vaccine recipients per 6.8 million doses of OPV distributed, and one case of paralytic disease among household and community contacts of vaccinees per 6.4 million doses distributed. The greatest risk of paralysis occurs with the first dose of OPV. From 1980 through 1989, the reported overall frequency of paralysis was one case in 700,000 first doses and one case per 6.9 million subsequent doses. Persons with antibody deficiency disorders who are exposed to vaccine virus either by exposure to a vaccinee or by receiving the vaccine are at higher risk of acquiring paralytic disease. For previously unvaccinated adults, the risk is slightly higher than that in children (see also Epidemiology, p 379). Other than efforts to identify those with immunodeficiency, no procedures are currently available for identifying persons likely to experience this type of adverse reaction.

Vaccinees and their parents should be informed of the extremely small risk of vaccine-associated paralysis for vaccinees and their susceptible, close personal contacts.

No serious side effects of currently available IPV have been documented. Because IPV contains trace amounts of streptomycin and neomycin, hypersensitivity reactions in individuals sensitive to these antibiotics are possible.

Case Investigation and Epidemic Control. Each suspected case of poliomyelitis should be reported promptly to the state health department. Poliomyelitis should be considered in the differential diagnosis of all cases of acute flaccid paralysis. If the course is clinically compatible with poliomyelitis, specimens should be obtained for viral studies and an immediate epidemiologic investigation should be undertaken. If evidence implicates vaccine-derived poliovirus, no vaccination plan need be employed, as no outbreaks associated with vaccine virus in the United States have been documented. If evidence implicates wild-type poliovirus and possible transmission, a vaccination plan designed to contain spread should be employed. Within an epidemic area, OPV should be provided for all persons who have not been completely immunized or whose immunization status is unknown, with the exceptions noted in Precautions and Contraindications to Immunization (p 385).

---

[*]Risk estimates are from Strebel PM, Sutter RW, Cochi SL, et al. Epidemiology of poliomyelitis in the United States one decade after the last reported case of indigenous wild virus-associated disease. *Clin Infect Dis.* 1992;14:568-579.

Q Fever

Clinical Manifestations: Acute Q fever is usually characterized by abrupt onset of fever, chills, weakness, headache, and anorexia, as well as other nonspecific systemic symptoms; chronic Q fever occurs less frequently. Cough and chest pains can signify pneumonia, which occurs in about half the patients. Weight loss and weakness can be pronounced. Hepatosplenomegaly is frequently noted. The illness lasts 1 to 4 weeks, with a gradual resolution. Rash is unusual. Endocarditis and hepatitis are the major manifestations of chronic disease. Although the mortality from acute Q fever is less than 1%, mortality among patients with endocarditis is 30% to 60%.

Etiology: *Coxiella burnetii*, the cause of Q fever, is unique among rickettsiae because it undergoes a host-dependent phase variation.

Epidemiology: Animal infection is widespread, usually asymptomatic, and primarily involves a large variety of domestic farm animals (especially sheep, goats, and cows), but also cats, rodents, marsupials, and other species. Tick vectors may be important in maintaining animal reservoirs. Infectious organisms can persist in the environment for many years. Human disease is uncommon, but many infections are asymptomatic. The disease occurs endemically throughout the world, typically in areas where cattle are raised and sheep and goats are herded. The disease has been transmitted to humans by inhalation of aerosols spontaneously generated from infected material such as placental tissue from infected cats or animals on farms, and by exposure to infected animals or tissues on farms, ranches, or in research facilities. Some animal workers, ranchers, research laboratory workers, and persons in other occupations or with avocational interests that place them in close contact with infected animals or tissues have a heightened risk of disease. Q fever has occurred among flocks of sheep used as experimental subjects in medical research facilities, and transmission to research investigators and technical personnel has been documented. Handling of animal fetuses and products of conception is a major means of infection. Although seasonal trends are not obvious, in some areas the disease coincides with the lambing season in the early spring. Because the birth of farm animals, such as sheep, goats, and cows, is a somewhat controllable event, the disease can occur throughout the year in areas where planned animal births are permitted. Evidence for human intrauterine infection has been reported.

The **incubation period** can vary from 14 to 39 days but is usually between 14 and 22 days.

Diagnostic Tests: Isolation of *C burnetii* from blood is usually not attempted because of the hazard to laboratory workers. Specific antiphase I and antiphase II immunofluorescent, enzyme immunoassay (EIA), complement fixation, and immune adherence hemagglutination antibody tests using paired serum specimens are used diagnostically. Specific IgM, IgG, and IgA tests using immunofluorescence or EIA methods are available in reference and research laboratories. In research laboratories, immunoblotting techniques have been used to diagnose chronic Q fever. *Coxiella burnetii* infection does not cause a positive serum Weil-Felix test.

Treatment: Tetracycline or doxycycline is the drug of choice. Chloramphenicol is an alternative but its efficacy has not been proven. Tetracyclines should not be given to children younger than 9 years unless the benefit is greater than the risk of dental staining. Therapy should be initiated promptly and continued until the patient is afebrile for 2 to 3 days. In chronic Q fever, relapses necessitating repeated courses of antimicrobial therapy can occur. The organism can remain latent in tissues for years; treatment of chronic disease is extremely difficult. Treatment of chronic endocarditis is prolonged and appears to be more effective when tetracycline or doxycycline is combined with rifampin, trimethoprim-sulfamethoxazole, or a quinolone. In patients younger than 18 years, quinolones are usually contraindicated. Relapses can occur after discontinuation of treatment.

Isolation of the Hospitalized Patient: No special precautions are recommended.

Control Measures: Experimental vaccines for domestic animals and laboratory workers are promising but not commercially available. Recommendations have been made to reduce the risk of infection in research facilities involving sheep.* Special safety practices are recommended for nonpropagative laboratory procedures involving *C burnetii* and for all propagative procedures, necropsies of infected animals, and manipulation of infected human and animal tissues. Otherwise, no specific management is recommended for persons who have been exposed. Flash pasteurization of milk at 71.6°C (161.1°F) for 15 seconds or 62.9°C (145.2°F) for 30 minutes destroys the organism, but the epidemiologic role of milk in transmission is uncertain.

Rabies

Clinical Manifestations: Infection with rabies virus characteristically produces an acute illness with rapidly progressive central nervous system manifestations, including anxiety, dysphagia, and convulsions, and almost invariably progresses to death. Some patients may present with paralysis.

Etiology: Rabies virus is an RNA virus classified in the *Rhabdovirus* family.

---

*Bernard KW, Parham GL, Winkler WG, Helmick CG. Q fever control measures: Recommendations for research facilities using sheep. *Infect Control.* 1982;3:461-465; and Harrison RJ, Vugia DJ, Ascher MS. Occupational health guidelines for control of Q fever in sheep research. *Ann NY Acad Sci.* 1990;590:283-290

Epidemiology: A large animal reservoir of sylvatic rabies exists in the United States, including skunks, bats, raccoons, foxes, and other species. In some areas, these wild animals infect domestic dogs, cats, and ferrets. Rabies in small rodents, rabbits, and hares is rare, but in some areas where raccoon rabies is spreading (eg, the mid-Atlantic and northeast states), an increasing number of woodchucks have been found to be rabid. The virus is present in saliva and is transmitted by bites or by licking of mucosa or open wounds. Most rabies cases in humans throughout the world result from dog bites in areas in which canine rabies is enzootic. Although experimental evidence has shown that dogs can harbor the virus in their saliva for as long as 14 days before the appearance of recognizable illness, most dogs and cats become ill within 5 days of virus shedding, and no case of human rabies in the United States has been attributed to a dog or cat that has remained healthy throughout the standard 10-day period of confinement. Airborne transmission has been reported in the laboratory and in bat-infested caves. Transmission has also occurred by transplantation of corneas from patients dying of undiagnosed rabies. Person-to-person transmission by bite has not been documented, although the virus has been isolated from the saliva of patients.

The **incubation period** in humans ranges from 5 days to more than 1 year; 2 months is the average. Recently, incubation periods of many years have been confirmed by antigenic typing of strains.

Diagnostic Tests: Infection in animals can be diagnosed by demonstration of virus-specific fluorescent antigen in brain tissue. Suspected rabid animals should be killed in a manner that does not render brain tissue unfit for examination. Virus can be isolated from brain, saliva, and other tissues in suckling mice or in tissue culture. However, virus isolation takes much longer than fluorescent microscopy of brain tissue. The diagnosis in suspected human cases sometimes can be made premortem or postmortem by fluorescent microscopy of skin biopsies from the nape of the neck, by isolation of the virus from the saliva or cerebrospinal fluid (CSF), or by detection of antibody in the serum and CSF in unvaccinated persons. The laboratory should be consulted before submission of specimens so that appropriate materials can be collected and transport arranged.

Treatment: Once symptoms have developed, no drug or vaccine improves the prognosis. Only three patients with human rabies have survived with intensive, supportive care; all other patients have succumbed despite treatment.

Isolation of the Hospitalized Patient: Strict isolation is recommended for the duration of the illness despite the absence of a proven risk of transmission to human contacts. Those attending the patient should be aware of the possible hazards of contamination with saliva. If the patient has bitten someone, or his saliva has contaminated an open wound or mucous membrane, the involved area should be thoroughly washed and immunization of the contact started (see Care of Exposed Persons, p 392).

Control Measures:

Case Reporting. All patients who are suspected of having rabies should be reported promptly to public health authorities.

Exposure Risk and Decisions to Give Immunoprophylaxis. Exposure to rabies results from a break in the skin caused by the teeth or claws of a rabid animal or by the contamination of scratches, abrasions, or mucous membranes with saliva from a rabid animal. The decision to immunize an exposed individual ordinarily should be made in consultation with the local health department, which can provide information on the risk of rabies in a particular area for each species of animal, and in accordance with the guidelines in Table 3.41 (p 391). In the United States, skunks, raccoons, and bats are more likely to be infected than other animals, but foxes, coyotes, cattle, dogs, and cats occasionally are infected. Bites of rodents (such as squirrels and rats) or lagomorphs (rabbits and hares) rarely require specific antirabies prophylaxis. Additional factors must be considered when deciding if immunization is indicated. An unprovoked attack is more suggestive of a rabid animal than a bite during attempts to feed or handle an animal. Properly immunized dogs and cats have only a minimal chance of developing rabies. However, in rare instances, rabies has developed in properly vaccinated animals, including unusual pets, especially ferrets.

Rabies postexposure prophylaxis is recommended for all persons bitten or scratched by wild or domestic animals that may be infected. Exposures other than bites or scratches rarely result in infection. However, postexposure treatment is recommended for persons who report having an open wound or mucous membrane contaminated with saliva or other potentially infectious material (eg, brain tissue) from a rabid animal. Since the size of bites by bats may be small in comparison to those inflicted by terrestrial animals, postexposure treatment for physical contact with bats when a bite or mucous membrane exposure cannot be excluded may be prudent. Treatment should always be initiated as soon as possible after bites or scratches by known or suspected rabid animals occur.

Postexposure prophylaxis is also recommended for persons who report a possibly infectious exposure (eg, bite, scratch, or open wound or mucous membrane contaminated with saliva or other infectious material) to a human with rabies. However, exposure to a human with rabies has never been implicated as a means of rabies transmission except after cornea transplantation from donors who died of unsuspected rabies encephalitis. Casual contact with an infected person (eg, by touching a patient) or contact with noninfectious fluids or tissues (eg, urine or feces) does not alone constitute an exposure and is not an indication for prophylaxis (see Care of Hospital Contacts, p 392).

Handling of Suspect Animal. A suspect dog or cat that has bitten a human should be captured, confined, and observed by a veterinarian for 10 days. Any illness in the animal should be reported immediately to the local health department. If the animal develops signs of rabies, it should be killed and its head removed and shipped under refrigeration (iced, not frozen) to a qualified laboratory for examination.

Other biting animals, including ferrets and wild animals, that might have exposed a person to rabies should be reported immediately to the local health department. Prior vaccination of an animal may not preclude the

TABLE 3.41—Rabies Postexposure Prophylaxis Guide,
United States, 1991

Animal Type	Evaluation and Disposition of Animal	Postexposure Prophylaxis Recommendations
Dogs and cats	Healthy and available for 10 days observation	Do not begin prophylaxis unless animal develops symptoms of rabies*
	Rabid or suspected rabid†	Immediate vaccination‡ and RIG§
	Unknown (escaped)	Consult public health officials for advice
Skunks, raccoons, bats, foxes, and most other carni- vores; woodchucks	Regarded as rabid unless geographic area is known to be free of rabies or until animal proven negative by laboratory tests.†	Immediate vaccination‡ and RIG§
Livestock, ferrets, rodents, and lago- morphs (rabbits and hares)	Consider individually	Consult public health officials. Bites of squirrels, hamsters, guinea pigs, gerbils, chipmunks, rats, mice, other rodents, rabbits, and hares almost never require antirabies treatment.

*During the 10-d holding period, treatment with RIG§ and vaccine should be initiated at the first sign of rabies in the biting dog or cat. The symptomatic animal should be killed immediately and tested.

†The animal should be killed and tested as soon as possible. Holding for observation is not recommended. Vaccination is discontinued if immunofluorescent test of the animal is negative.

‡See text.

§RIG = Rabies Immune Globulin (Human).

necessity for euthanasia and testing if the period of virus shedding is unknown for that species. Management of animals other than dogs and cats depends on the species, the circumstances of the bite, and the epidemiology of rabies in the area.

Because clinical signs of rabies in a wild animal cannot be interpreted reliably, a suspect wild mammal (or bat) should be killed at once and its brain examined for evidence of rabies. The exposed person need not be treated if examination of the brain by fluorescent antibody procedures is negative for rabies.

Care of Hospital Contacts. Immunization of hospital contacts of a patient with rabies should be reserved for persons who were bitten or whose mucous membranes or open wounds have come in contact with the saliva, CSF, or brain tissue of a patient with rabies (see Care of Exposed Persons, below). Other hospital contacts of a patient with rabies do not require immunization.

Care of Exposed Persons.

Local Care. The immediate objective of postexposure treatment is to prevent virus from entering neural tissue. Prompt and thorough local treatment of all bites and scratches is essential, as virus may remain localized to the area of the bite for a variable time. All wounds should be thoroughly flushed and cleaned with soap and water. Quaternary ammonium compounds (such as Zephiran), which were recommended in the past, are no longer considered superior to soap. The need for tetanus prophylaxis and measures to control bacterial infection should also be considered. The wound, if possible, should not be sutured.

Immunoprophylaxis. After local care is completed, concurrent use of both passive and active immunoprophylaxis is required for optimal therapy (see Table 3.41, p 391). Wherever possible, human rather than equine products should be used for passive immunization, and human diploid cell or fetal rhesus lung diploid vaccine should be used for active immunization. Physicians can obtain expert counsel from their local or state health departments.

Active Immunization. Human diploid cell vaccine (HDCV)[*] or rhesus diploid cell vaccine, Rabies Vaccine Adsorbed (RVA),[†] 1.0 mL, is given intramuscularly in the deltoid area on the first day of treatment, and repeat doses are given on days 3, 7, 14, and 28. A sixth dose is recommended in some European countries but not in the United States, as five doses appear to be equally protective. Serologic testing after HDCV immunization generally has not been necessary, but it has been advised for recipients who may be immunosuppressed.

Care should be taken to ensure that the vaccine is administered intramuscularly. Intradermal vaccine is not advised for postexposure treatment. Because antibody responses in adults who received vaccine in the gluteal area have sometimes been less than in those who were injected in the deltoid muscle, the latter site should always be used, except in infants.

• *Adverse reactions and precautions with HDCV.* Reactions primarily reported in adults after vaccination with HDCV are less common than with previously available vaccines. Reactions are uncommon in children. In a study using five doses of HDCV, local reactions such as pain, erythema, and swelling or itching at the injection site were reported in approximately 25% of the recipients; mild systemic reactions such as headache, nausea, abdominal pain, muscle aches, and dizziness were reported in about 20% of the recipients. Several cases of neurologic illness resembling Guillain-Barré syndrome that resolved without sequelae in 12 weeks, and a focal, subacute, central nervous system disorder temporally associated with

---

[*]Manufactured by Pasteur Merieux Vaccins and available in the United States from Connaught Laboratories, Inc, Swiftwater, PA.
[†]Manufactured by the Michigan Department of Public Health and available from SmithKline Beecham, Philadelphia, PA.

HDCV have been reported. The rate of neurologic abnormalities after HDCV is approximately 1 in 150,000.

Immune-complex-like reactions in persons receiving booster doses of HDCV have been observed. The reaction, characterized by onset 2 to 21 days postinoculation, presents with a generalized urticaria and can include arthralgia, arthritis, angioedema, nausea, vomiting, fever, and malaise. These illnesses were in no instances life threatening. Current estimates suggest that this immune-complex-like illness can occur in as many as 6% of adults receiving booster doses as part of a pre-exposure immunization regimen; it is rare in persons receiving primary immunization, which includes most children receiving vaccine in the United States. All serious, systemic, neuroparalytic or anaphylactic reactions to the rabies vaccine should be reported immediately (see Reporting of Adverse Reactions, p 30).

If the patient has a serious allergic reaction to HDCV, the RVA vaccine produced in rhesus diploid cells can be given on the same schedule as HDCV.

Although the safety of the use of rabies vaccine during pregnancy is known only through sporadic experiences, pregnancy should not be considered a contraindication to the use of vaccine after exposure.

• *Nerve tissue vaccines.* Nerve tissue vaccines are not licensed in the United States, but are available in many areas of the world. These preparations induce neuroparalytic reactions in between 1:2,000 and 1:8,000 recipients. Immunization with nerve tissue vaccine should be discontinued if meningeal or neuroparalytic reactions develop. Corticosteroids can be used for treatment of complications, but they should be used only for life-threatening reactions because they definitely increase the risk of rabies in experimentally inoculated animals.

Passive Immunization. Rabies Immune Globulin (Human) (RIG)* should be used concomitantly with the first dose of vaccine for postexposure prophylaxis to bridge the time between onset of treatment and active antibody production by the vaccinee. The exception to the concomitant use of vaccine and RIG is the patient previously immunized with HDCV (or another rabies vaccine if the patient is known to have developed serum antibody); these patients should be given two doses of vaccine only, one immediately (day 0) and the other on day 3. If vaccine is not immediately available, RIG should be given alone and vaccination started later. If RIG is not immediately available, vaccine should be given followed by RIG when obtained in the first 8 days after the beginning of treatment. If administration of both vaccine and RIG are delayed, both should be used regardless of the interval between exposure and treatment; but every effort should be made to give RIG as soon as possible after exposure.

The recommended dose of RIG is 20 IU per kilogram of body weight. Approximately one half of the antibody preparation is used to infiltrate the wound(s); the remainder is given intramuscularly. Rabies IG is supplied in 2-mL (300 IU) and 10-mL (1,500 IU) vials. Passive antibody can inhibit the response to rabies vaccines; therefore, the recommended dose should not be

---

*Available from Connaught Laboratories, Inc, Swiftwater, PA, and from Miles, Inc, West Haven, CT.

exceeded. Vaccine should never be administered in the same parts of the body or with the same syringe used to give RIG. Rabies IG is virtually free of hypersensitivity reactions.

Rabies IG is not recommended for the following exposed persons: (1) those who previously received postexposure prophylaxis with HDCV or RVA; (2) those who received a three-dose, intramuscular, pre-exposure regimen of HDCV or RVA; (3) those who received a three-dose, intradermal, pre-exposure regimen of HDCV with the Merieux product (distributed by Connaught) in the United States; and (4) those who have a documented adequate rabies titer after previous vaccination with any other rabies vaccine. These persons should receive two 1.0-mL doses of HDCV or RVA; doses are given on the day of exposure and on day 3.

- *Complete postexposure antirabies treatment*, including RIG, should be given if an exposed person immunized previously with vaccines other than HDCV has not had previous documentation of a serum antibody response.

Pre-exposure Control Measures, Including Immunization. The relatively low frequency of reactions to HDCV has made practical pre-exposure immunization for persons in high-risk groups, such as veterinarians, animal handlers, certain laboratory workers, children living in areas where rabies is a constant threat, and persons traveling to live in areas where rabies is common. Others, such as spelunkers, whose vocational or avocational pursuits in exploring caves result in frequent exposures to dogs, cats, foxes, skunks, or bats, should also be considered for pre-exposure prophylaxis.

Rabies Vaccine Adsorbed (RVA) is licensed for intramuscular administration only. Both intramuscular (1.0 mL) and intradermal (0.1 mL) dosage forms of HDCV are available. The latter is cheaper and only slightly less immunogenic. The schedule is the same for both routes of administration: three injections given on days 0, 7, and 28. This series of immunizations has resulted in the development of antibodies in virtually 100% of persons properly vaccinated. For this reason, routine serologic testing for rabies antibody is no longer indicated. The preferred site of administration for intradermal vaccine is the skin over the deltoid area.

Persons who are taking chloroquine or related drugs, such as mefloquine, should receive HDCV by the intramuscular route. A single case of rabies immunization failure in an individual living in a foreign country who was vaccinated intradermally has been reported; failure was probably related to the immunosuppressive effect of the concurrent administration of chloroquine for malaria prophylaxis.

Serum antibody titers decline by 2 years after the primary series given intramuscularly. Booster vaccination with HDCV (1.0 mL intramuscularly or 0.1 mL intradermally) or with RVA intramuscularly will produce an effective anamnestic response. However, significant allergic reactions have been associated with booster vaccination in about 6% of individuals; therefore, boosters are not routinely recommended unless the risk of exposure to rabies virus is likely to be continuous or frequent. This group includes veterinarians, animal handlers, and laboratory workers exposed to high concentrations of rabies virus (eg, in certain research or production laboratories). In these persons, rabies serum antibody titers should be determined at 6-month intervals, and booster doses of vaccine should be administered as appropriate to maintain antibody concentrations. The Centers for Disease Control and Prevention currently specifies complete virus neutralization at a 1:5 or greater titer by the rapid fluorescent-focus inhibition test as acceptable. The World Health Organization specifies 0.5 IU/mL or more as acceptable.

Public Health. A variety of approved public health measures, including immunization of dogs, cats, and ferrets, and the elimination of stray dogs and selected wildlife, are used to control rabies in animals. Unvaccinated dogs, cats, or other pets bitten by a known rabid animal should be destroyed immediately. If the owner is unwilling to have this done, the animal should be vaccinated and placed in strict isolation for 6 months. If the animal has a current vaccination (within 1 to 3 years, depending on the vaccine administered and local regulations), it should be revaccinated and restrained by leashing and confinement for 90 days.

Physicians should also urge parents and teachers to caution children against provoking or attempting to capture stray or wild animals as personal or family pets.

Rat-bite Fever

Clinical Manifestations: Rat-bite fever is characterized by fever of abrupt onset, chills, a maculopapular or petechial rash predominantly on the extremities, muscle pain, and headache. Specific clinical manifestations depend on the infecting organism. With *Streptobacillus moniliformis* infection (streptobacillary or Haverhill fever), the bite usually heals promptly, followed by nonsuppurative migratory polyarthritis or arthralgia in about 50% of the patients. Complications include soft-tissue and solid-organ abscesses, pneumonia, endocarditis, and pericarditis. With *Spirillum minus* infection, a period of initial apparent healing at the site of the bite is usually followed by ulceration, regional lymphangitis and lymphadenopathy, a distinctive rash of red or purple plaques, and, rarely, arthritic symptoms.

Etiology: Rat-bite fever is caused by either of two organisms: *S moniliformis*, a microaerophilic, Gram-negative, pleomorphic bacillus; and *S minus*, a small, Gram-negative, spiral organism with bipolar flagellar tufts.

Epidemiology: Rat-bite fever is a zoonotic illness. *Streptobacillus moniliformis* and *Spirillum minus* are found in upper respiratory tract secretions of infected animals. *Streptobacillus moniliformis* is transmitted by the bite of rats, squirrels, mice, cats, and weasels; by ingestion of contaminated food or milk products; and by contact with an infected animal. Haverhill fever refers to infection after ingestion of milk contaminated with *S moniliformis*. *Spirillum minus* is transmitted by the bite of rats and mice. On rare occasion, *S moniliformis* and *S minus* have been reported to be transmitted from person to person by a blood transfusion. Streptobacillary disease accounts for most cases of rat-bite fever in the United States; *S minus* infections occur primarily in Asia. Both infections are currently rare.

The **incubation period** for *S moniliformis* is usually 3 to 10 days; for *S minus* it is 7 to 21 days.

Diagnostic Tests: *Streptobacillus moniliformis* can be isolated from blood, joint fluid, or material from the bite lesion by inoculation into bacteriologic media enriched with horse serum. Since it is a fastidious organism, the laboratory should be notified that rat-bite fever is suspected.

Spirillum minus has not been recovered on artificial media. Organisms can be seen in blood smears by darkfield microscopy or on Wright-stained smears. *Spirillum minus* can be recovered from blood, lymph nodes, or local lesions by intraperitoneal inoculation of mice or guinea pigs.

Treatment: Procaine penicillin should be administered intramuscularly for 7 to 10 days for rat-bite fever caused by either agent. Initial intravenous penicillin G therapy for 5 days followed by oral penicillin V has been successful. Tetracycline, chloramphenicol, or streptomycin may be substituted in the patient who is allergic to penicillin. Tetracycline should not be given to children younger than 9 years of age unless the benefits of therapy are greater than the risks of dental staining. Patients with endocarditis should receive intravenous, high-dose penicillin G for at least 4 weeks. The addition of streptomycin initially may be useful.

Isolation of the Hospitalized Patient: No special precautions are recommended.

Control Measures: Exposed persons should be observed for symptoms. Rat control is important.

Respiratory Syncytial Virus

(See also Ribavirin Therapy of Respiratory Syncytial Virus, p 570)

Clinical Manifestations: Respiratory syncytial virus (RSV) causes acute respiratory illness in patients of any age. In infants and young children, it is the most important cause of bronchiolitis and pneumonia. During the first few weeks of life, particularly in preterm infants, respiratory signs can be minimal. Lethargy, irritability, and poor feeding, sometimes accompanied by apneic episodes, may be the major signs. Reinfection throughout life is common. Infection in older children and adults usually manifests as an upper respiratory tract illness, occasionally with bronchitis. Exacerbation of asthma or other chronic lung conditions is also common.

Etiology: Respiratory syncytial virus, a large, enveloped RNA virus, is a paramyxovirus. Two major strains (A and B) usually circulate concurrently.

The clinical and epidemiologic importance of this strain variation is yet to be determined.

Epidemiology: Humans are the only source of infection. Transmission is usually by direct or close contact with contaminated secretions, which may involve droplets or fomites. Virus can persist on environmental surfaces for many hours, and for one-half hour or more on the hands. Infection among hospital personnel can occur by self-inoculation with contaminated infant secretions. Hospital-acquired infections are frequent among both personnel and infants, and have significant impact on morbidity, mortality, and duration of hospitalization. Initial infection occurs most commonly during the first year of life. Severe illness can develop in infants and young children with compromised cardiac, pulmonary, or immune function. Immunodeficient children are also at risk for severe disease and can have prolonged viral shedding.

Respiratory syncytial virus usually occurs in annual epidemics during the winter and early spring, and it infects essentially all children during the first 3 years of life. Spread among household and child care contacts, including adults, is common. The period of viral shedding is usually 3 to 8 days, but it may be longer, especially in young infants in whom shedding may continue for as long as 3 to 4 weeks.

The **incubation period** ranges from 2 to 8 days; 4 to 6 days is most common.

Diagnostic Tests: Viral isolation from nasopharyngeal secretions is usually accomplished within 3 to 8 days. Respiratory syncytial virus is a relatively labile virus, and infectivity decreases rapidly at room temperature and after freeze-thawing. The laboratory should be consulted for optimal methods of collection and transport of specimens. Rapid diagnostic procedures, including immunofluorescent and enzyme immunoassay techniques, for the direct detection of viral antigen in clinical specimens are commercially available. The sensitivity of these assays in comparison to culture varies between 53% and 96%, but most are in the range of 80% to 90%. Serologic testing of acute and convalescent sera can be used to confirm infection; however, infection may not always be accompanied by detectable seroconversion, especially in young infants.

Treatment: Ribavirin, administered by small-particle aerosol for 12 to 20 hours each day, is recommended for hospitalized infants who have, or are at high risk for, severe RSV infection. (For specific indications and details of use, see Ribavirin Therapy of Respiratory Syncytial Virus Infection, p 570.)

Isolation of the Hospitalized Patient: Contact isolation precautions should be effective in preventing nosocomial transmission of RSV. The effectiveness of these measures, however, is dependent on compliance. In theory, strict attention to good hand washing practices should prevent transmission, but other measures, such as gloving, may help by improving staff compliance with hand washing between patients. During the peak RSV season, many infants and children hospitalized with respiratory symptoms will be infected with RSV and should be managed with contact isolation precautions. These precautions should include strict attention to good hand washing practices and wearing gowns when soiling of clothing may occur.

Control Measures: The control of nosocomial RSV is complicated by the continuing chance for introduction through infected patients, staff, and visitors. During large outbreaks, a variety of measures have been instituted and demonstrated to be effective, including (1) screening patients for RSV infection, (2) cohorting infected patients and staff, (3) excluding visitors with respiratory infections, and (4) excluding staff with respiratory illness or RSV infection from caring for susceptible infants. In several studies, the use of eye-nose goggles by staff decreased nosocomial RSV. These additional measures may be most important in preventing transmission to patients with compromised cardiac, pulmonary, or immune systems.

Rhinovirus Infections

Clinical Manifestations: Rhinovirus infections are usually the most frequent cause of the common cold in adults and a major cause in children. Rhinoviruses can also be involved in bronchitis, sinusitis, otitis media, and, perhaps, lower respiratory tract disease in young children. However, their role in the latter has not been proved. Rhinoviruses can precipitate asthmatic attacks.

Etiology: Rhinoviruses are RNA viruses classified as picodnaviruses. At least 100 antigenic types have been identified. Infection with one type appears to confer lasting type-specific immunity, but offers no protection against other types.

Epidemiology: Humans are the only known hosts. Transmission occurs by close person-to-person contact, respiratory droplets, fomites, and self-inoculation after contamination of the hands. Infections occur throughout the year, but peak activity is usually in the fall and spring. Several serotypes usually circulate simultaneously, but the prevalent types in a population tend to change from year to year. By adulthood, antibody to approximately one half of the serotypes has usually developed. Household spread is common. The period of communicability is variable, but it tends to correlate with the presence of clinical symptoms and the amount of virus shed. Rhinoviruses are usually shed from nasopharyngeal secretions for 7 days or less but shedding can be as long as 3 weeks.

The **incubation period** is approximately 2 to 5 days.

Diagnostic Tests: Inoculation of nasal secretions in appropriate tissue cultures for viral isolation is the best means of making a specific diagnosis. The large number of antigenic types makes serologic testing impractical.

Treatment: Symptomatic treatment only is given. However, placebo-controlled studies indicate that over-the-counter antihistamine/decongestant cold medications are ineffective, especially in children younger than 5 years of age.

Isolation of the Hospitalized Patient: Contact isolation precautions are advisable for hospitalized young children and infants. Respiratory secretions should be considered infectious for the duration of the illness (usually 7 days or less). Careful hand washing diminishes the possibility of nosocomial spread.

Control Measures: Frequent hand washing and hygienic measures in schools, households, and other settings where transmission is common may help reduce rhinovirus spread.

Rickettsial Diseases

The rickettsiae are pleomorphic bacteria, and most have arthropod vectors. Humans are incidental hosts and are not useful in propagating the organism in nature except for louse-borne epidemic typhus, for which humans are the principal reservoir and the human body louse is the vector. Except for members of the genera *Rochalimaea* and *Bartonella*, rickettsiae are obligate intracellular parasites and cannot be grown in cell-free media. They have typical bacterial cell walls and cytoplasmic membranes, and divide by binary fission. Their natural life cycles usually involve lower mammalian species as reservoirs (with the exception of *Rickettsia prowazekii*, the cause of epidemic typhus), and animal-to-human or vector-to-human transmission occurs as a result of environmental or occupational exposure.

Ticks are the vector for many of these diseases. Thus, control measures concern prevention of tick transmission of rickettsial agents to humans (see Control Measures for Prevention of Tick-Borne Infections, p 114).

Rickettsial infections have many features in common, including the following:

- Multiplication of the organism in an arthropod host (except Q fever).
- Intracellular replication (except *Rochalimaea* sp).
- Limited geographic and seasonal occurrence related to arthropod life cycles, activity, and distribution.
- Zoonotic diseases.
- Humans are incidental hosts (except for louse-borne typhus).
- Local, primary lesions occur with some rickettsial diseases.
- Fever, rash (except in Q fever and in most cases of ehrlichiosis), headache, myalgias, and respiratory symptoms are prominent features.
- Generalized capillary and small-vessel endothelial damage, thrombus formation, and tissue necrosis are common pathologic features (except in Q fever and cat scratch disease, which is currently considered to be a rickettsial infection).

- With the exception of Q fever, rickettsialpox, and *Rochalimaea* infections, nonspecific serum *Proteus* agglutinins (Weil-Felix reaction) develop during infection. However, their presence is frequently unreliable in diagnosis, since both false-positive and false-negative test results can occur.
- Group-specific serum antibodies are detectable in convalescence.
- Various serologic tests for detecting these antibodies, including indirect immunofluorescence, complement fixation, microagglutination, indirect hemagglutination, latex fixation, enzyme immunoassay, radioisotope precipitation, and radioimmunoassay, are available or in development in reference and research laboratories. The immunofluorescent test is recommended in most cases because of its relative simplicity, sensitivity, and specificity.
- Immunity after natural infection is usually of long duration against reinfection by the same agent (except in the case of scrub typhus caused by *Rickettsia tsutsugamushi*). Among the four different groups of rickettsial diseases, generally partial or complete cross-immunity is conferred by infections with rickettsiae within groups but not between groups.
- Infections usually respond to tetracyclines or chloramphenicol if given early and in adequate dosage, although these drugs are rickettsiostatic and not rickettsicidal. Tetracycline drugs should not be given to children younger than 9 years unless the benefits of therapy are greater than the risks of dental staining in comparison to the relative benefits and risks of alternative drugs.
- Treatment early in the course of illness can blunt serologic responses.
- Many rickettsial diseases, especially Rocky Mountain spotted fever and Q fever, are reportable to state and local health departments.

For details, the following chapters on rickettsial diseases should be consulted:

- Cat scratch disease (presumed, as of December 1993, to be a rickettsial infection)
- Ehrlichiosis
- Q fever
- Rickettsialpox
- Rocky Mountain spotted fever
- Endemic typhus
- Epidemic typhus

A number of other epidemiologically distinct but clinically similar tick-borne spotted-fever infections caused by rickettsiae have been recognized. The etiologic agents of some of these infections share the same group antigen as *Rickettsia rickettsii*; these include *Rickettsia conorii*, the etiologic agent of Boutonneuse fever (also known as Kenya tick-bite fever, African tick typhus, Mediterranean spotted fever, India tick typhus, and Marseille fever) endemic in southern Europe, Africa, and the Middle East; *Rickettsia sibericus*, the etiologic agent of Siberian tick typhus endemic in central Asia; and *Rickettsia australis*, the etiologic agent of Queensland tick typhus endemic in eastern Australia. All of these infections have clinical, pathologic, and epidemiologic features similar to those of Rocky Mountain spotted fever and are treated similarly, but they are usually milder and associated with a small indurated lesion that develops at the site of the tick bite ("tache noire"), with resultant eschar and regional lymph node enlargement. The specific diagnosis is confirmed serologically. These conditions are of importance among persons traveling to endemic areas.

Rickettsialpox

Clinical Manifestations: Rickettsialpox is characterized by generalized erythematous papulovesicular eruptions on the trunk, extremities (including face, palms, and soles), and mucous membranes after the appearance of a primary lesion at the site of the bite of the mouse mite vector. A black scab or eschar develops at the site about the time of fever onset. Systemic disease lasts about 1 week; manifestations can include chills, fever, headache, myalgias, anorexia, photophobia, and regional lymphadenopathy. The disease is self-limited, nonfatal, and without complications.

Etiology: Rickettsialpox is caused by *Rickettsia akari*, which is classified with the spotted-fever-group rickettsiae and antigenically is related to *Rickettsia rickettsii*.

Epidemiology: The natural host for *R akari* in the United States is *Mus musculus*, the common house mouse. The disease is transmitted by the mouse mite *Allodermanyssus sanguineous*. Disease risk is heightened in areas infested with mice. The disease was first recognized in apartment house dwellers in New York City and was found in large urban settings, paralleling the distribution of mice. The disease has also been recognized in Russia, Korea, and Africa. All age groups can be affected. No seasonal pattern of disease occurs. The disease is not communicable among humans. It is currently rare in the United States.

The **incubation period** is 9 to 14 days.

Diagnostic Tests: *Rickettsia akari* can be isolated from blood during the acute stage of disease, but this is not routinely attempted and should only be done in specialized laboratories. The Weil-Felix test for all Proteus OX agglutinins is negative. An indirect fluorescent antibody or complement fixation test for *R rickettsii* (the cause of Rocky Mountain spotted fever) will demonstrate fourfold change in antibody titers between acute and convalescent sera, since antibodies to *R akari* have extensive cross-reactivity with those against *R rickettsii*.

Treatment: Tetracycline or chloramphenicol will shorten the course of the disease; symptoms resolve within 48 hours of initiating antirickettsial therapy. Tetracyclines should not be given to children younger than 9 years unless the benefits of therapy are greater than the risks of dental staining. Treatment is effective when given for 3 to 5 days; relapse is rare.

Isolation of the Hospitalized Patient: No special precautions are recommended.

Control Measures: Disinfestation with residual insecticides and rodent control measures limit or eliminate the vector. No specific management of exposed persons is necessary.

Rocky Mountain Spotted Fever

Clinical Manifestations: Rocky Mountain spotted fever (RMSF) is a systemic, febrile illness with a characteristic rash usually occurring before the sixth day. Fever, headache, myalgia, toxicity, and nausea or vomiting are major clinical features. Abdominal pain and cough are noted less frequently. The rash initially is erythematous and macular, and later can become maculopapular and frequently petechial. Rash first appears on the wrists and ankles, spreading within hours proximally to the trunk. The palms and soles are typically involved. Although early development of a rash is a useful diagnostic sign, in some cases the rash fails to develop or develops only late in the illness. The disease can last as long as 3 weeks and can be severe with prominent central nervous system involvement; involvement of cardiac, pulmonary, gastrointestinal, renal, or other organs; disseminated intravascular coagulation; and shock leading to death.

Etiology: *Rickettsia rickettsii* is an obligate intracellular pathogen and a member of the spotted fever group of rickettsiae.

Epidemiology: The disease is transmitted to humans by the bite of ticks. Many small wild animals and dogs have antibodies to *R rickettsii*, but their exact role as natural hosts is not clear since ticks are both reservoirs and vectors of *R rickettsii*. In ticks, the agent is transmitted transovarially and between stages. Persons with occupational or recreational exposure to the tick vector (eg, pet owners, animal handlers, and outdoor persons) are at an increased risk of acquiring the organism. Persons of all ages, races, socio-economic status, and both sexes can be infected, but most cases occur in those younger than 15 years, probably because they are most frequently in tick habitats. Laboratory-acquired infection has occurred by accidental inoculation and aerosol contamination. Transmission has occurred on rare occasion by blood transfusion. Mortality is highest in males, in persons older than 30 years, in nonwhites, and in persons with no known tick bite or attachment. Delay in disease recognition because of the lack of history of tick bite and resulting delay in initiation of appropriate antimicrobial therapy can lead to death.

The disease is widespread in the United States. Most cases are reported in the south Atlantic, southeastern, and south central states. Focal sites in an affected area can account for much of the morbidity in an area. The dog tick (*Dermacentor variabilis*) is primarily responsible for transmission in these geographic areas, and summer is the season of highest prevalence. In the western United States, the upper Rocky Mountain states have the highest incidence; the vector is usually the wood tick (*Dermacenter andersoni*). The Lone Star tick (*Amblyomma americanum*) is a vector of *R rickettsii* in south central United States. Transmission parallels the tick season in a given geographic area. Spring and summer are the seasons of highest prevalence. The disease also occurs in Canada, Mexico, and Central and South America.

The **incubation period** is usually about 1 week but ranges from 1 to 14 days. It appears to be related to the size of the rickettsial inoculum.

Diagnostic Tests: Culture of *R rickettsii* is usually not attempted because of the dangers of transmission to laboratory personnel; only those laboratories with adequate biohazard containment equipment should attempt isolation of rickettsiae. The diagnosis can be established retrospectively by one of the multiple rickettsial group-specific serologic tests by the finding of a fourfold increase or decrease in antibody titer between acute and convalescent sera, as determined by indirect immunofluorescence, complement fixation, latex agglutination, indirect hemagglutination, or microagglutination tests. The indirect fluorescent antibody (IFA) and indirect hemagglutination (IHA) are the most sensitive and specific of these tests. Antibodies are detected by IFA 7 to 10 days after onset of illness. A microtiter enzyme immunoassay has been developed to characterize the IgM and IgG responses to *R rickettsii*. The complement fixation and microagglutination tests are highly specific for this disease, but they lack sensitivity, particularly if the patient has received early antibiotic treatment. Criteria for diagnosis with single convalescent serum specimens have been established. The nonspecific and insensitive Weil-Felix serologic reaction (Proteus OX-19 and OX-2 agglutinins) becomes positive 10 to 14 days after onset of the illness. No microbiologic test is readily available for rapid diagnosis early in the illness. However, *R rickettsii* have been identified by immunofluorescent staining of skin biopsy specimens obtained from the site of the rash. With adequate specimens, this method can be 70% sensitive and 100% specific, but it is not widely available.

In reference laboratories, polymerase chain reaction technology has been applied to detection of *R rickettsii* in blood during acute phase illness. Polymerase chain reaction has been found to be a specific but insensitive test.

Treatment: Early initiation of treatment based on clinical manifestations and epidemiologic considerations affords the highest likelihood of success in patients with suspected RMSF. Chloramphenicol or a tetracycline is the drug of choice. Tetracycline drugs should not be routinely given to children younger than 9 years of age. However, when comparing the benefits and risks of tetracycline and chloramphenicol in children younger than 9 years of age, some experts consider tetracycline to be the drug of choice for children of any age with presumed or proven RMSF. Therapy is continued until the patient is afebrile for at least 2 or 3 days. A usual course is 6 to 10 days.

Isolation of the Hospitalized Patient: No special precautions are recommended.

Control Measures: Control of ticks in their natural habitat is not practical. Avoidance of tick-infested areas is the best preventive measure. If a tick-infested area is entered, persons should wear protective clothing and apply tick/insect repellents to clothes and exposed body parts for added protection. They should be taught to thoroughly inspect themselves, their children (bodies and clothing), and pets for ticks after spending time outdoors during the tick season, and to remove ticks promptly (see Control Measures for Prevention of Tick-Borne Infections, p 114).

No licensed *R rickettsii* vaccine is currently available in the United States.

Rotavirus Infections

Clinical Manifestations: Infection can result in diarrhea, usually preceded or accompanied by emesis and low-grade fever. In severe cases, severe dehydration and acidosis may occur. Infection can also be accompanied by respiratory symptoms, such as cough and coryza. Neurologic symptoms occur in severe cases resulting from electrolyte imbalance or possibly direct viral infection of the central nervous system. Infection in immunocompromised children, including those with HIV infection, can result in a persistent infection associated with multisystem abnormalities.

Etiology: Rotaviruses (RV) are members of the family *Reoviridae* and are RNA viruses, with at least five distinct antigenic groups (A to E). Group A viruses are major causes of infantile diarrhea in the United States. At least six serotypes within group A have been identified. Groups B and C viruses can cause gastroenteritis in adults, especially in China and other parts of the world.

Epidemiology: Most human infections result from contact with infected humans. Rotavirus infections in animals occur in many species, but transmission from animals to humans has not been documented. Rotavirus in infected patients is present in high titer in stools, which is the only body specimen consistently positive. It can persist for as long as 10 days in normal hosts after the onset of symptoms. Transmission is believed to be by the fecal-oral route. Rotavirus can be found on toys and other surfaces in child care centers, indicating that fomites may serve as a mechanism of transmission. Respiratory transmission may also play a role in disease transmission. Spread within families and within institutions is common. Rotavirus is the most common cause of nosocomially acquired diarrhea in children and is an important cause of acute gastroenteritis in children attending child care. Common-source outbreaks have been reported.

Human RV infections occur throughout the world and are the single most common agent of diarrhea in infants younger than 2 years who require medical attention in developed countries. Death from dehydration, although unusual in developed countries, is a major cause of mortality in developing countries. Disease is most prevalent during the cooler months of the year in temperate climates. Seasonal variation in tropical climates is less pronounced. Although clinically apparent cases of gastroenteritis occur most commonly when infants are between 4 and 24 months old, serologic evidence of infection has been demonstrated in other age groups. Children can experience multiple infections. Infections in neonates are often asymptomatic. Although breast-feeding does not completely prevent infection, breast-fed infants may have milder RV illnesses. Serologic evidence of reinfection, frequently without clinical symptoms, is known to occur in adult contacts of RV-infected infants.

The **incubation period** is usually from 1 to 3 days.

Diagnostic Tests: Enzyme immunoassay (EIA) and latex agglutination assays for RV detection in stool are commercially available. Both assays are sensitive for the detection of RV antigens during symptomatic infection. However, EIAs are more sensitive for the detection of antigen late in the course of illness. Although the assays generally have high specificity, nonspecific reactions can occur in neonates and in persons with underlying intestinal pathology. These nonspecific reactions can be distinguished from true positives by the performance of confirmatory assays. In research laboratories, virus can also be identified in stool by electron microscopy and nucleic acid amplification techniques. Epidemiologic analysis of strains can be performed by determination of the viral RNA migration patterns on polyacrylamide gel electrophoresis. Strains can be further characterized by subgroup and serotype by other research techniques.

Treatment: No specific therapy is available. Oral or parenteral fluids are given to correct dehydration.* Orally administered human immunoglobulins have been used as an investigational therapy in a small number of immunocompromised patients with prolonged infections.

Isolation of the Hospitalized Patient: Strict adherence to enteric precautions is indicated for the duration of the illness. In view of the prolonged fecal shedding of low concentration of virus after recovery, continued enteric precautions for the duration of hospitalization should be considered if transmission to immunocompromised and other high-risk infants can occur.

Control Measures:

Child Care. General measures for interrupting enteric transmission in child care centers are recommended (see Children in Out-of-Home Child Care, p 83). Specific, effective control measures have not been established. Children with RV diarrhea in whom stool cannot be contained by diapers or toilet use should be excluded until the diarrhea ceases. Surfaces should be washed with soap and water. Disinfectants may also help prevent disease transmission resulting from contact with environmental surfaces.

Vaccines. Field trials of live-attenuated, orally administered Group A vaccines for safety and efficacy are in progress.

---

*For further information and detailed recommendations, see Duggan C, Santosham M, Glass RI. The management of acute diarrhea in children: oral rehydration, maintenance, and nutritional therapy. *MMWR.* 1992;41(RR-16):1-20

Rubella

Clinical Manifestations:

Postnatal Rubella. Rubella is usually a mild disease characterized by an erythematous, maculopapular, discrete rash, generalized lymphadenopathy (most commonly suboccipital, postauricular, and cervical), and slight fever. Transient polyarthralgia and polyarthritis occasionally occur in children and are common in adolescents and adults, especially females. Encephalitis and thrombocytopenia are rare complications.

Congenital Rubella. The most commonly described anomalies associated with congenital rubella are ophthalmologic (cataracts, microphthalmia, glaucoma, and chorioretinitis), cardiac (patent ductus arteriosus, peripheral pulmonary artery stenosis, and atrial or ventricular septal defects), auditory (sensorineural deafness), and neurologic (microcephaly, meningoencephalitis, and mental retardation). In addition, infants with congenital rubella are frequently growth-retarded and have radiolucent bone disease, hepatosplenomegaly, thrombocytopenia, jaundice, and purple skin lesions ("blueberry muffin" appearance). Mild forms of the disease can be associated with few or no obvious clinical manifestations at birth.

Etiology: Rubella virus is an RNA virus classified as a rubivirus in the *Togaviridae* family.

Epidemiology: Humans are the only source of infection. Postnatal rubella is transmitted chiefly through direct or droplet contact from nasopharyngeal secretions. The peak incidence of infection is in the late winter and early spring. Approximately 25% to 50% of infections are asymptomatic. The period of maximal communicability appears to be the few days before, and 5 to 7 days after, onset of the rash. Volunteer studies have demonstrated the presence of rubella virus in nasopharyngeal secretions from 7 days before to 14 days after the onset of the rash. A small number of infants with congenital rubella continue to shed virus in nasopharyngeal secretions and urine for 1 year or more and can transmit infection to susceptible contacts. In approximately 10% to 20% of these patients, virus can be isolated from the nasopharynx when the infant is 6 months old.

Before the widespread use of rubella vaccine, rubella was an epidemic disease, occurring in 6- to 9-year cycles, and most cases occurred in children. The incidence of rubella in the United States has declined by approximately 99% from the prevaccine era. The risk of acquiring rubella has declined sharply in all age groups, including adolescents and young adults. In the vaccine era, most cases have occurred in young, unvaccinated adults after outbreaks in colleges and occupational settings. Although the number of susceptible individuals has decreased since licensure of rubella vaccine, recent serologic surveys have indicated that approximately 10% of young adults are susceptible to rubella. This degree of susceptibility in young adults is the result of lack of vaccination, not waning immunity in immunized persons.

The **incubation period** for postnatal rubella ranges from 14 to 21 days, usually 16 to 18 days.

Diagnostic Tests: Rubella virus most consistently can be isolated from nasal specimens by inoculation of appropriate tissue culture. Throat swabs, blood, urine, and cerebrospinal fluid can also yield virus, particularly in congenitally infected infants. Serologic testing is also useful for confirming the presence of infection, especially in the absence of typical clinical manifestations. Acute and convalescent sera should be tested; a fourfold or greater rise in antibody titer or seroconversion is indicative of infection. Many virology laboratories can detect rubella-specific immunoglobulin M (IgM) antibody, the presence of which indicates recent postnatal infection or congenital infection in a newborn infant. Congenital infection can also be confirmed by stable or increasing serum concentrations of IgG rubella-specific antibody during a period of several months. Every effort should be made to establish a laboratory diagnosis when rubella infection is suspected in pregnant women or newborn infants. The diagnosis of congenital rubella infection in children older than 1 year is difficult; serology is usually not diagnostic and viral isolation, while confirmatory, is possible in only a small proportion of congenitally infected children of this age. The hemagglutination inhibition (HAI) rubella antibody test, which previously was the most frequently used method of serologic screening, has been generally supplanted by a number of equally or more sensitive assays for determining rubella immunity, including latex agglutination, fluorescence immunoassay, passive hemagglutination, hemolysis-in-gel, and enzyme immunoassay tests. Some persons in whom antibody has been absent by HAI testing have been found to be immune by more sensitive tests.

Treatment: Supportive.

Isolation of the Hospitalized Patient: For postnatal rubella, contact isolation is required for 7 days after the onset of the rash. Contact isolation is also required for congenitally infected infants and infants suspected of having congenital rubella. Infants with congenital rubella should be considered contagious until they are 1 year old, unless nasopharyngeal and urine cultures after 3 months of age are repeatedly negative for rubella virus.

Control Measures:

School and Child Care. Children with postnatal rubella should be excluded from school or child care for 7 days after the onset of the rash. Patients with congenital rubella in child care should be considered contagious until they are 1 year old, unless nasopharyngeal and urine cultures are negative for rubella. Mothers should be made aware of the potential hazard of their infants to susceptible, pregnant contacts.

Care of Exposed Persons. When a pregnant woman is exposed to rubella, a blood specimen should be obtained as soon as possible and tested for rubella antibody. An aliquot of sera should be stored frozen for possible repeat testing at a later time. The presence of antibody in a properly performed test around the time of exposure indicates that the individual is immune and not at risk. Those previously determined to be immune can also be reassured. If antibody is not detectable, a second blood specimen should be obtained 3 to 4 weeks later and tested concurrently with the first specimen. If antibody is present in the second but not the first specimen, infection is assumed to have occurred. If the test is negative, another blood specimen should be obtained 6 weeks after the exposure and also tested concurrently with the first specimen; a negative test indicates that infection has not occurred, and a positive test indicates that infection did occur.

To determine if the index patient has rubella, detection of rubella-specific serum IgM antibody or isolation of virus from nasal specimens can also be useful.

The routine use of immune globulin (IG) for postexposure prophylaxis of rubella in early pregnancy is not recommended. Administration of IG should be considered only if termination of the pregnancy is not an option. Limited data indicate that IG in a dose of 0.55 mL/kg may prevent or modify infection in an exposed, susceptible person. In one study, the attack rate of clinically apparent infection was reduced from 87% in control subjects to 18% in recipients of IG. However, the absence of clinical signs in a woman who has received IG does not guarantee that fetal infection has been prevented. In this study, 44% of the IG recipients were infected. Infants with congenital rubella are known to have been born to mothers who were given IG shortly after exposure.

Live rubella virus vaccine given after exposure does not prevent illness. However, immunization of exposed, nonpregnant persons may be indicated because if the current exposure does not result in infection, immunization will protect the individual in the future. Immunization of a person who is incubating natural rubella or who is already immune is not deleterious.

Rubella Virus Vaccine. The live-virus rubella vaccine currently distributed in the United States is the RA 27/3 strain of rubella virus grown in human diploid cell cultures. It contains no penicillin. Serum antibody is induced in more than 98% of the recipients.

Available data indicate that one dose confers long-term, probably lifelong, immunity in more than 90% of vaccinees. Two doses of rubella vaccine are now recommended in conjunction with the recently recommended two-dose measles immunization schedule (see Measles, p 312). Although primary rubella vaccine failures have not been a major problem, the potential consequences of rubella vaccine failure are substantial (ie, congenital rubella), and an additional dose of rubella vaccine should provide an added safeguard against such failures.

Vaccine Recommendations (see Table 3.42, p 409, for a summary). Rubella vaccine is administered in a single subcutaneous dose of 0.5 mL, either alone, as a combined preparation that also contains measles vaccine (MR), or in combination with measles and mumps vaccines (MMR), which is the usual formulation for rubella vaccination. Rubella vaccine can also be given simultaneously with other vaccines (see Simultaneous Administration of Multiple Vaccines, p 25).

Routine Childhood Immunization. Rubella vaccine is currently recommended to be administered in combination with measles and mumps vaccine (MMR) when a child is 12 months of age or older (see Tables 1.3 and 1.4, pp 23 and 24). A second dose of rubella vaccine administered as MMR is

TABLE 3.42—Indications and Contraindications for Rubella Vaccination

Indications	Contraindications
Children ≥12 mo (with measles and mumps vaccines [as MMR]) in a 2-dose schedule*	Pregnancy
	Immunodeficiency or immunocompromised condition†
Susceptible individuals in the following groups:	Recipient of IG or blood in past 3 mo‡
Prepubertal girls and boys	
Adults, especially premarital or postpartum women	
College students	
Child care personnel	
Health care personnel	
Military personnel	

*See Measles, p 312.
†Exception is HIV infection (see text for further discussion).
‡Rubella vaccine may be given postpartum concurrently or after the administration of anti-Rho (D) IG or blood products (see text for indications for subsequent testing for seroconversion). If rubella vaccine is given as MMR, longer intervals may be necessary (see p 318 and Table 3.30, p 319).

advised; the recommended age is determined by the measles vaccination schedule (see Measles, p 312). Clinical diagnosis of infection is usually unreliable and should not be accepted as evidence of immunity.

Special emphasis must continue to be placed on the immunization of postpubertal males and females, especially college students and military recruits. Those who are unimmunized or who have no serologic evidence of immunity to rubella should receive vaccine. Women should be informed of the theoretical risk to the fetus if they are pregnant or become pregnant within 3 months of vaccination (see Precautions and Contraindications, p 410, for further discussion). Specific recommendations are as follows:

• Postpubertal females who are not known to be immune to rubella should be immunized. They should not receive vaccine if they are known to be pregnant. Postpubertal females should be warned not to become pregnant for 3 months after receiving rubella vaccine.

• Premarital serologic screening for rubella immunity will enhance efforts to identify and vaccinate susceptible women before pregnancy.

• Prenatal or antepartum serologic screening for rubella immunity should be routinely undertaken. Rubella vaccine should be administered to susceptible women in the immediate postpartum period before discharge. Previous or simultaneous administration of Rho (D) Immune Globulin (Human) or blood products is not a contraindication to vaccination, but serologic testing should be done at least 8 weeks after vaccination in these cases in order to ascertain that seroconversion has occurred. MMR is an acceptable alternative for use in postpartum women if monovalent rubella vaccine is not available. Physicians can help ensure immunization of susceptible women by inquiring about the immune status of the mothers of their patients during visits for newborn infants and well-child care.

Breast-feeding is not a contraindication to postpartum immunization (for additional information, see Human Milk, p 73).

- A special effort should be made to be certain that all individuals are protected who plan to attend or work in educational institutions, child care centers, or other places where they are likely to be exposed to, or spread, rubella.
- Both male and female health care personnel who may be exposed to patients with rubella should be protected for their own benefit as well as for the prevention or transmission of rubella to pregnant patients.

Immunization should be performed unless documented evidence of rubella immunization or serologic evidence of naturally acquired immunity is provided.

Adverse Reactions.
- Five percent to 15% of susceptible children who receive rubella vaccine develop rash, fever, and/or lymphadenopathy 5 to 12 days after vaccination.
- Joint pain, usually in small peripheral joints, has been noted in approximately 0.5% of children. Arthralgia and arthritis tend to be more frequent (approximately 25%) in susceptible postpubertal females. Joint involvement usually begins 7 to 21 days after vaccination and is generally transient. After vaccination, persistent or recurrent arthralgic symptoms were reported in adult women by one group of investigators from Canada. However, data from the United States and other countries suggest that this adverse event is uncommon. An Institute of Medicine Committee concluded that the available evidence was consistent with a causal relationship between rubella vaccination and persistent arthritis, although the available data on current vaccine strains are limited.* The incidence of joint manifestations after vaccination is lower than that after natural infection at the corresponding age. In addition, in those reimmunized, the likelihood of these manifestations can be expected to be considerably less than that in previously immunized individuals, most of whom are already immune.
- Transient peripheral neuritic complaints, such as paresthesia and pain in the arms and legs, have also been reported, although rarely.
- Central nervous system manifestations and thrombocytopenia have been reported, but no causal relationship with vaccine has been established.

Precautions and Contraindications.
- *Pregnancy.* Rubella vaccine should not be given to pregnant women. If vaccine is inadvertently given, or if pregnancy occurs within 3 months of immunization, the patient should be counseled on the theoretical risks to the fetus. The maximal theoretical risk for the occurrence of congenital rubella is estimated to be 1.6%, based on data accumulated by the Centers for Disease Control and Prevention (CDC) from 226 susceptible women who received the current rubella vaccine (the RA27/3 strain) during the first

---

*Howson CP, Katz M, Johnston RB Jr, Fineberg HV. Chronic arthritis after rubella vaccination. *Clin Infect Dis.* 1992;15:307-312

trimester. Of the offspring, 2% had asymptomatic infection but none had congenital defects. In view of these observations, receipt of rubella vaccine in pregnancy is not ordinarily an indication for interruption of pregnancy.

Routine serologic testing of postpubertal women before immunization is not necessary. Serologic testing is a potential impediment to protection of these women against rubella because it requires two visits, one to identify susceptibles and one to administer vaccine. However, a sample of blood may be obtained before vaccination and stored for at least 3 months. If a woman becomes pregnant or has become pregnant after vaccination, the prevaccination specimen can be tested. Demonstration of rubella antibody in the prevaccine specimen indicates immunity and eliminates anxiety about fetal injury from rubella vaccine virus.

Vaccinating susceptible children whose mothers or other household contacts are pregnant does not cause a risk. Most vaccinees intermittently shed small amounts of virus from the pharynx 7 to 28 days after vaccination, but no evidence of transmission of the vaccine virus has been found in studies of more than 1,200 susceptible household contacts. Susceptible children, thus, should receive the vaccine.

- *Recent administration of immune globulin (IG).* Rubella vaccine should not be given in the 2 weeks before or the 3 months after the administration of IG or blood transfusion because of the possibility that antibody will neutralize vaccine virus and prevent a successful immunization. Since rubella vaccine is usually given as MMR, and high doses of IG (such as those given for the treatment of Kawasaki disease) can inhibit the response to the measles vaccine for longer intervals, rubella vaccination with MMR necessitates deferral for longer periods in such circumstances (see Measles, p 318 and Table 3.30, p 319). Rubella vaccine may be given to postpartum women at the same time as anti-Rho (D) IG (Rhogam) or after blood products are given, but these women should be tested 8 or more weeks later to determine if they have developed an active antibody response.
- *Altered immunity.* The following persons should not receive rubella vaccine: (1) patients with immunodeficiency diseases (except HIV infection); (2) patients receiving immunosuppressive therapy (such as those with leukemia, lymphoma, or generalized malignancy); (3) patients receiving large, systemic doses of corticosteroids, alkylating agents, antimetabolites, or radiation; and (4) otherwise immunocompromised persons. Patients with HIV infection should be vaccinated against measles using MMR and, thus, against rubella (see HIV Infection and AIDS, p 263).

  After cessation of immunosuppressive therapy, rubella vaccine is generally withheld for an interval of not less than 3 months. This interval is based on the assumption that immunologic responsiveness will have been restored in 3 months and the underlying disease for which immunosuppressive therapy was prescribed is in remission or under control. However, because the interval can vary with the intensity and type of immunosuppressive therapy, radiation therapy, underlying disease, and other factors, a definitive recommendation for an interval after cessation of immunosuppressive therapy when rubella vaccine can be safely and effectively administered is often not possible.

- *Febrile illness.* Children with minor illnesses with or without fever, such as upper respiratory tract infection, may be vaccinated (see Vaccine Safety and Contraindications, p 29). Fever per se is not a contraindication to immunization. However, if other manifestations suggest a more serious illness, the child should not be vaccinated until recovery has occurred.

Surveillance of Congenital Infections. Accurate diagnosis and reporting of the congenital rubella syndrome and vaccine complications are extremely important in assessing the control of rubella. All birth defects in which rubella infection is etiologically suspected should be thoroughly investigated and reported to the CDC through local or state health departments.

Salmonella Infections

Clinical Manifestations: *Salmonella* infections cause several clinical syndromes categorized as asymptomatic carriage, gastroenteritis, enteric fever, bacteremia, and focal infections (such as meningitis, osteomyelitis, and abscesses). These syndromes do not delineate mutually exclusive categories but represent the broad spectrum of illness caused by *Salmonella* in which overlap may exist. For example, gastroenteritis may be complicated by bacteremia and/or a metastatic focal infection. The most commonly recognized illness is gastroenteritis, in which diarrhea, abdominal cramps and tenderness, and fever are common manifestations. The site of infection is usually the small intestine, but colitis can occur.

Enteric fever is caused by *Salmonella typhi* and several other *Salmonella* serotypes. The onset of illness is typically gradual, with manifestations such as fever, constitutional symptoms (eg, headache, malaise, anorexia, and lethargy), abdominal pain and tenderness, hepatomegaly, splenomegaly, rose spots, and/or changes in mental status. Constipation may be an early feature. Diarrhea can occur later, usually in the second week of illness, and may not be a prominent symptom. Sustained or intermittent bacteremia can occur in both enteric fever and *Salmonella* bacteremia. Patients with bacteremia without focal infection have an illness characterized by fever without manifestations of enterocolitis or enteric fever. Recognizable focal infections ultimately may occur in as many as 10% of patients with *Salmonella* bacteremia.

Etiology: *Salmonella* organisms are Gram-negative bacilli in the family Enterobacteriaceae. One method of classification of *Salmonella* isolates is to differentiate them into one of the three following primary groups: *S typhi* (one serotype), *Salmonella choleraesuis* (one serotype), and *Salmonella enteritidis* (more than 2,000 serotypes). Current usage refers to each serotype as if it were a species (eg, *Salmonella typhimurium*). A second method of classification is based on somatic antigens and subdivides *Salmonella* organisms into groups A through I. The H (flagellar) antigen further delineates these groups into more than 2,000 serotypes. Most serotypes that cause human disease are in serogroups A-E. The most frequently reported human isolates in the United States in recent years have been *S typhimu-*

rium (group B), *Salmonella heidelberg* (B), *S enteritidis* (D), *Salmonella newport* (C2), *Salmonella infantis* (C1), *Salmonella agona* (B), *Salmonella hadar* (C2), and *Salmonella saint-paul* (B).

Epidemiology: The principal reservoirs for nontyphoidal *Salmonella* serotypes are animals, including poultry, livestock, reptiles, and pets. The major vehicles of transmission are foods of animal origin, including poultry, red meat, eggs, and unpasteurized milk. Many other food vehicles, such as fruits, vegetables, and rice, have been implicated. These vehicles are usually contaminated by contact with animal products or an infected human. Other modes of transmission include ingestion of contaminated water (primary route); contact with infected animals (eg, pet turtles); direct person-to-person transmission via the fecal-oral route; and contact with contaminated medications, dyes, and medical instruments. Ingestion of raw or improperly cooked shell eggs or raw milk, which may be contaminated even though certified, can produce severe disease. Unlike nontyphoidal *Salmonella*, *S typhi* is found only in humans. Cases of typhoid fever in the United States are usually acquired during foreign travel, from contact with a person who is a chronic carrier of *S typhi* or by consumption of food contaminated by a chronic carrier.

Age-specific attack rates for *Salmonella* infection are highest in those younger than 5 years of age and older than 70 years of age, and peak in the first year of life. Invasive infections and mortality are more frequent in infants, the elderly, and those with an underlying disease, particularly hemoglobinopathies (including sickle-cell disease), malignancy, acquired immune deficiency, and other immunosuppressive conditions. Most reported cases are sporadic in occurrence, but outbreaks in the home and in institutions are common. Nosocomial epidemics, including outbreaks of meningitis in newborn nurseries, have been reported. Typhoid fever, while uncommon in the United States, is endemic in many developing areas of the world.

The risk of transmission exists throughout the duration of fecal excretion. This period is variable. The median duration of excretion after infection with nontyphoidal *Salmonella* is longer in younger children than in older children or adults. Twelve weeks after infection, 45% of children younger than 5 years of age excrete *Salmonella* compared with 5% of older children and adults. The duration of excretion can be prolonged by antimicrobial therapy. Approximately 1% of patients continue to excrete *Salmonella* for more than 1 year.

The **incubation period** for gastroenteritis is from 6 to 72 hours. For enteric fever, the incubation period is from 3 to 60 days, but is usually 7 to 14 days.

Diagnostic Tests: Cultures of stool, blood, urine, and material from foci of infection, as indicated by the suspected *Salmonella* syndrome, should be obtained. Culture of a bone marrow aspirate may allow recovery of the organism causing enteric fever. Serologic tests for *Salmonella* agglutinins ("febrile agglutinins," the Widal test) may suggest the diagnosis of *S typhi* infection, but because of false-positive and false-negative results, these tests are not reliable.

Treatment:

- Antimicrobial therapy is usually not administered to patients with uncomplicated gastroenteritis caused by nontyphi *Salmonella* species because therapy does not shorten the duration of disease and can prolong the duration of excretion of *Salmonella* organisms.
- Antimicrobial therapy is warranted for *Salmonella* gastroenteritis occurring in patients with an increased risk of invasive disease and other complications, including infants younger than 3 months of age and patients with malignancies, hemoglobinopathies, acquired immune deficiency syndrome (AIDS) or other immunosuppressive illnesses, recipients of immunosuppressive therapy, persons with chronic gastrointestinal tract disease, or patients with severe colitis.

  Ampicillin, amoxicillin, trimethoprim-sulfamethoxazole, cefotaxime, or ceftriaxone is recommended for susceptible strains in patients for whom therapy is indicated. Strains acquired in developing countries often exhibit resistance to many antibiotics but are usually susceptible to ceftriaxone or cefotaxime, and to fluoroquinolones (eg, ciprofloxacin or ofloxacin). However, the fluoroquinolones are not approved by the Food and Drug Administration for use in patients younger than 18 years of age.
- In invasive *Salmonella* disease (such as typhoid, non-*S typhi* bacteremia, or osteomyelitis), appropriate drugs are chloramphenicol, ampicillin, amoxicillin, and trimethoprim-sulfamethoxazole. Cefotaxime, ceftriaxone, or a fluoroquinolone in adults is indicated if an ampicillin- or chloramphenicol-resistant organism is isolated or is strongly suggested by epidemiologic factors. Drug choice, route of administration, and duration are based on susceptibility of the organism, site of infection, host, and clinical response. For susceptible *S typhi*, administration of chloramphenicol, ceftriaxone, or cefotaxime for at least 14 days is recommended. In other infections in normal hosts without localization, such as bacteremia or enteric fever, patients should be treated for 14 days; whereas those with localized infection, such as osteomyelitis or abscess, and patients with bacteremia and AIDS should receive 4 to 6 weeks of therapy to prevent relapse. For *Salmonella* meningitis, ceftriaxone or cefotaxime is recommended, often for 4 weeks or longer.
- Chronic (more than 1 year) *S typhi* carriage may be eradicated in some patients by high-dose parenteral ampicillin, high-dose oral amoxicillin, ciprofloxacin (in adults only), or cholecystectomy.
- Antipyretics can cause precipitous declines in temperature and shock, and should be avoided in patients with enteric fever syndromes.
- Heparin should not be used to treat asymptomatic disseminated intravascular coagulation that occurs in many patients with enteric fever.
- Corticosteroids may be beneficial to patients with severe enteric fever, which is characterized by delirium, obtundation, stupor, coma, or shock. Steroids, however, should be reserved for critically ill patients in whom relief of the manifestations of toxemia may be life saving. The usual regimen is large doses of dexamethasone at an initial dose of 3 mg/kg, followed by eight doses of 1 mg/kg every 6 hours administered intravenously for 48 hours.

Isolation of the Hospitalized Patient: Enteric precautions should be used for the duration of illness. In patients with typhoid fever, enteric precautions should be continued until cultures of three consecutive stool specimens obtained after cessation of antimicrobial therapy are negative for *S typhi*.

Control Measures: Important measures include proper sanitation methods for food processing and preparation, sanitary water supplies, proper hand washing and personal hygiene, sanitary sewage disposal, exclusion of infected persons from handling food, prohibiting the sale of turtles for pets, reporting cases to appropriate health authorities, and investigating outbreaks. Eggs and other foods of animal origin should be cooked thoroughly. Raw eggs and food containing raw eggs should not be eaten. Notification of public health authorities and determination of serotype is of primary importance in the detection and investigation of outbreaks.

Child Care. Outbreaks of *Salmonella* infection are unusual in child care programs, and specific strategies for controlling it in child care have not been evaluated. General measures for interrupting enteric transmission in child care centers are recommended (see Children in Out-of-Home Child Care, p 83).

When *S typhi* disease is identified in a symptomatic child care attendee or staff member, stool specimens from other attendees and staff members should be cultured, and all infected persons should be excluded until three consecutive stool cultures are negative.

When species other than *S typhi* are identified in a symptomatic child care attendee or staff member with enterocolitis, older children and staff do not need to be excluded once they are asymptomatic. Asymptomatic contacts need not be cultured. If multiple symptomatic infected persons are identified, the decision to exclude these persons or cohort them in the program should be made in consultation with public health authorities. Antimicrobial therapy is not recommended for asymptomatically infected individuals, persons with uncomplicated enterocolitis, or those exposed to an infected individual.

Typhoid Vaccine. Resistance to infection with *S typhi* is enhanced by typhoid vaccination, but the degree of protection with currently available vaccines is limited and can be overcome by ingestion of a large bacterial inoculum. Two vaccines, as of December 1993, are available in the United States for civilian use; a third, an acetone-inactivated parenterally administered vaccine, is available only to the Armed Forces in the United States. Another vaccine, a Vi capsular polysaccharide, which is administered intramuscularly, is likely to be licensed for general use in the near future.

The two vaccines currently available to US civilians are (1) a parenteral heat-phenol-inactivated vaccine that has been widely used for many years, and (2) an orally administered, live-attenuated vaccine prepared from the Ty21a strain of *S typhi*. In field trials, Ty21a vaccine has been demonstrated to have similar efficacy to that of the parenteral vaccine, ranging from 42% to 96%. Since data are not available regarding its efficacy for children younger than 6 years of age and are limited concerning adverse reactions in this age group, the vaccine manufacturer recommends that the oral Ty21a vaccine should not be administered to children younger than 6 years of age.

Indications. In the United States, vaccination is recommended only for the following groups:
- *Travelers to areas where typhoid fever is endemic and a recognized risk of exposure will occur*. Risk is greatest for travelers to developing countries, especially Latin American, Asia, and Africa, who will be exposed to potentially contaminated food and drink. Such travelers need to be cautioned that typhoid vaccine is not a substitute for careful selection of food and drink.
- *Persons with intimate exposure to a documented typhoid fever carrier*, such as occurs with continued household contact.
- *Laboratory workers with frequent contact with S typhi*. The vaccine is not recommended for persons attending summer camps, for those in areas of natural disaster, or for control of common-source outbreaks.

Dosages. For primary vaccination, the following is recommended:
- Children 10 years of age or older, and adults:
  Oral Ty21a vaccine. One enteric-coated capsule is taken on alternate days for a total of four capsules. Each capsule should be taken with cool liquid, no warmer than 37°C, approximately 1 hour before meals. The capsules must be kept refrigerated and all four doses must be taken to achieve maximal efficacy.

OR

  Parenteral inactivated vaccine. The dose is 0.5 mL subcutaneously, given on two occasions, separated by 4 or more weeks. If time is insufficient for two doses of vaccine separated by 4 or more weeks to be given, three doses of the parenteral vaccine at weekly intervals are given. However, this schedule may be less effective.
- Children younger than 10 years of age:
  Oral Ty21a vaccine. Recommendations are the same for children 6 to 9 years of age and for adults. This vaccine is not recommended for children younger than 6 years of age.

OR

  Parenteral inactivated vaccine. The dose is 0.25 mL subcutaneously, given on two occasions, separated by 4 or more weeks.

Booster doses. In circumstances of continued or repeated exposure to *S typhi*, booster doses are recommended. If parenteral vaccine is used, booster doses should be given every 3 years. Even if more than 3 years have elapsed since the earlier vaccination, a single booster dose of parenteral vaccine is sufficient. When the heat-phenol-inactivated vaccine is used, less reaction follows booster vaccination by the intradermal route than by the subcutaneous route. (The acetone-inactivated parenteral vaccine should not be given by the intradermal route because of the potential for severe local reactions.) No data have been reported using oral live-attenuated vaccine as a booster. However, using the primary series of four doses of the oral vaccine as a booster for persons previously vaccinated with parenteral vaccine is a reasonable alternative to administration of a parenteral booster dose. The following routes and dosages of parenteral vaccine for booster vaccination are recommended:
- Children 10 years or older and adults: one dose, 0.5 mL subcutaneously or 0.1 mL intradermally.

- Children 6 months to 10 years: one dose, 0.25 mL subcutaneously or 0.1 mL intradermally.

The optimal booster schedule for persons who have received the oral Ty21a vaccine has not been determined. However, continued efficacy for 5 years after vaccination has been demonstrated. The manufacturer of Ty21a recommends revaccination with the entire four-dose series every 5 years. This recommendation may change as more data become available on the duration of protection produced by the Ty21a vaccine.

Adverse Reactions. Reported side effects with oral vaccine have been rare and consist of abdominal discomfort, nausea, vomiting, and rash or urticaria. In safety trials, adverse reactions occurred with equal frequency among groups receiving vaccine and placebo.

Parenteral, inactivated vaccines can produce several systemic and local adverse reactions, including fever (14% to 29%), headache (9% to 30%), and severe local pain and/or swelling (6% to 40%). Because of adverse reactions, 13% to 24% of vaccinees are reported to miss school or work. More severe reactions have been sporadically reported, including hypotension, chest pain, and shock.

Contraindications and Precautions. The only contraindication to parenteral typhoid vaccination is a history of severe local or systemic reactions after a previous dose. No data have been reported with parenteral, inactivated vaccine or oral vaccine in pregnant women. Since oral vaccine is a live-attenuated vaccine, it should not be administered to immunocompromised persons, including those known to be infected with HIV. Since the antimalarial mefloquine could potentially affect the immune response to the oral, live vaccine, administering oral vaccine at least 24 hours before or after a dose of mefloquine may be prudent.

Scabies

Clinical Manifestations: The disease manifests as an intensely pruritic, erythematous, papular eruption. Itching is most intense at night. In older children and adults, the sites of predilection are the interdigital folds, flexor aspects of the wrists, extensor surfaces of the elbows, anterior axillary folds, belt line, thighs, navel, penis, areolae, abdomen, intergluteal cleft, and buttocks. In infants younger than 2 years of age, the eruption is often vesicular and is likely to occur on the head, neck, palms, and soles, but these areas are usually spared in older children and adults. The distribution of typical scabies lesions does not parallel that of the adult female mite because the eruption is caused by the immature stages of the mite and sensitization to the proteins of the parasite.

The characteristic mite burrow appears as a grey or white, tortuous, thread-like line. Most burrows are obliterated by scratching long before a patient is seen by a physician. Excoriations are common. Occasionally, 2-to 5-mm red-brown nodules are present, particularly on covered parts of the body such as the genitalia, groin, and axilla. These scabies nodules are a granulomatous response to the dead mite parts and feces, and can persist for weeks and even months after effective treatment. Cutaneous secondary bacterial infection can occur, caused most commonly by *Streptococcus pyogenes* and *Staphylococcus aureus*.

Etiology: The mite *Sarcoptes scabiei* subspecies *hominis* is the cause of the disease.

Epidemiology: Humans are the source of the infection. Transmission occurs most often by close personal contact. Minimum contact with a patient with crusted scabies (Norwegian) can result in transmission because of the large number of mites in the exfoliating scales. Scabies can be transmitted as long as the patient remains infected and untreated, including the interval before symptoms develop.

Scabies occurs worldwide in cycles thought to be 15 to 30 years long. Scabies affects persons from all socioeconomic levels without regard to age, sex, or standards of personal hygiene. Scabies is endemic in many developing countries.

The **incubation period** in persons without previous exposure is usually 4 to 6 weeks. Persons who were previously infected develop symptoms 1 to 4 days after repeat exposure to the mite, but these reinfections are usually milder.

Diagnostic Tests: Diagnosis is confirmed by identification of the mite, the mites' eggs or scybala (feces) from skin scrapings of intact burrows, or papules from sites of predilection. Mineral oil, microscope immersion oil, or water applied to the skin facilitates collection of scrapings. A #15 scalpel is used to scrape along the entire length of the burrow (the mite is often found at one end of the burrow), and the scrapings and oil are placed on a slide under a cover slip and examined microscopically under low power.

Treatment: Infected children and adults should apply lotion or cream containing a scabicide over the entire body below the head. Because scabies can affect the head, scalp, and neck in infants and young toddlers, treatment of the entire head, neck, and body in this age group is required. The drug of choice, particularly for infants, young children, and pregnant or nursing women, is 5% permethrin, a synthetic pyrethroid (Elimite*). Alternative drugs are lindane (Kwell, Scabene) and crotamiton (Eurax). Permethrin should be removed by bathing after 8 to 14 hours, lindane after 8 to 12 hours, and crotamiton after 48 hours. Crotamiton is applied once daily for 2 to 5 days, but it is associated with frequent treatment failures.

The frequency of lindane applications should not exceed that recommended in order to avoid the possibility of neurotoxicity from absorption through the skin. Lindane should be used cautiously in young infants and pregnant women.

---

*This product differs in its concentration (5%) of permethrin from that used for the treatment of pediculosis (1%).

Isolation of the Hospitalized Patient: Contact isolation without a mask is recommended until the patient has been treated with an appropriate scabicide.

Control Measures:

- Prophylactic therapy is recommended for household members. Signs of scabies can appear as late as 1 to 2 months after exposure, during which time patients can transmit scabies. All members of the household should be treated at the same time to prevent reinfection. Bedding and clothing worn next to the skin should be laundered in a washer with hot water and a hot drying cycle. The parasites do not survive more than 3 to 4 days without contact with the skin. Clothing that cannot be laundered should be removed from the patient and stored from several days to a week or more to avoid reinfestation.
- Children should be allowed to return to child care or school after treatment has been completed.
- Epidemics and localized outbreaks may require stringent and consistent measures to treat contacts. Environmental disinfection is rarely warranted. Caretakers who have had prolonged skin-to-skin contact with infected patients may benefit from prophylactic treatment.
- Individuals with crusted scabies and their close contacts must be treated promptly and aggressively to avoid outbreaks.

Schistosomiasis

Clinical Manifestations: Initial entry of the infecting larvae (cercariae) through the skin is frequently accompanied by a transient, pruritic papular rash (cercarial dermatitis). After penetration, the organism enters the bloodstream, migrates through the lungs, and ultimately lodges in the venous plexus, draining either the intestines or the bladder (depending on the *Schistosoma* species). Four to 8 weeks after exposure, a serum sickness-like illness can develop, manifested by fever, malaise, cough, rash, abdominal pain, nausea, lymphadenopathy, and eosinophilia (Katayama fever). In acute infections with heavy infestation due to *Schistosoma mansoni* or *Schistosoma japonicum*, a mucoid, bloody diarrhea accompanied by tender hepatomegaly occurs. The severity of symptoms associated with chronic disease is related to the worm burden. Individuals with low to moderate worm burdens can be asymptomatic; heavily infected individuals can have a range of symptoms caused primarily by inflammation and fibrosis triggered by eggs produced by adult worms. Portal hypertension can develop and cause hepatosplenomegaly, ascites, and esophageal varices. Chronic involvement of the colon produces abdominal pain and bloody diarrhea. Other organ systems can be involved from eggs embolized to the lungs, causing pulmonary hypertension, or to the central nervous system, notably the spinal cord in *S mansoni* or *Schistosoma hematobium* infections. In *S hematobium* infections the bladder becomes inflamed and fibrotic. Symptoms include dysuria, urgency, terminal microscopic and gross hematuria, secondary urinary tract infections, and nonspecific pelvic pain.

Swimmer's itch (cercarial dermatitis) is caused by the larvae of other avian and mammalian schistosome species that penetrate human skin but do not complete the life cycle and do not cause chronic fibrotic disease. Manifestations include mild to moderate pruritus at the penetration site a few hours after exposure, followed in 5 to 14 days by an intermittent pruritic, sometimes papular, eruption. In previously sensitized individuals, more intense papular eruptions may occur for 7 to 10 days after exposure.

Etiology: The trematodes (flukes) *S mansoni, S japonicum, S hematobium,* and, rarely, *Schistosoma mekongi* and *Schistosoma intercalatum* cause the disease. All species have similar life cycles. Swimmer's itch is caused by multiple avian and mammalian species of *Schistosoma.*

Epidemiology: Humans are the principal hosts for the major species. Persistence of schistosomiasis depends on the presence of an appropriate snail as an intermediate host. Eggs excreted in stool (*S mansoni* and *S japonicum*) or urine (*S hematobium*) into fresh water hatch into motile miracidia, which infect snails. After development in the snails, cercariae emerge and penetrate the skin of humans encountered in the water. Children are frequently infected after infancy when they begin to explore the environment.

Schistosoma mansoni occurs throughout tropical Africa, in several Caribbean islands including Puerto Rico, and in Venezuela, Brazil, Suriname, and the Arabian peninsula. *Schistosoma japonicum* is found in China, the Philippines, and Indonesia. *Schistosoma hematobium* occurs in Africa and the eastern Mediterranean region. *Schistosoma mekongi* is limited to a small area of the Mekong delta in southeast Asia (Kampuchea and Laos). *Schistosoma intercalatum* is found in Central Africa. Children are frequently involved in transmission because of habits of promiscuous defecation, urination, and frequent wading in infected waters. Communicability lasts as long as live eggs are excreted in the urine and feces. Adults of the *S mansoni* species have been documented to live as long as 26 years in the human host. Thus, schistosomiasis can be diagnosed in patients many years after they have left the endemic areas.

Swimmer's itch occurs in all regions of the world after exposure to fresh, brackish, or salt water.

The **incubation period** is unknown.

Diagnostic Tests: Infection with *S mansoni* and other species (except *S hematobium*) is made by microscopic examination of concentrated stool specimens to detect characteristic eggs. In light infections, several specimens may have to be examined before eggs are found and biopsy of rectal mucosa may be necessary. The fresh tissue obtained should be compressed between two glass slides and examined under low power unstained for eggs. *Schistosoma hematobium* is diagnosed by examining filtered urine for eggs. Egg excretion peaks often between 12 noon and 3 pm. Biopsy of the bladder mucosa may be necessary. Serologic tests are available through the Centers for Disease Control and Prevention and may be particularly helpful in detecting light infections.

Swimmer's itch can be difficult to differentiate from other causes of dermatitis. A skin biopsy may demonstrate larvae but their absence does not exclude the diagnosis.

Treatment: The drug of choice for schistosomiasis caused by any species is praziquantel; the alternative drug for *S mansoni* is oxamniquine* (see Drugs for Parasitic Infections, p 574). For *S hematobium*, an alternative drug is metrifonate, which is available from the Drug Service of the Centers for Disease Control and Prevention (see Directory of Telephone Numbers, p 601). No satisfactory alternative drug for *S japonicum* is available.

Swimmer's itch is a self-limited disease that requires only symptomatic treatment of the urticarial rash.

Isolation of the Hospitalized Patient: No special precautions are recommended.

Control Measures: Elimination of the intermediate snail host is difficult to achieve in most areas. Thus, treatment of infected populations, sanitary disposal of human waste, and education about the source of infection are the key elements of current control measures. Travelers to endemic areas should be advised to avoid contact with freshwater streams and lakes.

Shigella Infections

Clinical Manifestations: In mild *Shigella* infections, clinical manifestations consist of watery or loose stools for several days, with minimal or no constitutional symptoms. Abrupt onset of fever, systemic toxicity, headache, and profuse watery diarrhea occur in patients with small bowel infection. Convulsions can occur. Abdominal cramps, tenderness, tenesmus, and mucoid stools with or without blood characterize large bowel disease (bacillary dysentery). Rare sequelae include bacteremia, Reiter's syndrome after *Shigella flexneri* infection, hemolytic-uremic syndrome from *Shigella dysenteriae* type 1 infection, colonic perforation, and fulminant toxic encephalopathy (ekiri syndrome), which can be lethal within 48 hours of onset.

Etiology: *Shigella* organisms are Gram-negative bacilli in the family Enterobacteriaceae. Four species (of more than 40 serotypes) have been identified. *Shigella sonnei* currently accounts for more than half the cases in the United States, and *S flexneri* accounts for a large percentage of the remainder.

---

*Available from Pfizer, Inc, New York, NY.

Shigella dysenteriae type 1 (the Shiga bacillus) is rare in the United States but widespread in rural Africa and the Indian subcontinent. *Shigella boydii* is uncommon.

Epidemiology: Feces of infected humans are the source. No animal reservoir is known. Predisposing factors include crowded living conditions, low hygienic standards, closed population groups with substandard environmental sanitation (eg, residential homes for retarded children), and travel to countries with low standards of food sanitation. Fecal-oral transmission from person-to-person contact is the common route by which children are infected. Other modes of transmission include ingestion of contaminated food or water, homosexual transmission, and contact with a contaminated, inanimate object. Houseflies are also vectors, causing physical transport of infected feces. Infection is most common in children 1 to 4 years old and is an important problem in child care centers in the United States. The risk of communicability exists until the organism is no longer present in feces. Even without antimicrobial therapy, convalescent carriage usually ceases within 4 weeks of the onset of illness. Chronic carriage (more than 1 year) is rare.

The **incubation period** varies from 1 to 7 days but is usually 2 to 4 days.

Diagnostic Tests: Culture of feces or rectal swab specimens should be performed. Blood should be cultured only in severely ill patients or in immunocompromised or malnourished patients since bacteremia is rare. A stool smear stained with methylene blue may reveal polymorphonuclear leukocytes and/or erythrocytes, a finding indicative of enterocolitis, which is consistent but not specific for *Shigella* infection.

Treatment:

- Antimicrobial therapy is effective in both shortening the duration of diarrhea and eliminating organisms from feces, and it is recommended for most patients with dysentery. Small bowel disease is often self-limited, lasting 48 to 72 hours, but may progress to dysentery. In cases of mild illness, the primary indication for treatment is to prevent further spread of the organism (although appropriate hand washing is likely to be equally effective).
- Antimicrobial susceptibility testing of clinical isolates is indicated since resistance to antimicrobial agents is common. Plasmid-mediated, multiple antimicrobial resistance has been identified in all *Shigella* species.
- For cases in which susceptibility is unknown or an ampicillin-resistant strain is isolated, the drug of choice is trimethoprim-sulfamethoxazole. Strains that are acquired in developing countries are often resistant to trimethoprim-sulfamethoxazole but susceptible to nalidixic acid, cefixime, ceftriaxone, cefotaxime, ciprofloxacin, and ofloxacin. The latter two are not recommended for use in persons younger than 18 years of age. For susceptible strains, ampicillin is effective. Amoxicillin is ineffective for the treatment of *Shigella* infections. Tetracycline is effective if the strain is susceptible and can be used for patients 9 years of age or older. The oral route is acceptable, except in seriously ill patients.
- Antimicrobial therapy should be administered for 5 days.

- Antidiarrheal compounds that inhibit intestinal peristalsis are contraindicated because they may prolong the clinical and bacteriologic course of disease.

Isolation of the Hospitalized Patient: Enteric precautions are indicated until diarrhea has stopped and cultures of three consecutive stool specimens obtained after cessation of antimicrobial therapy are negative.

Control Measures:

Child Care. General measures for interrupting enteric transmission (especially hand washing) in child care centers are recommended (see Children in Out-of-Home Child Care, p 83). Hand washing is the single most important control measure in decreasing transmission rates.

When *Shigella* infection is identified in a child care attendee or staff member, stool specimens from other symptomatic attendees and staff members should be cultured. Stool specimens from household contacts with diarrhea should also be cultured. All symptomatic individuals in whom *Shigella* is isolated from stool should receive antimicrobial therapy (see Treatment, p 422) and should no longer have diarrhea before readmission to the program. If several individuals are infected, cohort system should be considered until stool cultures are negative. Efforts should be made to prevent transfer of children to other child care centers in order to prevent spread of the infection.

General Control Measures. Strict attention to hand washing is essential to limit spread. Other important control measures include sanitary water supply, food processing, and sewage disposal; exclusion of infected persons as food handlers; prevention of food contamination by flies; and case reporting to appropriate health authorities (eg, hospital infection control officer and public health department).

Vaccination. Several investigational vaccines have been developed.

Staphylococcal Infections

Clinical Manifestations: *Staphylococcus aureus* causes a wide variety of suppurative infections, ranging from localized to invasive diseases. Localized diseases include furuncles, impetigo (bullous and nonbullous), and wound infections. *Staphylococcus aureus* is currently a leading cause of impetigo. Suppurative and/or invasive infections include septicemia, osteomyelitis, arthritis, endocarditis, and pneumonia. Meningitis is rare. *Staphylococcus aureus* also causes toxin-mediated diseases, such as toxic shock syndrome (see Staphylococcal Toxic Shock Syndrome, p 428), scalded skin syndrome, and food poisoning (see Staphylococcal Food Poisoning, p 427). Most staphylococcal abscesses and toxin-related diseases are caused by *S aureus*. Methicillin-resistant *S aureus* (MRSA) is not more virulent than methicillin-susceptible *S aureus* strains, but the former may be more difficult to treat because of multiple antibiotic resistance and resulting limited drug choices.

Coagulase-negative staphylococci, primarily *Staphylococcus epidermidis*, cause bacteremia in premature infants and immunocompromised patients and frequently cause infections of vascular access devices, cerebrospinal fluid shunts, and prosthetic heart valves, causing endocarditis. Coagulase-negative staphylococci can also cause urinary tract infections, especially in adolescent females.

Etiology: Staphylococci are Gram-positive cocci that appear microscopically as grape-like clusters. Staphylococci multiply aerobically and anaerobically; they are resistant to heat to 50°C (122°F), to high salt concentrations, and to drying; and they can survive on clothing and in dust.

Coagulase-negative staphylococci are classified in 11 species. Most infections are caused by *S epidermidis*. Slime production by *S epidermidis* is associated with invasiveness. *Staphylococcus saprophyticus* causes urinary tract infections.

Epidemiology: *Staphylococcus aureus* is a ubiquitous organism. Strains can be part of the normal human flora, and they colonize the anterior nares and moist body areas in approximately 30% of humans. Persons who have skin or draining staphylococcal lesions are highly contagious. Carriers can also transmit staphylococci. Infants who have been colonized while in the nursery can be the source of family spread. Person-to-person transmission is the usual mode of spread, occurring via the hands, nasal discharges, and, rarely, by aerosol. Communicability is as long as lesions or the carrier state persist. Infection is usually caused by the patient's endogenous *S aureus* strain.

Coagulase-negative staphylococci are ubiquitous on skin and mucosal surfaces. Person-to-person spread is the common mode of transmission. Infection is usually the result of invasion by a patient's endogenous strain. Foreign bodies, such as shunts, intravascular catheters, or prosthetic heart valves, predispose to infection with coagulase-negative staphylococci as well as to *S aureus*.

The **incubation period** is usually 1 to 10 days for bullous impetigo and the scalded skin syndrome. For other staphylococcal lesions, it is extremely variable. A long delay can occur between acquisition of the organism and onset of disease.

Diagnostic Tests: Gram-stained smears of material from lesions can provide presumptive evidence of infection. Isolation of organisms by culture of blood, tissue, pleural fluid, bones, or lesions is definitive. The positive coagulase test or mannitol fermentation differentiates *S aureus* from coagulase-negative staphylococci. When clusters of cases occur, examination of antibiotic susceptibility, plasmid typing, or phage-type patterns of the isolated strains can help determine the source of the outbreak.

Treatment:
Staphylococcus aureus.
- Serious infections require intravenous therapy with a penicillinase-resistant penicillin, such as nafcillin or oxacillin, because most *S aureus* strains in

the community and in hospitals produce penicillinase and are resistant to penicillin and ampicillin. First- or second-generation cephalosporins (eg, cephalothin or cefuroxime) or clindamycin are also useful. The newer expanded spectrum (third-generation) cephalosporins are usually not as active in vitro against staphylococci, and some may be inadequate for effective treatment. Some 5% to 10% of patients allergic to the penicillins will also be hypersensitive to the cephalosporins. Intravenous vancomycin can be used for *S aureus* strains resistant to the penicillinase-resistant penicillins, ie, MRSA, and for patients who are allergic to both penicillin and the cephalosporins. All *S aureus* strains are currently susceptible to vancomycin. The choice of antibiotics should be based on results of susceptibility tests.

- Duration of therapy for serious, invasive infections is often 3 weeks or more. After initial parenteral therapy and clinical response of the patient, completion of the recommended antibiotic course with an oral drug can be considered if good compliance and blood concentrations can be assured. **The exception to this guideline is endocarditis**.
- Drainage of abscesses is desirable and usually required.
- Skin and soft-tissue infection, such as impetigo or cellulitis due to *S aureus*, can usually be treated with oral penicillinase-resistant beta-lactam drugs, such as cloxacillin, dicloxacillin, or a cephalosporin. For superficial skin lesions, topical antibacterial therapy with mupirocin or bacitracin ointment and local hygiene may be sufficient. In situations where a patient or health care worker is found to be a chronic carrier of *S aureus*, including MRSA, topical mupirocin therapy can be effective in eradicating carriage.

Coagulase-Negative Staphylococci.
- Serious infections require intravenous therapy with antibiotics. Most strains causing infection are resistant to penicillin, in which case a semisynthetic penicillinase-resistant penicillin, such as nafcillin or oxacillin, can be used. Methicillin-resistant strains are common, especially in nosocomial infections. Most of these organisms are susceptible to vancomycin, the drug of choice for methicillin-resistant organisms. Rifampin and gentamicin are also effective, but rapid emergence of resistance limits their use. Use of either in combination with vancomycin can increase the antibacterial activity (ie, synergy).
- Intravenous vancomycin should be considered for initial treatment of all severe infections caused by coagulase-negative staphylococci.
- Removal of associated foreign bodies and drainage of abscesses is desirable and usually required.

Endocarditis, caused by either *S aureus* or, in patients with prosthetic cardiac valves, coagulase-negative staphylococci. Recommendations for antimicrobial treatment of endocarditis caused by either *S aureus* or coagulase-negative staphylococci have been formulated by the American Heart Association and should be consulted.[*]

---

[*]Bisno AL, Dismukes WE, Durack DT, et al. Antimicrobial treatment of infective endocarditis due to viridans streptococci, enterococci, and staphylococci. *JAMA*. 1989;261:1471-1477

Isolation of the Hospitalized Patient: For patients with exposed lesions (draining wounds, scalded skin syndrome, bullous impetigo, abscesses), contact isolation should be implemented. Patients infected or colonized with multiply-resistant staphylococci, including MRSA, can be managed by contact isolation to avoid transmission. Precautions should continue for the duration of illness. No special precautions are necessary for patients with other staphylococcal infections, such as bacteremia.

Control Measures:

1. Maximum precautions to avoid transmission of staphylococci via hands and clothing of personnel should be routine in hospitals. Careful hand washing before and after every patient contact is mandatory.

2. Carriers require no special treatment. Routine culturing of hospital personnel is not recommended. However, identification of carriers who disseminate a strain that has been implicated in epidemic disease in a closed population is necessary. Consideration should be given to removing these personnel from areas of patient contact and treating them with topical intranasal antibiotics, such as mupirocin, and in some cases with appropriate orally administered antibiotics. The goal of therapy in this instance is to eliminate carriage of an epidemiologically virulent strain. The carrier state can be very difficult to eradicate.

3. Epidemic *S aureus* disease in newborn nurseries presents special problems. Approaches include the following:

   • Infants with definite or suspected staphylococcal disease should be managed with contact precautions.

   • The cohorting of infants and staff should be instituted in the affected nursery. For example, all infants in a room should be discharged and the room carefully cleaned before new infants are admitted to that room. Staff, especially nursing staff, caring for one cohort should not care for another cohort, when more than one patient cohort is present.

   • Meticulous infection control techniques for patient contact should be re-emphasized. Careful hand washing by personnel is of paramount importance.

   • Cultures of infants (umbilicus and anterior nares) and personnel (nares and hands) should be obtained to determine prevalence of colonization and to identify staphylococcal strains involved in the outbreak for antimicrobial susceptibility testing, phage typing, or plasmid typing. Occasionally, personnel colonized with the outbreak strain will need to be removed from patient contact until carriage has been eliminated.

   • During epidemics, full-term infants may be bathed with hexachlorophene (3%) as soon after birth as possible and daily until they are discharged. The hexachlorophene should be thoroughly removed by washing after bathing. Care must be exercised in using hexachlorophene because systemic absorption can result in central nervous system damage. Hexachlorophene should not be used for routine bathing and should be used only for full-term infants.

   • Application of triple dye or bacitracin ointment to the umbilical stump of all infants twice daily throughout the nursery stay can also be helpful.

- In unusual circumstances, treatment with oral antistaphylococcal agents of all infants and personnel who are carriers may be necessary.
- Persons involved in hospital outbreaks should be observed and warned of the possibility of delayed disease and the potential for spread to family members.
- Surveillance in the nursery should be continued for several weeks after the epidemic has terminated.
- Surveillance of recently discharged infants for infections should be performed. Observation for disease in neonates, both in the nursery and at home for several weeks, is the most reliable index of *S aureus* outbreaks.

Staphylococcal Food Poisoning

Clinical Manifestations: Staphylococcal food poisoning is characterized by abrupt onset of severe abdominal cramps, nausea and vomiting, diarrhea, and, occasionally, low-grade fever. Its short incubation period, brevity of illness, and usual lack of fever help distinguish it from other types of food poisoning, except that caused by *Bacillus cereus*. Chemical food poisoning usually has a shorter incubation period. *Clostridium perfringens* food poisoning usually has a longer incubation period and infrequently is accompanied by vomiting, which is common in staphylococcal and *B cereus* food poisoning. Patients with food-borne *Salmonella* infection and *Shigella* infection often have fever, and the incubation period is longer.

Etiology: The enterotoxins produced by strains of *Staphylococcus aureus* and, rarely, *Staphylococcus epidermidis* are the cause. Of the eight immunologically distinct heat-stable enterotoxins (A,B,C_{1-3},D,E,F), enterotoxins A and D are the most common in the United States. Enterotoxin F is identical with the toxin associated with toxic shock syndrome (TSST-1) and has not been implicated in outbreaks of food poisoning.

Epidemiology: Illness is caused by preformed toxin present in food containing enterotoxigenic staphylococci. Contamination is usually by food handlers who may be healthy but colonized with this organism. Food products most commonly involved include filled pastries, egg and potato salads, poultry, and ham. The disease is not transmissible from person to person.

The **incubation period** is from 30 minutes to 7 hours.

Diagnostic Tests: Isolation of the same phage types of *S aureus* from stools or vomitus of affected persons, the vehicle of transmission, and the food handler responsible for contaminating the food is the method of diagnosis in an epidemic. Lesions on the hands of food handlers may be the source of contamination and should be cultured. Other possible sources that should be cultured include nose, throat, and rectum. The vomitus and stools of patients may contain the offending *S aureus* species and should also be cultured. Identification of enterotoxin or staphylococcal organisms in incriminated foods can be performed by the Food and Drug Administration, and phage typing of staphylococcal isolates can be performed by the Centers for Disease Control and Prevention.

Treatment: Antibiotics are not indicated.

Isolation of the Hospitalized Patient: No special precautions are recommended.

Control Measures: Optimum cooking and refrigeration of foods, particularly meat, dairy, and bakery products, will help to prevent the disease. Food handlers with staphylococcal infections should be excluded from food preparation.

Staphylococcal Toxic Shock Syndrome

Clinical Manifestations: Toxic shock syndrome (TSS) is an acute febrile illness with myalgia, vomiting, diarrhea, and pharyngitis; a diffuse macular erythroderma that desquamates; mucous membrane and conjunctival hyperemia; and multiorgan system involvement. The temperature usually is higher than 38.9°C (102°F). The erythematous, sunburn-like rash occurs during the acute phase, with desquamation of the skin, especially of the palms and soles, 7 to 10 days later. Hypotension and, in severe cases, shock and multiorgan system dysfunction can occur. The organ systems that can be involved include renal (abnormal urinalysis, elevated BUN, or serum creatinine concentrations), hepatic (elevated serum enzyme and bilirubin concentrations), hematologic (preponderance of immature and mature neutrophils in peripheral blood, and thrombocytopenia), and central nervous system (disorientation or alterations in consciousness without focal neurologic signs).

The case definition established by the Centers for Disease Control and Prevention is based on the following five major diagnostic criteria:
1. Fever of 38.9°C (102°F) or higher.
2. Presence of a diffuse macular erythroderma.
3. Desquamation 1 to 2 weeks after onset of illness, particularly of the palms and soles.
4. Hypotension, defined as a systolic blood pressure of 90 mm Hg or less for adults, and below the fifth percentile for children younger than 16 years of age; or an orthostatic drop in diastolic blood pressure of 15 mm Hg or more with a change from lying to sitting; orthostatic syncope; or orthostatic dizziness.
5. Involvement of three or more of the following organ systems: gastrointestinal, muscular, mucous membrane, renal, hepatic, hematologic, and central nervous system.

In addition, if blood and cerebrospinal fluid cultures are obtained, they must be negative. The only exception is that the blood cultures may be positive for *Staphylococcus aureus*. Serologic tests for Rocky Mountain spotted fever, leptospirosis, and measles also must be negative. ·

Toxic shock syndrome is probable when only four of the five major criteria are fulfilled. Patients who die before desquamation would have occurred, but whose illness is otherwise compatible with TSS, are considered definite cases. The syndrome can be confused with Kawasaki disease, scarlet fever, Rocky Mountain spotted fever, measles, leptospirosis, and other febrile, mucocutaneous diseases. Telogen effluvium, including hair thinning or patchy hair loss, and nail splitting, ridging, or loss, frequently occur 1 to 2 months after onset. Neuropsychologic sequelae have been reported but appear to be infrequent.

Etiology: In many patients the etiologic agent is TSS toxin-1-producing strains of *S aureus*; however, TSST-1-negative strains of *S aureus* have been implicated.

Epidemiology: Toxic shock syndrome became widely recognized in 1980, with the documentation of an increased risk of illness among menstruating women who used tampons. Since then, the incidence of menstrually associated cases and the proportion of TSS associated with menstruation has decreased. Disease occurs in males as well as females. Nonmenstrual TSS cases have been associated with cutaneous or subcutaneous lesions, childbirth or abortion, surgical wound infections, vaginal infections occurring at times other than during menstruation or the postpartum period, and other sources of focal staphylococcal infection, including sinusitis and pneumonia. On occasion, the source of infection may be unknown. Patients considered at risk for TSS include (1) menstruating women using tampons or other inserted vaginal devices; (2) persons (male and female) with focal *S aureus* infection; and (3) women using diaphragms or contraceptive sponges. The diagnosis should also be considered in persons with scarlet fever syndrome, and persons with fever and hypotension. Toxic shock syndrome is frequently a life-threatening or fatal disease; with treatment, the case fatality rate is 2% to 4%. No evidence of person-to-person transmission or identified common exposures has been found.

The median **incubation period**, based on postoperative TSS, is 2 days.

Diagnostic Tests: Because *S aureus* may be isolated from the anterior nares and vagina of 10% to 30% of healthy individuals, and approximately 30% of such strains can produce TSST-1, identification of TSST-1-producing *S aureus* is only presumptive evidence. The diagnosis is made on the basis of clinical criteria (see Clinical Manifestations, p 428).

Treatment:
- Management of the hypotensive patient depends on severity of the illness and its complications. Aggressive intravenous fluid replacement for hypovolemic shock is necessary; in some cases vasopressor agents are required.
- Antistaphylococcal antibiotics are recommended to eradicate the focus of toxin-producing *S aureus* and reduce the risk of a recurrent episode. Anti-

biotic therapy, however, does not necessarily affect the outcome of the acute illness.

- Any vaginal foreign bodies (eg, tampons, contraceptive sponges) or incision and wound packing (nonmenstrual) should be removed. Infected wounds should be explored and drained, even if the wound does not show prominent signs of inflammation.
- Additional types of therapy have been required in some patients to correct electrolyte and acid-base imbalance and to manage complications of prolonged shock, acute renal failure, adult respiratory distress syndrome, myocardial failure, and disseminated intravascular coagulation with thrombocytopenia. In severe cases, corticosteroid therapy or intravenous immune globulin may be of benefit.
- To decrease the risk of recurrence, menstruating patients should not use tampons during subsequent menstrual periods.

Isolation of the Hospitalized Patient: Drainage/secretion precautions are recommended for the duration of the illness.

Control Measures: None.

Group A Streptococcal Infections

Clinical Manifestations: The most common clinical illness produced by group A streptococcal (GAS) infection is acute pharyngitis or tonsillitis. Some patients, usually untreated, develop purulent complications, including otitis media, sinusitis, peritonsillar and retropharyngeal abscesses, and suppurative cervical adenitis. The significance of streptococcal upper respiratory tract disease is its acute morbidity and nonsuppurative sequelae, rheumatic fever, and acute glomerulonephritis. Scarlet fever occurs most commonly in association with pharyngitis, and, rarely, with pyoderma or an infected surgical or traumatic wound. It has a characteristic sandpaper-like rash, which is caused by one or more of the several erythrogenic exotoxins produced by GAS strains. Severe scarlet fever with systemic toxicity is rare today, but does occur. With this exception, the epidemiology, symptoms, sequelae, and treatment of scarlet fever are no different from those of streptococcal pharyngitis.

Toddlers (1 to 3 years old) with GAS respiratory infection frequently present with moderate fever with seromucoid rhinitis, and may have a protracted illness with fever, irritability, and anorexia. The classic clinical presentation of streptococcal upper respiratory tract infection as pharyngitis is uncommon in children younger than 3 years of age. Rheumatic fever is also uncommon in this group.

The second most common site of GAS infection is the skin. Streptococcal skin infections (ie, pyoderma and impetigo) can result in glomerulonephritis, which occasionally can occur in epidemics, but rheumatic fever is not a sequela of streptococcal pyoderma. Less commonly, GAS causes erysipelas, perianal cellulitis, vaginitis, bacteremia, pneumonia, endocarditis, pericarditis, septic arthritis, cellulitis osteomyelitis, myositis, puerperal sepsis, and, in neonates, omphalitis.

The GAS toxic shock syndrome caused by GAS is associated with hypotension (shock), renal impairment, coagulopathy (disseminated intravascular coagulation or thrombocytopenia), adult acute respiratory distress syndrome, rash and local tissue destruction, and a fatality rate as high as 30%. The occurrence of shock and multiorgan failure early in the course of GAS infection characterizes streptococcal toxic shock syndrome and helps differentiate it from other types of invasive group A streptococcal infection.

Etiology: More than 80 distinct M-protein types of group A beta-hemolytic streptococci (*Streptococcus pyogenes*) have been identified. Epidemiologic studies suggest an association between certain serotypes (eg, types 1, 3, 5, 6, 18, 19, and 24) and rheumatic fever, but a "rheumatogenic" factor has not been identified. Several serotypes (eg, 49, 55, 57) are clearly associated with pyoderma and acute glomerulonephritis. Pharyngitis-associated nephritis is often associated with other serotypes (eg, type 12). Groups C and G streptococci have been associated with pharyngitis, and occasionally nephritis, but do not cause rheumatic fever. The GAS toxic shock syndrome is believed to be a toxin-mediated disease.

Epidemiology: Pharyngitis usually results from contact with a person who has streptococcal pharyngitis. Fomites and household pets such as dogs have not been demonstrated to be vectors of GAS infection. Transmission of GAS infection, including outbreaks of pharyngitis such as occur in schools, almost always occurs by contact with respiratory secretions. Pharyngitis, impetigo, and their nonsuppurative complications may be associated with crowding, which is often present in socioeconomically disadvantaged populations. Close contact, such as occurs in schools, child care, and military installations, can facilitate transmission. Food-borne outbreaks have occurred and are a consequence of human contamination of food in conjunction with improper preparation or refrigeration procedures.

Streptococcal pharyngitis can occur at any age, but it is most frequent among school-aged children. Group A streptococcal pharyngitis and pyoderma are less frequent in adults than in children except during epidemics.

Geographically, both streptococcal pharyngitis and impetigo are ubiquitous. Impetigo is more common in tropical climates and in warm seasons, presumably in part because of antecedent insect bites and other minor skin trauma. However, impetigo occurs in all climates. Streptococcal pharyngitis occurs more frequently in the late fall, winter, and spring in temperate climates, presumably because of close person-to-person contact indoors, such as occurs in schools.

Throat culture surveys of asymptomatic children during school outbreaks of pharyngitis have yielded streptococcal prevalence rates as high as 15% to 30%. These children include carriers (those with no immune response to group A cellular and extracellular antigens), persons with asymptomatic infections, and those who have been treated for symptomatic infection without eradication of the organism. Pharyngeal carriage may persist for several months but is not associated with an appreciable risk of rheumatic fever or contagiousness.

Communicability of patients with streptococcal pharyngitis is highest during the acute infection, but gradually diminishes during a period of weeks in untreated individuals. Transmission by a carrier is unlikely, perhaps because of diminished numbers of organisms in the pharynx or the disappearance of bacteria from nasal secretions. The occurrence of transmission during the incubation period is uncertain.

Incidence rates of rheumatic fever in the United States have decreased for several decades, but outbreaks of rheumatic fever in the 1980s in both school-children and military populations in different geographic areas demonstrate that acute rheumatic fever can still occur. The reason(s) for these local outbreaks is not clear, but the introduction and spread of specific strains of streptococcal serotypes are likely factors.

The colonization of healthy skin by GAS precedes the development of streptococcal impetigo. The organism is acquired from others with impetigo, possibly by physical contact. In addition, individuals with streptococcal pharyngitis or upper respiratory tract carriage can infect their open skin lesions (eg, insect bites or burns) or those of others. Usually the upper respiratory tract becomes colonized after the skin lesions. Infections of surgical wounds, puerperal sepsis, and neonatal infections (which most often begin with omphalitis) usually result from contact transmission via hand carriage. At times, anal or vaginal carriers and persons with pyoderma or local suppurative infections can transmit infection, particularly to surgical or obstetrical patients and newborn infants, resulting in nosocomial outbreaks.

The **incubation period** of streptococcal pharyngitis is 2 to 5 days. For impetigo, a 7- to 10-day period between the acquisition of GAS on healthy skin and the development of lesions has been demonstrated.

Diagnostic Tests: The throat culture remains the test of choice for children with pharyngitis, since the clinical differentiation of viral and GAS pharyngitis is often impossible. A swab specimen, properly obtained by vigorous swabbing of the tonsils and posterior pharynx, should be cultured on sheep blood agar to confirm GAS infection. Latex agglutination, fluorescent antibody, coagglutination, and precipitation techniques are very accurate in differentiating group A from other beta-hemolytic streptococci. Appropriate use of bacitracin-sensitivity disks (containing 0.04 units) allows presumptive identification of GAS but is a less accurate method. False-negative cultures occur in fewer than 10% of symptomatic patients when the throat swab specimen is properly obtained. Recovery of GAS from the pharynx does not distinguish patients with streptococcal infection, as defined by a serologic antibody response, from streptococcal carriers who have pharyngitis resulting from other causes (ie, viral infection). The number of colonies of GAS on the agar does not reliably differentiate infection from carriage, since at least one third of patients with scant growth on culture will have GAS infection.

Tests for the rapid diagnosis of GAS performed on properly obtained throat swabs may be used as an adjunct to culture. Most of these tests are based on direct extraction of group A carbohydrate antigen from organisms obtained by throat swab. Although these tests vary in methodology, their sensitivities and specificities are comparable when carefully performed, including rigorous attention to technique and use of controls. The specificity of these tests is generally high, but the sensitivity has been reported to vary considerably and can be as low as 50% to 70%. The sensitivity is even lower when the number of organisms, which reflects the quantity of GAS antigen, is low. The accuracy of these tests may be most dependent on the quality of the throat swab specimen, which must contain pharyngeal and tonsillar secretions, and on the experience of the person who is performing the test. **Therefore, when a patient suspected of having GAS pharyngitis has a negative rapid streptococcal test, a culture should be obtained** to ensure that the patient does not have GAS infection. Because of the high specificity of these rapid tests, a positive test does not require throat culture confirmation.

Rapid diagnostic tests using new techniques, such as optical immunoassay and chemiluminescent DNA probes, have been developed. Although the initial data about the reliability and value of these tests are encouraging and indicate that these tests might be as sensitive and specific as the throat culture, they have not been extensively evaluated (particularly with respect to studies of asymptomatic patients, GAS serologic data in study patients, correlation of results with severity of clinical disease, and ease and reliability of tests performed in physician offices). Hence, until additional corroborative information becomes available, throat cultures continue to be indicated in patients with suspected GAS pharyngitis who have negative results with one of these newer tests. In the future, with improved technology and resulting sensitivity of these tests, changes may be made in the current recommendations for diagnosing GAS pharyngitis.

Indications for Cultures. Factors to be considered in the decision to obtain a throat culture in children with pharyngitis are the patient's age, clinical signs and symptoms, the season, and the family and community epidemiology. An important reason for culturing even those with classic findings is to establish the presence or absence of GAS, which may help in the management of contacts who subsequently become ill. Additionally, the most reliable means to diagnose GAS infection in individuals with suggestive but not classic findings is by culture. In children younger than 3 years, GAS infection is uncommon. However, outbreaks of streptococcal pharyngitis have been reported in child care settings.

Indications for culturing contacts vary according to circumstances. Siblings and all other household contacts of a child who has developed acute rheumatic fever, glomerulonephritis, or streptococcal toxic shock syndrome should have throat cultures taken and, if positive, should be treated regardless of whether the contact is currently or recently symptomatic. Pyoderma lesions should also be cultured for GAS in families in which one or more cases of acute nephritis or streptococcal toxic shock syndrome has occurred. In these circumstances, antibiotic treatment should focus on eradicating carriage. Household contacts of an index patient with streptococcal pharyngitis who have recent or current symptoms suggestive of streptococcal infection should be cultured. Culturing asymptomatic household contacts is not recommended except during outbreaks or in other unique epidemiologic situations, such as presence of a person in the family with rheumatic heart disease or streptococcal toxic shock syndrome.

Posttreatment throat cultures are usually indicated only in patients who are at high risk for rheumatic fever or who are symptomatic. Repeated courses of antibiotic therapy are not indicated in asymptomatic patients who continue to harbor GAS after appropriate antibiotic therapy, except for those who have or have had, or whose family members have or have had, rheumatic fever or rheumatic heart disease, or in other unique epidemiologic circumstances, such as outbreaks of rheumatic fever or acute nephritis.

Children in whom repeated episodes of documented GAS pharyngitis occur at short intervals present a special problem. These illnesses may be caused by the same serotypes (ie, a true relapse) or by heterologous serotypes (infection unrelated to the previous episode). In assessing such a situation, confirming that the cultured bacteria are GAS (ie, not beta-hemolytic streptococci of other serogroups) is important. Poor compliance with oral treatment and bacterial resistance to the prescribed antimicrobial should be excluded. In some areas, erythromycin resistance may occur, resulting in treatment failures. Culturing asymptomatic household members in most circumstances is usually not helpful. However, if multiple members have symptomatic pharyngitis or other GAS infection, such as impetigo or pyoderma, simultaneous cultures of all household members and treatment of all persons with positive cultures may be of value.

In schools, child care, or other environments where large numbers of persons are in close contact, GAS upper respiratory tract carriage in healthy children can be as high as 5% to 15% in the absence of an outbreak of streptococcal disease. Therefore, classroom or more widespread culture surveys are not routinely indicated and should be considered only if one or more cases of rheumatic fever, glomerulonephritis, or streptococcal toxic shock syndrome has occurred.

Cultures of impetiginous lesions are not routinely indicated, since they often yield both streptococci and staphylococci, and determination of the primary pathogen from culture results may not be possible.

Treatment:

Pharyngitis

- Penicillin V is the drug of choice for the treatment of GAS pharyngitis, except in penicillin-allergic individuals. Group A streptococci resistant to penicillin have not been documented. Ampicillin or amoxicillin are often used in place of penicillin V. Penicillin therapy prevents rheumatic fever, even when therapy is started as long as 9 days after the onset of the acute illness. Thus, for patients seen early in their illness, a brief delay for processing of the throat culture before therapy is started does not increase the risk of rheumatic fever. In all patients with acute rheumatic fever, a complete course of penicillin or other appropriate antibiotic for GAS pharyngitis should be given to eradicate GAS from the throat, even though the organism may or may not be recovered by the initial throat culture.

  The dose of orally administered penicillin V is 400,000 U (250 mg), three times daily for 10 days. With good compliance, oral penicillin totaling 800,000 U (500 mg/d) in two divided doses is effective. To prevent rheumatic fever, oral treatment with penicillin should be given for at least 10 days, regardless of the promptness of clinical recovery. Although different preparations of oral penicillin vary in absorption, their clinical efficacy is similar. Relapses may occur more frequently with oral penicillin than with intramuscularly administered benzathine penicillin G as a result of poor compliance with oral therapy.

- Intramuscular benzathine penicillin G, 600,000 U, is appropriate for children who weigh less than 60 lb (27.3 kg); for larger children and adults, the dose is 1,200,000 U. Intramuscular benzathine penicillin G ensures adequate blood concentrations and avoids the problem of compliance, but it is painful. Mixtures containing shorter-acting penicillins (eg, procaine penicillin) in addition to benzathine penicillin G have not been demonstrated to be superior to benzathine penicillin G alone, except in reducing discomfort from the injection. If such a mixture is used, it must contain benzathine penicillin G in the recommended doses. Although supporting data are limited, the combination of 900,000 U of benzathine penicillin G and 300,000 U of procaine penicillin G may be satisfactory for children who weigh less than 60 lb (27.3 kg). Less discomfort is associated with an intramuscular injection of benzathine penicillin G if the preparation is brought to room temperature before administration.
- Orally administered erythromycin is indicated for patients allergic to penicillin. Treatment should also be given for 10 days. Erythromycin estolate (20 to 40 mg/kg/d in two to four divided doses) or erythromycin ethyl succinate (40 to 50 mg/kg/d in three to four divided doses) is effective in treating streptococcal pharyngitis; the maximal dose is 1 g/d. Although GAS strains resistant to erythromycin have been prevalent in some areas of the world (eg, Asia and Finland), and have resulted in treatment failures, they remain uncommon in most areas of the United States.
- A 10-day course of a narrow-spectrum ("first-generation"), oral cephalosporin is an acceptable alternative, particularly for individuals allergic to penicillin. However, as many as 15% of penicillin-allergic persons are also allergic to cephalosporins. A cephalosporin should not be administered to patients with immediate, anaphylactic-type hypersensitivity to penicillin. The additional cost of cephalosporins and their wider range of antibacterial activity compared with penicillin preclude recommending them for routine use in persons with GAS pharyngitis who are not allergic to penicillin.
- Tetracyclines and sulfonamides should **not** be used for treating GAS pharyngitis. Many strains are resistant to tetracycline, and sulfonamides do not eradicate GAS, although sulfonamides are effective for continuous prophylaxis in preventing recurrent rheumatic fever (see Secondary Prophylaxis of Rheumatic Fever, p 438).
- Although some studies suggest that beta-lactamase-producing upper respiratory tract flora may interfere with the efficacy of penicillin in treatment of GAS pharyngitis, antibiotic therapy of GAS pharyngitis directed against these organisms remains controversial and is usually not necessary in patients with acute pharyngitis. However, beta-lactamase-resistant and antistaphylococcal drugs, such as amoxicillin-clavulanate, narrow-spectrum cephalosporins, dicloxacillin, and clindamycin, can be beneficial in the retreatment of patients with recurrent GAS pharyngitis who have failed penicillin treatment.

- Asymptomatic pharyngeal carriers of GAS appear to be at little risk for developing nonsuppurative sequelae of streptococcal infection or for spreading infection to those who live and work around them; they usually do not warrant antibiotic treatment. However, GAS carriers present a difficult diagnostic problem when they develop symptomatic upper respiratory tract infection because differentiation between acute streptococcal infection or chronic carriage in a patient with a viral infection is usually not possible at the time the patient presents. In these circumstances, a single course of therapy is reasonable.
- Children in families with multiple episodes of documented, symptomatic GAS pharyngitis over many weeks pose special treatment considerations. The entire family should be cultured simultaneously (see Indications for Cultures, p 433). Those harboring GAS should be treated (preferably with intramuscularly administered benzathine penicillin G) and recultured 3 to 4 weeks later. If they are still harboring GAS, a second course of treatment should be given. Some physicians may elect to treat all family members in select circumstances, such as a large family with repeated and prolonged intrafamily transmission, especially if members are at risk of complications of GAS infection.

  Several other antibiotic regimens have been evaluated and appear effective in eradicating the organism in these circumstances. These regimens include 10 days of (1) clindamycin, (2) amoxicillin-clavulanate, (3) dicloxacillin, and (4) penicillin therapy with rifampin given concurrently during the last 4 days. In these circumstances, one of these drugs may be more effective than penicillin and could be recommended in situations where eradication is especially important (ie, rheumatic fever, streptococcal toxic shock syndrome, or outbreak situations). Persons so treated should be recultured after this second treatment; if one or more persons still harbor GAS but are asymptomatic, no further treatment is necessary (except in persons with present or past rheumatic fever, those with a family history of rheumatic heart disease, or in outbreaks).

Streptococcal Impetigo
- Local antibacterial preparations, such as bacitracin or mupirocin ointment, may be useful in limiting person-to-person spread of GAS impetigo. With multiple lesions or impetigo in multiple family members, child care groups, or athletic teams, GAS impetigo should be treated systemically with antibiotic regimens, as recommended for pharyngitis. **However, since episodes of impetigo are frequently caused by *Staphylococcus aureus*, children with impetigo usually should be treated with an antibiotic active against both GAS and *S aureus*.**

Other Infections.
- High-dose, parenteral, and often prolonged (2 to 4 weeks) treatment is required for infections such as endocarditis, pneumonia, septicemia, meningitis, arthritis, osteomyelitis, and streptococcal toxic shock syndrome.
- The drug of choice is penicillin G.

Nonsuppurative Sequelae. Acute rheumatic fever and acute glomerulonephritis are serious nonsuppurative sequelae of GAS infections. During epidemics, as many as 3% of untreated patients with acute streptococcal pharyngitis may develop rheumatic fever. With endemic infections, the attack rates are lower but still constitute a risk. The risk of rheumatic fever can be virtually eliminated by adequate treatment of the antecedent GAS infection; however, cases of rheumatic fever even after alleged appropriate therapy do occur. The prevention of acute nephritis, especially that following pyoderma, by antimicrobial treatment is less certain. Suppurative sequelae, such as peritonsillar abscesses and cervical adenitis, are usually prevented by prompt therapy with penicillin of the primary infection. Severe infections, such as the streptococcal toxic shock syndrome, may follow respiratory tract or skin infection, but whether severe infection can be prevented by early therapy is unknown.

Isolation of the Hospitalized Patient: Drainage/secretion precautions are recommended for patients with pharyngitis. For patients with pneumonia, contact isolation is indicated. In both cases, these measures are continued until 24 hours after the initiation of effective therapy. For burns with secondary GAS infections and for all widespread or draining cutaneous infections, contact isolation or drainage/secretion precautions, depending on the extent of the infection, should be observed for at least 24 hours after the start of effective therapy.

Control Measures: The most important means of controlling GAS disease and its sequelae is prompt identification and treatment of infections.

School and Child Care. Children with streptococcal pharyngitis or skin infections should not return to school or child care until at least 24 hours after beginning antimicrobial therapy, and until they are afebrile. Close contact with other children during this time should be avoided if possible.

Care of Exposed Persons. Contacts of documented cases of streptococcal infection who have recent or current clinical evidence of a streptococcal infection should have appropriate cultures obtained and should be treated if the culture is positive. Rates of GAS acquisition are higher among sibling contacts (25%) than among parent contacts in nonepidemic settings; rates as high as 50% for sibling contacts and 20% for parent contacts have been reported during epidemics. More than half of those contacts who acquire the organism will become ill. Asymptomatic acquisition of GAS may pose some risk of nonsuppurative complications, as studies indicate that as many as one third of patients with rheumatic fever had no history of recent streptococcal infection and another third had minor respiratory infections that were not brought to medical attention. However, asymptomatic family contacts usually need not be cultured except in unusual epidemiologic circumstances or when the contacts are at risk for developing complications of infection (see Indications for Cultures, p 433). Short courses (fewer than 10 days) of antibiotics for contacts are inappropriate. In some circumstances, such as a large family with documented, repeated intrafamily transmission during a prolonged period and contacts at risk of complications, physicians may elect to treat all family members (see Treatment, p 434). Cultures should be obtained in these circumstances to identify those individuals harboring the organism. However, these circumstances arise infrequently.

Chemoprophylaxis. For children with repeated episodes of documented GAS pharyngitis occurring at short intervals, some experts recommend oral penicillin prophylaxis during the time of year of greatest risk. The dosage is the same as for secondary prophylaxis of rheumatic fever.

Secondary Prophylaxis of Rheumatic Fever. Patients who have a well-documented history of rheumatic fever (including cases manifested solely by Sydenham's chorea) and those who show documented evidence of rheumatic heart disease should be given continuous antibiotic prophylaxis to prevent recurrent attacks (secondary prophylaxis) because asymptomatic and symptomatic GAS infections can result in a rheumatic recurrence. Continuous prophylaxis should be initiated as soon as the diagnosis of rheumatic fever or rheumatic heart disease is made. Secondary prophylaxis should be long term, perhaps for life, in patients with rheumatic heart disease.

The risk of recurrence declines with the interval from the most recent attack, and patients without rheumatic heart disease are at a lower risk of recurrence than those with cardiac involvement. These considerations influence the duration of secondary prophylaxis in adults but should not alter the practice of secondary prophylaxis in children, adolescents, and young adults. Secondary prophylaxis should be continued for 5 or more years or at least until the individual is 21 years of age. Prophylaxis should continue for life in patients with rheumatic heart disease, even after prosthetic valve replacement, because these patients remain at risk for recurrence of rheumatic fever. When streptococcal infections occur in family members of rheumatic fever patients, infected persons should be treated rapidly with an appropriate antibiotic (see Indications for Cultures, p 433, and Treatment, p 434).

The following three regimens for secondary prophylaxis are effective:

1. Benzathine penicillin G, 1,200,000 U, intramuscularly, once every 3 or 4 weeks.
2. Penicillin V, orally, 250 mg twice a day.
3. Sulfisoxazole, orally, 1 g once a day for patients weighing 60 lb (27.3 kg) or more, and 0.5 g once a day for patients weighing less than 60 lb.

The intramuscular regimen has been proven to be the most reliable because the success of oral prophylaxis depends primarily on patient compliance, although inconvenience and the pain of injection may cause some patients to discontinue intramuscular prophylaxis. In some countries, and in situations where the risk of GAS infection is high, benzathine penicillin G is given every 3 weeks because of greater effectiveness. In the United States, every 4 weeks appears adequate in most patients. Oral sulfisoxazole is as effective as oral penicillin for secondary prophylaxis.

Allergic reactions to oral penicillin are similar to those with intramuscular penicillin, but they are usually less severe and occur less frequently. These reactions also occur less often in children than in adults. Anaphylaxis is extremely rare in patients receiving oral penicillin. Severe allergic reactions in patients receiving continuous benzathine penicillin G prophylaxis are also rare. Anaphylaxis and death have been reported, but usually in patients with severe rheumatic heart disease. Most of these severe reactions, hence, may result from vasovagal responses rather than anaphylaxis. Reactions include a serum sickness-like reaction, characterized by fever and joint pains, which can be mistaken for an acute rheumatic fever recurrence.

Sulfisoxazole reactions are infrequent and usually minor; blood counts may be advisable after 2 weeks of prophylaxis, as leukopenia has been reported. Prophylaxis with sulfisoxazole in late pregnancy is contraindicated because of interference with fetal bilirubin metabolism. Febrile mucocutaneous syndromes (erythema multiforme, Stevens-Johnson syndrome, or epidermal necrolysis) have been associated with penicillin as well as sulfonamides. When an adverse event occurs with any of these therapeutic regimens, the drug should be stopped immediately and an alternative drug selected. For the rare patient allergic to both penicillin and sulfonamides, erythromycin (250 mg twice daily) may be used.

Bacterial Endocarditis Prophylaxis. Patients with rheumatic valvular heart disease also require additional short-term antibiotic prophylaxis at the time of certain procedures (including dental and surgical procedures) to prevent the possible development of bacterial endocarditis (see Prevention of Bacterial Endocarditis, p 525). Patients who have had rheumatic fever without evidence of valvular heart disease do not need prophylaxis for prevention of endocarditis. Penicillin, ampicillin, or amoxicillin should not be used for endocarditis prophylaxis in patients who are receiving oral penicillin for secondary rheumatic fever prophylaxis because of relative resistance to penicillins and aminopenicillins of viridans streptococci in the oral cavity in such patients. Erythromycin is the alternative antibiotic recommended for such patients.

Group B Streptococcal Infections

Clinical Manifestations: Group B streptococci are a major cause of perinatal bacterial infections, including endometritis, amnionitis, and urinary tract infections in parturient women and systemic and focal infections in infants from birth until 3 or more months of age. Two distinct forms of invasive disease occur in neonates. Early-onset disease is often characterized by respiratory distress, apnea, shock, pneumonia, and, occasionally, meningitis, and its onset usually occurs within the first 24 hours of life (range, 0 to 6 days). Late-onset disease, which typically occurs at 3 to 4 weeks of age (range, 7 days to 3 months), is frequently manifested as occult bacteremia or meningitis; other focal infections, such as osteomyelitis, septic arthritis, and cellulitis, can also occur. Group B streptococci also cause infections in adults, particularly those with diabetes, malignancy, or other immunocompromising conditions.

Etiology: Group B streptococci (*Streptococcus agalactiae*) are divided into the seven following serotypes: Ia, Ib/c, Ia/c, II, III, IV, and V. All serotypes are associated with infections in newborn infants and in adults. Serotype III is the predominant cause of early-onset meningitis and late-onset infections.

Epidemiology: Group B streptococci (GBS) are common inhabitants of the gastrointestinal and the genitourinary tracts. Less commonly, they colonize the pharynx. The colonization rate in pregnant women and newborn infants ranges from 5% to 35%. Colonization during pregnancy is usually constant but may be intermittent. Neonatal GBS disease has an incidence of one to five cases per 1,000 live births; the incidence varies considerably among hospitals. Early-onset disease occurs in approximately one infant per 100 to 200 colonized women. Transmission from mother to infant occurs in utero shortly before delivery or during delivery. After delivery, person-to-person transmission can occur. Although uncommon, GBS can be acquired in the nursery from colonized infants or hospital personnel (probably via hand contamination), or in the community. The risk of early-onset disease is increased in preterm infants born at less than 37 weeks gestation, in those born after the amniotic membranes have been ruptured for more than 18 hours, and in infants born of women with intrapartum fever or chorioamnionitis, multiple births (such as twins), or GBS bacteriuria. Low or absent concentration of type-specific serum antibody also appears to be a predisposing factor. The period of communicability is unknown, but it may extend throughout the duration of colonization or of disease. Infants can remain colonized for several months after birth and after treatment of symptomatic infections.

The **incubation period** of early-onset disease is less than 6 days. In late-onset disease the incubation period from GBS acquisition to disease is unknown. Onset usually occurs from 7 days to 3 months of age.

Diagnostic Tests: Gram-positive cocci in fluids that are ordinarily sterile (cerebrospinal, pleural, joint fluid, or urine) provide presumptive evidence of infection. Cultures of blood and body fluids are necessary to establish the diagnosis. Serotype identification by type-specific antisera is available in reference laboratories. Group B streptococci antigen may be detected in biologic fluids (serum, cerebrospinal fluid, and urine) by latex particle agglutination or other rapid tests; positive tests in symptomatic infants constitute presumptive evidence of infection. The sensitivity and specificity of rapid diagnostic tests are variable, and false-positive results occur in a minimum of 5% to 8% of urine samples, especially bagged urine specimens that become perineally contaminated during collection. A positive test in an asymptomatic infant, thus, is not diagnostic of invasive infection, and testing of urine by this method is not a reliable screening test for neonatal GBS septicemia in asymptomatic infants.

Treatment:
- Penicillin or ampicillin plus an aminoglycoside is the initial treatment of choice for a newborn infant with presumptive, invasive, life-threatening infection.
- Penicillin G or ampicillin alone can be given when GBS is identified in a focus of infection, and clinical and microbiologic response has been documented. Before so doing, however, some experts advise determination of the susceptibility of the organism to penicillin or ampicillin.
- The recommended dosage of penicillin G for meningitis for infants 7 days or younger is 250,000 to 400,000 U/kg/d, intravenously, in three divided doses; for infants more than 7 days old, 400,000 U/kg/d, in four divided doses, intravenously, is recommended. For ampicillin, the recommended

dosage for infants with meningitis age 7 days or younger is 200 mg/kg/d in three divided doses, intravenously; for infants more than 7 days old, 300 mg/kg/d in four to six divided doses, is recommended. The optimal dose, however, is unknown.

- For meningitis, some experts believe that a second lumbar puncture at approximately 24 hours after initiation of therapy to document bacteriologic cure has prognostic importance. Additional lumbar punctures and other studies are often indicated if response to therapy is in doubt after 36 to 72 hours of treatment. Consultation with an expert in infectious diseases may be useful.
- For infants with bacteremia without a defined focus, treatment should be continued for at least 10 days. For infants with uncomplicated meningitis, 14 to 21 days of treatment is usually satisfactory, but longer periods of treatment may be necessary for infants with prolonged or complicated courses. Osteomyelitis requires longer treatment depending on the severity of infection, response to treatment, and complications. Treatment duration should be guided by the patient's clinical and bacteriologic responses.
- Treatment of the twin of an index case is indicated because of the high frequency of coinfection in both infants.

Isolation of the Hospitalized Patient: No special precautions are recommended except during a nursery outbreak of GBS disease (see Control Measures, below).

Control Measures:

Chemoprophylaxis. Recommendations for prevention of early-onset neonatal GBS infection are as follows:
- Screening of all pregnant women for GBS at 26 to 28 weeks gestation is a method upon which effective, selective intrapartum chemoprophylaxis can be based.
- If GBS cultures are performed, a single swab of the lower vagina and anorectum should be placed into selective broth medium, transported to the laboratory, and subcultured onto solid media for optimal detection.
- Antepartum treatment of asymptomatic women for GBS regardless of maternal colonization status is not recommended except for those with GBS bacteriuria.
- At hospital admission, such as for preterm labor or premature rupture of membranes, women who have no prenatal GBS culture result available may be tested for GBS, either by rapid antigen test (if an appropriate test is available) or by culture.
- Maternal GBS carriers, identified either antepartum or intrapartum, with one or more risk factors, should be given intrapartum intravenous ampicillin (2 g initially; 1 to 2 g every 4 to 6 hours) or penicillin G (5 mU every 6 hours) until delivery; penicillin-allergic women may be given clindamycin or erythromycin intravenously. Risk factors include (1) preterm labor at less than 37 weeks gestation; (2) premature rupture of membranes at less than 37 weeks gestation; (3) fever during labor; (4) multiple births (such as twins); and (5) rupture of membranes beyond

18 hours at any gestation. When membranes have been ruptured for 12 hours, an assessment of the likely duration of labor should be made so that chemoprophylaxis can be initiated if rupture is considered likely to extend beyond 18 hours. If maternal GBS colonization status is unknown, chemoprophylaxis may be appropriate for one or more of the aforementioned risk factors.

- Previous delivery of a sibling with invasive GBS disease warrants intrapartum maternal chemoprophylaxis in each subsequent pregnancy.
- Management of infants whose mothers are receiving chemoprophylaxis should be based on the clinical findings and gestational age of the infants.
- As maternal GBS chemoprophylaxis is implemented in an area, active surveillance and assessment of the benefits of these strategies by public health agencies should be performed so that future approaches might be modified to enhance safety and efficacy.

Neonatal Infection Control. Routine cultures of infants to determine GBS colonization are not recommended. Epidemiologic evaluation of late-onset cases in a special care nursery may be required to exclude a nosocomial source.

Nursery Outbreak. Cohorting of ill and colonized infants and the use of a gown and gloves during an outbreak are recommended. Other methods of control (eg, treatment of asymptomatic carriers with penicillin or treatment of the umbilical cord with triple dye or hexachlorophene) are impractical or ineffective. Routine hand washing by personnel caring for infants colonized or infected with GBS is recommended to prevent spread to other infants.

Non-Group A or B Streptococcal and Enterococcal Infections

Clinical Manifestations: Streptococci of groups other than A or B may be associated with invasive disease in newborn infants, older children, and adults. Urinary tract infection, endocarditis, upper and lower respiratory tract infections, and meningitis are the principal clinical syndromes.

Etiology: Streptococci of groups D, C, G, and *Enterococcus* species are common pathogens. The two most common enterococcal species are *Enterococcus fecalis* and *Enterococcus faecium.* Streptococcal groups F, H, and K are also potential pathogens. Nongroupable streptococci, such as viridans and anaerobic streptococci (peptostreptococci), can be pathogenic in a variety of infections.

Epidemiology: The common habitats in humans of these streptococcal groups are skin (C, F, and G), oropharynx (C, F, G, H, and K), gastrointestinal tract (D and *Enterococcus,* F and G), and vagina (C and D, and *Enterococcus,* F, and G). The normal habitats of different species of viridans streptococci include the oropharynx, teeth surfaces, skin, and intestinal and genitourinary tracts. Intrapartum transmission probably causes early-onset neonatal infections.

The **incubation period** and the period of communicability are unknown.

Diagnostic Tests: Microscopic examination of fluids that are ordinarily sterile can yield presumptive evidence of infections by Gram-positive cocci. The diagnosis is established by culture and serogrouping of the isolate, using group-specific antisera.

Treatment: Enterococci and occasional strains from some streptococcal groups (eg, C and G) are less susceptible to penicillin than are most other streptococcal isolates. Enterococci are not susceptible to cephalosporins, and strains resistant to ampicillin or vancomycin have been identified. In invasive enterococcal infections, including endocarditis and meningitis, ampicillin and vancomycin, in combination with an aminoglycoside (usually gentamicin), should be administered until in vitro susceptibility is known and appropriate combination therapy can be selected. Ampicillin and gentamicin may be required for optimum treatment of groups C, F, and G severe infections. In other infections, penicillin G or ampicillin alone is given.

Endocarditis. Guidelines for antimicrobial therapy have been formulated by the American Heart Association's Council on Cardiovascular Disease in the Young and should be consulted for appropriate regimens and details of therapy.[*]

Isolation of the Hospitalized Patient: No special precautions are recommended unless ampicillin- or vancomycin-resistant enterococcal infection is documented. In this situation, contact isolation should be instituted for the duration of the patient's hospitalization.

Control Measures: Patients with valvular or congenital heart disease should receive antibiotic prophylaxis to prevent streptococcal and enterococcal endocarditis at the time of dental and selected other surgical procedures (see Prevention of Bacterial Endocarditis, p 525).

Strongyloidiasis
(Strongyloides stercoralis)

Clinical Manifestations: Infection can be manifested by eosinophilia only. Hence, strongyloidiasis warrants consideration whenever hypereosinophilia (more than 30%), without an obvious clinical correlation, is found, especially if the patient has resided in an endemic area. Infective larvae first

---

[*]Bisno AL, Dismukes WE, Durack DT, et al. Antimicrobial treatment of infective endocarditis due to viridans streptococci, enterococci, and staphylococci. *JAMA.* 1989;261:1471-1477

entering the body can produce transient pruritic papules at the site of penetration of the skin, usually on the feet. Larval migration through the lungs can cause pneumonitis, with coughing productive of blood-streaked sputum. The intestinal phase of infection can be accompanied by vague abdominal pain, distention, vomiting, and diarrhea that consists of mucoid, voluminous stools. Malabsorption has been reported. Larval migration from defecated stool can result in pruritic skin lesions in the perianal area, buttocks, and upper thighs. The lesions may present as migrating, pruritic, serpiginous, erythematous tracks called "cutaneous larva currens." In immunocompromised patients, complications include disseminated strongyloidiasis (caused by hyperinfection), diffuse pulmonary infiltrates, and septicemia from Gram-negative bacilli.

Etiology: *Strongyloides stercoralis* is a nematode (roundworm).

Epidemiology: Strongyloidiasis is endemic in the tropics and subtropics, including the southern and southwestern United States, wherever suitable moist soil and improper disposal of human waste coexist. Humans are the principal hosts. Dogs, cats, and other animals can also be reservoirs. Transmission involves penetration of the skin by infective larvae, either from autoinfection or contact with infected soil. Infections rarely can be acquired from intimate skin contact or from inadvertent coprophagia, such as from ingestion of contaminated food scavenged from garbage. Because some larvae mature into the infective forms in the colon, autoinfection is common. Asymptomatic infection, especially in healthy hosts, is common. In immunocompromised patients, autoinfection is more frequent and causes hyperinfection with resulting disseminated strongyloidiasis, wherein the patient's organs and tissues are suffused with larvae, and the number of adult worms in the small intestine is extraordinarily high. In addition, because these larvae penetrate the wall of the colon, bacteremia and meningitis caused by enteric flora can occur. Even mild immunosuppression associated with treatment with corticosteroids can precipitate hyperinfection. The period of communicability lasts as long as the patient is infected, which can be several decades.

The **incubation period** is not known.

Diagnostic Tests: Stool examination discloses the characteristic larvae, but several specimens may have to be examined before a positive one is found. Examination of duodenal contents obtained by a commercially available string test (Enterotest*) or direct aspirate is more likely to demonstrate larvae. Serodiagnosis can be helpful but is only available in a few reference laboratories, and false negatives do occur. The enzyme immunoassay test for antibodies is positive in approximately 85% of cases; however, cross-reaction with the antigens of filarial worms also occurs and limits the specificity of serodiagnosis. Hypereosinophilia (more than 30%) is common. In disseminated strongyloidiasis, larvae can be found in the sputum.

---

*Available from Hedeco, Palo Alto, CA.

Treatment: Thiabendazole* (see Drugs for Parasitic Infection, p 574) is curative in most patients. Side effects of nausea, vomiting, and malaise are common. Treatment may have to be repeated or prolonged in the hyperinfection syndrome. Relapses occur and should be treated. Albendazole is widely used in countries other than the United States because the drug is highly efficacious in the treatment of strongyloidiasis and has few reported side effects. The drug is available from the manufacturer[†] on a compassionate-use protocol, and its approval by the Food and Drug Administration in the United States may occur in the near future. Thiabendazole and albendazole are contraindicated in pregnancy. Ivermectin, in a single dose, has been reported to be effective in this infection.

Isolation of the Hospitalized Patient: No special precautions are recommended. However, protective gloves should be worn when handling waste products or body secretions.

Control Measures: Sanitary disposal measures for human waste should be followed. Education about the risk of infection through bare skin is important.

For the patient who has an immunologic defect or who requires immunosuppressive therapy and is from an endemic region, examination of the stool and, possibly, duodenal fluid and respiratory secretions for *S stercoralis* should be considered before immunosuppressive therapy is started. Serologic tests appear to be the most sensitive for diagnosis, but they do not distinguish between past and current infection, and results from a reference laboratory may not be immediately available. If a patient's status requires the initiation of immunosuppressive therapy before the results of diagnostic tests can be obtained, then the risks of empiric antiparasitic therapy for strongyloidiasis must be weighed against the risks of a disseminated infection.

Syphilis

Clinical Manifestations:

Congenital Syphilis. Infection can result in stillbirth; it can be asymptomatic, especially in the first weeks of life; or it may have multisystem manifestations, including osteitis, hepatitis, lymphadenopathy, pneumonitis, mucocutaneous lesions, anemia, and hemorrhage. Late manifestations of congenital syphilis can involve the central nervous system, bones, teeth, eyes, skin, and/or cartilage.

Acquired Syphilis. Infection can be divided into three stages. The primary stage appears as one or more painless, indurated ulcers (chancre) of the skin and mucous membranes at the site of inoculation, most commonly on the genitalia. The secondary stage is characterized by a polymorphic rash,

---

*Available from Merck & Co, West Point, PA.
[†]SmithKline Beecham, Philadelphia, PA.

which is most frequently maculopapular, generalized, and classically involves the palms and soles. In moist areas around the vulva or anus, hypertrophic papular lesions (condyloma lata) can occur. Generalized lymphadenopathy, fever, malaise, splenomegaly, sore throat, headache, and arthralgia can be present. A variable latent period follows, which can be interrupted by recurrences of symptoms of secondary syphilis. The tertiary stage can be marked by aortitis, various manifestations of neurosyphilis, or gummatous changes of the skin, bone, or viscera. These commonly occur 15 years or more after the primary infection.

Etiology: *Treponema pallidum* is a thin, motile spirochete.

Epidemiology: Syphilis occurs throughout the world but is most frequent in large urban areas. The incidence of both acquired and congenital syphilis has dramatically increased in the United States since 1986. In the pediatric age group, the disease is most common in adolescents. In adults in the United States, infection in males is two times more common than in females, but the difference is diminishing. In HIV-infected adults, syphilis is common and the risk of neurologic complications may be increased.

Congenital syphilis is contracted from an infected mother via transplacental transmission of *T pallidum* at any time during pregnancy or at birth. In women with untreated early syphilis, 40% of pregnancies result in spontaneous abortion, stillbirths, or perinatal deaths. Untreated syphilis, at any stage of the disease, can be transmitted to the fetus; the rate of transmission is almost 100% during the secondary stage and slowly decreases with increasing duration of disease. The moist secretions of congenital syphilis are highly infectious. Organisms are rarely found in lesions more than 24 hours after treatment has begun.

Acquired syphilis is contracted almost always through sexual contact from direct contact with ulcerative lesions of the skin or mucous membranes of infected persons. Sexual abuse must be suspected in any young child with acquired syphilis. Open, moist lesions of the primary or secondary stages teem with spirochetes. Infectious lesions usually do not occur more than 1 year after infection, but relapses with infectious secondary lesions have occurred as many as 4 years later.

The **incubation period** for acquired primary syphilis is typically about 3 weeks, but ranges from 10 to 90 days after exposure.

Diagnostic Tests: Definitive diagnosis is achieved by identifying spirochetes by microscopic darkfield examination or direct fluorescent antibody tests of lesion exudate or tissue. Specimens should be scraped from moist, mucocutaneous lesions or aspirated from a regional lymph node. Since false-negative microscopic results are common, serologic testing, follow-up, and often repeated testing are necessary. Specimens from mouth lesions require direct fluorescent antibody techniques to distinguish *T pallidum* from nonpathogenic treponemes.

Presumptive diagnosis is possible using two types of serologic tests, ie, (1) nontreponemal tests and (2) treponemal tests. Neither type of test alone is sufficient for diagnosis.

The nontreponemal tests for syphilis include the VDRL slide test, the rapid plasma reagin (RPR) test, and the automated reagin test (ART). These tests measure antibody directed against lipoidal antigen from *T pallidum* and/or its interaction with host tissues. These tests are inexpensive and rapidly performed, and provide quantitative results, which are helpful indicators of disease activity and are useful for follow-up after treatment. Nontreponemal tests may be falsely negative, ie, nonreactive, in early primary, latent acquired, and late congenital syphilis.

A reactive nontreponemal test from a patient with typical lesions usually indicates the need for treatment. However, any reactive nontreponemal test should be confirmed by one of the specific treponemal tests to exclude a false-positive test, which can be caused by infectious mononucleosis, connective tissue disease, tuberculosis, endocarditis, and abuse of injectable drugs. Treatment should not be delayed pending the treponemal test results in symptomatic patients or patients at high risk of infection. A sustained fourfold decrease in titer of the nontreponemal test with treatment demonstrates adequate therapy; a similar titer increase after treatment suggests reinfection or relapse. The quantitative nontreponemal test usually becomes nonreactive after successful therapy within 1 year in primary syphilis, and within 2 years in secondary syphilis.

Treponemal tests include the fluorescent treponemal antibody absorption (FTA-ABS) test, the microhemagglutination test for *T pallidum* (MHA-TP), and the *T pallidum* immobilization (TPI) test. Positive FTA-ABS and MHA-TP tests usually remain reactive for life, even with successful therapy.

Treponemal tests are also not 100% specific for syphilis; positive reactions occur in subjects with other spirochetal diseases such as yaws, pinta, leptospirosis, rat-bite fever, and Lyme disease. Nontreponemal tests can be used to differentiate Lyme disease from syphilis, as the VDRL is uniformly nonreactive in Lyme disease.

Usually a nontreponemal test is obtained; if reactive, it is followed by a treponemal test. The probability of syphilis is high in a sexually active patient whose serum is reactive on **both** a nontreponemal and a treponemal test.

In summary, the nontreponemal antibody tests (VDRL, RPR, and ART) are useful for screening; the treponemal tests (FTA-ABS, MHA-TP) are used to establish a provisional diagnosis. Quantitative nontreponemal antibody tests are used to assess the adequacy of therapy and to detect reinfection and relapse.

Testing During Pregnancy. All women should be screened for syphilis early in pregnancy with a nontreponemal test (eg, VDRL or RPR) and preferably again at delivery. In areas of high prevalence and in patients considered at high risk for syphilis, nontreponemal tests should also be done at the beginning of the third trimester (28 weeks). For those treated during pregnancy, follow-up serology is necessary to assess the efficacy of therapy.

Evaluation of Newborn Infants for Congenital Infection. No newborn should leave any hospital without determination of the syphilis serologic status of his or her mother. Testing should have been done at least once during pregnancy and preferably at delivery as well. An infant should be evaluated for congenital syphilis if he or she is born to a mother with positive nontreponemal tests confirmed by a positive treponemal test and who has one or more of the following conditions:

- Syphilis untreated or inadequately treated (see Treatment, p 450).
- Syphilis during pregnancy treated with a nonpenicillin regimen.
- Syphilis during pregnancy treated with an appropriate penicillin regimen, but one which did not have the expected decrease in nontreponemal antibody titer after therapy.
- Syphilis treated less than 1 month before delivery (since treatment failures occur and the efficacy of treatment cannot be assumed).
- Syphilis treatment not documented.
- Syphilis treated before pregnancy, but with insufficient serologic follow-up during pregnancy to assess the response to treatment and current infection status.

Infants born to women with any of the preceding conditions should be evaluated for syphilis. The infant's evaluation should include the following:

- Physical examination.
- Quantitative nontreponemal serologic test for syphilis.
- Cerebrospinal fluid VDRL, analysis for cells, and protein concentration.
- Long-bone roentgenograms (unless the diagnosis has been otherwise established).
- If available, determination of antitreponemal immunoglobulin M (IgM) antibody by a testing method recognized by the Centers for Disease Control and Prevention (CDC) either as a standard or provisional method.
- Other clinically indicated tests (eg, chest roentgenogram).

The VDRL or RPR test is commonly used to evaluate newborn infants for congenital infection with *T pallidum*. Serum from the infant is preferred to cord blood, since cord blood can produce false-positive and false-negative results.

A guide for interpretation of the results of nontreponemal and treponemal serologic tests for syphilis in mothers and their infants is given in Table 3.43 (p 449). A nonreactive VDRL in both the infected mother and infant can occur in a neonate with congenital syphilis if the mother acquired the disease late in pregnancy or in the case of a prozone phenomenon. Alternatively, the mother's test can be reactive and the infected infant's test nonreactive, depending on the timing of maternal and fetal infection. A mother who has been treated appropriately for syphilis during pregnancy can still transfer both nontreponemal and treponemal antibodies to the fetus, resulting in positive VDRL and FTA-ABS tests in the newborn infant. The neonate's VDRL titer in these circumstances is usually less than or equal to the mother's titer and reverts to negative in 4 to 6 months, whereas a positive FTA-ABS test from passively acquired antibody may not become negative for 1 year or longer. A reactive antitreponemal IgM antibody test on the infant's serum by a method considered reliable by the CDC is specific for congenital syphilis and, thus, can be useful, but, as of December 1993, no IgM tests are commercially available in the United States. Thus, in an asymptomatic infant at birth, distinguishing between early infection and passive transfer of antibody from a previously treated mother remains difficult or impossible.

In an infant with clinical or roentgenographic findings (eg, metaphysitis of the long bones) suggestive of congenital syphilis, a positive VDRL and/

TABLE 3.43—Guide for Interpretation of the Syphilis Serology of Mothers and Their Infants

Nontreponemal Test (eg, VDRL, RPR, ART, RST, EIA)		Treponemal Test (eg, MHA-TP, FTA-ABS)		Interpretation*
Mother	Infant	Mother	Infant	
−	−	−	−	No syphilis or incubating syphilis in the mother and infant
+	+	−	−	No syphilis in mother (false-positive nontreponemal test with passive transfer to infant)
+	+ or −	+	+	Maternal syphilis with possible infant infection; or mother treated for syphilis during pregnancy; or mother with latent syphilis and possible infection of infant†
+	+	+	+	Recent or previous syphilis in the mother; possible infection in infant
−	−	+	+	Mother successfully treated for syphilis before or early in pregnancy; or mother with Lyme disease, yaws, or pinta (ie, false-positive serology)

*Table presents a guide and not the definitive interpretation of serologic tests for syphilis in mothers and their newborn infants. Other factors that should be considered include the timing of maternal infection, the nature and timing of maternal treatment, quantitative maternal and infant titers, and serial determination of nontreponemal test titers in both mother and infant.
†Approximately 20% of mothers with latent syphilis have nonreactive nontreponemal tests.

or FTA-ABS test in serum strongly supports the diagnosis regardless of the therapy the mother received during the pregnancy.

Cerebrospinal Fluid Tests. Cerebrospinal fluid (CSF) should be examined in all infants born to mothers with syphilis during pregnancy, and in all patients with suspected or proven congenital syphilis, with suspected neurosyphilis, or with acquired, untreated syphilis of more than 1 year's duration. The CSF abnormalities in patients with neurosyphilis include increased protein concentration and leukocyte cell count, and a reactive VDRL. However, because of the wide range of normal values for CSF cell counts and protein concentrations in the newborn, results are often uninterpretable. If CSF test results cannot exclude infection in an infant evaluated for congenital syphilis, the infant should be treated. In patients beyond the neonatal period, normal CSF findings differentiate latent syphilis from asymptomatic neurosyphilis in individuals with acquired, untreated syphilis of more than 1 year's duration. The RPR, FTA-ABS, and MHA-TP tests should not be used for CSF evaluation. Cerebrospinal fluid VDRL test results should be interpreted cautiously since a negative VDRL does not exclude neurosyphilis and the CSF VDRL can be positive in an uninfected newborn with a transplacentally acquired, high-serum VDRL titer.

Treatment: Parenteral penicillin G remains the preferred drug for syphilis at any stage. Recommendations for penicillin G and duration of therapy vary, depending on the stage of the disease and its clinical manifestations. Parenteral penicillin G is the only documented effective therapy for patients who have syphilis during pregnancy and for those with neurosyphilis, and it is strongly recommended whenever possible in HIV-infected patients.

Patients with penicillin allergy should almost always be treated with penicillin, after desensitization if necessary, or should be managed in consultation with an expert. Skin testing for penicillin allergy can be useful for some patients in some circumstances. Skin testing with the major and minor determinants can reliably identify individuals at high risk for reacting to penicillin; currently, only the major determinant (penicilloyl-poly-L-lysine) and penicillin G are available commercially. Testing with the major determinant of penicillin G is estimated to miss 3% to 6% of penicillin-allergic patients who are at risk for serious or fatal reactions. Thus, a cautious approach to penicillin therapy is advised when the patient cannot be tested with all of the penicillin skin test reagents.

Congenital Syphilis: Newborn Infants (see also Table 3.44, p 451). Infants should be treated for congenital syphilis if they have proven or highly probable disease, as is demonstrated if (1) they have physical or roentgenographic evidence of active disease; (2) their serum quantitative nontreponemal titer is at least four times higher than the mother's titer; (3) their CSF VDRL is reactive or the CSF cell count and/or protein concentration is abnormal; or (4) they have a positive antitreponemal IgM antibody test performed by a test method deemed reliable by the CDC. If an asymptomatic infant has a nontreponemal test that is higher than but less than four times the mother's titer, some experts recommend treatment if follow-up cannot be assured. When an infant is evaluated for congenital syphilis, if test results cannot exclude infection, the infant should be treated. Similarly, an infant who warrants evaluation for congenital syphilis (see Evaluation of Newborn Infants for Congenital Infection, p 447) but cannot be fully evaluated should be treated.

In infants with proven or highly probable disease, aqueous crystalline penicillin G is preferred. The dosage should be based on chronologic, not gestational, age. The recommended dosage is 100,000 to 150,000 U/kg/d (given every 8 to 12 hours), intravenously, to complete a 10- to 14-day course. Alternatively, some experts recommend aqueous procaine penicillin G (50,000 U/kg/d, intramuscularly), for a minimum of 10 days. If more than 1 day of therapy is missed, the entire course should be restarted.

TABLE 3.44—Recommended Treatment of Neonates (≤4 Weeks of Age) With Proven or Possible Congenital Syphilis

Clinical Status	Antimicrobial Therapy*
Proven or highly probable disease	Aqueous crystalline penicillin G, IV, for 10-14 d[†]
Asymptomatic, normal CSF and radiographic examination— maternal treatment:	
None, inadequate,[‡] undocumented, failed, or reinfected	Aqueous crystalline penicillin G, IV, for 10-14 d[†]
Erythromycin	Clinical, serologic follow-up, and benzathine penicillin G, IM, single dose[§]
Adequate therapy but given less than 1 mo before delivery, or mother's response to treatment is not demonstrated by a fourfold decrease in titer of a nontreponemal serologic test	Clinical, serologic follow-up, and benzathine penicillin G, IM, single dose[§]

*See text for drug dosage and details.
[†]Some experts recommend aqueous procaine penicillin G, IM, for 10-14 d.
[‡]See text below for definition (includes those in whom sequential serologic tests on the mother do not demonstrate a 4-fold or greater decrease in a nontreponemal antibody titer).
[§]Some experts recommend aqueous crystalline or procaine penicillin G, as for proven or highly probable disease. Other experts would follow the infant without giving antibiotic therapy if both clinical and serologic follow-up can be assured.

Asymptomatic infants born to mothers who received appropriate penicillin treatment for syphilis during pregnancy and responded with a documented fourfold decrease in their VDRL, RPR, or ART titer are at minimal risk for congenital syphilis. However, these infants should be examined carefully, preferably monthly, until their nontreponemal serologic test results are negative.

Infants whose mothers received inadequate treatment for syphilis during pregnancy require special consideration. Maternal treatment for syphilis during pregnancy is deemed inadequate for this purpose in the following circumstances: (1) the mother's penicillin dose is unknown, undocumented, or inadequate; (2) the mother received erythromycin for syphilis; (3) treatment was given within 30 days of the infant's birth; or (4) the mother's response to treatment has not been established by demonstrating a fourfold fall in titer of a nontreponemal serologic test for syphilis.

Asymptomatic infants born to mothers whose treatment for syphilis may have been inadequate, as defined by one or more of these criteria, should be fully evaluated, including CSF examination and roentgenograms (see Evaluation of Newborn Infants for Congenital Infection, p 447). Some experts would treat all such infants with aqueous crystalline penicillin G (or aqueous procaine penicillin G) for 10 days. However, if the infant's evaluation, including CSF findings and roentgenograms, is normal, many experts would treat infants in specific circumstances given in Table 3.44 (p 451) with a single dose of 50,000 U/kg of benzathine penicillin G intramuscularly. In the case in which maternal response to treatment has not been demonstrated but the mother received an appropriate regimen of penicillin therapy more than 1 month before delivery, the infant's evaluation is normal, and both clinical and serologic follow-up can be ensured, some experts would follow the infant without giving antibiotic therapy. The Committee's recommendations for these different circumstances are given in Table 3.44 (p 451).

Congenital Syphilis: Older Infants and Children. Because of the difficulty in establishing the diagnosis of neurosyphilis, infants diagnosed after 4 weeks of age should be treated with aqueous crystalline penicillin, 200,000 to 300,000 U/kg/d, intravenously (administered every 6 hours), for 10 to 14 days. This regimen should also be used to treat children older than 1 year who have late and previously untreated congenital syphilis. Some experts suggest also giving such patients three doses of benzathine penicillin G, 50,000 U/kg, intramuscularly, weekly for 3 weeks, after 10 to 14 days of intravenous aqueous penicillin. If the patient has minimal clinical manifestations of disease, CSF examination is normal, and the CSF VDRL is negative, some experts would treat with three doses of benzathine penicillin G, 50,000 U/kg, intramuscularly, only.

Syphilis in Pregnancy. Regardless of the stage of pregnancy, patients should be treated with penicillin according to the dosage schedules appropriate for the stage of syphilis as recommended for nonpregnant patients. For penicillin-allergic patients, no proven alternative therapy has been established. A pregnant woman with a history of penicillin allergy should be treated with penicillin after desensitization. In some patients, skin testing may be helpful. Desensitization should be performed in consultation with an expert and only in facilities where emergency assistance is available.

Tetracycline is not recommended for pregnant women because of potential adverse effects on the fetus. Erythromycin treatment of syphilis during pregnancy cannot be considered reliable to cure infection in a fetus.

Early Acquired Syphilis (primary, secondary, latent syphilis of less than 1 year's duration). Benzathine penicillin G, intramuscularly, in a total dose of 50,000 U/kg, not to exceed 2.4 million units, is the preferred treatment.

For patients allergic to penicillin, tetracycline (adult dose, 500 mg, orally, four times a day) or doxycycline (adult dose 100 mg, orally, twice daily) usually should be given for 2 weeks. The clinical experience with doxycycline is less, but patient adherence to a regimen requiring twice daily doses is likely to be better. Tetracycline or doxycycline should not be given to children younger than 9 years unless the benefits of therapy are greater than the risks of dental staining. Drugs other than penicillin and tetracycline do not have proven efficacy in the treatment of syphilis. For penicillin-allergic patients, if follow-up can be ensured, erythromycin (500 mg, orally, four times daily) for 14 days, or ceftriaxone regimens of 8 to 10 days, in consultation with an expert, can be given. For penicillin-allergic patients for whom follow-up cannot be ensured, especially children younger than 9 years of age, consideration must be given to hospitalization and desensitization followed by administration of penicillin G.

Syphilis of More Than 1 Year's Duration (except neurosyphilis). Benzathine penicillin G, at a dose of 50,000 U/kg, intramuscularly, weekly (not to exceed 2.4 million units) for 3 successive weeks, can be used. In patients who are allergic to penicillin, either tetracycline (adult dose, 500 mg, orally, four times a day) or doxycycline (adult dose, 100 mg, orally, twice daily) for 4 weeks should be given only if a CSF examination has excluded neurosyphilis. Tetracycline or doxycycline ordinarily should not be given to children younger than 9 years of age unless the benefits of therapy are greater than the risks of dental staining. Examination of the CSF (VDRL, protein concentration, and cell count) is mandatory for those with suspected or symptomatic neurosyphilis, those who have concurrent HIV infection, those who have failed treatment, and those receiving antibiotics other than penicillin. Cerebrospinal fluid examination is recommended for all patients with syphilis for more than 1 year to exclude asymptomatic neurosyphilis.

Neurosyphilis. The recommended regimen for adults is aqueous crystalline penicillin G, 12 to 24 million units daily (2 to 4 million units every 4 hours), intravenously, for 10 to 14 days. Many authorities recommend following this regimen with benzathine penicillin G, 2.4 million units, intramuscularly, given weekly for 3 successive weeks. In children, aqueous crystalline penicillin G, 200,000 to 300,000 U/kg/d (50,000 U/kg every 4 to 6 hours) for 10 to 14 days, in doses not to exceed the adult dose, is recommended, possibly followed by benzathine penicillin, 50,000 U/kg per dose (not to exceed 2.4 million units) in three weekly doses.

An alternative regimen, if outpatient compliance can be ensured, is aqueous procaine penicillin G, 2.4 million units, intramuscularly, daily, plus probenecid, 500 mg, orally, four times a day. Both should be given for 10 to 14 days, possibly followed by benzathine penicillin G, 2.4 million units, intramuscularly, given weekly for 3 successive weeks.

If the patient has a history of allergy to penicillin, consideration should be given to desensitization, and the patient should be managed in consultation with an expert.

Other Considerations.
- Mothers of infants with congenital syphilis should be tested for HIV.
- All recent sexual contacts of persons with acquired syphilis should be evaluated (see Control Measures, p 455).
- All patients with syphilis should be tested for HIV infection.
- For HIV-infected patients with syphilis, careful follow-up is essential. Patients infected with HIV who have early syphilis may be at increased risk for neurologic complications and higher rates of treatment failure with the currently recommended regimens. Nevertheless, such risk, although not precisely defined, is probably small. No therapy, however, has been demonstrated to be more effective in preventing the development of neurosyphilis than that recommended for patients without HIV infection.

Follow-up and Retreatment.
Congenital Syphilis. Infants should have careful follow-up evaluations at 1, 2, 4, 6, and 12 months of age. Serologic nontreponemal tests should be performed 3, 6, and 12 months after the conclusion of treatment, or until they become nonreactive. Nontreponemal antibody titers should decline by 3 months of age and should be nonreactive by 6 months of age if the infant was

not infected and the initially positive serologic test reflected transplacentally acquired maternal antibody. Patients with persistent, stable titers, including those with low titers, should be considered for retreatment.

Infants with congenital neurosyphilis and initially positive CSF VDRL tests or abnormal or uninterpretable CSF cell counts and/or protein concentrations should undergo repeat clinical evaluation and CSF examination at 6-month intervals until their CSF examination is normal. A reactive CSF VDRL at 6 months is an indication for retreatment. Abnormal CSF findings, including persistent changes on serial examinations at age 2 years, warrant retreatment.

Early Acquired Syphilis. Pregnant women with syphilis should have quantitative nontreponemal serologic tests performed monthly for the remainder of their pregnancy. Other patients with early acquired syphilis should return for repeat quantitative nontreponemal tests at 3, 6, and 12 months after the conclusion of treatment. Patients with syphilis for more than 1 year should also undergo serologic testing 24 months after treatment. Careful follow-up serologic testing is particularly important in patients treated with antibiotics other than penicillin.

Retreatment. In the following circumstances, retreatment is indicated:
- The clinical signs or symptoms of syphilis persist or recur.
- A sustained, fourfold increase in the titer of a nontreponemal test occurs; in a pregnant woman, a fourfold increase in titer alone is an indication for retreatment.
- An initially high-titer nontreponemal test fails to decrease fourfold within a year; in a pregnant woman with primary or secondary syphilis, it fails to decrease fourfold within a 3-month period; or in a pregnant woman with latent syphilis, it fails to decrease fourfold within 6 months.

Retreated patients should be treated with the schedules recommended for patients with syphilis for more than 1 year. In general, only one retreatment course is indicated. The possibility of reinfection or concurrent HIV infection should always be considered when retreating patients with early syphilis.

The CSF should be examined before retreatment unless evidence indicates that the patient has been reinfected and again requires treatment for early syphilis. Patients with neurosyphilis must have periodic serologic testing in follow-up, clinical evaluation at 6-month intervals, and repeat CSF examinations for at least 3 years or until CSF examination is normal.

Isolation of the Hospitalized Patient: Drainage/secretion precautions in addition to the routinely recommended universal precautions are indicated for all infants with suspected or proven congenital syphilis until therapy has been administered for at least 24 hours. Parents, visitors, and medical staff should use gloves when handling the infant. Because moist, open lesions and possibly blood are contagious in all forms of syphilis, these precautions are also required for primary and secondary syphilis with skin and mucous membrane lesions. Precautions are not indicated otherwise, ie, for those with tertiary syphilis or those who are seropositive but have no lesions.

Control Measures:

- All women should be screened for syphilis early in pregnancy and preferably at delivery. Women at high risk for syphilis should also be screened at 28 weeks (see Diagnostic Tests, p 446).
- Education about sexually transmitted diseases, treatment of sexual contacts, reporting of each case to local public health authorities for contact investigation and appropriate follow-up, and serologic screening of high-risk populations are indicated.
- All recent sexual contacts of a person with acquired syphilis should be identified, examined, serologically tested, and treated appropriately. Sexual contacts within the last 3 months who are seronegative are at high risk for early syphilis and should be treated for early acquired syphilis. Every effort, including physical examination and serologic testing, should be made to establish a diagnosis in these patients.
- All individuals, including hospital personnel, who have had close, unprotected contact with a patient with early congenital syphilis before identification of the disease or during the first 24 hours of therapy should be examined clinically for the presence of lesions 2 to 3 weeks after contact. Serologic testing should be performed and repeated 3 months after contact, or sooner if symptoms occur.

Tapeworm Diseases
(Taeniasis and Cysticercosis)

Clinical Manifestations:

Taeniasis: Mild gastrointestinal symptoms, such as nausea, diarrhea, and pain, can occur. Tapeworm segments can be seen migrating from the anus or feces.

Cysticercosis: Manifestations depend on the location and numbers of cysts of the pork tapeworm and the host response. Cysts may be found anywhere in the body. Subcutaneous cysts produce palpable nodules, and ocular involvement can cause visual impairment. Cysts in the brain (neurocysticercosis) can cause seizures, behavioral disturbances, obstructive hydrocephalus, and other neurologic symptoms. The host reaction to degenerating cysts can produce signs and symptoms of meningitis. Cysts in the spinal column can cause gait disturbance, pain, or transverse myelitis.

Etiology: Taeniasis is caused by intestinal infection by the adult tapeworm, *Taenia saginata* (beef tapeworm) or *Taenia solium* (pork tapeworm). Usually only one adult worm is present in the intestine. Cysticercosis is caused by the larval form of *T solium.*

Epidemiology: Taeniasis has a worldwide distribution, and prevalence rates are high in areas with poor sanitation and human fecal contamination where cattle graze or swine are fed. Most cases in the United States are imported from Mexico, Central and South America, Africa, Asia,

Spain, and Portugal. Taeniasis is acquired by eating undercooked beef
(*T saginata*) or pork (*T solium*) that contains encysted larvae. Infection is
often asymptomatic.

Cysticercosis is acquired by ingesting the eggs of the pork tapeworm
T solium. The eggs hatch in the intestine and migrate to tissues throughout the
body including the central nervous system where cysts form. Although most
cases of cysticercosis in the United States are imported, cysticercosis has
been acquired from food handlers in the United States who acquired *T solium*
tapeworm infections in other countries.

The **incubation period** for taeniasis, the time from ingestion of the larvae
until segments are passed in the feces, is 2 to 3 months. For cysticercosis, it is
from months to years.

Diagnosis: Diagnosis of taeniasis (adult tapeworm infection) is based on
demonstration of the proglottids or ova in feces. Species identification of the
parasite is based on the different structures of the terminal gravid segments.
Diagnosis of neurocysticercosis is based primarily on computerized tomography (CT) or magnetic resonance imaging (MRI). Enhanced CT may be helpful in identifying spinal and intraventricular lesions. The enzyme-linked
immunotransfer blot assay to detect antibody to *T solium* is the antibody test
of choice and is available through the Centers for Disease Control and Prevention. Serum and cerebrospinal fluid (CSF) can be tested. The antibody
assays are rarely positive in children with solitary parenchymal lesions but
are often positive in those with inflamed lesions in contact with the subarach-
noid space. The test is slightly more sensitive with serum samples than with
CSF specimens.

Treatment (see also Drugs for Parasitic Infections, p 574):

Taeniasis: Niclosamide* and praziquantel* are each highly effective in
eradicating infection with the adult tapeworm.

Cysticercosis: Treatment of neurocysticercosis is based on the number of
lesions and presence or absence of inflammation as determined by CT or
MRI of the brain. Acutely inflamed, single, intraparenchymal cysts involute
rapidly (8 to 12 weeks) and, thus, rarely require therapy. Single, uninflamed
lesions often follow the same course if no treatment is indicated. Multiple,
uninflamed cysts require antihelmintic therapy since they may persist and
cause progressive neurologic symptoms. Praziquantel, given for 15 days, is
effective. It may be given with dexamethasone for 2 or 3 days to minimize
the vigorous inflammatory response often associated with chemotherapy, and
is indicated if neurologic symptoms develop during praziquantel therapy.
Albendazole† for 8 days is also effective but is not yet approved by the Food
and Drug Administration.

Intraventricular cysts and hydrocephalus may require surgical intervention.
Seizures may recur for months, and will require anticonvulsant medication
until patients have been seizure-free for 1 to 2 years.

---

*Available from Miles, Inc, West Haven, CT.
†Available from SmithKline Beecham, Philadelphia, PA.

Ocular cysticercosis is usually treated by surgical excision of cysts and not with antihelmintic drugs because of the inflammatory reaction that might occur. However, the effectiveness of albendazole is being studied.

Isolation of the Hospitalized Patient: No special precautions are indicated. However, since the eggs of *T solium* are infectious for man, careful hand washing and disposal of feces is recommended.

Control Measures: Avoid eating raw or undercooked beef or pork. Persons known to harbor the adult tapeworms of *T solium* should be immediately treated and have careful hand washing and disposal of fecal material until the infection is eradicated.

Food handlers who have recently emigrated from endemic countries should have a stool examination for detection of eggs and/or proglottids.

Other Tapeworm Infections (Including Hydatid Disease)

Most infections are asymptomatic, but nausea, abdominal pain, and diarrhea have been observed in persons who are heavily infested.

Hymenolepis nana. This tapeworm, also called "dwarf tapeworm," has its entire cycle within humans. Therefore, person-to-person transmission is possible. More problematic is autoinfection, which tends to perpetuate the infection in the host because the eggs can hatch within the intestine and reinitiate the cycle, leading to the development of new worms. This cycle makes eradicating the infection with niclosamide* difficult. If infection persists after treatment with niclosamide, praziquantel* should be administered. Repeat treatment may be necessary.

Dipylidium caninum. This tapeworm, with the dog or cat flea as its intermediate host, infects children when they inadvertently swallow a flea while playing with a pet. Diagnosis is made by finding the characteristic eggs or tapeworm segments in the stool. Treatment consists of niclosamide*; praziquantel* is an alternative choice and is given in the same doses as for *Taenia* infections.

Diphyllobothrium latum (and related species). This tapeworm, also called "fish tapeworm," has fish as one of its intermediate hosts. Consumption of infected raw, freshwater fish (including salmon) leads to the infection. The worm sometimes causes megaloblastic anemia. The diagnosis is made by recognition of the characteristic eggs or proglottids passed in the stool. Therapy with niclosamide* is effective; praziquantel* is an alternative. Both are given in a single dose. Hydroxocobalamin injections and folic acid supplements may be required.

Echinococcus granulosus and Echinococcus multilocularis. These tapeworms are the causes of hydatid disease. The distribution of *E granulosus* is related to sheep or cattle herding. Countries with the highest prevalence include

---

*Available from Miles, Inc, West Haven, CT.

Argentina, Greece, Italy, Lebanon, Romania, South Africa, Spain, Syria, Turkey, and the countries in the former Soviet Union. In the United States, small endemic foci exist in Arizona, California, New Mexico, and Utah. Dogs, coyotes, wolves, dingos, and jackals can become infected by swallowing protoscolices of the parasite within hydatid cysts in the organs of sheep or other intermediate hosts. Dogs pass embryonated eggs in their stools, and the sheep become infected by swallowing the eggs. If humans swallow echinococcus eggs, they can become inadvertent intermediate hosts and develop cysts in various organs, such as the liver, lungs, kidney, and spleen. These cysts grow slowly (1 cm in diameter per year) and eventually can contain several liters of fluid. If a cyst ruptures, anaphylaxis and multiple secondary cysts from seeding of protoscolices can result. Clinical diagnosis is frequently difficult. A history of contact with dogs in an endemic area is helpful. Space-occupying lesions can be demonstrated by roentgenograms or computed tomography of various organs. Serologic tests, available at the Centers for Disease Control and Prevention, are helpful, but they are not always positive. Surgical treatment is indicated in some patients and requires meticulous care to prevent spillage of the cyst contents. Injection of a 0.1% cetrimide solution into the cyst before attempted removal can minimize the risk of dissemination if spillage occurs. Treatment with albendazole* (10 mg/kg/d) for several months has been of benefit in many cases. This drug is not yet approved by the Food and Drug Administration.

Echinococcus multilocularis, a species whose life cycle involves foxes and rodents, causes the alveolar form of hydatid disease, which is characterized by invasive growth of the larvae in the liver with occasional metastatic spread. The alveolar form of hydatid disease is limited to the Northern hemisphere and is usually diagnosed in persons 50 years or older. The preferred treatment is surgical extirpation of the entire larval mass. In nonresectable cases, continuous treatment with mebendazole has been associated with clinical improvement.

Tetanus (Lockjaw)

Clinical Manifestations: Tetanus (lockjaw) is a neurologic disease with severe muscular spasms. It is caused by the neurotoxin produced by the anaerobic bacterium *Clostridium tetani* in a contaminated wound. Onset is gradual, occurring over 1 to 7 days, and progresses to severe generalized muscle spasms, which frequently are aggravated by any external stimulus. Severe spasms persist for 1 week or more and subside in a period of weeks in those who recover. Neonatal tetanus, a common cause of neonatal mortality in developing countries but rare in the United States, arises from contamination of the umbilical stump. Local tetanus is manifested by local muscle spasms in areas contiguous to a wound.

---

*Available from SmithKline Beecham, Philadelphia, PA.

Etiology: *Clostridium tetani*, the tetanus bacillus, is a spore-forming, anaerobic, Gram-positive bacillus that produces a potent exotoxin (tetanospasmin), which binds to central nervous system tissues.

Epidemiology: Tetanus occurs worldwide and is more frequent in warmer climates and months, in part because of the frequency of contaminated wounds. The organism, a normal inhabitant of soil and of animal and human intestines, is ubiquitous in the environment, especially at sites likely to have been contaminated by excreta. Wounds, recognized or unrecognized, are the sites at which the organism multiplies and elaborates toxin. Contaminated wounds, those with devitalized tissue and deep-puncture trauma, are at greatest risk. Neonatal tetanus is common in many countries where women do not receive tetanus immunizations. Widespread active immunization against tetanus has vastly modified the epidemiology of the disease in the United States. Tetanus is not transmissible from person to person.

The **incubation period** is 3 days to 3 weeks; the average is 8 days. In neonates it is usually 5 to 14 days. Shorter incubation periods historically have been associated with more heavily contaminated wounds, more severe disease, and a worse prognosis. Recent experience in the United States does not confirm such a relationship.

Diagnostic Tests: The offending wound should be cultured. However, etiologic confirmation is made infrequently by culture. The diagnosis is made clinically by excluding other possibilities.

Treatment:
- Tetanus Immune Globulin (TIG) (Human) is recommended for treatment. A single dose of 3,000 to 6,000 U is recommended; the optimum therapeutic dose has not yet been established. Preparations currently available must be given intramuscularly. Part of the dose should infiltrate locally around the wound, although the efficacy of this approach has not been proven. The result of studies on the benefit from intrathecal TIG are conflicting. The TIG formulation in use in the United States is not licensed or appropriate for intrathecal or intravenous use.
- In countries where TIG is not available, equine tetanus antitoxin (TAT) should be used. Tetanus antitoxin is administered as a single dose of 50,000 to 100,000 U after appropriate testing for sensitivity, and desensitization if necessary (see Sensitivity Tests for Reactions to Animal Sera, p 46, and "Desensitization" for Animal Sera, p 47). Part of this dose (20,000 U) should be given intravenously. Serum sickness occurs in 10% to 20% of recipients of equine serum.
- Immune Globulin Intravenous (IGIV) (Human) contains antibodies to tetanus and can be considered for treatment if TIG is not available. Approval by the Food and Drug Administration has not been given for this use and the dosage has not been determined.
- Parenteral penicillin G (100,000 U/kg/d, given at 4- to 6-hour intervals) or a tetracycline (which ordinarily should not be given to children younger

than 9 years) is effective in reducing the number of vegetative forms of the organism. Therapy for 10 to 14 days is recommended.

- All wounds should be properly cleaned and debrided when indicated, especially if extensive necrosis is present. In neonatal tetanus, wide excision of the umbilical stump is not indicated.
- Supportive care is of major importance.

Isolation of the Hospitalized Patient: No special precautions are recommended.

Control Measures:

Care of Exposed Persons (see Table 3.45, p 461). Less than 1% of the recently reported cases of tetanus in the United States have occurred in individuals with adequate, up-to-date immunization. After primary immunization with tetanus toxoid, antitoxin persists at protective levels in most persons for at least 10 years, and for a longer time after a booster immunization. Boosters need to be given as soon as possible after the injury.

- In the management of clean, minor wounds in those who have completed a primary series, ie, three doses of tetanus toxoid or receipt of a booster dose within 10 years, an additional dose of tetanus toxoid is not necessary.
- For other, more serious wounds (such as those contaminated with dirt, feces, soil, and/or saliva, puncture wounds, and those with devitalized tissue), a dose of tetanus toxoid should be given as soon as possible after the injury, according to the guidelines in Table 3.45 (p 461). Indications for TIG or antitoxin use in partially immunized persons with more serious wounds are also listed in Table 3.45 (p 461). If tetanus immunization is incomplete at the time of wound treatment, a dose should be given, and the series should be completed according to the primary immunization schedule. TIG should be administered for tetanus-prone wounds in AIDS patients, regardless of the history of tetanus immunizations.
- In usual practice, when tetanus toxoid is required for wound prophylaxis in a child 7 years or older, the use of Td instead of tetanus toxoid alone is advisable so that adequate levels of diphtheria immunity are also maintained. When a booster injection is indicated for wound prophylaxis in a child younger than 7 years, DTP or DTaP should be used unless pertussis vaccine is contraindicated (see Pertussis, p 364), in which case immunization with DT is recommended.
- Passive protection with TIG or antitoxin is not indicated for patients with clean, minor wounds, regardless of immunization status, or for patients with other wounds who have had three or more previous injections of tetanus toxoid. Patients with more serious wounds who have had less than three previous injections of tetanus vaccine should receive TIG or antitoxin as well as an additional dose of tetanus toxoid within 3 days. Intramuscular TIG is recommended in a dose of 250 U. Tetanus antitoxin is used if TIG is unavailable; the dose is 3,000 to 5,000 U intramuscularly, after appropriate testing of the patient for sensitivity (see Sensitivity Tests for Reactions to Animal Sera, p 46). If tetanus toxoid and TIG or TAT are given concurrently, separate syringes and sites should be used. Administration of TIG or TAT does not preclude initiation of teta-

TABLE 3.45—Guide to Tetanus Prophylaxis in Routine Wound Management

History of Adsorbed Tetanus Toxoid (Doses)	Clean, Minor Wounds		All Other Wounds*	
	Td†	TIG‡	Td†	TIG‡
Unknown or <3	Yes	No	Yes	Yes
≥3§	No‖	No	No¶	No

*Such as, but not limited to, wounds contaminated with dirt, feces, soil, and saliva; puncture wounds; avulsions; and wounds resulting from missiles, crushing, burns, and frostbite.

†For children <7 years old; DTP or DTaP (if ≥3 doses of DTP have been previously given) is preferred to tetanus toxoid alone; if pertussis vaccine is contraindicated, DT is given. For persons ≥7 years of age, Td is preferred to tetanus toxoid alone. Td = adult-type tetanus and diphtheria toxoids.

‡TIG = tetanus immune globulin.

§If only 3 doses of fluid toxoid have been received, then a fourth dose of toxoid, preferably an adsorbed toxoid, should be given.

‖Yes, if >10 years since last dose.

¶Yes, if >5 years since last dose. (More frequent boosters are not needed and can accentuate side effects.)

nus toxoid active immunization. Efforts should be made to both initiate immunization and arrange for its completion.

- Regardless of immunization status, all wounds should be properly cleaned and debrided. Wounds should receive prompt surgical treatment to remove all devitalized tissue and foreign material as an essential part of tetanus prophylaxis.

*Immunization.** Active immunization with tetanus toxoid is indicated for all persons (see Tables 1.3 and 1.4, pp 23 and 24). Adsorbed tetanus toxoid is preferred to fluid toxoid because immunity lasts longer. Recommendations for use are as follows:

- Immunization for children from 2 months to the seventh birthday (see Tables 1.3 and 1.4, pp 23 and 24) should consist of five doses of tetanus vaccine. The initial three doses are given as DTP vaccine, administered intramuscularly at 2-month intervals beginning at 2 months of age. A fourth dose, either of DTaP or DTP, is recommended 6 to 12 months after the third dose, usually at 15 to 18 months of age; if given before 15 months, DTP is given since DTaP is not currently licensed for use in children younger than 15 months. A fifth dose of DTaP or DTP is given before school entry (kindergarten or elementary school) at 4 to 6 years of age, unless the fourth dose was given after the fourth birthday.† Doses may be given concurrently with other vaccines (see Simultaneous Administration of Multiple Vaccines, p 25).

---

*Vaccines containing both tetanus and diphtheria toxoids in use in the United States, including DTP, DT, Td and DTaP, are adsorbed to aluminum salts.

†For further details on use of DTP and DTaP vaccines, see Pertussis (p 357).

- Children younger than 7 years in whom pertussis immunization is deferred or contraindicated (see Pertussis, p 364) should be immunized with DT. For children younger than 1 year, three doses of DT are given at 2-month intervals; a fourth dose of DT should be given approximately 6 to 12 months after the third dose, usually at 15 to 18 months of age; and the fifth dose of DT is given before school entry at 4 to 6 years of age. Children who have not received previous doses of DT, DTP, or DTaP and who are 1 year or older should receive two doses of DT approximately 2 months apart, followed by a third dose 6 to 12 months after the second dose to complete the initial series. DT may be given concurrently with other vaccines (see Simultaneous Administration of Multiple Vaccines, p 25). An additional dose is necessary before school entry when the child is 4 to 6 years old, unless the fourth dose was given after the fourth birthday.
- Children who have received one or two doses of DTP (or DT) in the first year of life and for whom further pertussis vaccination is contraindicated should receive additional doses of DT until a total of five doses of diphtheria and tetanus toxoids are received by the time of school entry. The fourth dose is administered 6 to 12 months after the third dose. The preschool (fifth) dose is omitted if the fourth dose was given after the fourth birthday.
- Children 7 years and older and adults not previously immunized should receive Td, ie, adult-type tetanus and diphtheria toxoids (see Table 1.4, p 24). The Td preparation contains not more than 2 Lf (flocculating units) of diphtheria toxoid, as compared to 6.7 to 12.5 Lf diphtheria toxoid in the DTP, DT, and DTaP preparations for use in infants and younger children. Because of the lower dose of diphtheria toxoid, Td is less likely than DTP, DTaP, or DT to produce reactions in older children and adults. Two doses of Td are given 1 to 2 months apart; a third dose should be given 6 to 12 months after the second.
- After the initial immunization series is completed, a booster dose of tetanus toxoid should be given intramuscularly every 10 years. This 10-year period is determined from the last dose administered irrespective of whether it was given earlier in routine childhood immunization or as part of wound management. Since the immunity conferred by adsorbed preparations of tetanus toxoid has proved to be of long duration, routine boosters at intervals more frequent than every 10 years are not indicated and may be associated with an increased incidence and severity of reactions.
- Prevention of neonatal tetanus can be accomplished by prenatal immunization of the previously unimmunized mother. Two doses should be administered at least 4 weeks apart and the second dose should be given at least 2 weeks before delivery. Booster immunization is not contraindicated during pregnancy.
- Additional measures include community immunization programs for adolescent girls and women of childbearing age and appropriate training of midwives.
- Active immunization against tetanus should always be undertaken during convalescence from tetanus because this exotoxin-mediated disease usually does not confer immunity.

- If more than 5 years have elapsed since the last dose, a booster of Td should be considered for persons who are going to summer camps or on wilderness expeditions where tetanus boosters may not be readily available.

Precautions and Contraindications. Severe anaphylactic reactions attributable to tetanus toxoid have been reported but are extremely rare. An immediate allergic reaction to toxoid-containing vaccine (eg, DTP or Td) that is severe or anaphylactic in type is a contraindication to further doses (see Pertussis, p 364).

Other Control Measures. Sterilization of hospital supplies will prevent the infrequent instances of tetanus that may occur in a hospital from contaminated sutures, instruments, or plaster casts.

Tinea Capitis
(Ringworm of the Scalp)

Clinical Manifestations: Fungal infection of the scalp can present with one of the following distinct clinical syndromes.
- Patchy areas of dandruff-like scaling, with either subtle or extensive hair loss. This form is easily confused with dandruff, seborrheic dermatitis, or atopic dermatitis.
- Discrete areas of hair loss studded by the stubs of broken hairs—so-called "black dot ringworm."
- Numerous discrete pustules or excoriations with little hair loss or scaling.
- Kerion—a boggy, inflammatory, mass surrounded by follicular pustules. Kerion may be accompanied by fever and local lymphadenopathy and is frequently misdiagnosed as impetigo or cellulitis.

Tinea capitis can be confused with many other diseases, including seborrheic dermatitis, psoriasis, alopecia areata, trichotillomania, folliculitis, impetigo, and lupus erythematosus.

Etiology: *Trichophyton tonsurans* is currently the cause of tinea capitis in more than 90% of cases in North and Central America. *Microsporum canis*, *Microsporum audouinii*, and *Trichophyton mentagrophytes* are now less common. The causative agents may vary in different geographic areas, but in general are adapted to infecting man or animals.

Epidemiology: *Trichophyton tonsurans* infection of the scalp is the result of person-to-person transmission. This organism remains viable on combs, brushes, couches, and sheets for long periods of time. *Trichophyton tonsurans* is occasionally cultured from the scalps of asymptomatic children, and it is readily cultured from asymptomatic family members of infected individuals. *Trichophyton tonsurans* tinea capitis occurs most commonly in children between the ages of 3 and 9, and it appears to be more common in black children.

Microsporum canis infection results from transmission from animals to humans. It is frequently the result of contact with household pets.

The **incubation period** is unknown.

Diagnostic Tests: Hairs for potassium hydroxide wet mount examination and for culture may be obtained by gentle scraping of a moistened area of the scalp with a curved scalpel. Broken "black dot" hairs should be obtained when possible. In cases of *T tonsurans* infection, microscopic examination of a potassium hydroxide wet mount preparation discloses numerous arthroconidia within the hair shaft. In *M canis* infection, spores surround the hair shaft. Diagnosis of tinea capitis can be confirmed by culture on Saboraud's agar supplemented with cycloheximide and chloramphenicol. Dermatophyte test medium (DTM), an alternative fungal culture medium, contains a phenol red indicator and will turn from yellow to red in the area surrounding a dermatophyte colony.

Wood's light examination of the hair of patients with *Microsporum* infection results in brilliant green fluorescence. However, because *T tonsurans* does not fluoresce under Wood's light, this diagnostic test is not helpful in most cases of tinea capitis.

Treatment: Tinea capitis must be treated with systemic antifungal therapy. Microsize griseofulvin is given orally, 10 to 20 mg/kg/d, in two divided doses. The dose of ultramicrosize griseofulvin is 5 to 10 mg/kg/d, also in two divided doses. Griseofulvin is given optimally after a meal containing fat (eg, peanut butter or ice cream). Four to six weeks of treatment is usually required. Ketoconazole is not as effective as griseofulvin in the treatment of tinea capitis. It should be reserved for patients with either griseofulvin allergy, or evidence of a fungal infection that is resistant to griseofulvin.

Topical antifungal medications are not effective in the treatment of tinea capitis. Selenium sulfide, 2.5%, shampoo, used twice weekly, decreases fungal shedding and may help to curb the spread of infection.

Isolation of the Hospitalized Patient: Drainage/secretion precautions are recommended.

Control Measures: Early treatment of infected persons is indicated, as is examination of siblings and other household contacts for evidence of tinea capitis. Ribbons, combs, and brushes should not be shared by family members. Barber tools should be cleaned and sterilized.

Children receiving treatment for tinea capitis may attend school. Hair cuts, shaving of the head, or wearing a cap during treatment are not necessary.

Tinea Corporis
(Ringworm of the Body)

Clinical Manifestations: Superficial tinea infections of the nonhairy (glabrous) skin involve the face, trunk, and limbs, but not the scalp, beard, groin, hands, and feet. The lesion is generally circular (hence, the term "ringworm"), slightly erythematous, and well demarcated with a scaly, vesicular, or pustular border. Pruritis is common. A frequent source of confusion in diagnosis is an alteration of appearance of lesions resulting from topical corticosteroid application. This atypical presentation has been termed "tinea incognita."

Etiology: The prime causes of the disease are fungi of the genera *Trichophyton*, especially *Trichophyton rubrum* and *Trichophyton mentagrophytes*; *Microsporum*, especially *Microsporum canis*; and *Epidermophyton floccosum*.

Epidemiology: The fungi occur worldwide and are transmissible by direct contact with infected humans, animals, or fomites. Fungi in the lesions are communicable.

The **incubation period** is unknown.

Diagnosis: The organisms can be identified by microscopic examination of the scrapings in a potassium hydroxide wet mount. They can be isolated by culture on Sabouraud's medium, supplemented with cycloheximide and chloramphenicol. Dermatophyte test medium (DTM) will turn from yellow to red in the area surrounding a dermatophyte colony and is a useful diagnostic aid.

Treatment: Topical application of miconazole, clotrimazole, haloprogin, econazole, tolnaftate, naftifine, or ciclopirox preparation twice daily, or ketoconazole, oxiconazole, or sulconazole preparation once daily, is recommended (see Topical Drugs for Superficial Fungal Infections, p 565). Although clinical resolution may be evident within 2 weeks, a minimum duration of 4 weeks is generally indicated. If the lesions are extensive or unresponsive to topical therapy, griseofulvin is administered orally for 4 weeks (see Tinea Capitis, p 463). Oral ketoconazole is occasionally used as an alternative to griseofulvin.

Isolation of the Hospitalized Patient: Drainage/secretion precautions are recommended.

Control Measures: Direct contact with known or suspected sources of infection should be avoided. Periodic inspections of contacts for early lesions and prompt therapy are recommended.

Tinea Cruris
(Jock Itch)

Clinical Manifestations: Tinea cruris is an extremely common superficial fungal disorder of the groin and upper thighs. The eruption is sharply marginated and usually is bilaterally symmetric. Involved skin is erythematous and scaly, and varies in color from red to brown; occasionally, it is accompanied by central clearing and a vesiculopapular border. In chronic infections, the margin can be subtle, and lichenification can be present. Tinea cruris may be extremely pruritic. It should be differentiated from intertrigo, seborrheic dermatitis, psoriasis, primary irritant dermatitis, allergic contact dermatitis (generally caused by the therapeutic agents applied to the area), or erythrasma (a superficial bacterial infection of the skin caused by *Corynebacterium minutissimum*).

Etiology: The fungi *Epidermophyton floccosum*, *Trichophyton rubrum*, and *Trichophyton mentagrophytes* are the causes. This infection is commonly seen in association with tinea pedis.

Epidemiology: Tinea cruris occurs predominantly in adolescent and adult males. Moisture, close-fitting garments, friction, and obesity are predisposing factors. Direct or indirect person-to-person transmission may occur.
    The **incubation period** is unknown.

Diagnostic Tests: The fungi responsible for tinea cruris may be detected by microscopic examination of a potassium hydroxide wet mount of scales and may be identified by fungal cultures. A characteristic, coral-red fluorescence under Wood's light can identify the presence of erythrasma and, thus, exclude tinea cruris.

Treatment: Topical application for 2 to 4 weeks of clotrimazole, haloprogin, econazole, miconazole, terbinafine, tolnaftate, or ciclopirox preparation gently rubbed into the affected areas and surrounding skin twice daily, or topical ketoconazole, naftifine, oxiconazole, or sulconazole preparation once daily, is effective (see Topical Drugs for Superficial Fungal Infections, p 565). Topical preparations of antifungal medication mixed with high-potency steroids should not be used because the steroids can cause striae and atrophy of the skin. Loose-fitting, washed, cotton underclothes to reduce chafing, as well as the use of a bland, absorbent powder can be helpful adjuvants to therapy. Griseofulvin orally for 2 to 4 weeks may be needed in unresponsive cases (see Tinea Capitis, p 463).

Isolation of the Hospitalized Patient: Drainage/secretion precautions are recommended.

Control Measures: Infections should be treated promptly. Potentially involved areas should be kept dry, and loose undergarments should be recommended.

Tinea Pedis
(Athlete's Foot, Ringworm of the Feet)

Clinical Manifestations: Tinea pedis consists of fine vesiculopustular or scaly lesions that are frequently pruritic. The lesions can involve all areas of the foot, but usually they are patchy in distribution, with a pre-disposition to fissures and scaling between the toes. Toenails may be infected and can be dystrophic. Tinea pedis (and many other fungal infections) can be accompanied by a hypersensitivity reaction to the fungi, with resulting vesicular eruptions on the palms and the sides of the fingers, and, occasionally, by an erythematous vesicular eruption on the extremities and trunk (the dermatophytid or "id" reaction). This condition must be differentiated from foot eczema, juvenile plantar dermatosis, and shoe dermatitis.

Etiology: Fungi of the genera *Microsporum*, *Epidermophyton*, and *Tricho-phyton*, especially *Trichophyton rubrum*, *Trichophyton mentagrophytes*, and *Epidermophyton floccosum*, are the causes.

Epidemiology: Tinea pedis is a common infection in adolescents and adults but is relatively uncommon in young children. It occurs worldwide. The fungi are acquired by contact with skin scales containing fungi or with fungi in damp areas, such as swimming pools, locker rooms, and shower rooms. It is communicable for as long as the infection is present.

The **incubation period** is unknown.

Diagnosis: Tinea pedis is usually diagnosed by the clinical manifestations and corroborated by microscopic examination of a potassium hydroxide wet mount of the cutaneous scrapings and appropriate fungal cultures. Infection of the nail must be verified by fungal culture.

Treatment: Topical application of miconazole, haloprogin, econazole, clotrimazole, ciclopirox, terbinafine, or tolnaftate preparation twice daily, or ketoconazole, naftifine, oxiconazole, or sulconazole preparation once daily, can be used for active infections (see Topical Drugs for Superficial Infections, p 565). Acute vesicular lesions may be treated with intermittent use of open, wet compresses (eg, Burrow's solution, 1:80). Micronized griseofulvin, similar to that used for tinea capitis (see Tinea Capitis, p 463), administered orally for 6 to 8 weeks, may be necessary for the treatment of severe, chronic, and recalcitrant forms of tinea pedis. "Id" reactions are treated by wet compresses, topical corticosteroids, occasionally systemic corticosteroids, and eradication of the primary source of infection. Recurrence is prevented by proper foot hygiene, which includes keeping the feet dry and cool, gentle cleaning, drying between the toes, the use of absorbent antifungal foot powder, frequent airing of affected areas, and avoidance of oc-clusive footwear and nylon socks or other fabrics that interfere with dissipation of moisture.

Treatment of most nail infections requires oral antifungal therapy with griseofulvin. Ketoconazole is an alternative. Treatment should be continued for 6 to 24 months or until the entire nail has regrown and is no longer infected.

Isolation of the Hospitalized Patient: Drainage/secretion precautions are recommended.

Control Measures: Treatment of patients with active infections should reduce transmission. Public areas conducive to transmission (eg, swimming pools) should not be used by those with active infection. Chemical foot baths are of no value and can facilitate spread of infection. Since recurrence after treatment is common, proper foot hygiene is important (see Treatment, p 467).

Tinea Versicolor (Pityriasis Versicolor)

Clinical Manifestations: Tinea (pityriasis) versicolor is a common, superficial disorder of the skin characterized by multiple scaling and oval macular and patchy lesions, usually distributed over the upper portions of the trunk, proximal areas of the arms, and neck. Facial involvement is particularly common in children. The lesions can be hypopigmented or hyperpigmented (fawn-colored or brown) and can be somewhat lighter than the surrounding skin. They fail to tan during the summer and during the winter are relatively darker—hence the term "versicolor." Common conditions confused with this disorder include pityriasis alba, postinflammatory hypopigmentation, vitiligo, melasma, seborrheic dermatitis, pityriasis rosea, and secondary syphilis.

Etiology: *Malassezia furfur* is the cause. This lipid-dependent fungus exists on normal skin in the yeast form and causes clinical lesions only when substantial hyphal forms develop.

Epidemiology: Tinea versicolor occurs worldwide. Although primarily a disorder of adolescents and young adults 15 to 30 years of age, it can also be seen in prepubertal children and, at times, infants. The fungus is transmitted by personal contact during periods of scaling.

Diagnosis: Scale scrapings examined microscopically in potassiumhydroxide wet mount preparation or stained with methylene blue or May-Grunwald-Giemsa stain disclose the pathognomonic clusters of yeast cells (as large as 8 μm in diameter) and short hyphal fragments. Growth of this yeast or culture requires a source of long-chain fatty acids, which may be accomplished by overlaying Sabouraud's medium with sterile olive oil

Treatment: Topical treatment with 2.5% selenium sulfide lotion is recommended. This preparation is applied in a thin layer covering the body surface from the face to the knees for 30 minutes, followed by monthly applications for 3 months (to help prevent recurrences). Patients should be warned that repigmentation will occur several months after successful treatment. Other preparations with therapeutic efficacy include sodium hyposulfite or thiosulfate in 15% to 25% concentrations (eg, Tinver lotion) applied twice daily for 2 to 4 weeks, or topical antifungal agents such as clotrimazole, econazole, haloprogin, ketoconazole, miconazole, or naftifine (see Topical Drugs for Superficial Fungal Infections, p 565). For persistent cases, oral ketoconazole for 3 days can be considered.

Isolation of the Hospitalized Patient: Drainage/secretion precautions are recommended.

Control Measures: Infected individuals should be treated.

Toxocariasis
(Visceral Larva Migrans;
Ocular Larva Migrans)

Clinical Manifestations: The severity of the symptoms of toxocariasis depends on the number of larvae ingested and the degree of allergic response. Most persons who are lightly infected are asymptomatic. Visceral larva migrans typically occurs in children 1 to 4 years old with history of pica, but it can also occur in older children. Characteristic manifestations include fever, leukocytosis, persistent eosinophilia, hypergammaglobulinemia, and hepatomegaly. Other manifestations include malaise, anemia, cough, and, in rare instances, pneumonia, myocarditis, and encephalitis. When ocular invasion (endophthalmitis or retinal granulomas) occurs, other evidence of the infection is usually lacking, suggesting that the visceral and ocular forms are distinct syndromes. Atypical forms of presentation include hemorrhagic skin rash and convulsions.

Etiology: Toxocariasis is caused by *Toxocara* species, which are common roundworms of dogs and cats (especially puppies or kittens), specifically *Toxocara canis* and *Toxocara cati* in the United States; most cases are caused by *T canis*. Other nematodes of animals can also cause this syndrome, although they rarely do.

Epidemiology: Humans are infected by the ingestion of eggs in soil containing infective larvae. A history of pica, particularly the eating of soil, is common. Direct contact with dogs is of secondary importance because eggs are not immediately infective when they are shed in the feces. Most reported cases are from North America and other developed countries, and involve children. Puppies in the household are the apparent source for most cases, but the eggs are found in many parks and public places, ie, wherever dogs and cats defecate.

The **incubation period** is unknown.

Diagnostic Tests: Hypereosinophilia and hypergammaglobulinemia associated with elevated titers of isohemagglutinins to the A and B blood group antigens are presumptive evidence. Microscopic identification of the larvae in a liver biopsy specimen is diagnostic, but this finding is infrequent. Hence, a negative liver biopsy for larvae does not exclude the diagnosis. An enzyme immunoassay for *Toxocara* serum antibodies, which is available at the Centers for Disease Control and Prevention, can provide presumptive evidence of toxocariasis. It is both specific and sensitive for the diagnosis of visceral larva migrans, but is less sensitive for the diagnosis of ocular larva migrans.

Treatment: Thiabendazole or diethylcarbamazine* (see Drugs for Parasitic Infections, p 574) is effective in reducing symptoms of visceral larva migrans, but the effectiveness of either drug for killing larvae has not been demonstrated. Significant toxicity has been observed with diethylcarbamazine. Albendazole, a drug not yet approved in the United States, has been used for therapy in other countries. In severe cases, where patients have myocarditis or involvement of the central nervous system, treatment with corticosteroids is indicated. Attention should be given to correcting the underlying causes of pica to prevent reinfection.

Antihelmintic treatment of ocular larva migrans is not effective; treatment involves injection of corticosteroids to reduce inflammation and surgery to repair secondary damage.

Isolation of the Hospitalized Patient: No special precautions are recommended.

Control Measures: Disposal of cat and dog feces is essential. Treatment of puppies and kittens with antihelmintics at 2, 4, 6, and 8 weeks of age prevents excretion of eggs by worms acquired transplacentally or through mother's milk. No specific management of exposed persons is recommended. Covering of sandboxes when not in use is helpful.

Toxoplasma gondii Infections (Toxoplasmosis)

Clinical Manifestations: In congenital toxoplasmosis, manifestations at birth can include a maculopapular rash, generalized lymphadenopathy, hepatomegaly, splenomegaly, jaundice, or thrombocytopenia. As a consequence of intrauterine meningoencephalitis, the infant can develop

---

*Available from Lederle Laboratories, Pearl River, NY.

cerebrospinal fluid abnormalities, hydrocephalus, microcephaly, chorioretinitis, and/or convulsions. Cerebral calcifications may be demonstrated on a roentgenogram or computerized tomography of the head. Some severely affected infants die in utero or within a few days of birth. However, congenital infection is usually asymptomatic at birth, although sequelae can become apparent several years later. Sequelae of congenital toxoplasmosis include mental retardation, learning disabilities, impaired vision, or blindness.

Isolated ocular toxoplasmosis most often occurs as a result of congenital infection but can result from acquired infection. Ocular disease can become reactivated years after the initial infection, both in healthy and immunocompromised individuals.

In acquired toxoplasmosis, infection is usually asymptomatic. When symptoms do develop, they are nonspecific and include malaise, fever, sore throat, and myalgia. Lymphadenopathy, frequently cervical, is the most common sign. A maculopapular rash and hepatosplenomegaly may also occur. The clinical course is usually benign and self-limited. Myocarditis and pneumonitis are rare complications.

Chronically infected immunodeficient patients, such as those with AIDS, can experience reactivated central nervous system disease or, less commonly, systemic toxoplasmosis. Although rare, infants who are born to HIV-infected mothers or mothers immunosuppressed for other reasons, and who are chronically infected with *Toxoplasma*, may acquire congenital toxoplasmosis as a result of reactivated maternal parasitemia.

Etiology: *Toxoplasma gondii* is a protozoan parasite.

Epidemiology: *Toxoplasma gondii* is worldwide in distribution and infects many species of warm-blooded animals. Members of the cat family are the definitive hosts. Cats acquire the infection when they are exposed to feces from an infected cat or when they feed on infected animals, such as mice or uncooked household meats. The parasite replicates sexually in the feline small intestine. For 2 to 4 weeks after primary infection, cats excrete the oocysts in their stools. After excretion, oocysts require a maturation phase (sporulation) of 24 to 48 hours in temperate climates before they are infective by the oral route. Infected animals (including sheep, pigs, and cattle) can have tissue cysts in their brain, myocardium, skeletal muscles, and other organs. The tissue cysts remain viable for the lifetime of the host. Humans become infected either by consumption of poorly cooked meat or by accidental ingestion of sporulated oocysts from soil or in contaminated food. Transmission by blood product transfusion and from infected organ donors (heart and bone marrow) has been documented. Except for such rare occurrences and transplacental infection from mother to fetus, toxoplasmosis is not communicable from person to person.

The **incubation period** of the acquired infection, based on a well-studied outbreak, is estimated to be approximately 7 days (with a range of 4 to 21 days).

Diagnostic Tests: Serologic tests are the primary means of diagnosis, but results must be carefully interpreted. Immunoglobulin G (IgG)-specific antibodies are commonly measured by the indirect immunofluorescence test or enzyme immunoassay (EIA). IgG-specific antibodies peak in concentration 1 to 2 months after infection and remain positive indefinitely. For determination of acute infection, the Centers for Disease Control and Prevention recommends a capture-EIA for IgM antibodies. Specific IgM antibodies can be detected 2 weeks after the infection, reach peak concentration in 1 month, decline thereafter, and usually become undetectable within 6 to 9 months. On rare occasion, IgM-specific antibodies are detectable for as long as 2 years in patients with toxoplasmosis. Tests to detect IgA antibodies, which fall to undetectable concentrations sooner than IgM antibodies, are useful for pregnant women and other patients for whom more precise information about the duration of infection is needed; these tests are available only through reference laboratories. Tests for specific IgM antibodies should be performed by an experienced laboratory; test kits used by some laboratories can give false-positive and false-negative results.

Seroconversion or a fourfold rise in specific IgG antibody titer suggests recently acquired infection, but the results can be misleading if serum specimens are not tested concurrently to control for day-to-day laboratory variability. Patients with seroconversion or a fourfold rise in IgG antibody titer should have specific IgM antibody determinations performed by a reference laboratory.

Prenatal. Fetal blood sampling and ultrasound examination can be used to make a prenatal diagnosis of congenital toxoplasmosis. If the diagnosis is unconfirmed at the time of delivery in an infant with suspected toxoplasmosis, ophthalmologic and neurologic examinations and computerized tomography of the head should be performed, and an attempt should be made to isolate *T gondii* from the placenta and cord blood, by mouse inoculation.

Postnatal. After birth, congenital toxoplasmosis can be diagnosed by the detection of *Toxoplasma*-specific IgM or IgA, the persistence of *Toxoplasma* IgG beyond 12 months of age, or the isolation of the organism by mouse inoculation. Blood should be sent to a reference laboratory that performs the mouse inoculation and the *Toxoplasma* IgM and IgA assays by the double-sandwich IgM EIA (DS-IgM EIA) or IgM Immunosorbent Agglutination Assay (ISAGA). DS-IgM EIA detects approximately 75% of infants with congenital infection. The sensitivity of both the immunofluorescent and capture-EIA assays for *Toxoplasma* IgM are significantly less than that of the DS-IgM and IgA EIA or ISAGA assays, and negative results with these tests do not exclude congenital infection. Circulating maternal *Toxoplasma* IgG antibodies in an uninfected infant usually become undetectable by 6 to 12 months of age.

HIV Infection. Patients with AIDS infected with *Toxoplasma* have variable titers of IgG antibody to *Toxoplasma* but rarely have IgM antibody. Seroconversion and fourfold rises in titer do not occur frequently, making serodiagnosis difficult. In such patients, characteristic clinical features of central nervous system disease, particularly if any detectable *Toxoplasma* antibody is present in serum, are sufficient for a presumptive diagnosis. Demonstration of *T gondii* organisms, antigen, or DNA in biopsied tissue, blood, or cerebrospinal fluid confirms the diagnosis. They may be necessary in patients who do not respond to a therapeutic trial.

Infants born to women who are infected with both HIV and *Toxoplasma* or to women who have evidence of primary *Toxoplasma* infection during gestation should be evaluated for congenital toxoplasmosis.

Diagnosis of ocular toxoplasmosis is based upon observation of characteristic retinal lesions in conjunction with serum IgG or IgM antibodies.

Treatment: Pyrimethamine and sulfonamides (specifically sulfadiazine*) act synergistically against *Toxoplasma*. The most widely accepted regimen for children and adults consists of oral pyrimethamine in a loading dose of 2 mg/kg/d in two divided doses for 1 to 3 days, followed by 1 mg/kg/d in a single dose for 4 weeks, plus oral sulfadiazine (or trisulfapyrimidines), 100 mg/kg/d (maximum 8 g/d) in three or four divided doses for at least 4 weeks. Folinic acid (calcium leucovorin) should be administered orally or parenterally (usually 5 to 10 mg/d) to patients receiving pyrimethamine to prevent hematologic toxicity. In patients with AIDS, maintenance therapy with these drugs is usually given to prevent relapse. An alternative therapy for *Toxoplasma* encephalitis in AIDS patients during the acute phase is clindamycin substituted for sulfadiazine, ie, a regimen of pyrimethamine and clindamycin. Clindamycin may also be used to treat ocular toxoplasmosis, usually in conjunction with sulfadiazine and pyrimethamine (with folinic acid). The use of corticosteroids in the management of ocular complications or central nervous system disease is controversial.

Infants born to mothers with primary *Toxoplasma* infection during pregnancy or *Toxoplasma* antibody-positive mothers with HIV infection are at high risk of congenital *Toxoplasma* infection. These infants should be considered for treatment irrespective of clinical manifestations. Because the diagnosis can take several months to confirm, physicians may initiate treatment based upon early findings while more definitive data are pending. Treatment regimens include pyrimethamine (with folinic acid), sulfadiazine,* and sometimes spiramycin.† The optimal dosage and duration of therapy of these drugs are uncertain, and consultation with experts should be sought. Spiramycin has been used effectively in Europe for the treatment of primary infection in pregnant women to reduce transmission of *T gondii* to the fetus.

Isolation of the Hospitalized Patient: No special precautions are recommended.

Control Measures: Cat litter should be disposed of daily (oocysts are not infective during the first 24 to 48 hours after passage). Domestic cats should be fed commercially prepared cat food, should be restricted from hunting

---

*As of 1993, sulfadiazine is no longer marketed in the United States. Until a domestic source of the drug is re-established, the drug may be obtained from the Division of Parasitic Diseases at the Centers for Disease Control and Prevention (see Directory of Telephone Numbers, p 601).

†Available only as an investigational drug in the United States through the Food and Drug Administration (see Directory of Telephone Numbers, p 601).

wild rodents, and should not be allowed to eat raw or partially cooked kitchen scraps. All red meats should be cooked thoroughly before human consumption. Pregnant women with negative or unknown *Toxoplasma* titers should avoid contact with cat feces, should not do gardening or yard work in areas to which cats have access, and should not eat undercooked meat.

Trichinosis
(Trichinella spiralis)

Clinical Manifestations: The clinical spectrum of infection is highly variable, ranging from inapparent infection to fulminating, fatal illness. The severity of the disease is proportional to the infective dose. During the first week after ingesting infected meat, the patient can experience abdominal discomfort, nausea, vomiting, and/or diarrhea. Two to 8 weeks later, as larvae migrate into tissues, fever, myalgia, periorbital edema, urticarial rash, and conjunctival and subungual hemorrhages can develop. In severe infections, myocardial failure, neurologic involvement, and pneumonitis can follow in 1 or 2 months.

Etiology: *Trichinella spiralis*, a nematode capable of infecting only warm-blooded animals, is the cause.

Epidemiology: The infection is enzootic worldwide in many carnivores, especially scavengers. The usual source of human infections is pork; bear meat and other wild carnivorous game can also be sources. Infection occurs as a result of ingestion of raw or insufficiently cooked meat containing encysted larvae of *T spiralis*. Feeding pigs uncooked garbage perpetuates the cycle of infection. In the United States, the incidence of the infection in humans has declined considerably, but infection occurs sporadically, often within a family or among friends who have prepared uncooked sausage from fresh pork. In North America, infection has also resulted from eating undercooked bear or walrus meat. The disease is not transmitted from person to person.

The **incubation period** is usually 1 to 2 weeks.

Diagnostic Tests: Eosinophilia approaching 70%, in conjunction with compatible symptoms and dietary history, suggests the diagnosis. Serologic tests are available through state laboratories and the Centers for Disease Control and Prevention. Serum antibody titers rarely become positive before the third week of illness. Testing paired sera is usually diagnostic. Beginning 2 weeks after infection, larvae can be seen on muscle biopsy. The tissue is best examined fresh, compressed between two microscope slides. Identification of larvae in suspect meat can be the most rapid source of diagnostic information.

Treatment: Mebendazole for 10 to 13 days is recommended (see Drugs for Parasitic Infections, p 574). Thiabendazole is an alternative drug. Although thiabendazole kills the adult worms in the small intestine, it appears ineffective against the encysted larvae. Corticosteroids alleviate symptoms of the inflammatory reaction and can be lifesaving when the central nervous system or heart is involved.

Isolation of the Hospitalized Patient: No special precautions are recommended.

Control Measures: Transmission to pigs can be reduced by not feeding them garbage, and by active rat control. Persons should be educated about the necessity of cooking pork thoroughly (until the meat is no longer pink). Freezing of pork at −23.3°C (−10°F) for 10 days kills the larvae. However, *Trichinella* organisms in Arctic wild animals can survive this procedure. Individuals known to have recently ingested contaminated meat should be treated with mebendazole (or thiabendazole).

Trichomonas vaginalis Infections (Trichomoniasis)

Clinical Manifestations: Infection with *Trichomonas* is frequently asymptomatic. The usual clinical picture in symptomatic female patients consists of a frothy vaginal discharge and mild vulvovaginal itching in postmenarcheal women. Dysuria and lower abdominal pain can occur. The vaginal discharge is frequently pale yellow to gray-green in color and has a fishy odor. Symptoms are frequently more severe just before or after menstruation. The vaginal mucosa can be edematous and the cervix can be inflamed, with petechiae ("strawberry cervix"), and can bleed easily. Infected males can develop urethritis or prostatitis, but the majority are asymptomatic. Recurrence or reinfection is common.

Etiology: *Trichomonas vaginalis* is a flagellated protozoan.

Epidemiology: *Trichomonas* infection is primarily a sexually transmitted disease and frequently coexists with other infections, particularly gonococcal infections. Although *T vaginalis* can be acquired without direct sexual contact, its presence in a prepubertal child should raise the question of sexual abuse. *Trichomonas vaginalis* can also be found in newborns, who acquire it during birth.

The **incubation period** is 4 to 20 days (average, 1 week).

Diagnostic Tests: Diagnosis is usually made by examination of a wet mount preparation of the vaginal discharge. The lashing of the flagella and the motility of the organism are distinctive. Positive preparations are more frequent in symptomatic women and are directly related to the number of organisms. Culture of the organism and antibody tests using an enzyme immunoassay, or direct or indirect immunofluorescence techniques for demonstration of the organism, are possible but not generally indicated.

Treatment: Metronidazole is the treatment of choice, resulting in cure rates of approximately 95%. For prepubertal girls, 15 mg/kg/d in three divided doses (maximum dose, 250 mg) is recommended. In adolescents and adults, the dose is 2 g in a single dose. Patients should abstain from alcohol for 48 hours due to the disulfiram-like effects of the drug. Treatment failures should be retreated with metronidazole (120g in two divided doses for adolescents and adults) for 7 days. The sexual partner should be treated concurrently. Metronidazole should not be used in the first trimester of pregnancy. Patients may be treated after the first trimester. Effective alternatives to metronidazole therapy are not available.

Isolation of the Hospitalized Patient: No special precautions are recommended.

Control Measures: Measures to prevent sexually transmitted diseases, particularly the consistent use of condoms, are indicated.

Trichuriasis
(Whipworm Infection)

Clinical Manifestations: Abdominal pain, tenesmus, and bloody diarrhea with mucous can occur. Chronic infection associated with heavy infestation can be associated with rectal prolapse.

Etiology: *Trichuris trichiura*, the whipworm, is the agent. Adult worms are 30 to 50 mm in length, with a large thread-like anterior end that is embedded in the mucosa of the large intestine.

Epidemiology: The parasite has a worldwide distribution but is more common in the tropics and in areas of poor sanitation. In some areas of Asia, the prevalence is 50%. In the United States, trichuriasis has generally been limited to rural areas of the southeast and to migrants from tropical areas. Infections are usually asymptomatic. Eggs require a minimum of 10 days incubation in the soil before they are infectious. The disease is not communicable from person to person.

The **incubation period** is not known.

Diagnostic Tests: Eggs may be found on direct examination of the stool or using concentration techniques.

Treatment: Mebendazole for 3 days is usually effective in eradicating most of the worms.

Isolation of the Hospitalized Patient: No special precautions are necessary.

Control Measures: Proper disposal of fecal material is indicated.

African Trypanosomiasis (African Sleeping Sickness)

Clinical Manifestations: The rapidity and severity of clinical manifestations vary with the infecting species. With *Trypanosoma brucei gambiense* (West African) infection, a cutaneous nodule or chancre may appear at the site of parasite inoculation within a few days of an infective tsetse fly bite; however, systemic illness occurs months to years later. The systemic infection is characterized by intermittent fever, posterior cervical lymphadenopathy ("Winterbottom's sign") and a variety of nonspecific complaints including arthralgia, rash, pruritus, and edema. Months to years later, the central nervous system (CNS) can be invaded, producing a chronic meningoencephalitis characterized by behavioral changes, cachexia, headache, hallucinations, delusions, and somnolence. In contrast, in *Trypanosoma brucei rhodesiense* (East African) infection, generalized illness develops days to weeks after parasite inoculation. Acute manifestations include high fever, cutaneous chancre, myocarditis, hepatitis, anemia, and laboratory evidence of disseminated intravascular coagulation. Clinical meningoencephalitis can develop as early as 3 weeks after the onset of the untreated systemic illness. *Trypanosoma brucei rhodesiense* infection has a high fatality rate; without treatment, infected patients usually die within days to months of the clinical onset of disease.

Etiology: African trypanosomiasis is caused by subspecies of the *T brucei* complex (see Clinical Manifestations, above), which are extracellular protozoan hemoflagellates.

Epidemiology: Approximately 20,000 human cases occur annually worldwide, although only one or two cases, acquired in Africa, are reported every year in the United States. Transmission is confined to an area in Africa between the latitudes of 15° north and 20° south, corresponding precisely with the distribution of the tsetse fly vector (*Glossina* species). In East Africa, wild animals such as antelope, bushbuck, and hartebeest constitute the major reservoir of *T brucei rhodesiense*, whereas humans are postulated to be the sole reservoir of *T brucei gambiense* in West and Central Africa.

The **incubation period** in *T brucei rhodesiense* infection is 3 to 21 days, usually 5 to 14 days; in *T brucei gambiense* infection, it is usually longer and extremely variable, ranging from several months to years.

Diagnostic Tests: Diagnosis is made by identification of trypomastigotes in the blood, cerebrospinal fluid (CSF), or fluid aspirated from a chancre or lymph node. Concentration and Giemsa staining of the buffy coat layer of peripheral blood can aid in the diagnosis. *Trypanosoma brucei gambiense* is more likely to be found in lymph node aspirates. Although an increased concentration of IgM in either serum or CSF is considered characteristic of African trypanosomiasis, polyclonal hyperglobulinemia involving all classes of immunoglobulin is common.

Treatment: When no evidence of CNS involvement is present, the drug of choice for the acute hemolymphatic stage of infection is suramin. Pentamidine is an alternative drug for early infections caused by *T brucei gambiense*. Until recently, melarsoprol, a toxic parenteral arsenical compound, was the drug of choice for CNS involvement with both species of *T brucei*. However, eflornithine* has been demonstrated to be effective for CNS involvement caused by *T brucei gambiense*. Melarsoprol is still the drug of choice for CNS disease caused by *T brucei rhodesiense*. Suramin and melarsoprol are available in the United States from the Drug Service, Centers for Disease Control and Prevention (see Directory of Telephone Numbers, p 601).

Isolation of the Hospitalized Patient: Other than universal precautions, no special precautions are recommended.

Control Measures: Travelers to endemic areas should avoid known foci of sleeping sickness and/or tsetse infestation and minimize tsetse fly bites by use of protective clothing, bed netting, and insect repellants. Infected patients should not breast-feed or donate blood.

American Trypanosomiasis (Chagas' Disease)

Clinical Manifestations: The early phase of this disease is frequently asymptomatic. However, children are more likely to exhibit symptoms than adults. In some patients, a red nodule known as a chagoma develops at the site of the original inoculation, usually on the face or arms. The surrounding skin becomes indurated and later hypopigmented. Unilateral, firm edema of the eyelids, known as Romana's sign, is the earliest indication of the infection, but it is present in fewer than 50% of patients with signs of acute Chagas' disease. The edematous skin is violaceous in color, with conjunctivitis and enlargement of the ipsilateral preauricular lymph node. A few days after the appearance of Romana's sign, fever, generalized lymphadenopathy, and malaise develop. Acute myocarditis, hepatosplenomegaly, edema, and meningoencephalitis can follow. Serious sequelae consisting of cardiomyopathy and heart failure (the major cause of death), megaesophagus, and/or megacolon can develop many years after the initial

---

*Available from Marion Merrell Dow, Inc, Cincinnati, OH.

manifestations. Congenital disease is characterized by low birth weight, hepatomegaly, and meningoencephalitis, with convulsions and tremors.

Etiology: *Trypanosoma cruzi*, a protozoan hemoflagellate, is the cause.

Epidemiology: The parasites are transmitted through the feces of the insects of the triatomid family. These insects defecate while taking a blood meal. The bitten person is inoculated by inadvertently rubbing the insect feces containing the parasite into the site of the bite or mucous membranes of the eye or the mouth. The parasite can also be transmitted congenitally and through blood transfusion. Accidental laboratory infections can result from the handling of blood from infected persons or laboratory animals, the vectors, and vector excreta. The disease is limited to the Western hemisphere, predominantly Mexico and Central and South America. Although small mammals in the southern and southwestern United States harbor *T cruzi*, vector-borne transmission to humans is extremely rare in the United States. Several transfusion-associated cases have been documented in the United States. Infection is common in immigrants from Central and South America. The disease is a leading cause of death in South America where between 7 and 15 million people are infected.

The **incubation period** for the acute disease is 1 to 2 weeks. The chronic manifestations do not appear for years.

Diagnostic Tests: During the acute disease, the parasite is demonstrable in blood, either by Giemsa staining or by direct wet-mount preparation. In chronic infections, which are characterized by low-level parasitemia, parasites in the blood must be cultured on a special medium, inoculated into mice, or identified by xenodiagnosis. Serologic tests include complement fixation, indirect hemagglutination, indirect immunofluorescence, and enzyme-linked immunoassay.

Treatment: The acute phase of Chagas' disease is treated with nifurtimox* or benznidazole.† These drugs are not effective against the forms of the parasite usually found in the chronic phase of the disease.

Isolation of the Hospitalized Patient: Universal precautions should be scrupulously followed.

Control Measures: Education about the mode of spread and the methods of prevention should be made available in endemic areas. Homes should be examined for the presence of the vectors. If they are found, thorough disinfection is indicated. Vector control through use of effective insecticides, control of the rodent population on which the vectors feed, and elimination of

---

*Available from the Drug Service, Centers for Disease Control and Prevention (see Directory of Telephone Numbers, p 601).
†Available from Roche, Nutley, NJ.

habitats of the vectors is recommended. Screens on windows and doors exclude the insect vectors. Blood and serologic examinations should be performed on household members with a similar exposure to the vector as that of a known patient.

Blood donors in endemic areas must be screened by serologic tests. Blood recipients can be protected in endemic areas by treatment of the donated blood with gentian violet at a dilution of 1:4,000.

Infected patients should not donate blood.

Tuberculosis

Clinical Manifestations: Most infected children are asymptomatic when the tuberculin reaction is found to be positive. The primary complex of tuberculous infection is usually not demonstrable on chest roentgenogram, and in most immunologically healthy children with primary tuberculosis, the infection does not immediately progress to disease. Early clinical manifestations occurring 1 to 6 months after initial infection can include one or more of the following: lymphadenopathy of the hilar, mediastinal, cervical, or other nodes; pulmonary involvement of a segment or lobe, occasionally with consolidation; atelectasis; pleural effusion; miliary tuberculosis; and tuberculous meningitis. Other clinical presentations that can occur later after initial infection include tuberculosis of the middle ear and mastoid, bones, joints, and skin. Extrapulmonary disease (eg, miliary, meningeal, renal, bone, or joint) occurs in approximately 25% of children younger than 15 years of age with tuberculosis. Tuberculosis of the kidney and reactivation or adult-type pulmonary tuberculosis are rare in young children but can occur in adolescents.

Etiology: The agent is *Mycobacterium tuberculosis*, an acid-fast bacillus (AFB). Human disease caused by *Mycobacterium bovis*, the agent of bovine tuberculosis, has been identified in the United States, while *Mycobacterium africanum* is rare. Other mycobacteria rarely cause pulmonary disease in immunocompetent children but may cause lymphadenopathy (see Diseases due to Nontuberculous Mycobacteria, p 500).

Epidemiology: Tuberculous disease ("tuberculosis") is differentiated from tuberculous infection by the presence of clinical manifestations. In patients with infection, the tuberculin skin test is positive but the chest roentgenogram is normal and no signs or symptoms consistent with tuberculosis are present. Patients with disease have manifestations of pulmonary or extrapulmonary infection indicated either by chest roentgenograms or by clinical signs and symptoms. The interval between initial tuberculous infection and the onset of disease may be several weeks or many years. In adults, the distinction between infection and clinical disease is usually clear, but in young children the two stages are often less distinct. Infants and children who are exposed to adult contacts with infectious tuberculosis comprise a group of individuals at high risk for disease from recent infection. The majority of adults with tuberculosis had initially been infected years before (ie, they have reactivation disease).

Case rates of tuberculosis for all ages are highest in urban, low-income areas, and in nonwhite racial and ethnic groups, among whom more than two thirds of reported cases in the United States now occur. Foreign-born persons account for more than one quarter of cases. Specific groups with the highest rates of infection and disease are minority groups (ie, first-generation immigrants from high-risk countries, Hispanics, blacks, Asians, American Indians, and Alaskan natives), the homeless, and residents of correctional facilities.

Although infected children of all ages are at increased risk for developing tuberculous disease, infants and postpubertal adolescents are at highest risk in the United States. Other risk factors for progression of infection to disease include recent close contact with an infected person; recent skin test conversion; immunodeficiency, particularly that caused by HIV infection; intravenous drug use; certain diseases and medical conditions, specifically Hodgkin's disease, lymphoma, diabetes mellitus, chronic renal failure, malnutrition, and immunosuppression induced by drugs (including daily steroid therapy).

Transmission of tuberculosis is usually by inhalation of droplet nuclei produced by an adult or adolescent with infectious pulmonary tuberculosis. The duration of infectivity of an adult receiving effective treatment depends on the drug susceptibilities of the organism, the degree of sputum acid-fast smear positivity, and cough frequency. Although infectivity usually lasts only a few weeks, it may last longer, especially if the adult patient is nonadherent with medical therapy or is infected with a resistant strain. If the sputum is negative on repeated smears and if the cough has disappeared, the person is considered noninfectious. The majority of adult and adolescent patients are considered to be noninfectious within a few weeks of starting appropriate therapy to which the infecting organism is susceptible. Children with primary pulmonary tuberculosis are usually not contagious because their lesions are small, discharge of bacilli is minimal, and cough is minimal or nonexistent.

The portal of entry is usually the respiratory tract. Skin, gastrointestinal tract, and mucous membranes have been implicated in a few cases. On rare occasions, tuberculosis is transmitted from mother to fetus transplacentally or by infected amniotic fluid.

The **incubation period** from infection to development of a positive reaction to a tuberculin skin test is about 2 to 10 weeks. The risk for developing disease is highest in the first 2 years after infection. However, months to years may elapse between infection and disease. In most instances, untreated infection becomes dormant and never progresses to clinical disease in the healthy host.

Diagnostic Tests: Isolation of tubercle bacilli by culture from early-morning gastric washings, or from sputum, pleural fluid, cerebrospinal fluid (CSF), urine, or other body fluids establishes the diagnosis. In a young child, the best culture material for the diagnosis of pulmonary tuberculosis is usually an early-morning gastric aspirate.

Since *M tuberculosis* is a slow-growing microorganism, recovery may take as long as 10 weeks by older culture methods and 2 to 3 weeks by the radiometric method. Even with optimal culture techniques, the organism is isolated from fewer than 50% of children with pulmonary tuberculosis. Identification of isolated *M tuberculosis* in the laboratory can be more rapid if DNA probes are combined with radiometric techniques. Attempts should be made to demonstrate AFB in sputum and/or body fluids by the Ziehl-Neelsen method or by auramine-rhodamine staining and fluorescence microscopy. Histologic examination and demonstration of AFB in specimens from lymph node, pleura, liver, bone marrow biopsies, or other tissues can be valuable for diagnosis.

Bacteriophage typing and restriction fragment length polymorphism analysis (a DNA fingerprinting technique), available through the Centers for Disease Control and Prevention (CDC), can be useful in epidemiologic studies.

Identification of a source case should be very actively pursued to support the diagnosis, determine possible drug resistance in the source case (which will influence the choice of drugs in the patient), and find all infected or diseased persons. A chest roentgenogram showing hilar lymph node enlargement with or without segmental atelectasis suggests the possibility of tuberculous disease. Culture material should always be obtained when (1) no source case isolate is available; (2) the source case isolate is drug resistant; (3) the child is immunocompromised (especially with HIV infection); or (4) the child has extrapulmonary disease.

Tuberculin Testing. The skin test is the only practical tool for diagnosing tuberculous infection in asymptomatic individuals. A positive reaction signifies infection with *M tuberculosis*. In most children, tuberculin reactivity first appears 3 to 6 weeks, and occasionally as long as 3 months, after initial infection. Tuberculin reactivity caused by *M tuberculosis* infection usually continues for the individual's lifetime, even after preventive chemotherapy is given.

To achieve significant progress in reducing the number of future cases of tuberculosis, identification of groups at high risk for infection (see Epidemiology, p 480), testing those persons with a Mantoux tuberculin skin test, evaluation of persons infected with disease, and providing appropriate therapy to persons with infection or disease are necessary. As a result, effective strategies for controlling infection and disease have evolved, ranging from periodic routine screening of the entire population (in which most individuals are at low risk) to aggressive identification and annual skin testing of high-risk groups. The CDC and the American Thoracic Society (ATS) do not recommend routine skin testing in low-risk groups in communities with a low prevalence of tuberculosis except for one-time testing during childhood for epidemiologic assessment of tuberculous infection in the area. For children in low-risk groups, the Academy previously had suggested two alternatives: (1) no testing or (2) skin tests at three times during childhood (at 12 to 15 months, 4 to 6 years, and 14 to 16 years). In accordance with the changing epidemiology of tuberculosis and public health strategies, the recommendations have been revised (see p 485).

Skin Tests. The two major techniques for tuberculin skin testing are the Mantoux test and multiple puncture tests (MPT). The Mantoux test uses a standardized antigen containing 5 tuberculin units of purified protein derivative (PPD), administered intradermally. The MPTs have been used widely because of the speed and ease with which they can be administered, even by unskilled personnel. The antigens in these tests are either PPD or Old Tuberculin (OT).

Several problems with MPTs severely limit their usefulness. First, the exact dose of tuberculin antigen introduced into the skin cannot be standardized. As a result, MPTs are not intended to be used as diagnostic tests. The need for a subsequent Mantoux test in a person with a positive MPT leads to the second problem, the booster phenomenon. Boosting represents an increase in reaction to a skin test caused by repetitive tests in a person previously infected with mycobacteria. The incidence of the booster phenomenon increases with age and is greater in geographic areas where exposure to nontuberculous mycobacteria is common or in children previously vaccinated with bacillus Calmette-Guerin (BCG). Third, the MPTs have variable and, in some populations, high rates of false-positive and false-negative results compared with the Mantoux test. Although some studies have demonstrated sensitivities of 95% to 99% for various MPTs, other studies have yielded false-positive rates of 10% to 15% and false-negative rates of 10% to 30% in various populations. Fourth, the widespread use of MPTs has led to the practice of allowing parents to interpret the skin tests and report the results to the physician's office by telephone or mail, resulting in inaccurate reading of the results. No other screening test used in pediatrics has been interpreted routinely by nonprofessionals.

A major reason that periodic skin testing with MPTs is no longer a useful strategy for the general population is the variable incidence of infection and disease, which is still low in most areas of the United States. Multiple puncture tests have a reported sensitivity of 68% to 97%, and a specificity of 40% to 90% for correlation with a Mantoux reaction of 10 mm or greater. As an example of the frequency of misleading results, if the prevalence of infection is 1% and 100,000 children are screened using MPTs, which have a sensitivity and specificity of 90%, the number of true positives would be 900 while the false positives would be 9,900, giving a positive predictive value of 8%. Therefore, 10,800 children would require two additional visits for the placement of a confirming Mantoux test and for the subsequent reading of the test. The MPTs, thus, are not appropriate tests to use for diagnosis, and their use should be severely restricted, if not eliminated. Furthermore, the efficiency and cost-to-benefit ratio of a strategy using MPTs followed by Mantoux testing compared to using the Mantoux alone in low-risk patients would have to be evaluated for each clinical setting.

Special Considerations. Previous BCG vaccination is never a contraindication to tuberculin testing. Recommendations for considering a Mantoux test reaction as positive are the same irrespective of previous BCG vaccination. No reliable method exists for distinguishing tuberculin reactions caused by BCG vaccination from those caused by natural infection. Many persons who receive BCG vaccine never have a reactive tuberculin skin test. In those with a reaction, the size of induration is often less than 10 mm and wanes after 3 to 5 years. For example, induration of 10 mm or greater in a BCG-vaccinated child from a country with a high prevalence of tuberculosis indicates likely infection with *M tuberculosis* and necessitates further diagnostic evaluation and, usually, preventive chemotherapy.

A negative Mantoux test never excludes tuberculous infection or disease. Approximately 10% of immunocompetent children with culture-documented tuberculosis do not react initially to 5 tuberculin units (TU) of PPD. Host-related factors, such as young age, poor nutrition, immunosuppression including HIV infection, viral infection (especially measles, varicella, and influenza), and severe, disseminated tuberculosis can decrease tuberculin reactivity. Many adults coinfected with HIV and *M tuberculosis* have anergy for tuberculin. Coinfected children are also frequently anergic.

Control skin tests to assess anergy are indicated only in patients with suspected or proven immunosuppression and in those with possible severe, disseminated disease. Their use in otherwise healthy children with pulmonary disease and in annual tuberculin skin testing of high-risk children is unwarranted. In addition, standardized and reliable skin tests for assessing anergy in infants and children are generally not available.

Other strengths of PPD skin test antigens (1 or 250 TU) should not be used.

Interpretation of the Mantoux Test Results (see Table 3.46, p 485). Interpretation of the skin test reaction depends on the purpose for which the test was given and on the consequences of false classification. Classification of test responses is based on epidemiologic and clinical factors. The appropriate cutoff size of induration indicating a positive reaction varies with the person tested and with related epidemiologic factors. In areas of the United States where nontuberculous mycobacteria are common, only 5% of children in the general population who have a 5- to 9-mm area of induration to a Mantoux tuberculin skin test are infected with *M tuberculosis*. However, a child with the same reaction who is in contact with an adult with infectious tuberculosis has an almost 50% chance of infection. The critical information is whether the child is likely to have been exposed to an adult with tuberculosis.

All current guidelines (CDC, ATS, and AAP) accept 15 mm or greater of induration as positive in any person. A reaction of 5 mm or greater is interpreted as positive by the CDC and ATS in the following groups: (1) persons who have had close recent contact with individuals who have infectious tuberculosis; (2) persons who have chest roentgenograms consistent with old healed tuberculosis; and (3) persons with HIV infection or with risk factors for HIV infection who have an unknown HIV status. The Academy also includes those children with clinical evidence of tuberculosis, and those with immunosuppression from causes other than HIV infection. A tuberculin reaction of 10 mm or greater is considered positive in other high-risk groups. These definitions of a positive reaction are listed in Table 3.46 (p 485).

Interpreting the Mantoux test results according to these guidelines necessitates special consideration. First, classifying children by risk group requires the willingness and ability of medical personnel to obtain a thorough history of the child and of adults caring for the child. Second, children with identical reactions may be evaluated differently, depending on the risk factors for tuberculosis. Third, the physician must have knowledge of the tuberculosis case rates and characteristics of tuberculosis within his or her community.

TABLE 3.46—Definition of Positive Mantoux Skin Test (5TU-PPD) in Children*

Reaction ≥5 mm

Children in close contact with persons who have known or suspected infectious cases of tuberculosis:

- Households with active or previously active cases if (1) treatment cannot be verified as adequate before exposure, (2) treatment was initiated after period of child's contact, or (3) reactivation is suspected

Children suspected to have tuberculous disease:

- Chest roentgenogram consistent with active or previously active tuberculosis
- Clinical evidence of tuberculosis

Children with immunosuppressive conditions† or HIV infection

Reaction ≥10 mm

Children at increased risk of dissemination from:

- Young age: <4 y of age
- Other medical risk factors, including Hodgkin's disease, lymphoma, diabetes mellitus, chronic renal failure, and malnutrition

Children with increased environmental exposure:

- Born, or whose parents were born, in regions of the world where tuberculosis is highly prevalent
- Frequently exposed to adults who are HIV infected, homeless, users of intravenous and other street drugs, poor and medically indigent city dwellers, residents of nursing homes, incarcerated or institutionalized persons, and migrant farm workers

Reaction ≥15 mm

Children ≥4 y of age without any risk factors

---

*These recommendations should apply regardless of whether BCG has been previously administered.
†Including immunosuppressive doses of corticosteroids.

Recommendations for Skin Testing:

- Routine annual skin testing for tuberculosis (Mantoux) in children with no risk factors in low-prevalence communities is not indicated. In such settings, positive skin reactions are most likely to be falsely positive.
- Children at high risk (see Table 3.47, p 486) should be tested annually, using Mantoux tests. All results (positive or negative) should be read routinely by qualified medical personnel.

TABLE 3.47—Infants, Children, and Adolescents at High Risk for
M tuberculosis Infection

• Contacts of adults with infectious tuberculosis

• Those who are from, or have parents who are from, regions of the world with high prevalence of tuberculosis

• Those with abnormalities on chest roentgenogram suggestive of tuberculosis

• Those with clinical evidence of tuberculosis

• HIV-seropositive persons

• Those with immunosuppressive conditions

• Those with other medical risk factors: Hodgkin's disease, lymphoma, diabetes mellitus, chronic renal failure, malnutrition

• Incarcerated adolescents

• Children frequently exposed to the following adults: HIV-infected individuals, homeless persons, users of intravenous and other street drugs, poor and medically indigent city dwellers, residents of nursing homes, migrant farm workers

---

- Children who have no risk factors but who reside in high-prevalence regions and children whose history for risk factors is incomplete or unreliable may receive periodic Mantoux tests, such as at 1, 4 to 6, and 11 to 16 years of age. Such a decision should be based on the local epidemiology of tuberculosis.
- A Mantoux test is considered positive at a reaction of 5 mm or greater for the highest risk groups (see Table 3.46, p 485):
  – Children in close contact with persons who have known or suspected infectious cases of tuberculosis.
  – Children suspected to have disease based on clinical and/or roentgenographic evidence.
  – Children with underlying host factors that indicate extremely high risk for severe tuberculosis, including immunosuppressive conditions and HIV infection.
- A Mantoux test is considered positive at a reaction of 10 mm or more for children younger than 4 years of age, for those with medical diseases (other than immunosuppression) who are at increased risk for dissemination, or for those at increased risk for disease because of environmental exposure (see Table 3.46, p 485).
- A Mantoux test is considered positive at a reaction of 15 mm or greater for all children including those with no risk factors.
- Tuberculin skin testing can be done at the same time that measles vaccine (ie, usually MMR) is given. If testing is indicated in a child who does not have clinical or roentgenographic manifestations suggestive of tuberculosis, and cannot be done concurrently, testing should be postponed for 4 to 6 weeks.

Treatment (see Table 3.48, p 488) for summary):

Prevention of Disease. Isoniazid (INH) given to persons who have tuberculosis infection without disease (ie, no clinical or roentgenographic manifestations) provides substantial protection (54% to 88% efficacy) against development of active disease for at least 20 years. Among children, efficacy approaches 100% with appropriate adherence to therapy. All infants, children, and adolescents who have a positive tuberculin test but no evidence of clinical tuberculosis and who have never received antituberculous therapy should receive INH alone (if INH resistance is not suspected), unless a specific contraindication exists. Isoniazid in this circumstance is therapeutic for the infection and preventive against development of disease. A chest roentgenogram should be obtained at the time preventive therapy is initiated; if the roentgenogram is normal and the child remains asymptomatic, it need not be repeated.

Preventive INH therapy should be initiated in recent contacts, especially HIV-positive contacts, of persons with infectious tuberculosis, once clinical disease has been excluded, even if the tuberculin skin test reaction is negative (see Preventive Therapy for Contacts, p 498). In addition, persons known to be anergic who are from a population with a high prevalence of tuberculosis should be considered for preventive therapy.

Duration of Preventive Chemotherapy. The optimal duration for tuberculous infection remains unknown. In early studies, children received INH for 1 year. Data in adults indicate that after 6 months of continuous medication, a 65% reduction in disease is achieved compared to a 75% reduction with 12 months of treatment. In adults, 6 to 12 months of preventive therapy with INH is now recommended in most cases.

In infants and children, the recommended duration of INH is 9 months. The exceptions are patients with HIV infection, for whom a minimum of 12 months is recommended. Isoniazid is given daily, 10 mg/kg (maximum 300 mg), in a single dose. In situations where adherence with daily preventive therapy cannot be assured, twice weekly directly observed therapy with INH can be considered, preferably after completion of 1 month of daily therapy. **Direct observation means that a health care worker is present when INH is given to the patient.** Each dose of INH in the twice-weekly regimen is 20 to 30 mg/kg, not to exceed a daily maximum of 900 mg.

Preventive Therapy for Contacts of Patients With INH-Resistant M tuberculosis. Possible INH resistance should always be considered, particularly in children from population groups in which drug resistance is high, especially in foreign-born children from countries with a high prevalence of drug-resistant tuberculosis. For contacts who are likely to have been infected by an index case with INH-resistant but rifampin-susceptible organisms, and in whom the consequences of the infection are likely to be severe (eg, children younger than 4 years of age), rifampin (10 mg/kg, maximum 600 mg, given daily in a single dose) should be given in addition to INH (10 mg/kg, maximum 300 mg, given daily in a single dose) until susceptibility test results on the isolate from the index case are available. If the index case is known or proven to be excreting organisms resistant to INH, the INH should be discontinued and rifampin given for a total of 9 months. Isoniazid alone should be given if no proof of exposure to INH-resistant organisms is found. Optimal therapy for children with tuberculous infection caused by organisms resistant

TABLE 3.48—Recommended Treatment Regimens for Drug-Susceptible Tuberculosis in Infants, Children, and Adolescents

Infection or Disease Category	Regimen*,†	Remarks
Asymptomatic infection (positive skin test, no disease):		If daily therapy is not possible, twice weekly therapy may be used for 9 mo.
Isoniazid-susceptible	9 mo of I daily	
Isoniazid-resistant	9 mo of R daily	
Pulmonary (including hilar adenopathy)	**6-mo regimen (standard):** 2 mo of I,R, and Z daily, followed by 4 mo of I and R daily	If possible drug resistance is a concern, another drug (ethambutol or streptomycin‡) should be added to the initial 3-drug therapy until drug susceptibility is determined. The 2-drug 9-mo regimen should not be used.
	OR 2 mo of I,R, and Z daily, followed by 4 mo of I and R twice weekly	Drugs can be given 2 or 3 times per wk under direct observation in the initial phase if nonadherence is likely.
	9-mo regimen (alternative): 9 mo of I and R daily	For hilar adenopathy, regimens consisting of 6 mo of I and R daily, and 1 mo of I and R daily, followed by 5 mo of I and R twice weekly, have been successful in areas where drug resistance is rare.
	OR 1 mo of I and R daily, followed by 8 mo of I and R twice weekly	
Meningitis, disseminated (miliary), and bone/joint	2 mo of I,R,Z, and S‡ daily, followed by 10 mo of I and R daily	Streptomycin‡ is given in initial therapy until drug susceptibility is known.
	OR 2 mo of I,R,Z, and S‡ daily, followed by 10 mo of I and R twice weekly	For patients who may have acquired tuberculosis in geographic areas where resistance to streptomycin is common, capreomycin (15-30 mg/kg/d) or kanamycin (15-30 mg/kg/d) may be used instead of streptomycin.
Extrapulmonary other than meningitis, disseminated (miliary), or bone/joint	Same as for pulmonary disease	See "Pulmonary."

*I=isoniazid; R=rifampin; Z=pyrazinamide; S=streptomycin.
†Duration of therapy is longer in HIV-infected persons.
‡As of December 1993, available from Pfizer Streptomycin Program, Pfizer Pharmaceuticals, New York, NY (800/254-4445).

to isoniazid and rifampin is unknown. In deciding on therapy in this different circumstance, consultation with an expert is advised.

Treatment of Active (Current) Disease. The goal of treatment is to achieve sterilization of the tuberculous lesion in the shortest possible time. Achievement of this goal maximizes patient adherence, reduces treatment cost, and minimizes development of resistant organisms. The major problem limiting successful treatment is poor adherence in taking medications. Chemotherapy of tuberculosis is also complicated by two characteristics of mycobacteria, specifically (1) spontaneous emergence of drug-resistant mutants, and (2) persistence of viable mycobacteria as a result of their slow, intermittent growth.

The treatment of children with tuberculosis historically has been based on treatment regimens used in adults. The encouraging results of 6-month and 9-month treatment regimens in adults and children with both pulmonary and extrapulmonary tuberculosis have led to use of these shorter regimens in children. Published data with the 6-month and 9-month regimens in children in the United States and in developing countries are now available.

A 6-month regimen consisting of INH, rifampin, and pyrazinamide for the first 2 months and INH and rifampin for the remaining 4 months as standard therapy is recommended for treatment of fully susceptible *M tuberculosis* disease, including pulmonary, pulmonary with hilar adenopathy, and hilar adenopathy in infants, children, and adolescents with a positive tuberculin skin test. Drug susceptibilities of strains can be determined by susceptibility patterns of isolates from adult contacts and local endemic rates of single- and multiple-drug resistance. When initial drug resistance is suspected, either ethambutol or streptomycin[*] should be added as the fourth drug to the initial regimen until drug susceptibility results are available (see Chemotherapy for "Drug-Resistant" Tuberculosis, below). In children with hilar adenopathy without drug resistance, a 6-month regimen of only INH and rifampin may be adequate. Drug susceptibility studies on the initial isolate or that recovered from the adult contact should be performed in all cases.

In the 6-month regimen with triple-drug therapy, INH, rifampin, and pyrazinamide are given daily for the first 2 months. After this 2-month period, a regimen of INH and rifampin given twice weekly is acceptable if administration is directly observed (see Table 3.48, p 488, for doses). **Direct observation means that a health care worker or other responsible, mutually agreed upon individual is present when medications are administered to the patient. If the reliability of self-administration of medications is in doubt, directly observed, twice-weekly therapy administered by a health care professional must be provided.**

Chemotherapy for "Drug-Resistant" Tuberculosis. In the United States and Canada the incidence of drug resistance in previously untreated patients with tuberculosis has been relatively low, but drug resistance is now an increasing problem. For example, in certain areas the incidence of resistance to INH can be as high as 30%. Drug resistance is most common in (1) foreign-born persons from high-risk areas such as Asia, Africa, and Latin America; (2) New York City and several other cities where hospital-based outbreaks of drug-

---

[*]As of December 1993, available from Pfizer Streptomycin Program, Pfizer Pharmaceuticals, New York, NY (800/254-4445).

resistant tuberculosis have been documented; (3) the homeless; (4) those previously treated for tuberculosis; and (5) children with tuberculosis whose adult source case is in one of these groups. For all cases of childhood tuberculosis, the drug susceptibility of the *M tuberculosis* isolate from the adult source case and/or the child should be sought. If the child is at risk for isoniazid resistance, streptomycin* or ethambutol should be added to the initial phase of all chemotherapy regimens until susceptibility results are known. Treatment should always include at least two bactericidal drugs to which the organism is susceptible. Bactericidal drugs include INH, rifampin, streptomycin,* pyrazinamide, and high-dose ethambutol (25 mg/kg/d). In cases of tuberculosis with INH- and/or rifampin-resistant strains, 6-month chemotherapy regimens are not recommended. Twelve to 18 months of therapy is usually necessary to effect a cure. Consultation with an expert in tuberculosis is strongly advised in treating children with drug-resistant disease.

Extrapulmonary Tuberculosis. In general, extrapulmonary tuberculosis, including cervical lymphadenopathy, can be treated with the same regimens as pulmonary tuberculosis. Exceptions may be bone and joint disease, disseminated (miliary) disease, and meningitis, for which current data are inadequate to support a 6-month course of therapy. For these severe forms of drug-susceptible extrapulmonary tuberculosis, daily treatment with INH, rifampin, pyrazinamide, and, usually, streptomycin* for the first 1 or 2 months, followed by INH and rifampin administered daily or twice weekly under direct observation, is recommended for a total of 12 months of therapy. Four drugs are given initially to protect against the possibility of drug resistance and the severe consequences of treatment failure (see Chemotherapy for "Drug-Resistant" Tuberculosis, p 489). Based on personal experience and currently unpublished data, however, some experts recommend a treatment duration of 6 to 9 months for all forms of extrapulmonary tuberculosis.

Pyrazinamide is especially useful in disseminated and meningeal tuberculosis because it achieves better CSF concentrations than either streptomycin or ethambutol. In cases of severe tuberculosis with vomiting or obtundation, INH or rifampin (Rifadin-IV†) can be given intramuscularly or intravenously. The dose is the same as the oral dose.

Tuberculosis and HIV Infection. Adult patients with HIV infection have an increased incidence of tuberculosis. Manifestations in these patients can be unusual and can include extrapulmonary involvement of multiple organs. The clinical manifestations and roentgenographic appearance of tuberculosis in children with HIV infection tend to be similar to those in immunocompetent children. A negative tuberculin test caused by HIV-related immunosuppression can also occur. Specimens for culture should be obtained in all suspected cases in children, since infection with atypical mycobacteria is also common, and results of mycobacterial drug susceptibility testing provide important information for therapeutic decisions. Appropriate specimens include respiratory secretions, gastric aspirates, blood, urine, stool, bone marrow, liver, lymph node, or other tissue as indicated clinically.

---

*As of December 1993, available from Pfizer Streptomycin Program, Pfizer Pharmaceuticals, New York, NY (800/254-4445).
†Available from Marion Merrel Dow, Kansas City, MO.

Most HIV-infected adult patients with drug-susceptible tuberculosis respond well to antituberculosis drugs. However, optimal therapy of tuberculosis in children with HIV infection has not yet been established. Therapy always should include at least 3 drugs initially, and should be continued for a minimum of 9 months. Isoniazid, rifampin, and pyrazinamide with or without ethambutol or an aminoglycoside should be given for at least the first 2 months. A fourth drug may be needed for disseminated disease and whenever drug-resistant disease is suspected. Consultation with an expert who has experience in managing patients with HIV infection is advised.

Testing for HIV should be performed on all children with tuberculous disease with pre- and posttest counseling.

Tuberculosis in Pregnancy and Lactation. Tuberculosis in pregnancy should be managed in concert with an expert in the management of tuberculosis. During pregnancy, if active disease is diagnosed (positive bacteriology, or clinical or roentgenographic findings compatible with presumptive diagnosis), a 9-month regimen of INH and rifampin, supplemented by an initial course of ethambutol if drug resistance is suspected, is recommended. Pyrazinamide is usually not given because of inadequate data about teratogenesis. Hence, a 9-month course of therapy is necessary for drug-susceptible disease. When INH resistance is a possibility, INH, ethambutol, and rifampin are recommended initially. One of these drugs can be discontinued after 1 or 2 months, depending on results of susceptibility tests. If rifampin or INH is discontinued, treatment is continued for a total of 18 months; if ethambutol is discontinued, treatment is continued for a total of 9 months. Prompt initiation of chemotherapy is mandatory to protect both the mother and the fetus. If INH or rifampin resistance is documented, an expert in the management of tuberculosis should be consulted.

Asymptomatic pregnant women with positive tuberculin skin tests and normal chest roentgenograms should receive preventive therapy with INH for 9 months if they are HIV seropositive or have recently been in contact with an infectious person. For these individuals, preventive therapy should begin after the first trimester. In other circumstances in which none of these risk factors is present, although no harmful effects of INH to the fetus have been observed, preventive therapy can be delayed until after delivery.

For all pregnant women receiving INH, pyridoxine should be prescribed. Isoniazid, ethambutol, and rifampin appear to be relatively safe for the fetus. The benefit of ethambutol and rifampin for therapy of active disease in the mother outweighs the risk to the infant. Streptomycin* and pyrazinamide should not be used unless they are essential to control the disease.

Physicians who care for nursing mothers should be aware that INH is secreted in human milk. While potential hepatotoxicity in the infant is a concern, no adverse effects of INH on nursing infants have been demonstrated (see Human Milk, p 76).

Congenital Tuberculosis. Women who have only pulmonary tuberculosis are not likely to infect the fetus until after delivery, and congenital tuberculo-

---

*As of December 1993, available from Pfizer Streptomycin Program, Pfizer Pharmaceuticals, New York, NY (800/254-4445).

sis is extremely rare. In utero infections with tubercle bacilli, however, can occur after maternal bacillemia at different stages in the course of tuberculosis. Miliary tuberculosis can seed the placenta and thereby gain access to the fetal circulation. In women with tuberculous endometritis, transmission of infection can result from fetal aspiration of bacilli at the time of delivery. A third mode of transmission is ingestion of infected amniotic fluid in utero.

If an infant is suspected of having congenital tuberculosis, a Mantoux skin test (5 TU PPD), chest roentgenogram, lumbar puncture, and appropriate cultures should be performed promptly. Regardless of the skin test results, treatment of the infant should be initiated promptly with INH, rifampin, pyrazinamide, and streptomycin* or kanamycin. The mother should be evaluated for the presence of pulmonary or extrapulmonary (including uterine) tuberculosis. If the physical examination or chest roentgenogram support the diagnosis of tuberculosis, the patient should be treated using the same regimen as used for tuberculous meningitis (see Extrapulmonary Tuberculosis, p 490). The drug susceptibilities of the organism recovered from the mother and/or infant should be determined.

Steroids. Adjuvant treatment with corticosteroids in treating tuberculosis is controversial. Corticosteroids have been used for therapy of children with tuberculous meningitis to reduce vasculitis, inflammation, and, as a result, intracranial pressure. Data indicate that dexamethasone may lower mortality and long-term neurologic impairment. The administration of corticosteroids should be considered in all children with tuberculous meningitis and also may be considered in children with pleural and pericardial effusions (to hasten reabsorption of fluid), severe miliary disease (to mitigate alveolocapillary block), and endobronchial disease (to relieve obstruction and atelectasis). Corticosteroids should be given only when accompanied by appropriate antituberculosis therapy. Consultation with an expert in the treatment of tuberculosis should be obtained when steroid therapy is considered.

Evaluation and Monitoring of Therapy in Children and Adolescents. The duration of antituberculosis therapy is based on the patient's clinical and roentgenographic response, smear and culture results, and susceptibility studies of the *M tuberculosis* isolate from the patient or the suspect source case. With directly observed therapy, clinical evaluation is an integral component of each visit for drug administration. Careful monitoring of the clinical and bacteriologic responses to therapy on a monthly basis in sputum-positive patients is important. For bacteriologically confirmed, sputum-negative pulmonary tuberculosis, chest roentgenograms should be obtained after 2 or 3 months of therapy to evaluate response. Even with successful 6-month regimens, hilar adenopathy may require as long as 2 to 3 years for roentgenographic resolution, and a normal roentgenogram is not a necessary criterion to discontinue therapy. Follow-up roentgenograms beyond the termination of successful chemotherapy are usually not necessary except to document resolution of adenopathy or to help evaluate clinical deterioration.

---

*As of December 1993, available from Pfizer Streptomycin Program, Pfizer Pharmaceuticals, New York, NY (800/254-4445).

If therapy has been interrupted, the date for completion of therapy will need to be extended. Although guidelines cannot be provided for every situation, factors to consider in establishing the date for completion include the following: (1) the length of the interruption; (2) the time during therapy (early or late) in which interruption occurred; and (3) the patient's clinical, roentgenographic, and bacteriologic status before, during, and after interruption. Consultation with an expert is advised.

Untoward effects of INH therapy in children are rare. The incidence of hepatitis during INH therapy is so low in otherwise healthy infants, children, and adolescents that routine determination of serum aminotransferase concentrations is not recommended. However, in children with severe tuberculosis, especially meningitis and disseminated disease, liver function tests should be monitored during the first several months of treatment. Other indications for liver function tests include (1) concurrent or recent liver disease; (2) high daily dose of INH (more than 10 mg/kg/d) in combination with rifampin and/or pyrazinamide; (3) pregnancy or within 6 weeks postpartum; (4) clinical evidence of hepatotoxicity; or (5) hepatobiliary tract disease from other causes. In most other circumstances, monthly clinical evaluations for 3 months, followed by evaluation every 1 to 3 months to observe for signs or symptoms of hepatitis or other adverse effects of drug therapy, is an appropriate schedule for follow-up. Alternatively, some experts recommend routine clinical evaluation every 4 to 6 weeks throughout the course of therapy.

In all cases, frequent physician-patient contact to assess drug adherence, efficacy, and toxicity is an important aspect of management. If adherence becomes suspect, directly observed therapy should be instituted.

Immunizations. Patients who are receiving treatment for tuberculosis can be given measles vaccine or other live-virus vaccines as otherwise indicated, unless they are receiving corticosteroids, are severely ill, or have specific vaccine contraindications.

Specific Drugs. Antituberculosis drugs kill or inhibit the multiplication of drug-susceptible tubercle bacilli, thereby arresting the progression of tuberculosis and preventing most complications of early, primary disease. Chemotherapy does not cause rapid disappearance of already caseous or granulomatous lesions (eg, mediastinal lymphadenitis with endobronchial breakthrough). Dosage schedules and possible adverse reactions of major antituberculous drugs are summarized in Tables 3.49 and 3.50 (pp 494 and 495).

Isoniazid is bactericidal, rapidly absorbed, and penetrates well into body fluids, including CSF. It is metabolized in the liver and excreted primarily through the kidneys. The drug is well tolerated by children, who can be given relatively larger doses (according to body surface area or weight) than adults. In children given therapeutic doses, peripheral neuritis or convulsions caused by inhibition of pyridoxine metabolism is rare. The incidence of hepatitis in children and adolescents is low (see Evaluation and Monitoring of Therapy in Children and Adolescents, p 492).

Children receiving INH usually do not need pyridoxine supplements unless they have nutritional deficiencies. Pyridoxine is recommended for children and adolescents on meat- and milk-deficient diets, those with nutritional deficiencies, breast-feeding infants, and women during pregnancy (see Tuberculosis in Pregnancy and Lactation, p 491).

TABLE 3.49—Commonly Used Drugs for the Treatment of
Tuberculosis in Infants, Children, and Adolescents

Drugs	Dosage Forms	Daily Dose (mg/kg/d)	Twice Weekly Dose (mg/kg per dose)	Maximum Dose	Adverse Reactions
Ethambutol	Tablets: 100 mg 400 mg	15–25	50	2.5 g	Optic neuritis (reversible), decreased visual acuity, decreased red-green color discrimination, gastrointestinal disturbance, hypersensitivity
Isoniazid*	Scored tablets: 100 mg 300 mg Syrup: 10 mg/mL	10–15†	20-30	Daily: 300 mg Twice weekly: 900 mg	Mild hepatic enzyme elevation, hepatitis,† peripheral neuritis, hypersensitivity
Pyrazinamide	Scored tablets: 500 mg	20–40	50	2 g	Hepatotoxicity, hyperuricemia
Rifampin*	Capsules: 150 mg 300 mg Syrup: formulated in syrup from capsules	10–20	10–20	600 mg	Orange discoloration of secretions/urine, staining of contact lenses, vomiting, hepatitis, "flu-like" reaction, and thrombocytopenia; may render birth-control pills ineffective
Streptomycin‡ (IM administration)	Vials: 1 g 4 g	20–40	20–40	1 g	Ototoxicity, nephrotoxicity, skin rash

*Rifamate is a capsule containing 150 mg of isoniazid and 300 mg of rifampin. Two capsules provide the usual adult (>50 kg body weight) daily doses of each drug.

†When isoniazid is used in combination with rifampin, the incidence of hepatotoxicity increases if the isoniazid dose exceeds 10 mg/kg/d.

‡As of December 1993, available from Pfizer Streptomycin Program, Pfizer Pharmaceuticals, New York, NY (800/254-4445).

Rifampin is a bactericidal antituberculosis agent. Tubercle bacilli initially resistant to rifampin remain uncommon in most areas of the United States. For infants and young children, the contents of the capsules can be suspended in syrup of wild cherry or sprinkled on applesauce. Rifampin is excreted in bile and urine and can cause orange urine, sweat, and/or tears. It can also cause discoloration of soft contact lenses and render oral contraceptives ineffective. Hepatotoxicity occurs rarely.

Pyrazinamide is bactericidal and attains therapeutic CSF concentrations and in macrophages. In doses of 30 mg/kg/d or less, it is seldom hepatotoxic and is well tolerated by children.

TABLE 3.50—Less Commonly Used Drugs for Treatment of Drug-Resistant Tuberculosis in Infants, Children, and Adolescents*

Drugs	Dosage Forms	Daily Dose (mg/kg/d)	Maximum Dose	Adverse Reactions
Capreomycin	Vials: 1 g	15–30 (IM)	1 g	Ototoxicity, nephrotoxicity
Ciprofloxacin	Tablets: 250 mg 500 mg 750 mg	Adults: 500–1500 mg total per day, given in 2 divided doses	1.5 g	Theoretical effect on growing cartilage, gastrointestinal tract disturbance, rash, headache
Cycloserine	Capsules: 250 mg	10–20	1 g	Psychosis, personality changes, convulsions, rash
Ethionamide	Tablets: 250 mg	15–20, given in 2 or 3 divided doses	1 g	Gastrointestinal disturbance, hepatotoxicity, allergic reactions
Kanamycin	Vials: 75 mg/2 mL 500 mg/2 mL 1 g/3 mL	15–30 (IM)	1 g	Auditory toxicity, nephrotoxicity, vestibular toxicity
Ofloxacin	Tablets: 200 mg 300 mg 400 mg	Adults: 400–800 mg total per day	800 g	Theoretical effect on growing cartilage, gastrointestinal tract disturbance, rash, headache
Para–amino salicylic acid (PAS)	Tablets: 500 mg	200–300, given in 3 or 4 divided doses	10 g	Gastrointestinal tract disturbance, hypersensitivity, hepatotoxicity

*These drugs should be used in consultation with an expert in tuberculosis.

*Streptomycin** is a bactericidal drug. Resistance in tubercle bacilli is relatively common, particularly among immigrants from developing areas such as those in Southeast Asia. Therapeutic CSF concentrations are achieved only in meningitis. Streptomycin is usually prescribed for only 4 to 8 weeks and for no longer than 12 weeks because the incidence of vestibular and cochlear damage correlates with increasing total dose. If streptomycin is not available, kanamycin or capreomycin are alternatives.

Ethambutol is well absorbed, diffuses well, and is excreted in the urine. At 15 mg/kg/d, it is bacteriostatic only and its main role is to prevent emergence of drug-resistant organisms. Because the population of tubercle bacilli is usually smaller in primary tuberculosis than in adult-type tuberculosis, development of secondary resistance during treatment of primary disease is rare. A dose of 25 mg/kg/d is necessary for bactericidal activity and can be used in

*As of December 1993, available from Pfizer Streptomycin Program, Pfizer Pharmaceuticals, New York, NY (800/254-4445).

older children in whom appropriate ophthalmologic evaluation is possible. Since ethambutol can cause reversible optic neuritis, recipients should be monitored monthly for visual acuity, visual fields, and red-green color discrimination. Because cooperation is essential for performance of these tests, use of ethambutol in young children whose visual acuity cannot be monitored requires careful consideration of the risks and benefits.

The less commonly used antituberculosis drugs, their doses, and side effects are listed in Table 3.50 (p 495). Ethionamide is a bacteriostatic antituberculosis drug that is well tolerated by children, achieves therapeutic CSF concentrations, and is useful in drug-resistant cases. Other drugs that previously have had limited usefulness because of minimal effectiveness, toxic properties, or both should be used only after appropriate consultation has been obtained. In cases of drug resistance or if patients cannot tolerate other drugs, cycloserine, kanamycin, and capreomycin may be helpful (see Table 3.50, p 495). Several quinolones (ofloxacin and ciprofloxacin) have antituberculous activity and can be used in special circumstances. Since these compounds are approved by the Food and Drug Administration for use only in individuals 18 years of age and older, their use in younger patients necessitates careful assessment of the potential risks and benefits.

All of the foregoing therapeutic agents can be responsible for major toxic effects. **The cautions listed in the package insert for each drug should be followed.** Consultation with an expert is advised when the conventional antituberculosis regimens are considered.

Of the antituberculosis drugs listed in Tables 3.49 and 3.50 (pp 494 and 495), the only two that are approved by the Food and Drug Administration for use in children are INH and streptomycin.[*] Nevertheless, the Committee supports the appropriate use of other drugs as recommended here.

Management of the Newborn Infant Whose Mother (or Other Household Contact) Has Tuberculosis. Management of a newborn infant whose mother (or other household contact) is suspected of having tuberculosis is based on individual considerations. If possible, separation of the mother (or contact) and infant should be minimized. Differing circumstances and resulting recommendations are as follows:

1. *Mother (or other household contact) with a positive tuberculin skin test reaction and no evidence of current disease.* Investigation of other members of the household or extended family to whom the infant may later be exposed is indicated. If no evidence of current disease is found in the mother or extended family, the infant should be tested with a Mantoux skin test (5 TU PPD) at 3 to 4 months of age. When the family cannot be promptly tested, consideration should be given to administering INH (10 mg/kg/d) to the infant until skin testing and other evaluation of the family has excluded contact with a case of active tuberculosis. The infant does not need to be hospitalized during this time if adequate follow-up can be arranged, but adherence with medication administration should be closely monitored. The mother should also be considered for INH preventive therapy.

---

[*]As of December 1993, available from Pfizer Streptomycin Program, Pfizer Pharmaceuticals, New York, NY (800/254-4445).

2. *Mother with untreated (newly diagnosed) disease or disease that has been treated for 2 or more weeks and who is judged to be noncontagious at delivery.* Careful investigation of household members and extended family is mandatory. A chest roentgenogram and Mantoux tuberculin test should be performed on the infant at 3 to 4 months and at 6 months of age. Separation of the mother and infant is not necessary if adherence with treatment for the mother and infant is assured. The mother can breast-feed. The infant should receive INH even if the tuberculin skin test and chest roentgenogram do not suggest clinical tuberculosis, since cell-mediated immunity of a degree sufficient to mount a significant reaction to tuberculin skin testing may develop as late as age 6 months in an infant infected at birth. Isoniazid can be discontinued if the Mantoux skin test is negative at 3 or 4 months of age, the mother is adherent and has a satisfactory clinical response to treatment, and no other family members have infectious tuberculosis. The infant should be examined carefully at monthly intervals. If nonadherence is documented, the mother has AFB-positive sputum (on smear), and supervision is impossible, the infant should be separated from the ill family member and bacillus Calmette-Guerin (BCG) vaccine may be considered for the infant. However, the response to the vaccine in infants may be delayed and inadequate for prevention of tuberculosis.

3. *Mother has current disease and is suspected to be contagious at the time of delivery.* The mother and infant should be separated until the infant is receiving therapy or the mother is confirmed to be noncontagious. Otherwise, management is the same as when the disease is judged to be noncontagious to the infant at delivery (see #2 in this section).

4. *Mother has hematogenously spread tuberculosis (eg, meningitis, miliary disease, or bone involvement).* The infant should be evaluated for congenital tuberculosis (see Congenital Tuberculosis, p 491). If clinical and roentgenographic findings do not support the diagnosis of congenital tuberculosis, the infant should be separated from the mother until she is judged to be noncontagious. The infant should be given INH until 3 or 4 months of age, at which time the Mantoux skin test should be repeated. If the skin test is positive, INH should be continued for a total of 12 months. If the skin test is negative and the chest roentgenogram is normal, then INH may be discontinued, depending on the status of the mother and whether there are other cases of infectious tuberculosis in the family. The infant should continue to be examined carefully at monthly intervals. Management guidelines are further detailed in #2 in this section.

Isolation of the Hospitalized Patient: Most children with tuberculosis need not be isolated and can be hospitalized on an open ward if they are receiving chemotherapy. Children and adolescents with infectious pulmonary tuberculosis, ie, those whose sputum smears show AFB, should be on AFB (tuberculosis) isolation precautions until effective chemotherapy has been initiated, their sputum smears show a diminishing number of organisms, and their cough is abating.

Family members should be managed with AFB (tuberculosis) isolation precautions when visiting until they are demonstrated not to have infectious tuberculosis.

Control Measures:

Child Care and Schools. Children with tuberculous infection or disease can attend school or child care if they are receiving chemotherapy (see Children in Out-of-Home Child Care, p 81). They can return to regular activities as soon as effective chemotherapy (based on clinical, bacteriologic, and roentgenographic signs) has been instituted, clinical symptoms have disappeared, and an acceptable plan for completing the course of therapy has been developed.

Management of Contacts Including Epidemiologic Investigation. Children younger than 4 years of age with positive tuberculin skin tests or with clinical tuberculous disease should be the starting point for epidemiologic investigation, which is best accomplished with assistance from the local health department. Close contacts of the tuberculin-positive child should be skin tested, and persons with a positive reaction should be investigated for the presence of tuberculosis. Since children with primary tuberculosis are usually not contagious, their contacts are not likely to be infected unless they also have been in contact with the adult source. After the presumptive adult source for the child's disease is identified, other contacts of that person should be skin tested to identify those needing antituberculosis treatment. Chest roentgenograms of tuberculin-positive contacts should be obtained, and treatment for disease or preventive therapy should be started.

Preventive Therapy for Contacts. Persons exposed to a potentially infectious case of tuberculosis, especially persons with impaired immunity, and all household contacts younger than 4 years of age who are exposed to any adult with active tuberculosis should undergo tuberculin skin testing, should have a chest roentgenogram, and should be given INH preventive therapy even if the skin test is negative once clinical disease is excluded. Candidates for preventive therapy if skin test is negative include recent contacts, household contacts, and persons known to be anergic from populations with a high prevalence of tuberculosis (see Prevention of Disease, p 487). Infected persons can have a negative skin test because tuberculin cellular reactivity has not yet developed or because of anergy. If an HIV-infected person is anergic, aggressive contact investigation and attempts to isolate the organism should be undertaken. Preventive therapy may be considered for HIV-infected persons who are tuberculin negative but belong to groups in which the prevalence of tuberculosis infection is high. Persons who are not anergic should be retested 12 weeks after contact has been broken. If the skin test is still negative, INH can be discontinued. If the skin test becomes positive, INH is continued for a total of 9 months.

Care of Exposed Newborn (see p 496).

*Bacillus Calmette-Guerin Vaccine (BCG).** Bacillus Calmette-Guerin vaccines are live attenuated strains of *Mycobacterium bovis* that have been developed from multiple substrains cultured for many years in different labora-

---

*BCG vaccine (Tice strain) in the United States is available from Organon, Inc, West Orange, NJ.

tories. In controlled field trials in humans, efficacy has been shown in some, but not all, trials.

The one vaccine strain currently licensed in the United States* for prevention of tuberculosis is derived from the original strain of *M bovis*, but additional culture passages have occurred since efficacy field trials were last conducted in the United States in 1955. Unfortunately, no satisfactory laboratory test for efficacy is available. Therefore, the efficacy of the current vaccine is unknown.

Indications. The administration of BCG vaccine should be considered only for uninfected children who are at unavoidable risk of exposure and for whom other methods of prevention and control, including INH preventive therapy, have failed or are not feasible. Recommended vaccine recipients include the following: (1) infants and children whose tuberculin skin tests are negative and who live in households with repeated exposure to persistently untreated or ineffectively treated patients with sputum-positive tuberculosis or who are continuously exposed to persons with *M tuberculosis* resistant to INH and rifampin; and (2) infants and children in groups in which an excessive rate of new infections can be demonstrated and the usual surveillance and treatment have failed or are not feasible (eg, in groups without a source of regular health care). Experts should be contacted when considering its use as well as other control strategies.

When the vaccine is given, care should be taken to observe the precautions and directions for administration in the package insert. The freeze-dried vaccine should be reconstituted, protected from exposure to light, refrigerated when not in use, and administered within 8 hours of reconstitution.

Bacillus Calmette-Guerin vaccine may be given to infants from birth to 2 months of age without tuberculin testing, if the infant is known not to have been exposed; thereafter, BCG is given only to children who have negative Mantoux tests. PPD testing should be repeated 2 to 3 months after vaccination, and vaccination should be repeated if the patient is still skin-test negative.

Adverse Reactions. Bacillus Calmette-Guerin vaccine rarely causes serious complications. Side effects occur in 1% to 10% of vaccinated persons and include ulceration at the vaccine site and regional lymphadenitis. Severe complications include severe or prolonged ulceration at the vaccination site, and lupus vulgaris. Rare complications have been osteomyelitis with some vaccine strains, and disseminated, even fatal BCG infection in persons with impaired immunity.

Contraindications. Bacillus Calmette-Guerin should not be given to persons who have burns, skin infections, cellular or combined immunodeficiencies, or symptomatic HIV infection. It should also not be given to persons who are receiving therapy with immunosuppressive agents (including corticosteroids) or are otherwise immunodeficient. In areas of the United States where the risk of tuberculosis is low, BCG should not be given to children with known or suspected asymptomatic HIV infection. In populations in which the risk of tuberculosis is high, however, the World Health Organization has recom-

---

*BCG vaccine (Tice strain) in the United States is available from Organon, Inc, West Orange, NJ.

mended that asymptomatic HIV-infected children receive BCG at birth or shortly thereafter.

Although no untoward effects of BCG on the fetus have been observed, vaccination during pregnancy is not prudent. Malnutrition is not considered a contraindication.

Data about whether INH inhibits multiplication (and therefore effectiveness) of BCG are conflicting. Isoniazid, which has well-documented efficacy, should not be preempted by BCG, which does not have such efficacy.

Reporting of Cases. Reporting of cases of clinical tuberculosis is mandated by law in all states. Physicians should assist in a search for a source case and others infected by the source case. Usually adults or adolescents, such as members of the household (including parents, grandparents, teenage siblings, servants, boarders, baby-sitters, and frequent visitors) or other adults with whom the child has frequent contact are source cases.

Diseases Caused by Nontuberculous Mycobacteria
(Atypical Mycobacteria, Mycobacteria Other Than Tuberculosis)

Clinical Manifestations: Several different syndromes are caused by nontuberculous mycobacteria (NTM). In children, the most common of these syndromes is cervical lymphadenitis. Less common infections are osteomyelitis, cutaneous infection, otitis media, and pulmonary disease. Disseminated infections are almost always associated with severe congenital or acquired immunodeficiency syndromes characterized by defects in cell-mediated immunity, such as AIDS. Characteristic manifestations are fever, sweats, weight loss, and anemia.

Etiology: Of the many species of NTM that have been identified, only a small number account for most of the infections caused by these organisms. The species most frequently encountered in children are *Mycobacterium avium* complex (MAC) (including *M avium* and *Mycobacterium intracellularae*), *Mycobacterium scrofulaceum*, *Mycobacterium kansasii*, and *Mycobacterium marinum* (see Table 3.51, p 501). Infection in patients with HIV infection is caused by MAC. *Mycobacterium fortuitum* and *Mycobacterium chelonei* are frequently referred to as "rapid-growing" mycobacteria because they grow sufficiently in the laboratory to be identified in days, whereas other NTM and *Mycobacterium tuberculosis* take weeks to grow. The *M fortuitum* and *M chelonei* strains have occasionally been implicated in wound, soft-tissue, pulmonary, and middle ear infections. Other mycobacterial species, which are usually not pathogenic, have caused infections in immunocompromised hosts or have been associated with the presence of a foreign body.

TABLE 3.51—Nontuberculous Mycobacterial Species That Most Commonly Cause Disease in Children

Organism	Syndrome
M avium complex (MAC), including Battey bacillus	Lymphadenitis, pulmonary infection, disseminated disease in AIDS and other immunocompromised hosts
M scrofulaceum	Lymphadenitis
M kansasii	Lymphadenitis, pulmonary infection
M marinum	Cutaneous infection ("swimming pool granuloma")
M fortuitum	Lymphadenitis, cutaneous infection
M chelonei	Cutaneous infection, pulmonary infections, otitis media

Epidemiology: Because infections caused by NTM are not reportable in most areas, systematic data concerning their incidence and distribution are fewer than data for infections caused by *M tuberculosis*. In the past, as the incidence of tuberculosis decreased, the relative proportion of mycobacterial infections caused by NTM increased. Since the epidemic of HIV infection, however, the incidence of both tuberculosis and MAC infections has increased.

Many NTM species are ubiquitous and are found in soil, food, water, and animals. Most infections appear to be acquired by aspiration or inoculation of the organisms from these natural sources. Skin testing surveys using purified protein derivative (PPD) antigens derived from various NTM indicate that infections occur worldwide. In the United States, a survey in the 1960s suggested that NTM infection is more common in the southeastern and south central areas, but it occurs in all regions. Although many persons are exposed to NTM, only a few of these exposures lead either to long-term colonization or to overt clinical infection. The MAC colonization of the respiratory tract or gastrointestinal tract is common in persons with HIV infection. The usual portals of entry for NTM infection are believed to be abrasions in the skin (eg, for the cutaneous lesions caused by *M marinum*); the oropharyngeal mucosa (the presumed portal for cervical lymphadenitis); the gastrointestinal or respiratory tract for MAC; and the respiratory tract (including tympanostomy tubes) for otitis media and rare cases of mediastinal adenitis and of endobronchial disease. Most infections remain localized at the portal of entry or in regional lymph nodes. Severe pulmonary disease and dissemination to distal sites occur primarily in immunocompromised hosts, especially in persons with AIDS. No evidence for person-to-person transmission of NTM exists, but appropriate studies, especially in the case of HIV-infected and other immunosuppressed patients, have not been performed. Cases of otitis media caused by *M chelonei* have been associated with use of contaminated equipment and water. A water-borne route of transmission has been incriminated for MAC in immunodeficient hosts.

The **incubation period** is not known.

Diagnostic Tests: Definitive diagnosis of disease caused by NTM requires isolation and identification of the infecting organism. Caution must be exercised in the interpretation of cultures obtained from sites that are not necessarily sterile, such as from gastric washings, a draining sinus tract, or a single urine specimen. Caution in ascribing illness to the isolated NTM is especially warranted if the species cultured is usually nonpathogenic (eg, *Mycobacterium gordonae*) and if only a few colonies are recovered from a single specimen. Repeated isolation of numerous colonies of a single species is more likely to indicate disease than transient colonization. Most reliable for diagnostic purposes is the recovery of NTM from sites that are otherwise sterile, such as cerebrospinal fluid, pleural fluid, bone marrow, blood, lymph node aspirates, middle ear or mastoid aspirates, or surgically excised tissue. Use of the Du Pont Isolator* system has increased the sensitivity of blood cultures.

Patients with NTM infection can have false-positive tuberculin skin tests, since tuberculin preparations (PPD) derived from *M tuberculosis* share a number of antigens with NTM species. These false-positive tests occur in otherwise healthy children who have no history of exposure to *M tuberculosis* but may have been sensitized by exposure to NTM in the environment. Those cross-reactions that usually, but not always, result in Mantoux skin test reactions to PPD measuring less than 10 mm of induration can be more common than "true-positive" tuberculin reactions in populations with a low prevalence of tuberculosis and a high prevalence of NTM infections.

For both clinical and public health reasons, differentiating *M tuberculosis* infection from NTM infections is important. Studies in children have shown that dual Mantoux tests with standard PPD (for *M tuberculosis*) and PPD-Battey are sometimes helpful in distinguishing tuberculous from nontuberculous infections. Skin tests using PPD derived from different NTM species, however, are not commercially available.

A large reaction (15 mm or greater) to a standard (5 TU PPD) intradermal tuberculin skin test is more indicative of infection with *M tuberculosis*; a reaction of less than 10 mm suggests NTM infection in the patient with cervical adenitis or other syndromes consistent with NTM disease, a normal chest roentgenogram, nonreactive PPD tests in other family members, and no likely exposure to a case of infectious tuberculosis. The identification of family members with positive tuberculin reactions increases the likelihood of *M tuberculosis* infection in the index case. Negative results on tuberculin testing, chest roentgenogram, and investigation of contacts is consistent with possible NTM infection.

Disseminated MAC disease should prompt a search for an underlying predisposing factor, usually HIV infection. Tests of immune function and a search for other opportunistic pathogens (eg, *Pneumocystis carinii*) are indicated. Patients with disseminated MAC disease should be evaluated for HIV infection.

---

*Available from Du Pont, Wilmington, DE

Treatment: Many NTM are relatively resistant in vitro to antituberculosis drugs. In vitro resistance, however, does not necessarily correlate with clinical response. No controlled therapeutic trials have been performed in NTM infections. The approach to therapy should consider the following factors: (1) the species causing the infection, (2) the results of drug susceptibility testing, (3) the site(s) of infection, (4) the nature of the patient's underlying disease (if any), and (5) the frequent need to treat a patient presumptively for tuberculosis while awaiting culture reports that subsequently reveal NTM infection.

For the common problem of NTM lymphadenitis in otherwise healthy children, especially when the disease is caused by M scrofulaceum or MAC, chemotherapy usually offers little benefit, and surgical excision alone is frequently the most effective treatment.

Cutaneous infections with M marinum can require a combination of medical and surgical debridement. Minocycline has been successfully used for M marinum sporotrichoid skin infections; other tetracyclines can also be given. Tetracyclines, however, should not be given to children younger than 9 years of age unless the benefits of therapy are greater than the risks of dental staining. The combination of rifampin and ethambutol, or trimethoprim-sulfamethoxazole may also be effective.

Infections caused by M kansasii usually respond well to treatment with rifampin, ethambutol, and isoniazid, although the organism may be resistant in vitro to one or more of these agents.

Multidrug therapy is indicated in patients with AIDS and in other immunocompromised persons with disseminated MAC infection. Clinical isolates of MAC are usually resistant to most of the approved antituberculosis drugs. A 1992 United States Public Health Service Task Force concluded that although studies have not yet identified an optimal regimen or confirmed that any regimen produces sustained benefit for AIDS patients with disseminated MAC infection, the available information justifies treatment.* The following was recommended by the Task Force:

- Treatment regimens, except in clinical trials, should include at least two drugs.
- Every regimen should contain either azithromycin or clarithromycin; many experts prefer ethambutol as a second drug. Many clinicians have added one or more of the following as second, third, or fourth agents: clofazimine, rifabutin, rifampin, ciprofloxacin, and, in some situations, amikacin.
- Therapy should continue for the lifetime of the patient if clinical and microbiologic improvement is observed.
- Patients receiving therapy should be monitored as follows:
  - Clinical manifestations of disseminated MAC, such as fever, weight loss, and night sweats, should be monitored several times during the initial weeks of therapy. Microbiologic response, as assessed by blood culture every 4 weeks during initial therapy, can also be helpful in interpreting the efficacy of a therapeutic regimen.

---

*Centers for Disease Control and Prevention. Recommendations on prophylaxis and therapy for disseminated Mycobacterium avium complex for adults and adolescents infected with human immunodeficiency virus. MMWR. 1993;42(RR-9):17-20

- Most patients who ultimately respond show substantial clinical improvement in the first 4 to 6 weeks of therapy. Elimination of the organisms from blood cultures may take somewhat longer, often requiring 4 to 12 weeks.

The Task Force also recommended that patients with HIV infection and CD4 T-lymphocyte counts of less than 100/mm³ should receive lifetime prophylaxis with oral rifabutin (adult dose, 300 mg daily). This conclusion was based on two controlled trials that demonstrated that rifabutin reduced the frequency of MAC bacteremia by approximately 50%. These recommendations on therapy and prophylaxis were considered appropriate for both children and adults, but in young children an adjustment for age is necessary in interpreting T-lymphocyte counts (see HIV Infections and AIDS, p 261).

Ciprofloxacin is active in vitro against *M fortuitum* and, to a lesser extent, against MAC, and may have a role in treating some patients with infections caused by these organisms. Fluoroquinolones, however, should not be given to individuals younger than 18 years of age except in circumstances in which no other drug is available and the benefits of therapy are greater than the risks, such as children with AIDS who have disseminated infection.

Isolates of rapid-growing mycobacteria (*M fortuitum*, *M chelonei*) should be tested in vitro against antituberculous agents, as well as against other drugs (such as amikacin, imipenem, cefoxitin, ciprofloxacin, erythromycin, and doxycycline) to which they frequently are susceptible and which have been used with some clinical success. Details regarding choice of drugs, dosages, and duration should be reviewed with a consultant experienced in the management of these infections.

Additional information concerning treatment of NTM infections can be obtained from the Division of Tuberculosis Control, Centers for Disease Control and Prevention (see Directory of Telephone Numbers, p 601).

Isolation of the Hospitalized Patient: No special precautions are recommended.

Control Measures: No control measures are known, other than chemoprophylaxis in certain patients with HIV infection (see Treatment, p 503) and use of sterile equipment for middle ear instrumentation, including otoscopic equipment for prevention of *M chelonei* otitis media. No specific management of exposed persons is necessary.

Tularemia

Clinical Manifestations: Tularemia is usually characterized by high fever and severe, influenza-like constitutional symptoms of chills, myalgia, and, in older children, headache. However, clinically mild tularemia has been recognized increasingly. Onset is frequently abrupt and conforms to one of the specific tularemic syndromes. The ulceroglandular syndrome, the most common, is characterized by (1) a primary, painful maculopapular lesion at the portal of entry, with subsequent ulceration and slow healing; and (2) painful, acutely inflamed lymph nodes, which may drain spontaneously. Other disease syndromes are the following: oculoglandular (severe conjunctivitis and lymph node involvement), oropharyngeal (severe exudative pharyngitis), glandular (wherein no skin or mucous membrane lesion is present), typhoidal (high fever, hepatomegaly, and splenomegaly), and pneumonia.

Etiology: *Francisella tularensis*, the causative agent, is a small, Gram-negative coccobacillus.

Epidemiology: Sources of the organism include approximately 100 species of wild mammals (eg, rabbits, hares, muskrats, squirrels, and deer); at least nine species of domestic animals (eg, sheep, cattle, and cats); blood-sucking arthropods that bite these animals (eg, ticks, deerflies, and mosquitoes); and water contaminated by infected animals. In the United States, major reservoirs include rabbits and ticks. Ticks are the most important vectors. Infected animals and arthropods are infective for prolonged periods: frozen, killed rabbits can remain infective for more than 3 years. Persons at risk are those with direct occupational or indirect recreational exposure to infected animals or their habitat, such as rabbit hunters and trappers, those with tick or insect bites, and laboratory technicians working with *F tularensis* (which is highly infectious). Transmission is by bites of infected arthropods, direct contact with infected animals, ingestion of contaminated water or inadequately cooked meat, or inhalation of contaminated particles. Person-to-person transmission has not been documented. Organisms may be found in the blood during the first 2 weeks of the disease and in lesions for up to 1 month if untreated.

The **incubation period** ranges from 1 to 21 days; most cases occur 3 to 5 days after exposure.

Diagnostic Tests: A fourfold or greater rise in the serum *F tularensis* agglutinin titer is frequently evident after the second week of illness and is considered diagnostic. A single convalescent titer of 1:160 or greater is consistent with recent or past infection. Tube titers are more reliable than slide tests; nonspecific cross-agglutination with *Brucella*, *Proteus*, and heterophile antibodies can cause false-positive antibody titers to *F tularensis*. Cultures of blood, skin, ulcers, lymph node drainage, gastric washings, and respiratory secretions require special media or guinea pig inoculation. However, some commercial supplemented chocolate agar can support growth of *F tularensis*. Therefore, the laboratory should be informed that *F tularensis* is suspected, since the risk of infection in laboratory personnel is a potential hazard when cultures are performed. The indirect fluorescent anti- body test for ulcer exudate or aspirate can be useful but is not generally available.

Treatment: For many years, streptomycin* was the recommended drug of choice for treatment of tularemia. However, treatment with gentamicin

---

*As of December 1993, available from Pfizer Streptomycin Program, Pfizer Pharmaceuticals, New York, NY (800/254-4445).

appears to be equally effective and its advantage is that tests are readily available to monitor drug concentrations during therapy. With either drug, the duration of therapy is usually 6 to 10 days; the longer course is given for more severe illness.

The alternative drugs include tetracycline (which ordinarily should not be given to children younger than 9 years of age or to pregnant women) and chloramphenicol. Both of these compounds are more likely to result in clinical relapses.

Isolation of the Hospitalized Patient: Drainage/secretion precautions should be used until the lesions stop draining. Respiratory isolation should be considered for patients with pneumonic tularemia.

Control Measures:
- Persons at risk should minimize opportunities for insect bites by wearing protective clothing, by frequent inspection and removal of ticks from the skin and scalp, and by using insect repellents (see Control Measures for Prevention of Tick-Borne Infections, p 114).
- Children should be discouraged from handling sick or dead rabbits and rodents.
- Rubber gloves should be worn by hunters or trappers when handling the carcasses of wild rabbits and other potentially infected animals.
- Game meats should be thoroughly cooked.
- Face masks and rubber gloves should be worn by those working with cultures or infective material in the laboratory.
- Drainage/secretion precautions should be used for handling contaminated articles.
- Interstate or interarea shipment of infected animals should be prohibited.
- A live attenuated vaccine (available through the Centers for Disease Control and Prevention) is recommended for those repeatedly exposed to the organism, such as laboratory research technicians.

Endemic Typhus
(Murine Typhus)

Clinical Manifestations: Endemic typhus resembles epidemic typhus but is usually milder, has a less acute onset, and has less severe systemic symptoms. In young children, the disease is mild. Fever can be accompanied by persistent headache and myalgias. The rash is typically macular or maculopapular, appears during days 3 to 5 of illness, lasts 4 to 8 days, and tends to remain discrete, with sparse lesions and no hemorrhage. The disease seldom lasts longer than 2 weeks, and visceral involvement usually does not occur. The disease is rarely fatal.

Etiology: Endemic typhus is caused by *Rickettsia typhi* (formerly *Rickettsia mooseri*), an organism antigenically similar to *Rickettsia prowazekii*.

Epidemiology: Rats, in which infection is inapparent, are the natural hosts. Opossums can also be infected and serve as a reservoir. The vector for transmission to rats and, occasionally and accidentally, to humans is the rat flea (usually *Xenopsylla cheopis*). The disease is worldwide in distribution, affects all races, tends to occur more commonly in adults and in males, and is most common from April to October. The disease occurs infrequently in the United States; most cases occur in focal areas in southern California, the southeastern Gulf Coast and southern border states, and Hawaii. Exposure to rats and their fleas is the major risk factor, although a history of such exposure is frequently absent in infected patients.

The **incubation period** is 6 to 14 days.

Diagnostic Tests: Serum agglutinins against *Proteus* OX-19 peak 2 to 3 weeks after the onset of disease, but these tests lack sensitivity and specificity. Indirect fluorescent antibody, latex agglutination, or complement fixation antibody concentrations peak at a similar or slightly later time. A fourfold titer change between acute and convalescent serum specimens is diagnostic but can also occur in patients with epidemic typhus. Serologic differentiation between these diseases is possible but not routinely done. Isolation of the organism in culture is possible but is not routinely attempted because it is hazardous and requires specialized facilities and experienced personnel.

Treatment: A single dose of doxycycline (5 mg/kg; maximum 200 mg) is the treatment of choice. Although doxycycline generally should not be given to children younger than 9 years, the risk of dental staining from a single dose of doxycycline is minimal. Other tetracyclines and chloramphenicol are also effective drugs.

Isolation of the Hospitalized Patient: No special precautions are recommended.

Control Measures: Rat fleas should be controlled by appropriate insecticides, preferably before the use of rodenticides, because the flea will seek alternate hosts when rats are not available. Rat populations should then be controlled by appropriate means. A vaccine is no longer available in the United States. No treatment is recommended for exposed persons. The disease should be reported to public health departments.

Epidemic Typhus
(Louse-Borne Typhus)

Clinical Manifestations: In epidemic typhus, the onset of high fever, chills, and diffuse aching, accompanied by severe headache and malaise, is usually abrupt. Influenza-like illness is frequently suspected. The rash appears 4 to 7 days later, beginning on the trunk and spreading to the limbs. A concentrated eruption is present in the axillae. The rash is maculopapular, becomes petechial or hemorrhagic, then develops into brownish, pigmented areas. The face, palms, and soles are usually not affected. Mental changes are common, and delirium or coma can occur. Myocardial and renal failure occur when the disease is severe. Illness varies from moderately severe to fatal (10% to 40% mortality rate). When untreated, it typically lasts 2 weeks and ends by lysis of fever and subsidence of symptoms. In untreated cases, mortality is uncommon in children, ranges from 10% to 40% in adults, and increases with increasing age. Brill-Zinsser disease is a relapse of louse-borne typhus that occurs years after the initial episode. Stress or an unknown factor serves to reactivate the rickettsiae. The recrudescent illness is similar to the primary infection but generally is milder and of shorter duration.

Etiology: *Rickettsia prowazekii* is the cause.

Epidemiology: Humans are the major source of the organism, which is transmitted from person to person by the body louse, *Pediculus humanus* subspecies *corporis*. All ages and races and both sexes are affected. Poverty, crowding, poor sanitary conditions, lack of bathing, and poor personal hygiene contribute to the spread of lice, and, hence, the disease. Currently, cases of typhus are rarely reported but have occurred throughout the world, including Asia, Africa, some parts of Europe, and Central and South America. Typhus is common during the winter when conditions favor person-to-person transmission of the vector, the body louse. Rickettsiae are present in the blood and tissues of patients during the early febrile phase but not in secretions. Direct person-to-person spread of the disease does not occur in the absence of the vector. Cases in humans have been associated with contact with infected flying squirrels in the United States, their nests, or their ectoparasites. Squirrel-related disease appears to be a milder illness than louse-borne epidemic typhus.

The **incubation period** is 1 to 2 weeks.

Diagnostic Tests: *Rickettsia prowazekii* can be isolated from blood by inoculation into guinea pigs and mice or the yolk sac of embryonated hens' eggs, but because isolation is dangerous, it is rarely attempted. Serum agglutinins against *Proteus* OX-19 reach peak titers 2 to 3 weeks after the onset of disease, but an indirect fluorescent antibody or complement fixation antibody test is preferred. A fourfold change in antibody titer between acute and convalescent serum specimens is diagnostic of either epidemic or endemic typhus (see Endemic Typhus, p 507). An antibody absorption test can often differentiate the two diseases but is not routinely available.

Treatment: Tetracycline or chloramphenicol, given intravenously or orally, is the treatment of choice for louse-borne typhus. Therapy is given until the patient is afebrile for at least 7 days; the usual duration is 7 to 10 days. Tetracycline drugs are usually contraindicated for children younger than 9 years of age unless the benefits are clearly greater than the risks of dental staining. Cream and gel pediculocides containing pyrethrins (0.16% to 0.33%) and piperonyl butoxide (2% to 4%), crotamiton (10%), or lindane (1%) can be used for delousing. Convulsions have been reported in children receiving excessive doses of topical lindane.

Isolation of the Hospitalized Patient: No special precautions are recommended.

Control Measures: Thorough delousing in epidemic situations, particularly among exposed contacts of cases, is recommended. Several applications may be needed because the lice eggs are resistant to most insecticides. Washing clothes in hot water kills lice and eggs. During epidemics, insecticides dusted onto the clothes of louse-infested populations are effective in louse control efforts. In some circumstances, preventing flying squirrels from living in human dwellings by sealing their access ports is recommended. A vaccine is no longer available in the United States. Cases should be reported to public health departments.

Ureaplasma urealyticum Infections

Clinical Manifestations: The most common syndrome associated with *Ureaplasma urealyticum* is nongonococcal urethritis (NGU). The etiology of NGU remains uncertain but *U urealyticum* has been more frequently isolated from patients with NGU than from appropriate controls in several well-designed studies. Without treatment, the disease continues for 1 to 3 months.

Ureaplasma urealyticum has been isolated from nasopharyngeal secretions and endotracheal aspirates of infants 3 months or younger with pneumonia. It may be a cause of lower respiratory tract disease in neonates and young infants. In women, *U urealyticum* has been isolated in pure culture from Bartholin gland abscesses, tubo-ovarian and pelvic abscesses, and salpingitis. Whether *U urealyticum* is associated with low birth weight or neonatal central nervous system infections is uncertain. A recent multicenter US study failed to demonstrate any relation to low birth weight.

Etiology: Ureaplasmas and the Mycoplasmas form the family *Mycoplasmataciae*. The genus *Ureaplasma* contains a single species, *U urealyticum*, which includes at least 16 serotypes.

Epidemiology: The principal reservoir of the human *U urealyticum* is the genital tract of sexually active adults. Colonization is found in approximately one half of sexually active adults, can be prolonged, but is rare in prepubertal children and in those not sexually active.

Transmission during delivery is likely from an asymptomatic infected mother to her newborn. *Ureaplasma urealyticum* may colonize the throat, eyes, umbilicus, and perineum of newborns. *Ureaplasma urealyticum* has been isolated from the lower airways and lung biopsies of preterm infants with pneumonia and chronic lung disease.

The **incubation period** of NGU after sexual transmission is 10 to 20 days.

Diagnostic Tests: The *U urealyticum* organism can be cultured in urea-containing broth. However, most experts regard cultures as having limited utility except in research. Because carriage of *U urealyticum* is common in sexually active people, its presence on culture does not identify acute infection. No rapid diagnostic tests are currently available.

Treatment: For older children, adolescents, and adults, tetracycline is the drug of choice. Erythromycin is the preferred antimicrobial agent for children younger than 9 years of age and in men with urethritis caused by tetracycline-resistant strains. However, efficacy studies have been performed only in adult patients with NGU, and definitive evidence of the efficacy of these antibiotics in infants and children is lacking.

Isolation of the Hospitalized Patient: No special precautions are recommended.

Control Measures: Partners of infected sexually active persons may be contacted so they may be offered treatment.

Varicella-Zoster Infections

Clinical Manifestations: Primary infection with varicella-zoster virus (VZV) results in chickenpox. Chickenpox is manifest by a generalized, pruritic, vesicular rash, with mild fever and mild systemic symptoms. A variety of complications can occur, including bacterial superinfection, thrombocytopenia, arthritis, hepatitis, encephalitis or meningitis, and glomerulonephritis. Reye syndrome can also follow some cases of chickenpox. In immunocompromised children, progressive varicella characterized by continuing eruption of lesions and a high fever into the second week of the illness can occur. Encephalitis, pancreatitis, hepatitis, or pneumonia can develop. Chickenpox is often more severe in immunocompromised patients and in adults. Pneumonia, although rare in normal children, is the most common complication in older individuals. Children with AIDS can develop chronic chickenpox with new lesions appearing during a period of months.

The virus persists in a latent form after the primary infection. Reactivation results in herpes zoster ("shingles"). Grouped vesicular lesions appear in the distribution of one to three sensory dermatomes, sometimes accompanied by pain localized to the area. Systemic symptoms are few. Zoster occasionally can become generalized in immunocompromised patients, with lesions appearing outside the primary dermatomes and with visceral complications.

Fetal infection after maternal varicella in the first or early second trimester of pregnancy occasionally results in varicella embryopathy, which is characterized by limb atrophy and scarring of the skin of the extremity (the congenital varicella syndrome). Central nervous system and eye manifestations can also occur. Children who were exposed to VZV in utero can develop inapparent varicella and subsequent zoster early in life without having had extrauterine varicella. Severe varicella of the newborn infant with fatality rates as high as 30% can result when an infant's mother develops varicella from 5 days before to 2 days after delivery.

Etiology: Varicella-zoster virus is a herpesvirus.

Epidemiology: Humans are the only source of infection for this highly contagious virus. Person-to-person transmission occurs primarily by direct contact with patients with varicella or zoster, occasionally by airborne spread from respiratory secretions, and, rarely, from zoster lesions. In utero infection can also occur. Introduction of a VZV infection into a household usually results in infection of nearly all susceptible persons. Children who acquire their infection at home (secondary family cases) generally have more severe disease than that in the index case. Nosocomial transmission is well documented in pediatric units, but transmission is extremely rare in newborn nurseries.

At present, most reported cases of chickenpox occur in children younger than 10 years of age, but varicella in adolescents and young adults may be becoming more common. Immunity is generally lifelong. Symptomatic reinfection is rare in healthy persons, although asymptomatic reinfection does occur. Varicella is most common during the late winter and early spring. Asymptomatic primary infection is unusual.

Immunocompromised individuals with either primary (varicella) or recurrent (zoster) infection are at increased risk of severe disease. Other groups of pediatric patients who may experience unusually severe disease or a higher rate of complications include children in the first year of life, adolescents, pregnant adolescents, and patients receiving systemic corticosteroids. Varicella may be more severe or result in increased complications in those with chronic cutaneous or pulmonary disorders or those receiving chronic salicylate therapy (which can result in an increased risk for Reye syndrome). The composite risk of the congenital varicella syndrome after infection of the mother during the first trimester of pregnancy in five studies was 2%. Congenital varicella can also occur if infection of the mother occurs early in the second trimester.

Patients are most contagious for 1 to 2 days before and shortly after the onset of the rash. Contagiousness, however, can be for as long as 5 days after the onset of lesions, and in immunocompromised patients with progressive varicella, it probably lasts throughout the period of eruption of new lesions.

The **incubation period** is usually 14 to 16 days; some cases occur as early as 10 or as late as 21 days after contact. It may be short in immunocompromised patients, and it may be prolonged (for as long as 28 days) in recipients of Varicella-Zoster Immune Globulin (VZIG). Varicella in infants born to mothers with active varicella can develop between 1 and 16 days of life; the usual interval from onset of rash in the mother to onset in the neonate is 9 to 15 days.

Diagnostic Tests: Varicella-zoster virus can be isolated from vesicular lesions of otherwise healthy patients during the first 3 to 4 days of the eruption. Diagnosis can be accomplished by immunofluorescent staining of vesicular scrapings, using commercially available monoclonal antibodies that will distinguish between VZV and herpes simplex virus. The demonstration of multinucleated giant cells containing intranuclear inclusions in lesions (Tzanck smear) is less accurate than the immunofluorescent staining technique. Infection can be confirmed by testing acute- and convalescent-phase sera for VZV antibody. Serologic tests include enzyme immunoassay (EIA), latex agglutination (LA) or indirect fluorescent antibody (IFA), and fluorescent antibody-to-membrane antigen (FAMA) assays. These tests are reliable in determining immune status in healthy hosts but are not necessarily reliable in immunocompromised persons (see Care of Exposed Persons, p 514). The complement-fixation test is not sufficiently sensitive to be reliable in determining susceptibility in either case.

Treatment: Both intravenous acyclovir and vidarabine are effective in treating varicella or zoster in immunocompromised patients. However, acyclovir is less toxic, more effective, and the usual drug of choice. Therapy initiated early in the course of the illness maximizes efficacy. Although VZIG given shortly after exposure can prevent or modify the course of disease, VZIG is not effective in therapy once disease is established (see Care of Exposed Persons, p 514).

Oral acyclovir given to otherwise healthy children with varicella within 24 hours of the onset of rash results in a modest decrease in the duration and magnitude of fever and in the number and duration of skin lesions. However, therapy with oral acyclovir is not recommended routinely for treatment of uncomplicated varicella in the otherwise healthy child. This recommendation is based on the marginal therapeutic effect, cost of the drug, difficulty in initiating the drug in the first 24 hours of illness, and potential unforeseen dangers of treating large numbers of children who are at low risk of developing complications. Oral acyclovir should be considered for otherwise healthy persons at increased risk of moderate to severe varicella, such as those older than 12 years, those with chronic cutaneous or pulmonary disorders, those receiving chronic salicylate therapy, and persons receiving short or intermittent courses of corticosteroids, or aerosolized corticosteroids. For recommendations on dosage and duration of therapy, see Antiviral Drugs (p 567). Some experts would also consider use of oral acyclovir in secondary household cases in whom the disease is usually more severe. These recommendations do not necessarily apply to infants (children younger than 12 months of age), since data are insufficient regarding the safety or efficacy of acyclovir therapy for infants.

Oral acyclovir is not recommended in the pregnant adolescent or adult with uncomplicated varicella, since the risks and benefits to the fetus and mother are mostly unknown. Intravenous acyclovir should be considered for the pregnant patient with serious complications of varicella. Oral acyclovir usually should not be used to treat immunocompromised children with varicella. However, some experts have used oral acyclovir in highly selected, immunocompromised patients perceived to be at lower risk of developing severe varicella and in whom careful follow-up is assured. Acyclovir should not be used in exposed persons in an attempt to prevent varicella (see Care of Exposed Persons, p 514).

Children with varicella should not receive salicylates because adminis- tration of salicylates to such children increases the risk of subsequent Reye syndrome. Acetaminophen may be used for control of fever.

Isolation of the Hospitalized Patient: Strict isolation is indicated for patients with varicella for a minimum of 5 days after the onset of the rash and for the duration of the vesicular eruption, which in immunocompromised patients can be a week or longer. Patients should be placed in negative pres- sure rooms, if available. Exposed, susceptible patients should be in strict iso- lation from 8 until 21 days after the onset of the rash in the index patient. Those who received VZIG should be kept in isolation until 28 days after exposure.

Neonates born to mothers with active varicella should be placed in isola- tion at birth and, if still hospitalized, until 21 or 28 days of age, depending on whether they received VZIG. Infants with varicella embryopathy do not require isolation.

Immunocompromised patients who have zoster (localized or disseminated) and normal patients with disseminated zoster should remain in strict isolation for the duration of the illness. For normal patients with localized zoster, drainage/secretion precautions are indicated until all lesions are crusted.

Control Measures:

Hospital Exposure. If an inadvertent exposure in the hospital by an infected patient, health care worker, or visitor occurs, the following control measures should be employed:

- Those personnel and patients who have been exposed (see Table 3.52, p 514) and are susceptible to varicella should be identified.
- Varicella-Zoster Immune Globulin should be administered to appropriate candidates (see Table 3.53, p 515).
- All exposed, susceptible patients should be discharged as soon as possible.
- All exposed, susceptible patients who cannot be discharged should be placed in strict isolation from day 8 to day 21 after the onset of the rash in the index patient. For those who have received VZIG, strict isolation should be continued until day 28.
- All susceptible, exposed staff should be either furloughed or excused from patient contact from day 8 to day 21 after the onset of the rash in the index case. For those who have received VZIG or are immunocompromised, this interval should be until day 28.

Child Care and School. Children with uncomplicated chickenpox who have been excluded from school or child care may return on the sixth day after the onset of the rash. In mild cases with only a few lesions and rapid res- olution, children may return sooner if all lesions are crusted. Immunocom- promised and other children with a prolonged course should be excluded for the duration of the vesicular eruption.

Exclusion of children with zoster whose lesions cannot be covered is based on similar criteria. Those who are excluded may return after the lesions have

TABLE 3.52—Types of Exposure to Varicella or Zoster for Which VZIG Is Indicated*,†

• Household: Residing in the same household.

• Playmate: Face-to-face‡ indoor play.

• Hospital:
  Varicella:

  a) In same 2- to 4-bed room, or adjacent beds in a large ward,

  b) Face-to-face‡ contact with an infectious staff member or patient, or

  c) Visit by a person deemed contagious.

  Zoster: Intimate contact (eg, touching or hugging) with a person deemed contagious.

• Newborn infant: Onset of varicella in the mother 5 days or less before delivery or within 48 h after delivery. VZIG is not indicated if the mother has zoster.

---

*Patients should meet criteria of both significant exposure and candidacy for receiving VZIG, as given in Table 3.53 (p 515).

†VZIG should be administered within 96 h (preferably sooner) after exposure.

‡Experts differ in the duration of face-to-face contact that warrants the administration of VZIG. However, the contact should be nontransient. Some experts suggest a contact of 5 or more min as constituting significant exposure for this purpose; others define close contact as more than 1 h.

crusted. Lesions that are covered appear to pose little risk to susceptible individuals. Older children and staff members with zoster should be instructed to wash their hands if they touch potentially infectious lesions.

Care of Exposed Persons.

Chemoprophylaxis. Oral acyclovir is not recommended. Prophylactic use to prevent acquisition of infection by a contact has not been adequately studied and could result in an alteration of the incubation period and/or of the immune response to VZV infection.

Passive Immunoprophylaxis. Susceptible individuals at high risk of developing severe varicella should be given VZIG, which is a licensed product and can be obtained by calling the local office of the American Red Cross Blood Services.

The decision of whether to administer VZIG depends on the following three factors: (1) the likelihood that an individual will develop complications of varicella if infected; (2) the probability that a given exposure to varicella or zoster will result in infection; and (3) the likelihood that the exposed person is susceptible to varicella.

Household exposure to varicella poses an almost certain risk of infection; other types of exposure are less likely to result in infection. Exposure more than 5 days after the appearance of the first lesion in healthy patients poses a relatively low risk. Persons with a history of varicella are usually considered immune. However, persons without such a history may also be immune. In deciding whether a person with a negative history of varicella is likely to be

TABLE 3.53—Candidates for VZIG, Provided Significant Exposure* Has Occurred

---

Immunocompromised children without history of chickenpox.†

Susceptible, pregnant women.

Newborn infant whose mother had onset of chickenpox within the 5 d before delivery or within the 48 h after delivery.

Hospitalized premature infant (≥28 wk gestation) whose mother has no history of chickenpox.

Hospitalized premature infants (<28 wk gestation or ≤1,000 g), regardless of maternal history.

---

*See text and Table 3.52 (p 514) for additional discussion.
†Immunocompromised adolescents and adults are likely to be immune, but if susceptible, they should also receive VZIG.

susceptible, careful questioning about (1) history of varicella in other siblings (particularly younger siblings), (2) whether the patient attended an urban school, (3) previous exposure to patients with chickenpox or zoster, and (4) other clues can be helpful.

In healthy persons, serologic testing to determine immune status is reliable. However, in immunocompromised patients, the use of serologic tests to determine immune status is not necessarily reliable. Children with malignancies receiving immunosuppressive therapy who have low concentrations of serum VZV antibodies (detectable by sensitive assays) at the time of exposure, and children with a negative history of disease have contracted varicella. Many of these patients may have had passively acquired antibodies from recent transfusions of blood or blood products. Hence, a carefully obtained history of chickenpox should be the primary consideration in the determination of VZV immunity in immunocompromised patients. Administration of VZIG to exposed immunocompromised children with no history of varicella is usually advisable.

Patients receiving monthly treatments of high-dose intravenous immunoglobulin (IGIV, 100 to 400 mg/kg) are likely to be protected and probably do not require VZIG if the last dose of IGIV was given in the 3 weeks before exposure.

Administration and Dose. VZIG is given by intramuscular injection. It contains between 10% and 18% globulin; thimerosal 1:10,000 is included as a preservative. One complete vial (approximate volume, 1.25 mL) containing 125 U is given for each 10 kg of body weight (and is the minimum dose). The maximum suggested dose is 625 U (ie, five vials). For maximal effectiveness, VZIG should be given within 48 hours of, and not more than 96 hours after, exposure.

Use of VZIG in patients with a bleeding diathesis should be avoided, as with other intramuscular injections, if possible. VZIG should never be given intravenously. Local discomfort after intramuscular injection, the most frequent adverse effect, is common.

Indications. The following susceptible persons should receive VZIG (see also Tables 3.52 and 3.53, pp 514 and 515):

- *Immunocompromised individuals* should receive VZIG if they (1) have had a household exposure, (2) shared a hospital room containing four or fewer beds or adjacent beds in a large ward, (3) had a face-to-face contact with an infectious staff member or patient while an inpatient (see Table 3.52, p 514), or (4) played indoors with children who are contagious for chickenpox. Exposed immunocompromised older adolescents and adults known to be susceptible should also receive VZIG. Older adolescents and adults who are immunocompromised, while likely to be immune, should also receive VZIG, if susceptible. Hospitalized patients who have been exposed should be discharged before the eighth day after exposure, if possible. If not possible, they should be placed in strict isolation.

- *Varicella-susceptible pregnant women* may be at higher risk for serious complications than adults in general. Hence, VZIG is indicated for these women after exposure. A major concern is the risk to the fetus of the congenital varicella syndrome when a woman develops varicella-zoster infection, especially during the first half of pregnancy, but whether the fetus will be protected against the development of malformations if VZIG is given to a pregnant, susceptible woman after exposure is unknown. VZIG could conceivably result in asymptomatic maternal infection, but not protect the fetus. Antibody administered to a pregnant woman in the 5 days before delivery is unlikely to be absorbed and transported across the placenta in sufficient quantities to appreciably protect the infant. Therefore, administration of VZIG to the newborn infant is recommended.

- *Newborns*. VZIG (125 U) should be given as soon as possible after delivery to infants whose mothers have had onset of varicella from 5 days before to 2 days after delivery. Approximately one half of these infants can be expected to develop varicella even if VZIG is given, but the disease is often modified. Nevertheless, VZIG recipients should be followed closely.

  For healthy, full-term infants exposed postnatally to varicella, including those whose mothers' rash developed more than 48 hours after delivery, VZIG is not indicated because infants who develop varicella under these conditions are not known to be at any greater risk for complications of chickenpox than older children.

  Although nosocomial transmission of varicella in newborn nurseries is extremely rare, VZIG (125 U) is indicated for some hospitalized, preterm infants because of the poor transfer of antibody across the placenta early in pregnancy. These infants include (1) those born before 28 weeks of gestation (and/or who weigh less than 1,000 g) who still require hospitalization for treatment of prematurity or related conditions and are exposed to varicella or zoster; and (2) preterm infants born after 28 weeks gestation who are exposed in the hospital and whose mothers have negative history of infection (see Table 3.53, p 515).

- *Subsequent exposures and follow-up of VZIG recipients*. Since the administration of VZIG can cause the infection to be asymptomatic, testing of recipients 2 months or later after administration of VZIG for infection from chickenpox to ascertain their immune status may be considered. However, whether asymptomatic infection after VZIG administration confers lasting protection is not clear. Thus, even for the immunocompromised patient in whom asymptomatic infection has been documented, VZIG should be given after subsequent recognized varicella exposures.

The duration for which VZIG recipients are protected against chickenpox is unknown. If a second exposure occurs more than 3 weeks after administration of VZIG in a recipient who did not develop varicella, another dose of VZIG should be given.

• *Normal adults*. VZIG can be given to healthy, susceptible adults after exposure to varicella, but it is not routinely recommended by the Committee in this circumstance. It was previously recommended for these persons because of the recognized increased severity of varicella in persons 13 years or older. However, acyclovir is now available (and recommended) for treating persons of this age with varicella. In the case of adults with negative or uncertain histories of chickenpox, most have a high probability of immunity.

Active Immunization. A live-attenuated varicella vaccine is likely to be licensed for use in healthy children in the United States in the near future. Recommendations from the Academy will be forthcoming at that time. Vaccine is currently available on a compassionate-use protocol for children with acute lymphocytic leukemia in remission who are 12 months to 17 years.*

Vibrio Infections (Except Cholera)

Clinical Manifestations: *Vibrio* species are associated with the following three major clinical syndromes: diarrhea, septicemia, and wound infection. Diarrhea is most frequent, characterized by acute onset of watery stools and crampy, abdominal pain. Approximately one half of those afflicted will have low-grade fever, headache, and chills; about 30% will have vomiting. Spontaneous recovery follows in 2 to 5 days. Bacteremia is rare.

Infection can develop in contaminated wounds. Skin infections in compromised patients can cause extensive and rapid tissue necrosis. Patients with immunodeficiency or liver disease are susceptible to septicemia from bowel or skin infections, often resulting in shock, bullous or necrotic skin lesions, and death.

Etiology: Vibrios are facultatively anaerobic, motile, Gram-negative bacilli that are tolerant of salt. The most important noncholera *Vibrio* species associated with diarrhea is *Vibrio parahaemolyticus*; other species associated with gastrointestinal tract infection include *Vibrio cholerae non-01*, *Vibrio mimicus*, *Vibrio hollisae*, *Vibrio fluvialis*, and *Vibrio furnissii*. *Vibrio vulnificus* causes septicemia and wound infections in immunocompromised patients, especially those with liver disease. *Vibrio parahaemolyticus*, *Vibrio damsela*,

---

*To obtain the vaccine, contact the Varivax Coordinating Center, Bio-Pharm Clinical Services, Inc, 4 Valley Square, Blue Bell, PA 19422 (215/283-0897).

and *Vibrio alginolyticus* are also associated with wound infections. *Vibrio alginolyticus* has been associated with otitis externa.

Epidemiology: Noncholera vibrios are commonly found in seawater, increasing quantitatively during the summer. Most infections occur in summer and fall. Enteritis is usually acquired from seafood eaten raw or undercooked, especially oysters, crabs, and shrimp. Disease is probably not communicable from person to person. Wound infections commonly result from exposure of abrasions to contaminated seawater or from punctures resulting from handling of contaminated shellfish. Persons with increased susceptibility to infection with *Vibrio* species include those with liver disease, low gastric acidity, and immunodeficiency, including persons with HIV infection.

The median **incubation period** of enteritis is 23 hours, with a range of 5 to 92 hours.

Diagnostic Tests: These organisms can be isolated from stool or vomitus of patients with diarrhea, from blood, and from wound exudates. Because identification of the organism requires special techniques, laboratory personnel should be notified when *Vibrio* infection is suspected.

Treatment: Most episodes of diarrhea are mild and self-limited, and do not require treatment other than oral rehydration. Antibiotic therapy may benefit those with severe diarrhea or wound infections. Most organisms are susceptible to tetracycline (which usually should not be given to patients younger than 9 years), cefotaxime, gentamicin, and chloramphenicol.

Isolation of the Hospitalized Patient: Enteric precautions are indicated for the duration of diarrheal illness. Contact isolation precautions should be used for draining wounds.

Control Measures: Seafood should be cooked adequately, and if not ingested immediately, it should be refrigerated. Uncooked mollusks and crustaceans should be handled with care. Abrasions suffered by ocean bathers should be rinsed with clean, fresh water. Persons with liver disease or immunodeficiency should be warned to avoid eating raw oysters.

Yersinia enterocolitica and *Yersinia pseudotuberculosis* Infections (Enteritis and Other Illnesses)

Clinical Manifestations: *Yersinia* organisms cause several syndromes as well as a wide variety of uncommon presentations. The clinical manifestations depend on age and health of the host.

The most common manifestation of infection with *Yersinia enterocolitica* is enterocolitis with fever and diarrhea, often containing leukocytes, blood, and mucus. This syndrome occurs most often in young children. A pseudoappendicitis syndrome (fever, abdominal pain, right lower quadrant tenderness, and leukocytosis) occurs primarily in older children and young adults. Focal infections, abscess formation (such as hepatic and splenic), and bacteremia occur most often in patients with predisposing conditions such as excessive iron storage. Other manifestations of infection include pharyngitis, meningitis, osteomyelitis, pyomyositis, conjunctivitis, pneumonia, acute proliferative glomerulonephritis, and primary cutaneous infection. Postinfectious sequelae observed with *Y enterocolitica* include erythema nodosum and reactive arthritis, and occur most often in adults.

The major triad of infection caused by *Yersinia pseudotuberculosis* is fever, rash, and abdominal symptoms. Acute abdominal pain syndromes are most common, resulting from mesenteric adenitis, appendicitis, or terminal ileitis. Other findings can include diarrhea, erythema nodosum, septicemia, and sterile pleural and joint effusions. The rash is usually scarlatiniform. Clinical features can mimic those of Kawasaki disease.

Etiology: *Yersinia enterocolitica* and *Y pseudotuberculosis* are Gram-negative bacilli; 34 serotypes of *Y enterocolitica* and five serotypes of *Y pseudotuberculosis* are recognized. Differences in virulence exist among various sero types of *Y enterocolitica*.

Epidemiology: The reservoirs of the organisms are animals, including rodents (*Y pseudotuberculosis*) and swine (*Y enterocolitica*). Infection is believed to be transmitted by the ingestion of contaminated food, especially uncooked pork products and unpasteurized milk, or water; by direct or indirect contact with animals; by transfusion with packed red cells; and possibly by fecal-oral, person-to-person transmission. Bottle-fed infants can be infected if their caretakers are simultaneously handling raw pork intestines (chitterlings). *Yersinia enterocolitica* appears to be isolated more frequently in cooler climates and more frequently in winter than in summer. Patients with excessive iron storage syndromes have unusual susceptibility to *Yersinia* bacteremia. The period of communicability is unknown; it is probably for the duration of excretion of the specific organisms, which averages 6 weeks after diagnosis.

The **incubation period** is typically 4 to 6 days, varying from 1 to 14 days.

Diagnostic Tests: *Yersinia enterocolitica* and *Y pseudotuberculosis* can be recovered from throat swabs, mesenteric lymph nodes, peritoneal fluid, and blood. Stool cultures are generally positive during the first 2 weeks of illness, regardless of the nature of the gastrointestinal manifestations. *Yersinia enterocolitica* has been isolated from synovial fluid, bile, urine, cerebrospinal fluid, sputum, and wounds. Because laboratory identification of organisms from stool requires special techniques, laboratory personnel should be notified that *Yersinia* infection is suspected. Pathogenic strains of *Y enterocolitica* are usually pyrazinamidase-negative. Infection can be confirmed by demonstrating serum antibody titer rises after infection, but these tests are generally available only in reference or research laboratories. Cross-reactions of these antibodies with *Brucella*, *Vibrio*, *Escherichia coli*, *Salmonella*, and *Rickettsia* species lead to false-positive *Y enterocolitica* and *Y pseudotuberculosis* titers. In patients with thyroid disease, persistently elevated *Y enterocolitica* antibody titers can result from antigenic similarity of the organism with antigens of the thyroid epithelial cell membrane.

Treatment: Both *Y enterocolitica* and *Y pseudotuberculosis* are susceptible to aminoglycosides, cefotaxime, tetracycline (which usually should not be given to children younger than 9 years of age), chloramphenicol, and trimethoprim-sulfamethoxazole. *Yersinia enterocolitica* isolates typically are resistant to the first-generation cephalosporins and to most penicillins. Patients with septicemia or sites of infection other than the gastrointestinal tract and compromised hosts with enterocolitis should receive antibiotic therapy. Benefit from antibiotic therapy in patients with enterocolitis, the pseudoappendicular syndrome, or mesenteric adenitis, other than reduced duration of excretion of the organism in stool, has not been established.

Isolation of the Hospitalized Patient: For patients with enterocolitis, enteric precautions are indicated for the duration of illness.

Control Measures: Ingestion of uncooked meat, contaminated water, or unpasteurized milk should be avoided. Persons handling pork intestines should not simultaneously care for infants.

SECTION 4

ANTIMICROBIAL PROPHYLAXIS
Antimicrobial Prophylaxis

Antimicrobial agents are commonly prescribed to prevent infections in infants and children. The efficacy of the prophylactic use of these agents has been documented for some conditions but is unsubstantiated for most. Chemoprophylaxis is directed at different targets: specific pathogens, infection-prone body sites, and vulnerable patients. Effective prophylaxis is more readily achieved with specific pathogens and certain body sites.

Specific Pathogens

Prophylaxis is feasible if the physician can recognize situations associated with an increased risk of serious infection with a specific pathogen and select an antimicrobial agent that will eliminate the pathogen from persons at risk, with minimal adverse effects. For some pathogens that initially colonize the upper respiratory tract, elimination of the carrier state can be difficult and requires the use of an antibiotic, such as rifampin, which achieves effective concentrations in nasopharyngeal secretions. This property is lacking among antibiotics ordinarily used to treat infections caused by such pathogens. Table 4.1 (p 522) lists examples of pathogens amenable to antimicrobial prophylaxis in children and provides information about documented efficacy. In cases where prophylaxis is recommended, the regimen is described in the chapter on the specific disease in Section 3.

Infection-Prone Body Sites

Prevention of infection of vulnerable body sites may be possible if (1) the period of risk is defined and brief, (2) the expected pathogens have predictable antibiotic susceptibility, and (3) the site is accessible to antibiotics. Examples of infection-prone body sites amenable to chemoprophylaxis are listed in Table 4.2 (p 524). More detailed discussions of the prevention of surgical wound infection, bacterial endocarditis, and neonatal ophthalmia are given where relevant in Section 4.

Otitis media recurs less frequently in otitis-prone children treated prophylactically with antibiotics. Studies have demonstrated that either daily amoxicillin or sulfisoxazole is effective.

Protection afforded the urinary tract by chemoprophylaxis is critically dependent on the rate of emergence of antibiotic resistance in the gastrointestinal tract flora, the usual source of bacteria that invade the bladder. The long-term effec-

TABLE 4.1—Examples of Specific Pathogens Amenable to
Antimicrobial Prophylaxis

Pathogen	Disease to Be Prevented	Antimicrobial Agent	Efficacy
Bacteria			
Bordetella pertussis	Secondary cases of pertussis in household contacts	Erythromycin	Established
Chlamydia trachomatis	Urogenital infections in exposed persons	Tetracycline,* erythromycin	Proposed
Corynebacterium diphtheriae	Diphtheria in unimmunized contacts	Penicillin, erythromycin	Proposed
Haemophilus influenzae type b	Secondary cases of systemic infection in close contacts <1 y and those aged 12 to 47 mo who are not fully immunized	Rifampin	Established for household contacts
Mycobacterium tuberculosis	Overt pulmonary or metastatic infection	Isoniazid	Established
Neisseria gonorrhoeae	Urogenital infections in exposed persons	Ceftriaxone	Established
Neisseria meningitidis	Meningococcemia in exposed, susceptible persons	Rifampin, ceftriaxone, ciprofloxacin†	Established
Streptococcus pneumoniae	Fulminant pneumococcal infection in persons with asplenia	Penicillin	Established for penicillin V in children with sickle-cell anemia
Group A streptococcus	Recurrent rheumatic fever	Penicillin, sulfonamide	Established
Group B streptococcus	Neonatal infection	Ampicillin (intrapartum)	Established
Treponema pallidum	Syphilis in exposed persons	Penicillin	Established
Vibrio cholerae	Cholera in close contacts of a case	Tetracycline*	Proposed
Yersinia pestis	Plague in household contacts or persons exposed to pneumonic disease	Tetracycline,* sulfonamide	Proposed

TABLE 4.1—Examples of Specific Pathogens Amenable to Antimicrobial Prophylaxis *(continued)*

Pathogen	Disease to Be Prevented	Antimicrobial Agent	Efficacy
Fungi			
Pneumocystis carinii	Pneumonia in compromised host	Trimethoprim-sulfamethoxazole, pentamidine aerosol	Established (data in adults only)
Parasites			
Plasmodium species (malaria)	Overt infection (chloroquine-sensitive) in endemic areas	Chloroquine	Established
Viruses			
Influenza A	Influenza in persons at risk for complications	Amantadine	Established

*Tetracycline can cause dental staining in children younger than 9 y.
†Not recommended for use in children and adolescents younger than 18 y.

tiveness of nitrofurantoin and trimethoprim-sulfamethoxazole is explained by the minimal effect of these drugs on the development of resistant flora. Both drugs are concentrated in urine, and adequate inhibitory activity can be obtained with less than the usual therapeutic dose. Use of a single dose at bedtime has been successful.

Chemoprophylaxis of human and animal bite wounds has become common practice even though dog bites, the most common wound, become infected in only 5% of cases. Prophylaxis is recommended for wounds that cannot be adequately debrided or irrigated, for deep wounds of the hand, and for facial wounds where excess scarring from infection would be unacceptable.

Vulnerable Hosts

Most attempts to prevent infection in vulnerable patients have been foiled by the rapid replacement of initial bacteria by others resistant to antibiotics. Table 4.3 (p 524) lists circumstances in which antibiotics are frequently given to prevent infection.

TABLE 4.2—Examples of Infection-Prone Body Sites Amenable to Antimicrobial Prophylaxis

Body Site	Infection to Be Prevented	Agents Used	Efficacy
Conjunctivae	Neonatal gonococcal ophthalmia	1% silver nitrate,* 0.5% erythromycin,* 1% tetracycline*; penicillin	Established
Abnormal heart valve	Bacterial endocarditis (ie, after dental extraction)	Penicillin, others	See Prevention of Bacterial Endocarditis (p 525)
Surgical wound	Postoperative wound infection	Appropriate for expected contaminants	See Antimicrobial Prophylaxis in Pediatric Surgical Patients (p 535)
Middle ear	Recurrent otitis media	Sulfisoxazole, ampicillin	Established
Urinary tract	Recurrent urinary infection	Trimethoprim-sulfamethoxazole, nitrofurantoin	Established
Human/animal bite wound	Wound infection, cellulitis	Penicillin, amoxicillin-clavulanate	Proposed

*Topical administration

TABLE 4.3—Examples of Chemoprophylaxis for the Vulnerable Host

Infection to Be Prevented	Agents Used	Efficacy
Pneumocystis carinii pneumonia in immuno-compromised host	Trimethoprim-sulfamethoxazole, pentamidine aerosol	Established (data in adults only)
Fulminant bacteremia in persons with anatomic or functional asplenia	Penicillin, amoxicillin, trimethoprim-sulfamethoxazole	Established for penicillin V in infants and young children with sickle-cell anemia
Bacterial infection in persons with chronic granulomatous disease	Trimethoprim-sulfamethoxazole	Proposed

Prevention Of Bacterial Endocarditis

Recommendations by the American Heart Association*

Surgical and dental procedures and instrumentations involving mucosal surfaces or contaminated tissue commonly cause transient bacteremia that rarely persists for more than 15 minutes. Blood-borne bacteria may lodge on damaged or abnormal heart valves or on the endocardium or the endothelium near congenital anatomic defects, resulting in bacterial endocarditis or endarteritis. Although bacteremia is common following many invasive procedures, only a limited number of bacterial species commonly cause endocarditis. It is impossible to predict which patient will develop this infection or which particular procedure will be responsible.

Certain cardiac conditions are more often associated with endocarditis than others (Table 4.4, p 526). Furthermore, certain dental and surgical procedures are much more likely to initiate the bacteremia that results in endocarditis than are other procedures (Table 4.5, p 527). Prophylactic antibiotics are recommended for patients at risk for developing endocarditis who are undergoing those procedures most likely to produce bacteremia with organisms that commonly cause endocarditis.

Prophylaxis is most effective when given perioperatively in doses that are sufficient to assure adequate antibiotic concentrations in the serum during and after the procedure. To reduce the likelihood of microbial resistance, it is important that prophylactic antibiotics be used only during the perioperative period. They should be initiated shortly before a procedure (1 to 2 hours), and should not be continued for an extended period (no more than 6 to 8 hours). In the case of delayed healing, or of a procedure that involves infected tissue, it may be necessary to provide additional doses of antibiotics.

This statement represents recommended guidelines to supplement practitioners in the exercise of their clinical judgment and is not intended as a standard of care for all cases. It is impossible to make recommendations for all clinical situations in which endocarditis may develop. Practitioners must exercise their own clinical judgment in determining the choice of antibiotics and number of doses that are to be administered in individual cases or special circumstances. Furthermore, because endocarditis may occur in spite of appropriate antibiotic prophylaxis, physicians and dentists should maintain a high index of suspicion regarding any unusual clinical events (such as unexplained fever, weakness, lethargy, or malaise) following dental or other surgical procedures in patients who are at risk for developing bacterial endocarditis.

Because no adequate, controlled clinical trials of antibiotic regimens for the prevention of bacterial endocarditis in humans have been done, recommen-

---

*A statement from the Committee on Rheumatic Fever, Endocarditis, and Kawasaki Disease of the Council on Cardiovascular Disease in the Young of the American Heart Association. Prepared by Dajani AS, Bisno AL, Chung KJ, et al. Reprinted with permission from *JAMA*. 1990;264:2919-2922. Copyright 1990, American Medical Association.

TABLE 4.4—Cardiac Conditions*

Endocarditis Prophylaxis Recommended

Prosthetic cardiac valves, including bioprosthetic and homograft valves

Previous bacterial endocarditis, even in the absence of heart disease

Most congenital cardiac malformations

Rheumatic and other acquired valvular dysfunction, even after valvular surgery

Hypertrophic cardiomyopathy

Mitral valve prolapse with valvular regurgitation

Endocarditis Prophylaxis Not Recommended

Isolated secundum atrial septal defect

Surgical repair without residua beyond 6 mo of secundum atrial septal defect, ventricular septal defect, or patent ductus arteriosus

Previous coronary artery bypass graft surgery

Mitral valve prolapse without valvular regurgitation†

Physiologic, functional, or innocent heart murmurs

Previous Kawasaki disease without valvular dysfunction

Previous rheumatic fever without valvular dysfunction

Cardiac pacemakers and implanted defibrillators

---

*This table lists selected conditions but is not meant to be all-inclusive.

†Individuals who have a mitral valve prolapse associated with thickening and/or redundancy of the valve leaflets may be at increased risk for bacterial endocarditis, particularly men who are 45 years of age or older.

dations are based on in vitro studies, clinical experience, data from experimental animal models, and assessment of both the bacteria most likely to produce bacteremia from a given site and those most likely to result in endocarditis. The substantial morbidity and mortality in patients who have endocarditis and the paucity of controlled clinical studies emphasize the need for continuing research into the epidemiology, pathogenesis, prevention, and therapy of endocarditis.

The current recommendations are an update of those made by the committee* in 1984. They incorporate new data and include opinions of national and international experts.

STANDARD PROPHYLACTIC REGIMEN FOR DENTAL, ORAL, AND UPPER RESPIRATORY TRACT PROCEDURES

Poor dental hygiene and periodontal or periapical infections may produce bacteremia even in the absence of dental procedures. Individuals who are at risk for developing bacterial endocarditis should establish and maintain the best possible oral health to reduce potential sources of bacterial seeding. Dentists should make

---

*Committee on Rheumatic Fever, Endocarditis, and Kawasaki Disease of the Council on Cardiovascular Disease in the Young of the American Heart Association.

TABLE 4.5—Dental or Surgical Procedures*

Endocarditis Prophylaxis Recommended

Dental procedures known to induce gingival or mucosal bleeding, including professional cleaning

Tonsillectomy and/or adenoidectomy

Surgical operations that involve intestinal or respiratory mucosa

Bronchoscopy with a rigid bronchoscope

Sclerotherapy for esophageal varices

Esophageal dilatation

Gallbladder surgery

Cystoscopy

Urethral dilatation

Urethral catheterization if urinary tract infection is present[†]

Urinary tract surgery if urinary tract infection is present[†]

Prostatic surgery

Incision and drainage of infected tissue[†]

Vaginal hysterectomy

Vaginal delivery in the presence of infection[†]

Endocarditis Prophylaxis Not Recommended[‡]

Dental procedures not likely to induce gingival bleeding, such as simple adjustment of orthodontic appliances or fillings above the gum line

Injection of local intraoral anesthetic (except intraligamentary injections)

Shedding of primary teeth

Tympanostomy tube insertion

Endotracheal intubation

Bronchoscopy with a flexible bronchoscope, with or without biopsy

Cardiac catheterization

Endoscopy with or without gastrointestinal biopsy

Cesarean section

In the absence of infection for urethral catheterization, dilatation and curettage, uncomplicated vaginal delivery, therapeutic abortion, sterilization procedures, or insertion or removal of intrauterine devices

*This table lists selected procedures but is not meant to be all-inclusive.

[†]In addition to prophylactic regimen for genitourinary procedures, antibiotic therapy should be directed against the most likely bacterial pathogen.

[‡]In patients who have prosthetic heart valves, a previous history of endocarditis, or surgically constructed systemic-pulmonary shunts or conduits, physicians may choose to administer prophylactic antibiotics even for low-risk procedures that involve the lower respiratory, genitourinary, or gastrointestinal tracts.

every attempt to reduce gingival inflammation in patients who are at risk by means of brushing, flossing, fluoride rinse, chlorhexidine gluconate mouth rinse, and professional cleaning before proceeding with routine dental procedures. Chlorhexidine that is painted on isolated and dried gingiva 3 to 5 minutes prior to tooth extraction has been shown to reduce postextraction bacteremia. Other agents such as povidone-iodine or iodine and glycerin may also be appropriate. Furthermore, irrigation of the gingival sulcus with chlorhexidine prior to tooth extraction has been shown to reduce postextraction bacteremia in adults. Application of chlorhexidine may be used as an adjunct to antibiotic prophylaxis, particularly in patients who are at high risk and/or have poor dental hygiene.

Antibiotic prophylaxis is recommended with all dental procedures likely to cause gingival bleeding, including routine professional cleaning. If a series of dental procedures is required, it may be prudent to observe an interval of 7 days between procedures to reduce the potential for the emergence of resistant strains of organisms. If possible, a combination of procedures should be planned in the same period of prophylaxis. Edentulous patients may develop bacteremia from ulcers caused by ill-fitting dentures; therefore, denture wearers should be encouraged to have periodic examinations or to return to the practitioner if soreness develops. When new dentures are inserted, it is advisable to have the patient return to the practitioner to correct any overextension that could cause mucosal ulceration. Because the spontaneous shedding of primary teeth or simple adjustment of orthodontic appliances does not present a significant risk of endocarditis, antibiotic prophylaxis is not necessary in these situations. Similarly, endotracheal intubation is not an indication for antibiotic prophylaxis unless it is associated with another procedure for which prophylaxis is recommended.

Alpha-hemolytic (viridans) streptococci are the most common cause of endocarditis following dental procedures, and prophylaxis should be specifically directed against these organisms. Certain upper respiratory tract procedures, such as tonsillectomy and/or adenoidectomy, bronchoscopy with a rigid bronchoscope, and surgical procedures that involve the respiratory mucosa, may also cause bacteremia with organisms that commonly cause endocarditis and have similar antibiotic susceptibilities to those producing bacteremia following dental procedures. Therefore, the same regimen is recommended for these procedures as is recommended for dental procedures. Endocarditis has not been reported in association with insertion of tympanostomy tubes.

The recommended standard prophylactic regimen for all dental, oral, and upper respiratory tract procedures is amoxicillin (Table 4.6, p 529). The antibiotics amoxicillin, ampicillin, and penicillin V are equally effective in vitro against α-hemolytic streptococci; however, amoxicillin is now recommended because it is better absorbed from the gastrointestinal tract and provides higher and more sustained serum levels. The choice of penicillin V rather than amoxicillin as prophylaxis against α-hemolytic streptococcal bacteremia following dental, oral, and upper respiratory tract procedures is rational and acceptable.

Individuals who are allergic to penicillins (such as amoxicillin, ampicillin, or penicillin) should be treated with the provided alternative oral regimens. Erythromycin ethylsuccinate and erythromycin stearate are recommended because of more rapid and reliable absorption than other erythromycin formulations, resulting in higher and more sustained serum levels. For individuals who cannot

TABLE 4.6—Recommended Standard Prophylactic Regimen for Dental, Oral, or Upper Respiratory Tract Procedures in Patients Who Are at Risk*

Drug	Dosing Regiment
Standard Regimen	
Amoxicillin	3.0 g orally 1 h before procedure; then 1.5 g, 6 h after initial dose
Amoxicillin/Penicillin-Allergic Patients	
Erythromycin	Erythromycin ethylsuccinate, 800 mg, or erythromycin stearate, 1.0 g, orally 2 h before procedure; then half the
or	dose 6 h after initial dose
Clindamycin	300 mg orally 1 h before procedure and 150 mg 6 h after initial dose

*Includes those with prosthetic heart valves and other high risk patients.

†Initial pediatric doses are as follows: amoxicillin, 50 mg/kg; erythromycin ethylsuccinate or erythromycin stearate, 20 mg/kg; and clindamycin, 10 mg/kg. Follow-up doses should be one half the initial dose. **Total pediatric dose should not exceed total adult dose.** The following weight ranges may also be used for the initial pediatric dose of amoxicillin: <15 kg, 750 mg; 15 to 30 kg, 1500 mg; and >30 kg, 3000 mg (full adult dose).

tolerate either penicillins or erythromycin, clindamycin hydrochloride is the recommended alternative. Tetracyclines and sulfonamides *are not* recommended for endocarditis prophylaxis.

ALTERNATE PROPHYLACTIC REGIMENS FOR DENTAL, ORAL, AND UPPER RESPIRATORY TRACT PROCEDURES

Table 4.7 (p 530) lists alternate prophylactic regimens for individuals who may not be candidates to receive the standard prophylactic regimen. For individuals who are unable to take oral medications, a parenteral agent may be necessary. Ampicillin sodium is recommended because parenteral amoxicillin is not available in the United States. When parenteral administration is needed in an individual who is allergic to penicillin, clindamycin phosphate is recommended.

Individuals who have prosthetic heart valves, a previous history of endocarditis, or surgically constructed systemic-pulmonary shunts or conduits are at high risk for developing endocarditis, and endocardial infection in such individuals is associated with substantial morbidity and mortality. For this reason, previous recommendations of this committee emphasized the use of stringent prophylactic regimens, with a strong preference for the parenteral route of administration. In practice, there are substantial logistic and financial barriers to the use of parenteral regimens. Moreover, oral regimens have now been used in individuals who have prosthetic heart valves in other countries, and failures in prophylaxis have not been a problem. Consequently, this committee recommends the use of the standard prophylactic regimen (Table 4.6, above) in patients who have pros-

TABLE 4.7—Alternate Prophylactic Regimens for Dental, Oral, or Upper Respiratory Tract Procedures in Patients Who Are at Risk

Drug	Dosing Regimen*
Patients Unable to Take Oral Medications	
Ampicillin	Intravenous or intramuscular administration of ampicillin, 2.0 g, 30 min before procedure; then intravenous or intramuscular administration of ampicillin, 1.0 g, or oral administration of amoxicillin, 1.5 g, 6 h after initial dose
Ampicillin/Amoxicillin/Penicillin-Allergic Patients Unable to Take Oral Medications	
Clindamycin	Intravenous administration of 300 mg 30 min before procedure and an intravenous or oral administration of 150 mg 6 h after initial dose
Patients Considered High Risk and Not Candidates for Standard Regimen	
Ampicillin, gentamicin, and amoxicillin	Intravenous or intramuscular administration of ampicillin, 2.0 g, plus gentamicin, 1.5 mg/kg (not to exceed 80 mg), 30 min before procedure; followed by amoxicillin, 1.5 g, orally 6 h after initial dose; alternatively, the parenteral regimen may be repeated 8 h after initial dose
Ampicillin/Amoxicillin/Penicillin-Allergic Patients Considered High Risk	
Vancomycin	Intravenous administration of 1.0 g over 1 h, starting 1 h before procedure; no repeated dose necessary

*Initial pediatric doses are as follows: ampicillin, 50 mg/kg; clindamycin, 10 mg/kg; gentamicin, 2.0 mg/kg; and vancomycin, 20 mg/kg. Follow-up doses should be one half the initial dose. **Total pediatric dose should not exceed total adult dose.** No initial dose is recommended in this table for amoxicillin (25 mg/kg is the follow-up dose).

thetic heart valves and in the other high-risk groups. It is recognized that some practitioners may prefer to use parenteral prophylaxis in these high-risk groups of patients. Accordingly, an alternate regimen is also provided in Table 4.7, above.

REGIMENS FOR GENITOURINARY AND GASTROINTESTINAL PROCEDURES

Surgery, instrumentation, or diagnostic procedures that involve the genitourinary or gastrointestinal tracts may cause bacteremia. The rate of bacteremia that is found following urinary tract procedures is high if urinary tract infection is present. Although the risk that any particular patient will develop endocarditis is low, the genitourinary tract is second only to the oral cavity as a portal of entry for organisms that cause endocarditis. The instrumented gastrointestinal tract seems to be less important as a portal of entry for organisms that cause bacterial endocarditis than the oral cavity or genitourinary tract.

Bacterial endocarditis that occurs following genitourinary and gastrointestinal tract surgery or instrumentation is most often caused by *Enterococcus faecalis* (enterococci). Although Gram-negative bacillary bacteremia may follow these procedures, Gram-negative bacilli are only rarely responsible for endocarditis. Thus, antibiotic prophylaxis to prevent endocarditis that occurs following genitourinary or gastrointestinal procedures should be directed primarily against enterococci.

Table 4.8 (p 532) outlines the recommended regimens for prophylaxis for genitourinary or gastrointestinal tract procedures. The committee continues to recommend parenteral antibiotics, particularly in high-risk patients (eg, those with prosthetic heart valves or a previous history of endocarditis). In low-risk patients, an alternative oral regimen is provided.

SPECIFIC SITUATIONS AND CIRCUMSTANCES

Rheumatic Fever

Antibiotic regimens used to prevent the recurrence of acute rheumatic fever are inadequate for the prevention of bacterial endocarditis. Individuals who take an oral penicillin for secondary prevention of rheumatic fever or for other purposes may have viridans streptococci in their oral cavities that are relatively resistant to penicillin, amoxicillin, or ampicillin. In such cases, the physician or dentist should select erythromycin or another of the alternative regimens (listed in Tables 4.6 and 4.7, pp 529 and 530), instead of amoxicillin (or another penicillin) for endocarditis prophylaxis.

Patients Who Receive Anticoagulants

Intramuscular injections for endocarditis prophylaxis should be avoided in patients who receive heparin. The use of warfarin sodium is a relative contraindication to intramuscular injections. Intravenous or oral regimens should be used whenever possible.

Patients Who Have Renal Dysfunction

In patients who have a markedly compromised renal function, it may be necessary to modify or omit the second dose of gentamicin sulfate or vancomycin hydrochloride.

Patients Who Undergo Cardiac Surgery

Patients who have cardiac conditions (Table 4.4, p 526) that predispose them to endocarditis are at risk for developing bacterial endocarditis when undergoing open heart surgery. Similarly, patients who undergo surgery for placement of prosthetic heart valves or prosthetic intravascular or intracardiac materials are also at risk for the development of bacterial endocarditis. Because the morbidity and mortality of endocarditis in such patients are high, perioperative prophylactic antibiotics are recommended.

Endocarditis associated with open heart surgery is most often caused by *Staphylococcus aureus*, coagulase-negative staphylococci, or diphtheroids. Streptococci, Gram-negative bacteria, and fungi are less common. No single anti-

TABLE 4.8—Regimens for Genitourinary/Gastrointestinal Procedures

Drug	Dosing Regimen*
Standard Regimen	
Ampicillin, gentamicin, and amoxicillin	Intravenous or intramuscular administration of ampicillin, 2.0 g, plus gentamicin, 1.5 mg/kg (not to exceed 80 mg), 30 min before procedure; followed by amoxicillin, 1.5 g orally 6 h after initial dose; alternatively, the parenteral regimen may be repeated once 8 h after initial dose
Ampicillin/Amoxicillin/Penicillin-Allergic Patient Regimen	
Vancomycin and gentamicin	Intravenous administration of vancomycin, 1.0 g, over 1 h plus intravenous or intramuscular administration of gentamicin, 1.5 mg/kg (not to exceed 80 mg), 1 h before procedure; may be repeated once 8 h after initial dose
Alternate Low-Risk Patient Regimen	
Amoxicillin	3.0 g orally 1 h before procedure; then 1.5 g 6 h after initial dose

*Initial pediatric doses are as follows: ampicillin, 50 mg/kg; amoxicillin, 50 mg/kg; gentamicin, 2.0 mg/kg; and vancomycin, 20 mg/kg. Follow-up doses should be half the initial dose. **Total pediatric dose should not exceed total adult dose.**

biotic regimen is effective against all these organisms. Furthermore, prolonged use of broad-spectrum antibiotics may predispose to superinfection with unusual or resistant microorganisms.

Prophylaxis at the time of cardiac surgery should be directed primarily against staphylococci and should be of short duration. "First-generation" cephalosporins are most often used, but the choice of an antibiotic should be influenced by the antibiotic's susceptibility patterns at each hospital. For example, high prevalence of infection by methicillin-resistant *S aureus* in a particular institution should prompt consideration of vancomycin for perioperative prophylaxis. Prophylaxis with the chosen antibiotic should be started immediately before the operative procedure, repeated during prolonged procedures to maintain levels intraoperatively, and continued for no more than 24 hours postoperatively to minimize emergence of resistant microorganisms. The effects of cardiopulmonary bypass and compromised postoperative renal function on antibiotic levels in the serum should be considered, and doses timed appropriately before and during the procedure.

A careful preoperative dental evaluation is recommended so that required dental treatment can be completed before cardiac surgery whenever possible. Such measures may decrease the incidence of late postoperative endocarditis.

Status Following Cardiac Surgery

The same precautions should be observed in the years following most heart or valvular surgery that have been outlined for the patient who has not undergone a surgical procedure but is undergoing dental, gastrointestinal, genitourinary, or other procedures. The risk of developing endocarditis appears to continue indefinitely and is particularly significant for patients who have prosthetic heart valves. Furthermore, the morbidity and mortality that result from prosthetic valve endocarditis are high. Patients who have an isolated secundum atrial septal defect that has been surgically repaired, a ventricular septal defect, or patent ductus arteriosus do not seem to be at risk of developing endocarditis following a 6-month healing period after surgery. Data are insufficient to allow recommendations for prophylactic therapy after closure of these lesions by nonsurgical devices. There is no evidence that coronary artery bypass graft surgery introduces a risk for a patient's developing endocarditis. Therefore, antibiotic prophylaxis is not needed for this condition.

Cardiac Transplantation

There are insufficient data to support specific recommendations for patients who have had heart transplants. Some physicians place these patients in the category of people who will need prophylaxis, however.

Prevention of Neonatal Ophthalmia

Topical 1% silver nitrate, 0.5% erythromycin, and 1% tetracycline are considered equally effective for prophylaxis of ocular gonorrheal infection in newborn infants. Each is available in single-dose tubes. Silver nitrate causes more chemical conjunctivitis than the others but appears to be the best agent in areas where the incidence of penicillinase-producing *Neisseria gonorrhoeae* (PPNG) is appreciable. Published data on the efficacy of erythromycin prophylaxis against PPNG are not available, and only one study has demonstrated effectiveness of prophylactic tetracycline in an area with a high incidence of PPNG infections. However, silver nitrate and probably erythromycin are effective in preventing nongonococcal, nonchlamydial conjunctivitis in the first 2 weeks of life.

Neonatal chlamydial ophthalmia, although not as severe as gonococcal conjunctivitis, is common in the United States. In most areas, its frequency far surpasses that of gonococcal ophthalmia. The effectiveness of 0.5% erythromycin ophthalmologic ointment in the prevention of chlamydial conjunctivitis was demonstrated in one study, but it has not been confirmed in subsequent studies. *Chlamydia trachomatis* is also susceptible to tetracyclines, but results of studies of the clinical efficacy of tetracycline ointment in the prophylaxis of chlamydial conjunctivitis have been conflicting. Neither topical antibiotic regimen eliminates *C trachomatis* nasopharyngeal carriage or prevents pneumonia.

Specific recommendations for the prevention of neonatal ophthalmia are as follows:

- *Choice of drugs.* For prophylaxis of gonococcal ophthalmia neonatorum, a 1% silver nitrate solution in single-dose ampules or single-use tubes of an ophthalmic ointment containing 0.5% erythromycin or 1% tetracycline are each effective and acceptable. The effectiveness of erythromycin or tetracycline in the prevention of ophthalmia caused by PPNG is not established. No topical regimen has proven efficacy in preventing chlamydial conjunctivitis.

- *Administration.* Before administering local prophylaxis, each eyelid should be wiped gently with sterile cotton. Two drops of a 1% silver nitrate solution or a 1- to 2-cm ribbon of antibiotic ointment are placed in each lower conjunctival sac. The eyelids are then massaged gently to spread the ointment. After 1 minute, excess solution or ointment can be wiped away with sterile cotton. None of the prophylactic agents should be flushed from the eye after instillation. Critical studies have not evaluated the efficacy of silver nitrate prophylaxis with and without flushing, but anecdotal reports suggest that flushing may reduce the efficacy of prophylaxis. In addition, flushing probably does not reduce the incidence of chemical conjunctivitis.

  Prophylaxis should be given shortly after birth. Although some suggest that prophylaxis may be administered more effectively in the nursery than in the delivery room, the efficacy of delaying prophylaxis has not been studied. However, delaying prophylaxis for as long as 1 hour after birth is probably not likely to influence efficacy. **Hospitals in which prophylaxis is delayed should establish a check system to ensure that all infants are treated.**

- *Cesarean-section infants.* Infants born by cesarean section should receive prophylaxis against neonatal gonococcal ophthalmia. Although gonococcal and chlamydial infections are usually transmitted to the infant during passage through the birth canal, infection by the ascending route also occurs. The risk of these infections occurring in untreated infants born by cesarean section has not been determined.

- *Women with gonococcal infections.* Identification of women who have gonococcal infections by routine cultures and subsequent treatment of them is essential. Gonococcal infections in pregnant women, including those who are asymptomatic, have been associated with septic abortion, early and prolonged rupture of membranes, premature labor, and delivery of low-birth-weight infants. These infections can also result in scalp abscesses in infants receiving intrauterine fetal monitoring and in disseminated neonatal gonococcal infection. Failure to treat an infected woman before or at delivery can result in postnatal transmission of gonococcal infection to infants.

- *Neonates whose mothers have gonorrhea.* Newborn infants whose mothers have gonorrhea at the time of delivery should receive a single dose of ceftriaxone (125 mg; for low-birth-weight infants, 25 to 50 mg/kg) intravenously or intramuscularly, as occasional cases of gonococcal ophthalmia occur in infants managed by any of the current modes of prophylaxis.

- *Neonates with gonococcal ophthalmia or disseminated infection.* Newborns with clinical evidence of gonococcal ophthalmia or complicated (disseminated) gonococcal infection should be hospitalized, placed in isolation, and treated appropriately (see Gonococcal Infections, p 197). A penicillinase-resistant antimicrobial such as ceftriaxone should be used.

- *Pregnant women with chlamydial cervicitis.* Treatment of pregnant women who have chlamydial cervicitis can prevent neonatal chlamydial infection. Oral erythromycin is the only recommended treatment for these women; tetracycline is contraindicated (see *Chlamydia trachomatis*, p 156). Women whose infants develop chlamydial conjunctivitis and their sexual partners should receive treatment.

- *Neonates whose mothers have untreated chlamydial infection.* Newborn infants whose mothers have untreated chlamydial infection at the time of delivery should be treated with oral erythromycin (see *Chlamydia trachomatis*, p 156). Although the treatment of infants in this circumstance has not been evaluated in appropriate studies, oral erythromycin is probably effective in preventing chlamydial infection of the exposed infant. The minimum duration of such treatment has not been determined and 14 days is empirically recommended. Erythromycin may be poorly tolerated in neonates, in which case oral sulfonamides may be used after the immediate newborn period.

• *Identification of Chlamydia-positive women. Chlamydia*-positive women can be identified by screening with one of several rapid antigen detection tests (see *Chlamydia trachomatis*, p 155). Testing is warranted in areas of high prevalence and in women found to have other sexually transmitted diseases. Some experts advocate universal screening of pregnant women for *Chlamydia*.

Antimicrobial Prophylaxis in Pediatric Surgical Patients*

A major use of antimicrobial agents in hospitalized children is for prophylaxis against postoperative wound infections. In view of this frequent use and the emerging consensus on recommendations for prevention of surgical wound infections, guidelines for surgical antimicrobial prophylaxis in children have been developed. Prophylaxis is defined as the use of antimicrobial drugs in the absence of suspected or documented infection to reduce the incidence of infection.

Frequency of Antimicrobial Prophylaxis

In hospitalized patients, approximately one third of the courses of antimicrobial drugs are initiated for prophylaxis of infection after surgery or an invasive procedure such as cystoscopy or cardiac catheterization. The frequency and reasons for antimicrobial use have been studied primarily in general hospitals, but the patterns of use in children are similar to those in adults. Two studies demonstrated that prophylaxis accounts for approximately 75% of the use of antibiotics on pediatric surgical services. The efficacy of antimicrobial agents in lowering the incidence of postoperative infection after certain types of surgery has been amply demonstrated in controlled clinical trials. These and earlier studies in experimental animals have delineated the principles for effective use of antimicrobial agents in prophylaxis of wound infections, including choice of drugs and when and how long they are to be given.

---

*Adapted from American Academy of Pediatrics, Committee on Infectious Diseases, Committee on Drugs, and Section on Surgery. Antimicrobial prophylaxis in pediatric surgical patients. *Pediatrics.* 1984;74:437-439.

Inappropriate Antimicrobial Prophylaxis

Prophylaxis has been identified as a major cause of inappropriate use of antimicrobial agents in both adults and children. In a study of children younger than 6 years undergoing surgery, in which appropriateness of use was assessed on the basis of commonly accepted guidelines, prophylactic antimicrobials were administered inappropriately to 42% of children receiving preoperative antimicrobial(s), 67% receiving intraoperative antimicrobial(s), and 55% receiving postoperative antimicrobials. Similarly, in a large teaching hospital, 66% of antimicrobial use in children on surgical services was considered inappropriate for reasons of wrong drug, dose, time of initiation, duration, or lack of indication. These studies suggest that the use of antimicrobial agents in children undergoing surgery and other invasive procedures should be subject to periodic review.

Guidelines for Appropriate Use

Studies documenting that systemic prophylaxis reduces the incidence of surgical wound infections have been performed primarily in adults. Because the pathogenesis of these infections is the same in children, the principles of surgical prophylaxis in children should be similar. In the absence of studies in children, guidelines recommended by the American College of Surgeons, *The Medical Letter*,* the Veterans Administration Committee on Antimicrobial Drug Use, and the Centers for Disease Control and Prevention provide the only available standards for use of systemic prophylactic antibiotics in pediatric surgical patients. The following general principles are recommended as guidelines, with the understanding that studies in children may result in changes and that factors unique to children may justify exceptions.

Indications for Prophylaxis

Systemic prophylaxis is indicated when the benefits of preventing wound infection outweigh the risks of drug reactions and the emergence of resistant bacteria. The latter poses a potential risk not only to the recipient but also to other hospitalized patients, who may develop a nosocomial infection caused by antibiotic-resistant organisms. Procedures in which the benefits justify the risks incurred in antimicrobial prophylaxis are those associated with a significant risk of postoperative infection, and those in which the likelihood of infection may not be great but the consequences of infection can be catastrophic.

A major determinant of the probability of surgical wound infection is the number of microorganisms in the wound at the completion of the procedure. This fact allows the classification of surgical procedures (see the Addendum), based on an estimation of bacterial contamination and the risk of subsequent infection, into four broad categories: (1) clean wounds, (2) clean-contaminated wounds, (3) contaminated wounds, and (4) dirty and infected wounds. Within these categories, however, variation in the risk of infection is considerable.

---

*Antimicrobial prophylaxis in surgery. *The Medical Letter.* 1993;35:91-94

Recent data suggest that the use of a patient risk index, which in addition to classifying wounds as contaminated or dirty-infected also considers the American Society of Anesthesiologists' preoperative assessment score and the duration of the operation, is a better predictor of risk of surgical wound infection than is this classification.*

Clean Wounds.

In clean wound procedures, the benefits of systemic antimicrobial prophylaxis may not justify the potential risks associated with antimicrobial use, except in circumstances in which the consequences of infection may be major and life threatening, such as with implantation of a prosthetic foreign body (eg, insertion of a prosthetic heart valve), open-heart surgery for repair of structural defects, compromised immune status (such as patients receiving high doses of corticosteroids or chemotherapy for a malignancy), and body cavity exploration in neonates. Prophylaxis has been given in these circumstances, although studies establishing efficacy have not been performed. Systemic antimicrobial agents have also been empirically recommended for clean procedures in patients with infection at another site.

Clean-contaminated Wounds.

In clean-contaminated wound procedures, the degree of contamination is variable, and prophylaxis is limited to procedures with significant risk of wound contamination and infection. Based on data from adults, recommendations for prophylaxis for pediatric patients include the following: (1) many alimentary tract procedures, (2) selected biliary tract operations (eg, with obstructive jaundice), and (3) urinary tract surgery or instrumentation in the presence of bacteriuria or obstructive uropathy.

Contaminated; Dirty and Infected Wounds.

In contaminated and in dirty and infected wound procedures, such as those for a perforated abdominal viscus or a compound fracture, or if a major break in sterile technique has occurred, antimicrobial agents are indicated and are considered treatment rather than prophylaxis.

When Should Prophylactic Antibiotics Be Given?

Prophylaxis of infection requires effective drug concentrations in tissues during surgical procedures because bacterial contamination occurs intraoperatively. Except in patients undergoing cesarean section, the antimicrobial agent should be administered within 30 minutes of the surgical incision to ensure adequate tissue concentration at the time of possible contamination. For patients with cesarean section, it should be given after the umbilical cord is clamped.

---

*Culver DH, Horan TC, Gaynes RP, et al. Surgical wound infection rates by wound class, operative procedure, and patient risk index. *Am J Med.* 1991;91 (suppl 3B):152S-157S

For How Long Should Antibiotics Be Given?

A single antimicrobial dose that provides adequate tissue concentration throughout the procedure is usually sufficient. When surgery is prolonged or massive blood loss occurs, a second dose is advisable during the procedure. Postoperative doses of prophylactic drugs are generally unnecessary. These recommendations are based on studies in adults and may not necessarily apply to all pediatric patients, particularly neonates. However, inasmuch as the pathogenesis of wound infection does not differ with age, the recommendation for brief duration of prophylaxis is probably applicable to patients of all ages.

Which Antibiotics Should Be Given?

The choice of an antimicrobial is based on knowledge of the common bacteria causing infectious complications after the specific procedure, bacterial susceptibility to the drug, proved efficacy of the drug selected, and the safety of the drug. New, costly antimicrobial agents generally should not be used unless prophylactic efficacy has been proven superior to that of drugs of established benefit. The drugs should be active against the most likely pathogens, but they do not have to be active against every potential organism because effective prophylaxis appears to correlate with a decrease in the total number of pathogens rather than eradication of all organisms. Recommended doses and route of administration are based on the need to achieve therapeutic blood and tissue concentrations throughout the procedure; parenteral (usually intravenous) administration is usually necessary. For antimicrobial prophylaxis of patients undergoing colonic procedures, additional oral antibiotic prophylaxis should be given before the procedure but is not a substitute for adequate mechanical bowel preparation.

Physicians should be aware of potential interactions and/or adverse effects associated with prophylactic antimicrobials and other medications that the patient is receiving.

Conclusion

These guidelines for antimicrobial prophylaxis of surgical wound infections in children were originally developed by the Committee in collaboration with the Committee on Drugs and the Section on Surgery of the American Academy of Pediatrics in 1984.[*] They have been revised in accordance with recent data and recommendations. Because the benefit of systemic antimicrobial prophylaxis in many pediatric surgical procedures has not been established, additional studies in commonly performed surgical procedures in children (eg, insertion of neurosurgical shunts and orthopedic procedures) are needed. Pediatricians, pediatric surgeons, and surgical subspecialists should review the prophylactic use of anti-

---

[*]Adapted from American Academy of Pediatrics, Committee on Infectious Diseases, Committee on Drugs, and Section on Surgery. Antimicrobial prophylaxis in pediatric surgical patients. *Pediatrics.* 1984;74:437-439

microbial agents as part of the monitoring of antibiotic use in their hospitals, and they should use the guidelines given here to develop standards for anti-microbial use.

Addendum

Definitions of surgical wounds in the classification scheme are as follows:

Clean Wounds.

Clean wounds are uninfected operative wounds in which no inflammation is encountered, and the respiratory, alimentary, or genitourinary tract or the oropha-ryngeal cavity is not entered. The operative procedures are elective and the wounds are closed primarily, and, if necessary, drained with closed drainage. Operative incisional wounds that follow nonpenetrating (blunt) trauma should be included in this category if they meet the criteria.

Clean-contaminated Wounds.

In clean-contaminated operative wounds, the respiratory, alimentary, or geni-tourinary tract is entered under controlled conditions and without unusual con-tamination. Operations involving the biliary tract, appendix, vagina, and oropharynx are included in this category, provided that no evidence of infection is encountered and no major break in technique occurs.

Contaminated Wounds.

Contaminated wounds include open, fresh, accidental wounds; operative wounds in the setting of major breaks in sterile technique or gross spillage from the gastrointestinal tract; and incisions in which acute, nonpurulent inflammation is encountered.

Dirty and Infected Wounds.

Dirty and infected wounds include old traumatic wounds with retained devital-ized tissue and those that involve existing clinical infection or perforated viscera. This definition suggests that the organisms causing postoperative infection were present in the operative field before surgery.

SECTION 5

ANTIMICROBIALS AND RELATED THERAPY

Introduction

In some instances, drugs are recommended for specific indications other than those in the package insert approved by the Food and Drug Administration (FDA). An FDA-approved indication means that adequate and well-controlled studies were conducted and reviewed by the FDA. However, accepted medical practice often includes drug use that is not reflected in approved drug labeling. Lack of approval does not necessarily mean lack of efficacy but only that the appropriate studies either have not been done or have not been submitted to the FDA for approval. Lack of approval does not prevent a physician from using an available drug, and it does not imply improper use in so doing, provided that reasonable medical evidence justifies using it and prudence is exercised. The decision to prescribe a drug rests with the physician, who must weigh the risks and benefits of using the drug, whether or not it has specific FDA approval.

Some of the agents listed in the tables have not been approved by the FDA for use in pediatric patients. In some cases, application for pediatric use is currently pending FDA decision. However, the broad-spectrum fluroquinolones (such as ciprofloxacin), which are commonly prescribed for adults, are generally contraindicated for children because they cause cartilage damage in immature animals. Although no data indicate similar toxicity in young children, approval for these drugs for use in subjects younger than 18 years is unlikely in the next several years or more. Nevertheless, special situations arise in which ciprofloxacin or another of the quinolones might be considered for treatment of pediatric patients. One such situation is for infections caused by *Pseudomonas* strains that are resistant to multiple antibiotics or for which an orally administered antibiotic is preferred. In such instances, obtaining informed parental consent before use is prudent.

Tables of Antibacterial Drug Dosages

The various antimicrobials for which the following recommended doses are listed are those commonly used for the care of infants and children. The recommendations are separated into two tables—Table 5.1 (p 543) for newborn infants and Table 5.2 (p 545) for older infants and children—because the physiologic immaturity of the newborn infant and resulting different pharmacokinetics necessitate alteration in dosage regimens to achieve maximum efficacy and limit toxicity. The table for older infants and children provides recommendations for both mild and severe infections; that for newborn infants is not divided because infections in this age group, with a few exceptions, are always considered severe.

The recommended doses are not absolute and are intended only as a guide. Clinical judgment about the disease, alterations in renal or hepatic function, and other factors affecting pharmacokinetics, patient response, and laboratory results may dictate modifications of these recommendations in the individual patient. In some cases, monitoring of serum drug concentrations is recommended to avoid toxicity and to ensure therapeutic efficacy.

Package insert information should be consulted for such details as the diluent for reconstitution of injectable preparations, measures to be taken to avoid incompatibilities, and other precautions.

TABLE 5.1—Antibacterial Drugs for Newborn Infants: Dose (mg/kg or Units [U]/kg[a]) and Frequency of Administration[b]

Drug	Route	Infants <1 week old		Infants ≥1 week old	
		BW ≤2,000 g	BW >2,000 g	BW ≤2,000 g	BW >2,000 g
Aminoglycosides[c,d]					
amikacin	IV, IM	7.5 q 12 h	7.5-10 q 12 h	7.5-10 q 8 h	10 q 8 h
gentamicin	IV, IM	2.5 q 12 h	2.5 q 12 h	2.5 q 8 h	2.5 q 8 h
kanamycin	IV, IM	7.5 q 12 h	7.5-10 q 12 h	7.5-10 q 8 h	10 q 8 h
neomycin sulfate	PO only	25 q 6 h	25 q 6 h	25 q 6 h	25 q 6 h
tobramycin	IV, IM	2.5 q 12 h	2.5 q 12 h	2.5 q 8 h	2.5 q 8 h
Antistaphylococcal penicillins[e]					
methicillin	IV, IM	25 q 12 h	25 q 8 h	25 q 8 h	25 q 6 h
nafcillin	IV, IM	25 q 12 h	25 q 8 h	25 q 8 h	25 q 6 h
oxacillin	IV, IM	25 q 12 h	25 q 8 h	25 q 8 h	25 q 6 h
Aztreonam[f]	IV, IM	30 q 12 h	30 q 8 h	30 q 8 h	30 q 6 h
Cephalosporins					
cefotaxime	IV, IM	50 q 12 h	50 q 8 or 12 h	50 q 8 h	50 q 6 or 8 h
ceftazidime	IV, IM	50 q 12 h	50 q 8 or 12 h	30 q 8 h	30 q 8 h
ceftriaxone[c]	IV, IM	50 q 24 h	50 q 24 h	50 q 24 h	50-75 q 24 h
Chloramphenicol[g]	IV, PO	25 q 24 h	25 q 24 h	25 q 24 h	25 q 12 h

TABLE 5.1—Antibacterial Drugs for Newborn Infants: Dose (mg/kg or Units [U]/kg^a) and Frequency of Administration^b *(continued)*

| Drug | Route | Infants <1 week old | | Infants ≥1 week old | |
		BW ≤2,000 g	BW >2,000 g	BW ≤2,000 g	BW >2,000 g
Clindamycin	IV, IM, PO	5 q 12 h	5 q 8 h	5 q 8 h	5 q 6 h
Erythromycin	PO	10 q 12 h	10 q 12 h	10 q 8 h	10 q 8 h
Metronidazole^h	IV, PO	7.5 q 24 h	7.5 q 12 h	7.5 q 12 h	15 q 12 h
Penicillins					
ampicillin^e	IV, IM	25 q 12 h	25 q 8 h	25 q 8 h	25 q 6 h
mezlocillin	IV, IM	75 q 12 h	75 q 8 h	75 q 8 or 12 h	75 q 6 h
penicillin G^e	IV, IM	25,000 U q 12 h	25,000 U q 8 h	25,000 U q 8 h	25,000 U q 6 h
penicillin G, procaine	IM	50,000 U q 24 h	50,000 U q 24 h	50,000 U q 24 h	50,000 U q 24 h
ticarcillin	IV, IM	75 q 12 h	75 q 8 h	75 q 8 h	75 q 6 h
Vancomycin^c	IV	10 q 12–18 h	10 q 8–12 h	10 q 8 h	10 q 8 h

^{a}Unless otherwise listed, dosages are given as mg/kg.
^{b}Abbreviations: BW = body weight, IV = intravenous, IM = intramuscular, PO = oral, q = every.
^{c}Optimal dosage should be based on determination of serum concentrations, especially in low-birth-weight (<1,500 g) infants. In very-low-birth-weight infants (<1,000 g) once daily dosing or dosing every 18 h may be appropriate in the 1st wk of life.
^{d}Dosages for the aminoglycosides may differ from those recommended by the manufacturer in the package insert.
^{e}For meningitis, the recommended dosage should be doubled.
^{f}FDA approval pending (as of December 1993).
^{g}Drug should not be administered to hyperbilirubinemia neonates, especially those born prematurely.
^{h}Safety in infants and children has not been established.

TABLE 5.2—Antibacterial Drugs for Pediatric Patients Beyond the Newborn Period

| Drug Generic (Trade) | Route | Dosage per kg/d | | Comments |
		Mild to Moderate Infections	Severe Infections	
Aminoglycosides[a]				
amikacin (Amikin)	IV, IM	Inappropriate	15-22.5 mg in 2 or 3 doses (daily adult dose, 15 mg/kg; maximum, 1.5 g)	30 mg in 3 doses is recommended by some consultants.
gentamicin (Garamycin)	IV, IM	Inappropriate	3-7.5 mg in 3 doses (daily adult dose is the same)	
kanamycin (Kantrex)	IV, IM	Inappropriate	15-22.5 mg in 2-3 doses (daily adult dose, 1-1.5 g)	30 mg in 3 doses is recommended by some consultants.
neomycin (numerous)	PO only	100 mg in 4 doses	100 mg in 4 doses	For some enteric infections.
netilmicin (Netromycin)	IV, IM	Inappropriate	3-7.5 mg in 3 doses (daily adult dose is the same)	
paromomycin (Humatin)	PO	30 mg in 3 doses (maximum daily adult dose, 4 g)	Inappropriate	Possibly effective for *Cryptosporidium* infection.
streptomycin[b] (numerous)	IM	Inappropriate	20-40 mg in 2-3 doses (daily adult dose, 1-2 g)	

TABLE 5.2—Antibacterial Drugs for Pediatric Patients Beyond the Newborn Period *(continued)*

Drug Generic (Trade)	Route	Dosage per kg/d		Comments
		Mild to Moderate Infections	Severe Infections	
tobramycin (Nebcin)	IV, IM	Inappropriate	3-7.5 mg in 3 doses (daily adult dose, 3-5 mg in 3 doses)	
Aztreonam[c] (Azactam)	IV, IM	90 mg in 3 doses (daily adult dose, 3 g)	120 mg in 4 doses (maximum daily adult dose, 8 g)	Approval pending (as of December 1993) for use in infants and children.
Cephalosporins[c]				
cefaclor (Ceclor)	PO	20-40 mg in 2 or 3 doses (daily adult dose, 750 mg-1.5 g)	Inappropriate	A twice-daily regimen has been demonstrated to be effective for treatment of acute otitis media.
cefadroxil (Duricef, Utracef)	PO	30 mg in 2 doses (maximum daily adult dose, 2 g)	Inappropriate	
cefamandole (Mandol)	IV, IM	50-100 mg in 3-4 doses (daily adult dose, 1.5-3 g)	100-150 mg in 4-6 doses (daily adult dose, 4-12 g)	Inadequate CSF concentrations for treatment of meningitis.
cefazolin (Kefzol, Ancef)	IV, IM	25-50 mg in 2-4 doses (daily adult dose, 750 mg-2 g)	50-150 mg in 3 or 4 doses (daily adult dose, 4-6 g)	

cefixime (Suprax)	PO	8 mg in 1 or 2 doses (daily adult dose, 400 mg)	Inappropriate	Diarrhea occurs in 10%-15% of patients.
cefonicid (Monocid)	IV, IM	20-40 mg in 1 dose (maximum daily adult dose, 2 g)	No data available	Not approved for children.
cefoperazone (Cefobid)	IV, IM	100-150 mg in 2 or 3 doses (maximum daily adult dose, 4 g)	No data available	Not approved for children.
ceforanide (Precef)	IV, IM	20-40 mg in 2 doses (daily adult dose, 1-2 g)	Not established	Not approved for use in infants.
cefotaxime (Claforan)	IV, IM	75-100 mg in 3 or 4 doses (daily adult dose, 4-6 g)	150-225 mg in 3 or 4 doses (daily adult dose, 8-10 g)	A regimen of 75 mg/kg 3 times daily has been successfully used for therapy of meningitis.
cefoxitin (Mefoxin)	IV, IM	80-100 mg in 3-4 doses (daily adult dose, 3-4 g)	80-160 mg in 4-6 doses (daily adult dose, 6-12 g)	
cefpodoxime proxetil (Vantin)	PO	10 mg in 2 doses (maximum daily adult dose, 800 mg)	Inappropriate	
cefprozil (Cefzil)	PO	30 mg in 2 doses (maximum daily adult dose, 1 g)	Inappropriate	

TABLE 5.2—Antibacterial Drugs for Pediatric Patients Beyond the Newborn Period *(continued)*

Drug Generic (Trade)	Route	Dosage per kg/d		Comments
		Mild to Moderate Infections	Severe Infections	
ceftazidime (Fortaz, Tazicef, Tazidime)	IV, IM	75-100 mg in 3 doses (daily adult dose, 3 g)	125-150 mg in 3 doses (daily adult dose, 6 g)	Only cephalosporin with anti-*Pseudomonas* activity that has been approved for use in children.
ceftibuten (Cedax)	PO	9 mg in 1 dose (maximum daily adult dose: see package insert)	Inappropriate	Approval for use in children expected in 1994.
ceftizoxime (Cefizox)	IV, IM	100-150 mg in 3 doses (daily adult dose, 3-4 g)	150-200 mg in 3 doses (daily adult dose, 4-6 g)	
ceftriaxone (Rocephin)	IV, IM	50-75 mg in 1 or 2 doses (daily adult dose, 2 g)	80-100 mg in 1 or 2 doses (daily adult dose, 4 g)	For meningitis therapy, once-daily doses of 100 mg/kg (maximum) is now approved.
cefuroxime (Zinacef)	IV, IM	75-100 mg in 3 doses (daily adult dose, 2-4 g)	175-240 mg in 3 doses (daily adult dose, 4-6 g)	Activity in CSF is lower than that for cefotaxime or ceftriaxone.
cefuroxime axetil (Ceftin)	PO	30-40 mg in 3 doses (daily adult dose, 1-2 g)	Inappropriate	Available only in tablets. Suspension may be available in 1994.
cephalexin (Keflex)	PO	25-50 mg in 4 doses (daily adult dose, 1-4 g)	Inappropriate	

cephalothin (Keflin)	IV, IM	80-100 mg in 4 doses (daily adult dose, 2-4 g)	100-150 mg in 4-6 doses (daily adult dose, 8-12 g)	
cephapirin (Cefadyl)	IV, IM	40 mg in 4 doses (daily adult dose, 2 g)	40-80 mg in 4 doses (daily adult dose, 4-12 g)	
cephradine (Anspor, Velosef)	PO	25-50 mg in 2-4 doses (daily adult dose, 1-4 g)	Inappropriate	
(Velosef)	IV, IM	25-50 mg in 4 doses (daily adult dose, 2 g); 50-100 mg in 4 doses (daily adult dose, 2-8 g)		
loracarbef (Lorabid)	PO	30 (otitis) - 15 (other indications) mg in 2 doses (maximum daily adult dose, 800 mg)	Inappropriate	More stable in suspension than cefaclor.
Chloramphenicol (Chloromycetin)				
palmitate	PO	Inappropriate	50-75 mg in 4 doses (daily adult dose, 1-2 g)	Optimal dosage is determined by measurement of serum concentrations with resulting modifications to achieve therapeutic concentrations. Use only for serious infections because of the rare occurrence of aplastic anemia after administration.
succinate	IV	Inappropriate	50-100 mg in 4 doses (daily adult dose, 2-4 g)	

TABLE 5.2—Antibacterial Drugs for Pediatric Patients Beyond the Newborn Period *(continued)*

| Drug Generic (Trade) | Route | Dosage per kg/d | | Comments |
		Mild to Moderate Infections	Severe Infections	
Clindamycin (Cleocin)	IM, IV	15-25 mg in 3-4 doses (daily adult dose, 600 mg-1.2 g)	25-40 mg in 3-4 doses (daily adult dose, 1.2-2.7 g)	Good activity against anaerobes, especially *Bacteroides* species. Should not be used in the treatment of central nervous system infections.
	PO	20-30 mg in 4 doses (daily adult dose, 600 mg-1.8 g)	Inappropriate	
Fluoroquinolones				
ciprofloxacin (Cipro)	PO	Inappropriate	30 mg in 2 doses (daily adult dose, 1,000-1,500 mg)	Not approved for patients younger than 18 y.
Imipenem-cilastatinc,d (Primaxin)	IV, IM	60 mg in 4 doses (daily adult dose, 1-2 g)	60 mg in 4 doses (daily adult dose, 2-4 g)	Not to be used for therapy of meningitis.
Macrolides				
erythromycins (numerous)	PO	20-50 mg in 2-4 doses (daily adult dose, 1-2 g)	Inappropriate	Available in base, stearate, ethyl succinate, and estolate preparations.
	IV	Inappropriate	15-50 mg in 4 doses (daily adult dose, 1-4 g)	Administer in a continuous drip or by slow infusion over 60 min or longer. May cause cardiac arrhythmia.

Drug	Route			Comments
azithromycine (Zithromax)	PO	5-12 mg/kg once daily (maximum daily adult dose, 600 mg)	Inappropriate	A single 1-g dose can be used for chlamydial urethritis in adults.
clarithromycind (Biaxin)	PO	7.5 mg in 2 doses (maximum daily adult dose, 1 g)	Inappropriate	Approval for use in children younger than 12 y is pending (as of December 1993).
Methenamine mandelate (Mandelamine)	PO	50-75 mg in 3-4 doses (daily adult dose, 2-4 g)	Inappropriate	Should not be used for infants; urine pH must be adjusted to 5-5.5.
Metronidazole (Flagyl)	PO	15-35 mg in 3 doses (maximum daily adult dose, 1-2 g)	Inappropriate	Safety in children has not been established.
Nitrofurantoin (Furadantin)	PO	5-7 mg in 4 doses (daily adult dose, 200-400 mg)	Inappropriate	Should not be used for young infants; prophylactic dose is 1-2 mg/kg/d in one dose.
PENICILLIN				
Broad-spectrum penicillinsc				
ampicillin (numerous)	IV, IM		200-300 mg in 4 doses (daily adult dose, 6-12 g)	Ineffective against beta-lactamase-producing *Haemophilus influenzae*, *Staphylococcus aureus*, and *Moraxella catarrhalis*.
	PO	50-100 mg in 4 doses (daily adult dose, 2-4 g)	Inappropriate	Diarrhea occurs in approximately 20%.

TABLE 5.2—Antibacterial Drugs for Pediatric Patients Beyond the Newborn Period *(continued)*

Drug Generic (Trade)	Route	Dosage per kg/d		Comments
		Mild to Moderate Infections	Severe Infections	
amoxicillin (numerous)	PO	25-50 mg in 3 doses (daily adult dose, 750 mg-1.5 g)	Inappropriate	
amoxicillin-clavulanate (Augmentin)	PO	20-40 mg of amoxicillin in 3 doses (daily adult dose, 750 mg-1.5 g)	Inappropriate	Dosage based on amoxicillin component; should not be exceeded because of potential to cause diarrhea.
bacampicillin (Spectrobid)	PO	25-50 mg in 2 doses (daily adult dose, 1-2 g)	Inappropriate	Prodrug of ampicillin with excellent bioavailability.
cyclacillin (Cyclapen)	PO	50-100 mg in 3-4 doses (daily adult dose, 1-2 g)	Inappropriate	Less active in vitro than ampicillin against *H influenzae.*
mezlocillin (Mezlin)	IV, IM	50-100 mg in 4 doses (daily adult dose, 6-8 g)	200-300 mg in 4-6 doses (daily adult dose, 12-18 g)	Contains 1.85 mEq of Na per gram.
piperacillin[d] (Pipracil)	IV, IM	50-100 mg in 4 doses (daily adult dose, 6-8 g)	200-300 mg in 4-6 doses (daily adult dose, 12-18 g)	Contains 1.85 mEq of Na per gram.
ticarcillin (Ticar)	IV, IM	50-100 mg in 4 doses (daily adult dose, 2-4 g)	200-300 mg in 4-6 doses (daily adult dose, 12-24 g)	Contains 5.2 mEq of Na per gram.

Drug	Route			Comments
ticarcillin-clavulanate[c] (Timentin)	IV, IM	50-100 mg of ticarcillin in 4 doses (2-4 g)	200-300 mg of ticarcillin in 4 doses (12-24 g)	
Penicillin G and V[c,f]				
Penicillin G, crystalline K or Na (numerous)	IV, IM	25,000-50,000 U in 4 doses	100,000-400,000 U in 4-6 doses	1.68 mEq K or Na per 1,000,000 U; use Na salt for large IV doses.
Penicillin G, procaine (numerous)	IM	25,000-50,000 U in 1-2 doses	Inappropriate	Contraindicated in procaine allergy.
Penicillin G, benzathine (Bicillin, Permapen)	IM	<27.3 kg (60 lb): 600,000 U ≥27.3 kg: 1,200,000 U	Inappropriate	Major use is prevention of rheumatic fever by treatment and prophylaxis of streptococcal infections.
Penicillin G, potassium oral (numerous)	PO	25,000-50,000 U in 3 or 4 doses	Inappropriate	Variable absorption; optimal to administer unbuffered penicillin G at least 1 h before, or 2 h after meals.
Penicillin V (numerous)	PO	25,000-50,000 U in 3 or 4 doses	Inappropriate	1,600 U is equivalent to 1 mg; optimal to administer on empty stomach.
Penicillinase-resistant penicillins[c]				
methicillin (Staphcillin)	IV, IM	100-200 mg in 4 doses (daily adult dose, 4-8 g)	150-200 mg in 4-6 doses (daily adult dose, 4-12 g)	Methicillin-resistant staphylococci are usually resistant to all other semi-synthetic antistaphylococcal penicillins and synthetic antistaphylococcal cephalosporins. Interstitial nephritis (ie, hematuria) occurs in 0%-4% of patients.

TABLE 5.2—Antibacterial Drugs for Pediatric Patients Beyond the Newborn Period *(continued)*

| Drug Generic (Trade) | Route | Dosage per kg/d | | Comments |
		Mild to Moderate Infections	Severe Infections	
oxacillin (Prostaphlin, Bactocil)	IV, IM		150-200 mg in 4-6 doses (daily adult dose, 4-12 g)	Absorption of oral preparations is variable; administer at least 1 h before, or 2 h after meals.
	PO	100-200 mg in 4 doses (daily adult dose, 2-4 g)	Inappropriate	
nafcillin (Unipen, Natcil)	IV, IM	50-100 mg in 4 doses (daily adult dose, 2-4 g)	150-200 mg in 4-6 doses (daily adult dose, 4-12 g)	Serum concentrations after oral administration are low compared with those after other orally administered antistaphylococcal drugs.
	PO	50-100 mg in 4 doses (daily adult dose, 2-4 g)	Inappropriate	
cloxacillin (Tegopen, Cloxapen)	PO	50-100 mg in 4 doses (daily adult dose, 2-4 g)	Inappropriate	
dicloxacillin (Dynapen, Pathocil)	PO	25-50 mg in 4 doses (daily adult dose, 1-2 g)	Inappropriate	Excellent serum concentrations after oral administrations.

Polymyxins

Drug	Route			Comments
colistimethate (Coly-Mycin M)	IM	Inappropriate	2.5-5 mg in 4 doses (daily adult dose, 300 mg)	Limited-purpose drug.
colistin sulfate (Coly-Mycin S)	PO	5-15 mg in 3 doses	5-15 mg in 3 doses (daily adult dose, 200-300 mg)	Possible use for some enteric infections.
polymyxin B (Aerosporin)	IM	Inappropriate	2.5-4 mg in 4 doses	Limited-purpose drug (1 mg = 10,000 U).
	PO	10-20 mg in 3-4 doses	10-20 mg in 3-4 doses	Possible use for some enteric infections.

Sulfonamides

Drug	Route			Comments
sulfadiazine[g]	PO, IV	100-150 mg in 4 doses	100-150 mg in 4 doses	The first dose should be doubled; daily adult oral doses, 2-4 g; for IV, same dose as for children.
sulfisoxazole (Gantrisin)	PO, IV	100-150 mg in 4 doses	100-150 mg in 4 doses	
triple sulfonamides (numerous)	PO	120-150 mg in 4 doses	120-150 mg in 4 doses	
trimethoprim-sulfamethoxazole (Bactrim, Septra)	PO	8-12 mg trimethoprim-40-60 mg sulfamethoxazole in 2 doses (daily adult dose, 320 mg trimethoprim-1.6 g sulfamethoxazole)	20 mg trimethoprim-100 mg sulfamethoxazole in 4 doses (for use only in *Pneumocystis carinii* pneumonia)	For prophylaxis in immunocompromised patients, recommended daily dose is 5 mg trimethoprim-25 mg sulfamethoxazole per kg/d in 2 doses.

TABLE 5.2—Antibacterial Drugs for Pediatric Patients Beyond the Newborn Period *(continued)*

Drug Generic (Trade)	Route	Dosage per kg/d		Comments
		Mild to Moderate Infections	Severe Infections	
trimethoprim-sulfamethoxazole (Bactrim, Septra) *(cont.)*	IV	Inappropriate	20 mg trimethoprim-100 mg sulfa-methoxazole in 4 doses (for treatment of *Pneumocystis* infection)	Use intravenous formulation when oral formulation cannot be administered.
Tetracyclines (numerous)	IV	Inappropriate	10-25 mg in 2-4 doses (daily adult dose, 1-2 g)	Responsible for staining of developing teeth; use only in children 9 y or older except in circumstances in which benefits of therapy exceed risks and alternative drugs are less effective or toxic.
	PO	20-50 mg in 4 doses (daily adult dose, 1-2 g)	Inappropriate	
doxycycline (numerous)	PO, IV	2-4 mg in 1-2 doses (daily adult dose, 100-200 mg)	Inappropriate	Side effects similar to those of other tetracycline products.

| Vancomycin (Vancocin, Vancoled, Vancor) | IV | 40 mg in 4 doses (daily adult dose,[h] 1-2 g) | 40-60 mg in 4 doses (daily adult dose,[h] 2-4 g) | Some experts suggest a dose of 60 mg/kg/d for central nervous system or disseminated infections; dose should be given over at least 60 min. |

[a]Dosages for the aminoglycosides may differ from those recommended by the manufacturers (see package insert).

[b]As of December 1993, available from Pfizer Streptomycin Program, Pfizer Pharmaceuticals, New York, NY (800/254-4445).

[c]In patients with history of allergy to penicillin or one of its many congeners, alternative drugs are recommended. In some circumstances, a cephalosporin or other beta-lactam class drug may be acceptable. However, these drugs should not be used in patients with an immediate hypersensitivity (anaphylaxis) to penicillin because approximately 5% to 15% of penicillin-allergic patients will also be allergic to the cephalosporins.

[d]Not approved for use in patients younger than 12 y.

[e]Not approved for use in patients younger than 16 y.

[f]Patients with history of allergy to penicillin G or V should be considered for subsequent skin testing. Many such patients can be treated safely with penicillin, since only 10% of children with such history are proven allergic when skin tested.

[g]As of 1993, sulfadiazine is no longer marketed in the United States. Until a domestic source of the drug is re-established, the drug may be obtained from the Division of Parasitic Diseases at the Centers for Disease Control and Prevention (see Directory of Telephone Numbers, p 601).

[h]In adults, daily dose is given in 2-4 divided doses.

Dexamethasone Therapy for Bacterial Meningitis in Infants and Children

Case fatality rates for bacterial meningitis in infants and children in the United States are from 5% to 10%. As many as 20% of survivors have long-term sequelae, the most common of which is hearing impairment. The reported incidence of hearing loss after meningitis has ranged from 5% to 31% of patients, depending on the selection of patients, techniques used to assess hearing, and etiology. In one study from 1972 to 1977, hearing loss was documented in 31% of patients with *Streptococcus pneumoniae* meningitis, in 10% with *Neisseria meningitidis* meningitis, and in 6% with *Haemophilus influenzae* type b meningitis. Newer antimicrobial agents with superior bactericidal activity in cerebrospinal fluid (CSF) have not lowered morbidity and case fatality rates in comparison to that occurring with conventional antibiotic therapy.

The pathophysiologic events believed to contribute to adverse outcome from bacterial meningitis include alteration of cerebral capillary endothelial cells that comprise the blood-brain barrier, cytotoxic and vasogenic cerebral edema, and increased intracranial pressure. These events can lead to decreased cerebral perfusion pressure, resulting in diminution in cerebral blood flow and subsequent regional hypoxia and focal ischemia of brain tissue.

Because of its anti-inflammatory effects, corticosteroid therapy has been evaluated in experimental meningitis and in infants and children with meningitis. Dexamethasone produced significant decreases in intracranial pressure, brain edema, and lactate concentrations in CSF in experimental *H influenzae* type b and *S pneumoniae* meningitis. Additionally, dexamethasone administration was associated with lowered mortality and clinically evident neurologic sequelae in rabbits with experimental pneumococcal meningitis.

Results of double-blind, placebo-controlled trials of dexamethasone therapy for bacterial meningitis demonstrate decreased hearing loss and/or neurologic sequelae in dexamethasone recipients with *H influenzae* infection. Approximately 75% of patients in these studies were infected with this organism. No beneficial effect of dexamethasone on neurologic and audiologic outcome could be demonstrated in patients infected with *S pneumoniae* or *N meningitidis*. However, the limited number of patients with these infections in these studies have been inadequate to determine the effectiveness of dexamethasone in infants and children with pneumococcal or meningococcal meningitis. With the substantial decline in the incidence of *H influenzae* type b disease since the introduction of conjugate vaccination, the total number of cases of bacterial meningitis in infants and children has decreased and, as a result, the proportion of cases of bacterial meningitis caused by pneumococci and meningococci has increased substantially.

Adverse Effects

Dexamethasone therapy was not associated with delayed sterilization of CSF cultures in these studies. In approximately one fifth to two thirds of patients, secondary, low-grade fever occurred 24 to 48 hours after stopping dexamethasone, and lasted 24 to 36 hours. Rarely, dexamethasone recipients have developed gastrointestinal bleeding requiring blood transfusions on the second and third days of steroid treatment. However, whether the bleeding was a result of dexamethasone therapy is uncertain.

Recommendations

1. Dexamethasone therapy should be considered when bacterial meningitis in infants and children 6 weeks and older is diagnosed or strongly suspected on the basis of the CSF tests, including Gram-stained smears, after the physician has weighed the benefits and possible risks and before the etiology has been established.
2. Dexamethasone is recommended for treatment of infants and children with *H influenzae* meningitis.
3. Dexamethasone should be considered for the treatment of infants and children with pneumococcal or meningococcal meningitis. However, its efficacy for these infections is unproven, and some experts do not recommend its use.
4. The recommended dexamethasone regimen is 0.6 mg/kg/d in four divided doses, given intravenously, for the first 4 days of antibiotic treatment. A recent placebo-controlled trial indicates that a 2-day regimen of dexamethasone is also effective.
5. If dexamethasone is given, it should be administered as early as possible, preferably at the time of, or shortly after, the first dose of antibacterial therapy. Dexamethasone therapy when initiated more than 12 hours after the start of parenterally administered antimicrobial therapy is unlikely to be effective.
6. Dexamethasone should not be used for suspected or proven nonbacterial meningitis. If dexamethasone had been started before the diagnosis of nonbacterial meningitis was made, it should be discontinued.
7. "Partially treated" meningitis with negative cultures is not an indication for continued dexamethasone therapy.
8. If dexamethasone is used, all patients, not just those with severe disease, should be treated.
9. No data are currently available on which to base a recommendation concerning the use of dexamethasone for treatment of bacterial meningitis in infants younger than 6 weeks, or of meningitis in those with congenital or acquired abnormalities of the central nervous system, with or without a prosthetic device.
10. Measurements of hemoglobin concentrations and examinations of stool for blood should be performed regularly during dexamethasone therapy. If gross blood is found, dexamethasone therapy should be stopped and the patient should be observed closely for possible transfusion therapy.

Drugs of Choice for Invasive and Other Serious Fungal Infections

Table 5.3 (p 560) lists the drugs of choice for invasive and other serious fungal infections.

TABLE 5.3—Drugs of Choice for Invasive and Other Serious Fungal Infections

Disease	Intravenous		Oral, Absorbable		Intravenous or Oral	
	Amphotericin B	Miconazole	Flucytosine	Ketoconazole	Itraconazole*	Fluconazole*
Aspergillosis	P				A	
Blastomycosis	P			A	M	
Candidiasis: chronic, mucocutaneous	A	A	A	P		
Candidiasis: oropharyngeal, gastrointestinal	A (severe cases)	A	A	P		A
Candidiasis, systemic	P, S		S	A, M	A	A
Coccidioidomycosis	P				A	A
Cryptococcosis	C		C			A
Histoplasmosis	P			A	M	
Mucormycosis (phycomycosis, zygomycosis)	P					
Paracoccidioidomycosis (South American blastomycosis)	P (severe cases)	A		P	A	

*Efficacy and safety have not been established for children.
P=Preferred treatment in most cases.
M=For mild and moderately severe cases.
A=Efficacy less well established or alternative drug.
C=Combination recommended.
S=Combination recommended if infection is severe or central nervous system is involved.

Recommended Doses of Parenteral and Oral Antifungal Drugs

Table 5.4 lists recommended dosages of parenteral and oral antifungal drugs.

TABLE 5.4—Recommended Doses of Parenteral and Oral Antifungal Drugs

Drug	Route[a]	Dose (per day)	Adverse Reactions[b]
Amphotericin B[c]	IV	0.25 mg/kg (after test dose[d]) initially, increase as tolerated to 0.5-1 mg/kg; infuse as single dose over 4-6 h	Fever, chills, phlebitis, renal dysfunction, hypokalemia, anemia, cardiac arrhythmias, anaphylactoid reaction, hematologic abnormalities
	IT	0.025 mg, increase to 0.1-0.5 mg twice weekly	Radiculitis, sensory loss, and foot drop
Clotrimazole (troches)	PO (Topical)	10-mg tablet 5 times daily (dissolved slowly in mouth)	Nausea, vomiting, and increase in serum transaminase
Fluconazole	IV PO	Children[e]: 3-6 mg/kg/d Adults: 200 mg once, followed by 100 mg/d for oropharyngeal, esophageal candidiasis; 400 mg once, followed by 200-400 mg/d for cryptococcal meningitis (200 mg/d for maintenance in patients with AIDS)	Rash, nausea, abdominal pain, diarrhea, headache, and possible hepatotoxicity
Flucytosine	PO	50 to 150 mg/kg in 4 doses at 6-h intervals (adjust dose if renal dysfunction)	Bone marrow suppression; renal dysfunction can lead to drug accumulation; nausea, vomiting, increase in transaminases, BUN, and creatinine
Griseofulvin	PO	Ultramicrosize: 7.3 mg/kg, single dose; maximum dose, 375-750 mg Microsize: 15-20 mg/kg/d divided in 2 doses; maximum dose, 500-1,000 mg	Rash, leukopenia, proteinuria, paresthesias, gastrointestinal symptoms, and mental confusion
Itraconazole	PO	Children: dose not established; doses in children aged 3 to 16 y 100 mg/d have been reported. Adults: 200 mg once or twice daily	Nausea, epigastric pain, headache, edema, hypokalemia, increased serum aminotransferase, hypertension, adrenal insufficiency

TABLE 5.4—Recommended Doses of Parenteral and Oral
Antifungal Drugs *(continued)*

Drug	Route[a]	Dose (per day)	Adverse Reactions[b]
Ketoconazole	PO	Children: 3.3-6.6 mg/kg, once daily[f] Adults: 200-400 mg once daily	Rash, anaphylaxis, nausea, vomiting, abdominal pain, fever, gynecomastia, thrombocytopenia, hepatoxicity, and depression of endocrine function (dose-dependent, reversible), should not be given concurrently with terfenadine (an antihistamine)
Miconazole	IV	20 to 40 mg/kg/d, divided into 3 infusions 8 h apart; maximum 15 mg/kg per infusion. Infuse over 30-60 min	Phlebitis, rash, fever, nausea, anemia, hyponatremia, thrombocytopenia, and hyperlipemia
	IT	20 mg per dose for 3 to 7 d	
Nystatin	PO	Infants: 200,000 U, 4 times daily Children and adults: 400,000-600,000 U, 4 times daily	Nausea, vomiting, and diarrhea

[a]Abbreviations: IV = intravenous, IT = intrathecal, PO = oral.
[b]See package insert or listing in current edition of *Physicians' Desk Reference*. Montvale, NJ: Medical Economics.
[c]For details, see below.
[d]Test dose is 0.1 mg/kg, with maximum dose of 1 mg/kg (see below).
[e]For children 2 y and younger, the daily dose has not been established.
[f]Efficacy has not been established for children. A small number of children aged 3 to 13 y have been treated safely with this dosage.

Systemic Treatment With Amphotericin B

Amphotericin B is the most important antifungal drug. However, since it causes many major and minor adverse reactions, particularly nephrotoxicity, its parenteral use is primarily restricted to selected, potentially fatal fungal infections. Before using amphotericin B, the physician should consult the manufacturer's package insert for specific precautions, adverse reactions, and infusion information.

Amphotericin B is initially administered intravenously in a single test dose of 0.1 mg/kg (maximum, 1 mg) during a 20-minute to 4-hour period to assess the patient's febrile and hemodynamic responses. Temperature, pulse, respiration, and blood pressure should be carefully monitored during the infusion. The first therapeutic dose is 0.25 mg/kg administered over a 2- to 4-hour interval, and is given the same day as the test dose. Patients with severe reactions to the test dose should receive a lower dose. Subsequently, the dose is increased in daily increments of 0.1 to 0.25 mg/kg for 3 to 4 days until a total dose of 0.4 to 1 mg/kg is reached. In life-threatening situations, 0.25-mg/kg increments can be given in successive 2- to 4-hour infusions during a 12- to 24-hour period to achieve the maximum total daily dose of 1 mg/kg. Low doses of amphotericin B (eg, 0.1 to 0.3 kg/d) have been used successfully in infections such as *Candida* esophagitis.

The serum concentration is not significantly increased in patients with impaired renal function. Hemodialysis and peritoneal dialysis do not remove significant amounts of the drug.

In some illnesses, doses of 1.25 or 1.5 mg/kg may be necessary. The proper dose for preterm and newborn infants has not been determined, but the doses given here have been used successfully. Amphotericin B must be administered in 5% dextrose in water. The preparation should be discarded if the solution becomes turbid on addition of amphotericin B.

After completing 1 week of daily therapy, adequate serum concentrations of the drug can usually be maintained by administering double the daily dose (maximum 1.5 mg/kg) on alternate days.

The duration of therapy depends on the type and extent of the specific fungal infection.

Commonly observed adverse reactions include the following: fever (sometimes with shaking chills), nausea and vomiting, generalized body pains, pain at the intravenous administration site (phlebitis), abnormal renal function (hypokalemia, elevated serum creatinine and BUN concentrations, decreased creatinine clearance rate, and a diminished ability to concentrate urine), and anemia. An irreversible reduction in glomerular filtration rate often follows a therapeutic course of amphotericin B. Pretreatment with antipyretics can be helpful in alleviating febrile reactions. Hydrocortisone (25 to 50 mg in adults) can be added to the infusion to reduce febrile and other systemic reactions. Tolerance to the febrile reactions develops with time, allowing tapering and eventual discontinuation of the hydrocortisone. Some experts add heparin to the infusion to decrease phlebitis. Less common severe reactions include anuria, oliguria, hematologic abnormalities, hypomagnesemia, cardiovascular toxicity (arrhythmias, hypertension, and hypotension), anaphylactoid reactions, and convulsions and other neurologic symptoms.

For patients with central nervous system fungal infections who do not respond to intravenous therapy, consideration should be given to the concomitant administration of amphotericin B intrathecally, intraventricularly, or intracisternally. Preferably, injections should be given into the lateral ventricles through a cisternal Ommaya reservoir. The value of this approach has been clearly established only in coccidioidal meningitis, but it may be justified in the nonresponsive patient with other fungal infections, as cerebrospinal fluid concentrations of the drug are low or undetectable after intravenous administration of the drug. Amphotericin B may be administered twice weekly, or more frequently, in the lumbar, cisternal, or ventricular areas. The usual starting dose in adults is 0.1 mg three times a week; subsequent doses are increased by doubling until a maintenance dose of 0.5 mg is reached. Hydrocortisone (10 to 15 mg in adults) is added as required to relieve headaches. The solution should be freshly prepared and diluted with 2 to 10 mL of sterile 5% dextrose in water (10% dextrose in water for intralumbar injections) without preservatives. Before injection, the solution should be further diluted with spinal fluid so that the final concentration per milliliter is one tenth the dose. Duration of therapy depends on the clinical and mycologic responses. The spinal fluid should be cultured for fungi and bacteria as often as necessary. Nausea, vomiting, urinary retention, leg and back pain, headache, transitory radiculitis, sensory loss, and foot drop have been observed as a result of intrathecal therapy; permanent changes have also occurred.

Renal toxicity may be enhanced with the concomitant administration of amphotericin B and aminoglycosides, cyclosporine, cisplatin, or nitrogen mustard compounds.

Topical Drugs for Superficial and Fungal Infections

The recommended topical drugs for superficial and fungal infections are listed in Table 5.5 (p 565).

Antiviral Drugs

Table 5.6 (p 567) provides a list of drugs recommended for different viral infections.

TABLE 5.5—Topical Drugs for Superficial Fungal Infections

Drug	Strength	Formulation*	Brand Name(s)	Application(s) per Day	Adverse Reactions/Notes†
Amphotericin B	3%	C,L,O	Fungizone	2-4	Drying, local irritation, erythema, pruritus, burning; more effective topical preparations are now available
Ciclopirox	1%	C,L	Loprox	2	Irritation, erythema, burning
Clotrimazole	1%	C,L,S	Lotrimin‡ Mycelex‡	2	Erythema, stinging, blistering, peeling, edema, pruritus, hives, burning
Econazole	1%	C	Spectazole	2	Burning, pruritis, stinging, erythema
Haloprogin	1%	C,S	Halotex	2	Burning, irritation, erythema, scaling, pruritis, folliculitis
Ketaconazole	2%	C,Sh	Nizoral	1	Irritation, pruritis, stinging
Miconazole	2%	C,P,Su	Micatin‡ Monistat-Derm	2	Irritation, dermatitis
Naftifine	1%	C	Naftin	2	Burning, stinging, erythema, pruritis, irritation; fungicidal agent
Nystatin	100,000 U/mL	C,L,P,O,Su	Mycolog Mycostatin Mytrex Nilstat Nystatin Nystex (Others)	2	Rare adverse reactions; effective against yeast only

TABLE 5.5—Topical Drugs for Superficial Fungal Infections *(continued)*

Drug	Strength	Formulation*†	Brand Name(s)	Application(s) per Day	Adverse Reactions/Notes†
Oxiconazole	1%	C	Oxistat	1	Pruritis, burning, irritation, erythema
Sulconazole	1%	C,S	Exelderm	1-2	Pruritis, burning, stinging
Terbinafine	1%	C	Lamsil	1-2	Pruritis, irritation, burning
Tolnaftate	1%	C,P,S	Tinactin‡	2	Rare adverse reactions
Undecylenate	10%–20%	P,C,O,L	Caldesene‡ Cruex‡ Desenex‡ Others	2	Irritation
Other Remedies					
Benzoic acid (12%) and salicylic acid (3%)		S,O	Whitfield's ointment‡	2	Irritation, burning; potent keratolytic agent
Castellani's paint	—	S	—	1-2	Local irritation (contains basic fuchsin, phenol, resorcinol, acetone, alcohol)
Gentian violet‡	1%-2%	S	—	2	Staining
Selenium sulfide‡	1%	Sh	—	1	For tinea capitis§
Sodium thiosulfate	25%	S	Tinver	1-2	For tinea versicolor

*C=cream, F=foam, L=lotion, O=ointment, P=powder, S=solution, Sh=shampoo, Su=suppositories
†For use in pregnancy, see package insert.
‡Nonprescription drug.
§Primary therapy is oral griseofulvin.

TABLE 5.6—Antiviral Drugs

Generic (Trade Name)	Indication	Usually Recommended Dosage
Acyclovir[a] (Zovirax)	Genital herpes simplex virus (HSV) infection, first episode	Oral - 1,200 mg/d in 3 divided doses for 7-10 d.[b] IV - 15 mg/kg/d in 3 divided doses for 5-7 d.
	Genital HSV infection, recurrence	Oral - 1,200 mg/d in 3 divided doses or 1,600 mg/d in 2 divided doses for 5 d.[b]
	Recurrent genital HSV episodes in patient with frequent recurrences: Chronic suppressive therapy	Oral - 800-1,000 mg/d in 2-5 divided doses for as long as 12 continuous months.[b]
	HSV in immunocompromised host (localized, progressive, or disseminated)[c]	IV - For children <1 y, except neonates (see Neonatal HSV, p 568): 15-30 mg/kg/d in 3 divided doses for 7-14 d. Some experts also recommend this dose for children ≥1 y. IV - For children ≥1 y: 750 mg/m²/d in 3 divided doses for 7-14 d. Some experts recommend 1,500 mg/m²/d in 3 divided doses. Oral - 1,000 mg/d in 3-5 divided doses for 7-14 d.[b]
	Prophylaxis of HSV in immunocompromised HSV-seropositive patient[c]	Oral - 600-1,000 mg/d in 3-5 divided doses during risk period.[b] IV - 750 mg/m²/d in 3 divided doses during risk period.
	HSV encephalitis	IV - For children <1 y: 30 mg/kg/d in 3 divided doses for a minimum of 14 d. Some experts also recommend this dose for children ≥1 y. IV - For children ≥1 y: 1,500 mg/m²/d in 3 divided doses for 14-21 d. Some experts also recommend this dose for children <1 y.

TABLE 5.6—Antiviral Drugs *(continued)*

Generic (Trade Name)	Indication	Usually Recommended Dosage
	Neonatal HSV[c]	IV - 30 mg/kg/d in 3 divided doses for 14-21 d. Some experts recommend 45-60 mg/kg/d in 3 divided doses for term infants. For premature infants, 20 mg/kg/d in 2 divided doses is recommended for 14-21 d.
	Varicella or zoster in immunocompromised host	IV - For children <1 y: 30 mg/kg/d in 3 divided doses. Some experts also recommend this dose for children ≥1 y.
		IV - For children ≥1 y: 1,500 mg/m^2/d in 3 divided doses for 7-10 d.
	Zoster in immunocompetent host[c]	IV - Same as for zoster in immunocompromised host.
		Oral - 4,000 mg/d in 5 divided doses for 5-7 d for patients ≥12 y.[b]
	Varicella in immunocompetent host[d]	Oral - 80 mg/kg/d in 4 divided doses for 5 d, maximum dose 3,200 mg/d.
	Prophylaxis of cytomegalovirus (CMV) infection in immunocompromised host (eg, transplant recipient)[c]	Oral - 800-3,200 mg/d in 1-4 divided doses during risk period.[a,b]
		IV - 1,500 mg/m^2/d in 3 divided doses during risk period.
Amantadine (Symmetrel)	Influenza A: treatment and prophylaxis	Oral - See Influenza (p 277), including Table 3.24 (p 278).
Didanosine (DDI; formerly termed dideoxyinosine) (Videx)	Symptomatic HIV infection with intolerance of zidovudine; or clinical or immunologic deterioration during zidovudine therapy[e]	Oral - 200-300 mg/m^2/d in 2-3 divided doses.

Drug	Indication	Route - Dose
Foscarnet[a] (Foscavir)	CMV retinitis in patients with AIDS	IV - 180 mg/kg/d in 3 divided doses for 14-21 d, then 60-120 mg/kg once daily as maintenance dose.
	HSV infection resistant to acyclovir in immunocompromised host[c,e]	IV - 120 mg/kg/d in 3 divided doses until resolution of infection.
Ganciclovir (Cytovene)	Acquired CMV retinitis in immunocompromised host[f]	IV - 10 mg/kg/d in 2 divided doses for 14-21 d. For long-term suppression, 5 mg/kg/d for 5-7 d/wk.
	Prophylaxis of CMV in high-risk host[c]	IV - 10 mg/kg/d in 2 divided doses for 1 wk, then 5 mg/kg/d in 1 dose for 100 d.
Ribavirin (Virazole)	Treatment of respiratory syncytial virus (RSV) infection	Aerosol - Given by a small particle generator, in a solution of 6 g in 300 mL sterile water (20 mg/mL), for 12-20 h/d for 1-7 d; longer treatment may be necessary in some patients.
Rimantadine (Flumadine)	Influenza A: treatment and prophylaxis	Oral - See Influenza (p 277), including Table 3.24 (p 278).
Vidarabine (Vira-A)	Neonatal HSV[g]	IV - 15-30 mg/kg/d given in 1 dose during 12-24 h for 10-21 d.
	Varicella or zoster in immunocompromised host[c,g]	IV - 10 mg/kg/d given in 1 dose during 12-24 h for 5-10 d.
Zidovudine (formerly termed azidothymidine [AZT]) (Retrovir)	Symptomatic HIV infection[h]	Oral - For children <12 y: 720 mg/m²/d (maximum 800 mg/d) in 4 divided doses.[i] For children ≥12 y and adults: 500-600 mg/d in 3-6 divided doses.

[a] Dose should be decreased in patients with impaired renal function.
[b] Oral dosage of acyclovir in children should not exceed 80 mg/kg/d.
[c] Drug is not licensed for this indication or is investigational, as of December 1993.
[d] Selective indications; see Varicella-Zoster Infections (p 512).
[e] Indications and dosage for treatment of children are evolving.
[f] Some experts use ganciclovir in immunocompromised host with CMV gastrointestinal disease or with CMV pneumonitis (with or without CMV Immune Globulin Intravenous).
[g] Alternative to acyclovir, which is the usual drug of choice.
[h] Indications for treatment of children are evolving (see HIV Infection and AIDS, p 261).
[i] For infants, dose should be recalculated every 2 mo.

Use of Ribavirin in the Treatment of Respiratory Syncytial Virus Infection*

Ribavirin is an antiviral drug that was approved by the Food and Drug Administration in 1986 for aerosol treatment of serious respiratory syncytial virus (RSV) infections in hospitalized children. Ribavirin has a broad spectrum of antiviral activity in vitro, where it inhibits replication of RSV, influenza, parainfluenza, adenovirus, measles, Lassa fever, and Hantaan viruses. Proof of efficacy for human infection has been obtained in double-blind, placebo-controlled studies of RSV, Lassa fever, and Korean hemorrhagic fever. Presently, only anecdotal reports support the efficacy of this drug for treatment of measles or parainfluenza infection. Ribavirin treatment for RSV infections has been controversial because of the aerosol route of administration, concern for potential toxicity for exposed persons, cost, and the unpredictable and highly variable course of illness in the absence of specific therapy. These issues necessitate ongoing review of ribavirin therapy and the following updated recommendations by the American Academy of Pediatrics.

Background

RSV Disease

Respiratory syncytial virus is the most important cause of lower respiratory tract disease in infants and young children. Disease usually appears in yearly outbreaks in the winter or spring, and essentially all children become infected during their first 3 years of life. The number of infected infants who require hospitalization has been estimated to range from 1 to 50 per 1,000 in different locations. Currently, the mortality rate in hospitalized infants who previously were healthy is low (less than 1%). In infants with underlying diseases, however, the mortality can be much higher. Conditions that increase the risk of severe or fatal RSV infection are cyanotic or complicated congenital heart disease (including pulmonary hypertension); underlying pulmonary disease, especially bronchopulmonary dysplasia; prematurity; and immunodeficiency disease or therapy causing immunosuppression at any age.

Most previously healthy infants infected with RSV do not require hospitalization, and many who are hospitalized improve within a few days with supportive care and are discharged after a stay ranging from 3 to 5 days. Long-term sequelae of RSV infection are difficult to assess. Evidence recently has accumulated suggesting that some infected children develop long-term abnormalities in pulmonary function. Although these abnormalities may be subclinical in most children, some subjects have recurrent wheezing. Whether treatment of the initial respiratory syncytial virus infection can alter the rate or severity of such sequelae is unknown.

Ribavirin

Aerosolized ribavirin is the first specific drug available for treatment of RSV infections. It is a synthetic nucleoside analogue (1-β-D-ribafuranosyl-1,2,4-

---

*Reproduced from *Pediatrics*. 1993;92:501-504. References have been omitted but are given in the original publication.

triazole-3-carboxamide) resembling guanosine and inosine; it appears to interfere with the expression of messenger RNA and to inhibit viral protein synthesis. It is not significantly incorporated into host cell RNA or DNA.

Clinical Studies

Ribavirin is administered as aerosolized particles small enough (median aerosol diameter, 1 to 2 μm) to reach the lower respiratory tract. It is delivered via an oxygen hood, tent, or mask for 12 to 20 hours each day for a mean of 4 days. In controlled studies involving both healthy infants and those with underlying disease, clinical improvement was greater in ribavirin recipients than in placebo recipients. Ribavirin had a beneficial effect on some signs, such as retraction and rales, but not on others, such as fever and wheezing. However, these latter signs were present in only a minority of patients. Improvement in arterial blood oxygenation following ribavirin therapy has been substantial. In one study, the treated group had a mean arterial oxygen pressure (PaO_2) of 49.4 mm Hg at the start of therapy and 62.4 mm Hg at the end, a mean increase of 13 mm Hg, which was significantly greater than the comparable values for the placebo group (at the start and end of therapy 52 mm Hg and 56 mm Hg, respectively). The effect of therapy on persistence of virus in secretions differed in various studies.

No appreciable toxicity has been observed in any of the controlled trials, or in other follow-up studies. Although reversible bronchospasm has been observed occasionally (less than 0.1%), hyperactivity of the airways has not been demonstrated in studies of pulmonary function during administration of ribavirin aerosol. The effect of ribavirin aerosol on pulmonary function was examined in adult volunteers infected with RSV in a controlled, double-blind study. Serial pulmonary function tests, which included carbachol challenge, demonstrated no alterations in volunteers during ribavirin therapy or when tested 1 month later. The long-term effects of ribavirin on pulmonary function and on the sequelae of RSV infection require further investigation.

In a study of mechanically ventilated infants, most of whom were previously healthy, ribavirin treatment was safe and was associated with a reduced need for mechanical ventilation and supplemental oxygen, shorter duration of hospitalization, and cost-effectiveness.

One potential problem is deposition of the drug in the ventilator delivery system, which appears to be dependent on temperature, humidity, and electrostatic forces. This deposition can lead to malfunction or obstruction of the expiratory valve, resulting in inadvertently high positive end-expiratory pressures. The use of one-way valves in the inspiratory lines, a breathing circuit filter in the expiratory line, and frequent monitoring and filter replacement by trained staff have been effective in preventing these problems.

Experience with antiviral agents used to treat other viruses has raised the additional concern of development of resistance to ribavirin by RSV. To date, no change in susceptibility of any viral isolate to ribavirin has been observed, even with prolonged administration.

Safety for Health Care Personnel

Although mucous membrane irritation has been reported following exposure to ribavirin (especially in the eyes of contact lens wearers), it occurs in a small percentage of exposed personnel and is reversible. Reproductive and teratogenic toxicities were observed in pregnant rodents administered oral ribavirin. These effects were not reproduced in baboons and have not been reported in humans. Studies have indicated that although absorption of ribavirin can occur in health care personnel from environmental exposure, no deleterious effects have been reported. Concern about the safety of ribavirin has led some hospitals to apply strict precautions for use of ribavirin to minimize exposure of health care workers.

A review of animal and human data on ribavirin safety is summarized and interpreted as follows:

- In hamsters after a single oral dose of 2.5 mg/kg, and in rats after a daily oral dose of 10 mg/kg for 60 days or longer, fetal malformations have been noted. In rabbits, the species most sensitive to the effects of ribavirin, skeletal malformations were observed after daily oral administration of 0.1 to 0.3 mg/kg for 12 days. In contrast, seven pregnant baboons were treated orally with 60 to 120 mg/kg of ribavirin for 4 consecutive days, during the time of fetal organogenesis. The offspring of six of seven of these baboons showed no evidence of teratogenicity. The seventh animal aborted at day 45 (60-mg dose) but no traces of implantation were recovered, implying fetal death and resorption prior to organogenesis and prior to ribavirin therapy.
- Extrapolation from these animal experiments involving oral administration of ribavirin to circumstances of human exposure to ribavirin aerosol is difficult, especially in view of species differences in teratogenicity and the high doses administered.
- During treatment with aerosolized ribavirin, dissemination of the drug in the environment of the patient can occur, with the potential for inhalation by those caring for treated children. However, while 60% to 70% of the inhaled drug may be deposited in the airways, absorption from the respiratory tract into the circulation is minimal. In infants receiving aerosolized ribavirin, the mean peak plasma concentration was less than 1 μmol/L at a time when the peak concentrations in endotracheal secretions were greater than 1700 μmol/L.

Studies of health care personnel also have demonstrated minimal absorption. In one study of 19 nonpregnant nurses who were caring for infants receiving ribavirin by aerosol treatment via an oxygen tent, hood, or ventilator, nurses were exposed for a mean of 8 hours per day during a 3-day period (a total of 20 to 35 hours). Total air exchanges occurred 5.4 to 24 times per hour in the patients' rooms. Blood samples for analysis of ribavirin were obtained 1 day before exposure, 1 hour after the final exposure, and 3 to 5 days later; urine was collected before and 3 to 5 days after exposure. Ribavirin was not detected in any sample of plasma, erythrocytes, or urine. The lower limit of sensitivity of the radioimmunoassay used to measure ribavirin in the study was 0.02 μg/mL. In a similar study of health care personnel caring for infants treated with ribavirin, 90 samples of serum, urine, and erythrocytes were assayed for ribavirin. Ribavirin was detected in a concentration of 0.44 μg/mL in only one erythrocyte sample. (The minimum level of detection of the test used was 0.02 μg/mL.) The concurrent serum and urine samples were negative. No symptoms were reported by any health care workers in this study.

These findings and the lack of validated reports of adverse effects in human fetuses after 7 years of clinical use of the drug in the United States suggest that the teratogenic risk of ribavirin exposure in humans is extremely low. The National Institute for Occupational Safety and Health (NIOSH) recently conducted a study at a Florida Hospital, where the technique they employed consistently found small concentrations of ribavirin in the post-shift urine of nurses. No clinical findings were reported in association with these observations. NIOSH recommends review of work policies and institution of engineering controls in order to reduce environmental concentration of ribavirin in the patient's room.

Recommendations

Experience in more than 100,000 patients indicates that aerosolized ribavirin treatment for RSV infection is both safe and effective. As with other antiviral therapy, the maximum benefit will be derived by early treatment of high-risk patients. The route of administration, cost, and need for hospitalization support a strategy of selective use of ribavirin as follows:

- *Patients at high risk for complications from other conditions.* Ribavirin treatment is recommended for the following patients hospitalized with RSV lower respiratory tract disease:
  - Infants at high risk for severe or complicated RSV infection, including those with complicated congenital heart disease (including pulmonary hypertension); those with bronchopulmonary dysplasia, cystic fibrosis, and other chronic lung conditions; premature infants; children with immunodeficiency (especially those with AIDS or severe combined immunodeficiency disease); recent transplant recipients; and patients undergoing chemotherapy for malignancy.
  - Infants who are severely ill. Because severity of illness is often difficult to judge clinically in infants with RSV infection, determination of blood gas concentrations is often necessary. Values for PaO_2 of less than 65 mm Hg (ie, oximetry reading less than 90%) and increasing concentration of carbon dioxide arterial pressure ($PaCO_2$) are useful indicators of severity.
  - All patients mechanically ventilated for RSV infection.
- *Treatment for hospitalized infants.* Ribavirin treatment should also be considered for hospitalized infants who may be at increased risk of progressing from a mild to a more complicated course by virtue of young age (less than 6 weeks) or underlying condition, such as multiple congenital anomalies or certain neurologic or metabolic diseases (eg, severe cerebral palsy, myasthenia).
- *Diagnosis of RSV infection.* Rapid diagnostic techniques to identify RSV antigen in respiratory secretions should be performed when the child is admitted to the hospital (see Respiratory Syncytial Virus, p 397). Tissue culture isolation requires 3 to 5 days. If rapid tests are not available, patients in the recommended categories who have bronchiolitis or pneumonia clinically compatible with RSV infection and who are admitted during the RSV season (generally November to April) should be considered for ribavirin therapy. If the etiology of the infant's pulmonary disease is subsequently found to be an agent other than RSV, ribavirin therapy can be discontinued. If no agent is identified initially as the cause of the lower respiratory tract disease, but the most likely clinical diagnosis remains RSV infection and the infant is severely ill, continuation of treatment is

reasonable. Further diagnostic efforts to ascertain the causative agent should be undertaken, recognizing that false-negative rapid diagnostic test results have been noted in 5% to 20% of cases.

- *Administration.* Ribavirin is nebulized by a small-particle aerosol generator into an oxygen hood, tent, or mask from a solution containing 20 mg of ribavirin per milliliter of water. The generator is supplied with the drug by the manufacturer. The aerosol is administered for 12 to 20 hours per day, usually for 3 to 5 days depending on the patient's clinical course; a longer duration of therapy may be useful in immunodeficient patients. A recent study noted good patient tolerance and favorable ribavirin pharmacokinetics when a regimen of 60 mg/mL for 2 hours three times daily was used; however, the efficacy of this dosage has not been proven. Maximal therapeutic responses usually are noted after 2 to 4 days of treatment.

- *Isolation of patients.* Treatment with ribavirin does not eliminate the need for contact isolation of patients with RSV.

- *Precautions for health care personnel and visitors.* Health care personnel and visitors should be informed about the potential but unknown risks of environmental exposure to ribavirin. In-service education for hospital personnel is most effective just prior to the RSV season. While evidence of human teratogenicity is lacking, in view of the embryopathic effects in nonprimate animals, pregnant women should be advised not to care directly for patients who are receiving ribavirin. Several methods have been employed to lower environmental exposure. For example, aerosol administration should be stopped temporarily when the hood or tent is open. Also, the drug should be administered in well-ventilated rooms (at least six air changes per hour).

No additional precautions to protect patients, visitors, or hospital workers in the room are required. Masks designed to block absorption of 1- to 2-μg particulate droplets may reduce inhalation of ribavirin, but clinical studies are lacking. Standard surgical masks do not block particles of this size. Gloves and gowns are not essential since dermal absorption of ribavirin appears to be negligible. However, gloves and gown may lower the risk of nosocomial spread of RSV. Scavenger devices to lower the escape of aerosolized ribavirin into a room also can be used. Additional research and clinical experience are needed to establish more specific guidelines regarding occupational exposure.

Drugs For Parasitic Infections

The following tables (5.7, 5.8, and 5.9) are reproduced from the December 10, 1993, issue of *The Medical Letter* (1993;35:111-122).* They provide recommendations that are likely to be consistent in many cases with those of the Committee, as given in the chapters on specific diseases in Section 3. However, because the *Medical Letter* recommendations are developed independently and may occasionally differ from those of the Committee, both should be consulted. The Com-

---

*Reprinted from *The Medical Letter* with permission.

mittee thanks *The Medical Letter* for their courtesy in allowing this information to be reprinted.

In Table 5.7 (p 576), first-choice and alternative drugs with recommended adult and pediatric dosages for most parasitic infections are given. In each case, the need for treatment must be weighed against the toxic effects of the drug. A decision to withhold therapy may often be correct, particularly when the drugs can cause severe adverse effects. When the first-choice drug is initially ineffective and the alternative is more hazardous, a second course of treatment with the first drug before giving the alternative may be prudent. Adverse effects of some antiparasitic drugs are listed in Table 5.9 (p 596).

Several drugs recommended in Table 5.7 have not been approved by the Food and Drug Administration and, thus, are investigational (see footnotes). When prescribing an unapproved drug, the physician should inform the patient of the investigational status and adverse effects of the drug.

These recommendations are periodically (usually every other year) updated by *The Medical Letter.*

TABLE 5.7—Drugs for Treatment of Parasitic Infections

Infection		Drug	Adult Dosage*	Pediatric Dosage*
AMEBIASIS (*Entamoeba histolytica*)				
asymptomatic				
Drug of choice:		Iodoquinol[1]	650 mg tid x 20d	30-40 mg/kg/d in 3 doses x 20d
	OR	Paromomycin	25-30 mg/kg/d in 3 doses x 7d	25-30 mg/kg/d in 3 doses x 7d
Alternative:		Diloxanide furoate[2]	500 mg tid x 10d	20 mg/kg/d in 3 doses x 10d
mild to moderate intestinal disease				
Drugs of choice:[3]		Metronidazole	750 mg tid x 10d	35-50 mg/kg/d in 3 doses x 10d
	OR	Tinidazole[4]	2 grams/d x 3d	50 mg/kg (max. 2 grams) qd x 3d
severe intestinal disease				
Drugs of choice:[3]		Metronidazole	750 mg tid x 10d	35-50 mg/kg/d in 3 doses x 10d
	OR	Tinidazole[4]	600 mg bid x 5d	50 mg/kg (max. 2 grams) qd x 3d
Alternative:		Dehydroemetine[2]	1 to 1.5 mg/kg/d (max. 90 mg/d) IM for up to 5d	1 to 1.5 mg/kg/d (max. 90 mg/d) IM in 2 doses for up to 5d
hepatic abscess				
Drugs of choice:[3]		Metronidazole	750 mg tid x 10d	35-50 mg/kg/d in 3 doses x 10d
	OR	Tinidazole[4]	800 mg tid x 5d	60 mg/kg (max. 2 grams) qd x 3d
Alternatives:		Dehydroemetine[2]	1 to 1.5 mg/kg/d (max. 90 mg/d) IM for up to 5d	1 to 1.5 mg/kg/d (max. 90 mg/d) IM in 2 doses for up to 5d
		followed by chloro-quine phosphate	600 mg base (1 gram)/d x 2d, then 300 mg base (500 mg)/d x 2-3 wks	10 mg base/kg (max. 300 mg base)/d x 2-3 wks
AMEBIC MENINGOENCEPHALITIS, PRIMARY				
Naegleria				
Drug of choice:		Amphotericin B[5,8]	1 mg/kg/d IV, uncertain duration	1 mg/kg/d IV, uncertain duration
Acanthamoeba				
Drug of choice:		See footnote 7		

Ancylostoma duodenale, see HOOKWORM

ANGIOSTRONGYLIASIS

Angiostrongylus cantonensis
Drug of choice: Mebendazole[6,8,9]   100 mg bid x 5d

Angiostrongylus costaricensis
Drug of choice: Thiabendazole[6,8]   75 mg/kg/d in 3 doses x 3d (max. 3 grams/d)[10]   75 mg/kg/d in 3 doses x 3d (max. 3 grams/d)[10]

ANISAKIASIS (Anisakis)
Treatment of choice: Surgical or endoscopic removal

ASCARIASIS (Ascaris lumbricoides, roundworm)
Drug of choice: Mebendazole   100 mg bid x 3d   100 mg bid x 3d
    OR   Pyrantel pamoate   11 mg/kg once (max. 1 gram)   11 mg/kg once (max. 1 gram)
    OR   Albendazole   400 mg once   400 mg once

---

*   The letter d stands for day.

1.   Dosage and duration of administration should not be exceeded because of possibility of causing optic neuritis; maximum dosage is 2 grams/day.

2.   In the USA, this drug is available from the CDC Drug Service, Centers for Disease Control and Prevention, Atlanta, Georgia 30333; telephone: 404-639-3670 (evenings, weekends, and holidays: 404-639-2888).

3.   Treatment should be followed by a course of iodoquinol or one of the other intraluminal drugs used to treat asymptomatic amebiasis.

4.   A nitro-imidazole similar to metronidazole, but not marketed in the USA; tinidazole appears to be at least as effective as metronidazole and better tolerated. Ornidazole, a similar drug, is also used outside the USA.

5.   One patient with a Naegleria infection was successfully treated with amphotericin B, miconazole, and rifampin (JS Seidel et al, N Engl J Med, 306:346, 1982).

6.   An approved drug, but considered investigational for this condition by the U.S. Food and Drug Administration

7.   Strains of Acanthamoeba isolated from fatal granulomatous amebic encephalitis are usually sensitive in vitro to pentamidine, ketoconazole (Nizoral), flucytosine, and (less so) to amphotericin B (RJ Duma et al, Antimicrob Agents Chemother, 10:370, 1976). For treatment of keratitis caused by Acanthamoeba, concurrent topical use of 0.1% propamidine isethionate (Brolene – Rhône-Poulenc Rorer, Canada) plus neosporin, or oral itraconazole plus topical miconazole, have been successful (MB Moore and JP McCulley, Br J Ophthalmol, 73:271, 1989; Y Ishibashi et al, Am J Ophthalmol, 109:121, 1990). Topical polyhexamethylene biguanide has also been effective in a few patients with keratitis (JH Varga et al, Am J Ophthalmol, 115:466, 1993).

8.   Effectiveness documented only in animals

9.   Most patients recover spontaneously without antiparasitic drug therapy. Analgesics, corticosteroids, and careful removal of CSF at frequent intervals can relieve symptoms (J Koo et al, Rev Infect Dis, 10:1155, 1988). Albendazole, levamisole (Ergamisol), or ivermectin has also been used successfully in animals.

TABLE 5.7—Drugs for Treatment of Parasitic Infections *(continued)*

Infection	Drug	Adult Dosage*	Pediatric Dosage*
BABESIOSIS *(Babesia microti)* Drugs of choice:[11]	Clindamycin[6]	1.2 grams bid parenteral or 600 mg tid oral x 7d	20-40 mg/kg/d in 3 doses x 7d
	plus quinine	650 mg tid oral x 7d	25 mg/kg/d in 3 doses x 7d
BALANTIDIASIS *(Balantidium coli)* Drug of choice:	Tetracycline[6]	500 mg qid x 10d	40 mg/kg/d in 4 doses x 10d (max. 2 grams/d)[12]
Alternatives:	Iodoquinol[1,6]	650 mg tid x 20d	40 mg/kg/d in 3 doses x 20d
	Metronidazole[6]	750 mg tid x 5d	35-50 mg/kg/d in 3 doses x 5d
BAYLISASCARIASIS *(Baylisascaris procyonis)* Drug of choice:	See footnote 13		
BLASTOCYSTIS *hominis* infection Drug of choice:	See footnote 14		
CAPILLARIASIS *(Capillaria philippinensis)* Drug of choice:	Mebendazole[6]	200 mg bid x 20d	200 mg bid x 20d
Alternatives:	Albendazole	200 mg bid x 10d	200 mg bid x 10d
	Thiabendazole[6]	25 mg/kg/d in 2 doses x 30d	25 mg/kg/d in 2 doses x 30d
Chagas' disease, see TRYPANOSOMIASIS			
Clonorchis sinensis, see FLUKE infection			
CRYPTOSPORIDIOSIS *(Cryptosporidium)* Drug of choice:	See footnote 15		
CUTANEOUS LARVA MIGRANS (creeping eruption, dog and cat hookworm) Drug of choice:[16]	Thiabendazole	Topically and/or 50 mg/kg/d in 2 doses (max. 3 grams/d) x 2-5d[10]	Topically and/or 50 mg/kg/d in 2 doses (max. 3 grams/d) x 2-5d[10]
	OR Albendazole[17]	200 mg bid x 3d	200 mg bid x 3d
CYCLOSPORA infection[18] Drug of choice:	Trimethoprim-sulfamethoxazole[19]	TMP 160 mg, SMX 800 mg bid x 3 days	TMP 5 mg/kg, SMX 25 mg/kg bid x 3 days
CYSTICERCOSIS, see TAPEWORM infection			

***DIENTAMOEBA fragilis* infection**

Drug of choice:			
	Iodoquinol[1]	650 mg tid x 20d	40 mg/kg/d in 3 doses x 20d
OR	Paromomycin[6]	25-30 mg/kg/d in 3 doses x 7d	25-30 mg/kg/d in 3 doses x 7d
OR	Tetracycline[6]	500 mg qid x 10d	40 mg/kg/d (max. 2 grams/d) in 4 doses x 10d[12]

Diphyllobothrium latum, see TAPEWORM infection

***DRACUNCULUS medinensis* (guinea worm) infection**

Drug of choice:	Metronidazole[6,20]	250 mg tid x 10d	25 mg/kg/d (max. 750 mg/d) in 3 doses x 10d
Alternative:	Thiabendazole[6,20]	50-75 mg/kg/d in 2 doses x 3d[10]	50-75 mg/kg/d in 2 doses x 3d[10]

10. This dose is likely to be toxic and may have to be decreased.

11. Exchange transfusion has been used in severely ill patients with high (>10%) parasitemia (V Iacopino and T Earnhart, Arch Intern Med, 150:1527, 1990). One report indicates that azithromycin (*Zithromax*), 500-1000 mg daily, plus quinine may also be effective (LM Weiss et al, J Infect Dis, 168:1289, 1993). Concurrent use of pentamidine and trimethoprim-sulfamethoxazole has been reported to cure an infection with *B. divergens* (D Raoult et al, Ann Intern Med, 107:944, 1987).

12. Not recommended for use in children less than eight years old.

13. Drugs that could be tried include diethylcarbamazine, levamisole, and fenbendazole (KR Kazacos, J Am Vet Med Assoc, 195:894, 1989) and ivermectin. Steroid therapy may be helpful, especially in eye or CNS infection. Ocular baylisascariasis has been treated successfully using laser therapy to destroy intraretinal larvae.

14. Clinical significance of these organisms is controversial, but metronidazole 750 mg tid x 10d or iodoquinol 650 mg tid x 20d anecdotally have been reported to be effective (I Grossman et al, Am J Gastroenterol, 87:729, 1992; PFL Boreham and D Stenzel, Adv Parasitol, 32:2, 1993).

15. Infection is self-limited in immunocompetent patients. In HIV-infected patients with large-volume intractable diarrhea, octreotide (*Sandostatin*) 300-500 µg tid subcutaneously may control the diarrhea, but not the infection (JD Cello et al, Ann Intern Med, 115:705, 1991). Paromomycin may sometimes be helpful (K Armitage et al, Arch Intern Med, 152:2497, 1992). In unpublished clinical trials, azithromycin, 1250 mg daily for two weeks followed by 500 mg daily, has apparently been effective in some patients.

16. Several reports suggest that ivermectin, 150-200 µg/kg once, is also effective (E Caumes et al, Arch Dermatol, 128:994, 1992).

17. SK Jones et al, Br J Dermatol, 122:99, 1990; HD Davies et al, Arch Dermatol, 129:588, 1993

18. A newly described coccidian parasite, previously designated a cyanobacterium-like body, which causes severe self-limited diarrhea (YR Ortega et al, N Engl J Med, 328:1308, 1993; RP Bendall et al, Lancet, 341:590, 1993)

19. G Madico et al, Lancet, 342:122, 1993

20. Not curative, but decreases inflammation and facilitates removing the worm. Mebendazole 400-800 mg/d for 6d has been reported to kill the worm directly.

TABLE 5.7—Drugs for Treatment of Parasitic Infections *(continued)*

Infection	Drug	Adult Dosage*	Pediatric Dosage*
Echinococcus, see TAPEWORM infection			
Entamoeba histolytica, see AMEBIASIS			
ENTAMOEBA polecki infection			
Drug of choice:	Metronidazole[6]	750 mg tid x 10d	35-50 mg/kg/d in 3 doses x 10d
ENTEROBIUS vermicularis (pinworm) infection			
Drug of choice:	Pyrantel pamoate	11 mg/kg once (max. 1 gram); repeat after 2 weeks	11 mg/kg once (max. 1 gram); repeat after 2 weeks
OR	Mebendazole	A single dose of 100 mg; repeat after 2 weeks	A single dose of 100 mg; repeat after 2 weeks
OR	Albendazole	400 mg once; repeat in 2 weeks	400 mg once, repeat in 2 weeks
Fasciola hepatica, see FLUKE infection			
FILARIASIS			
Wuchereria bancrofti, Brugia malayi			
Drug of choice:[21]	Diethylcarbamazine[22]	Day 1: 50 mg, oral, p.c. Day 2: 50 mg tid Day 3: 100 mg tid Days 4 through 21: 6 mg/kg/d in 3 doses[23]	Day 1: 1 mg/kg. oral, p.c. Day 2: 1 mg/kg tid Day 3: 1-2 mg/kg tid Days 4 through 21: 6 mg/kg/d in 3 doses[23]
Loa loa			
Drug of choice:[24]	Diethylcarbamazine[22]	Day 1: 50 mg, oral, p.c. Day 2: 50 mg tid Day 3: 100 mg tid Days 4 through 21: 9 mg/kg/d in 3 doses[23]	Day 1: 1 mg/kg. oral, p.c. Day 2: 1 mg/kg tid Day 3: 1-2 mg/kg tid Days 4 through 21: 9 mg/kg/d in 3 doses[23]
Mansonella ozzardi			
Drug of choice:	See footnote 25		
Mansonella perstans			
Drug of choice:	Mebendazole[6]	100 mg bid x 30d	

Tropical Pulmonary Eosinophilia (TPE)

Drug of choice:	Diethylcarbamazine	6 mg/kg/d in 3 doses x 21d	6 mg/kg/d in 3 doses x 21d

Onchocerca volvulus

Drug of choice:	Ivermectin[2]	150 µg/kg oral once, repeated every 6 to 12 months	150 µg/kg oral once, repeated every 6 to 12 months

FLUKE, hermaphroditic, infection

***Clonorchis sinensis* (Chinese liver fluke)**

Drug of choice:	Praziquantel	75 mg/kg/d in 3 doses x 1d	75 mg/kg/d in 3 doses x 1d

***Fasciola hepatica* (sheep liver fluke)**

Drug of choice:[26]	Bithionol[2]	30-50 mg/kg on alternate days x 10-15 doses	30-50 mg/kg on alternate days x 10-15 doses

21. A single dose of ivermectin, 20-200 µg/kg, has been reported to be effective for treatment of microfilaremia (EA Ottesen et al, N Engl J Med, 322:1113, 1990; M Sabry et al, Trans R Soc Trop Med Hyg, 85:640, 1991; JW Mak et al, Am J Trop Med Hyg, 48:591, 1993).

22. Antihistamines or corticosteroids may be required to decrease allergic reactions due to disintegration of microfilariae in treatment of filarial infections, especially those caused by *Loa loa*.

23. For patients with no microfilariae in the blood or skin, full doses can be given from day one.

24. Diethylcarbamazine should be administered with special caution in heavy infections with *Loa loa* because rapid killing of microfilariae can provoke an encephalopathy (B Carme et al, Am J Trop Med Hyg, 44:684, 1991). Ivermectin or albendazole has been used to reduce microfilaremia (Y Martin-Prevel et al, Am J Trop Med Hyg, 48:186, 1993; AD Klion et al, J Infect Dis, 168:202, 1993). Apheresis has been reported to be effective in lowering microfilarial counts in patients heavily infected with Loa loa (EA Ottesen, Infect Dis Clin North Am, 7:619, 1993). Diethylcarbamazine, 300 mg once weekly, has been recommended for prevention of loiasis (TB Nutman et al, N Engl J Med, 319:752, 1988).

25. Diethylcarbamazine has no effect. Ivermectin, 150 µg/kg, may be effective (TB Nutman et al, J Infect Dis, 156:622, 1987).

26. Unlike infections with other flukes, *hepatica* infections may not respond to praziquantel. Limited data indicate that triclabendazole *(Fasinex)*, a veterinary fasciolide, is safe and effective in a single oral dose of 10 mg/kg (L Loutan et al, Lancet, 2:383, 1989; U Bechtel et al, Dtsch Med Wochenschr, 117:978, 1992).

TABLE 5.7—Drugs for Treatment of Parasitic Infections *(continued)*

Infection	Drug	Adult Dosage*	Pediatric Dosage*
FLUKE, hermaphroditic, infection *(continued)*			
Fasciolopsis buski (intestinal fluke)			
Drug of choice:	Praziquantel[6]	75 mg/kg/d in 3 doses x 1d	75 mg/kg/d in 3 doses x 1d
OR	Niclosamide[6]	a single dose of 4 tablets (2 g), chewed thoroughly	11-34 kg: 2 tablets (1 g) >34 kg: 3 tablets (1.5 g)
Heterophyes heterophyes (intestinal fluke)			
Drug of choice:	Praziquantel[6]	75 mg/kg/d in 3 doses x 1d	75 mg/kg/d in 3 doses x 1d
Metagonimus yokogawai (intestinal fluke)			
Drug of choice:	Praziquantel[6]	75 mg/kg/d in 3 doses x 1d	75 mg/kg/d in 3 doses x 1d
Nanophyetus salmincola			
Drug of choice:	Praziquantel[6]	60 mg/kg/d in 3 doses x 1d	60 mg/kg/d in 3 doses x 1d
Opisthorchis viverrini (liver fluke)			
Drug of choice:	Praziquantel	75 mg/kg/d in 3 doses x 1d	75 mg/kg/d in 3 doses x 1d
Paragonimus westermani (lung fluke)			
Drug of choice:	Praziquantel[6]	75 mg/kg/d in 3 doses x 2d	75 mg/kg/d in 3 doses x 2d
Alternative:[27]	Bithionol[2]	30-50 mg/kg on alternate days x 10-15 doses	30-50 mg/kg on alternate days x 10-15 doses
GIARDIASIS (*Giardia lamblia*)			
Drug of choice:	Metronidazole[6]	250 mg tid x 5d	15 mg/kg/d in 3 doses x 5d
Alternatives:[28]	Quinacrine HCl	100 mg tid p.c. x 5d	6 mg/kg/d in 3 doses p.c. x 5d (max. 300 mg/d)
	Tinidazole[4]	2 grams once	50 mg/kg once (max. 2 grams)
	Furazolidone	100 mg qid x 7-10d	6 mg/kg/d in 4 doses x 7-10d
	Paromomycin[29]	25-30 mg/kg/d in 3 doses x 7d	
GNATHOSTOMIASIS (*Gnathostoma spinigerum*)			
Treatment of choice:[30]	Surgical removal		
plus	Albendazole[31]	400-800 mg qd x 21d	
HOOKWORM infection (*Ancylostoma duodenale, Necator americanus*)			
Drug of choice:	Mebendazole	100 mg bid x 3d	100 mg bid x 3d
OR	Pyrantel pamoate[6]	11 mg/kg (max. 1 gram) x 3d	11 mg/kg (max. 1 gram) x 3d
OR	Albendazole	400 mg once	400 mg once
Hydatid cyst, see TAPEWORM infection			

Hymenolepis nana, see TAPEWORM infection

ISOSPORIASIS (*Isospora belli*)

Drug of choice:	Trimethoprim-sulfamethoxazole[6,32]	160 mg TMP, 800 mg SMX qid x 10d, then bid x 3 wks

LEISHMANIASIS (*L. mexicana, L. tropica, L. major, L. braziliensis, L. donovani* [Kala-azar])

Drug of choice:		Sodium stibogluconate[2]	20 mg Sb/kg/d IV or IM x 20-28d[33]
	OR	Meglumine antimonate	20 mg Sb/kg/d x 20-28d[33]
Alternatives:[34]		Amphotericin B[6]	0.25 to 1 mg/kg by slow infusion daily or every 2d for up to 8 wks
		Pentamidine isethionate[6]	2-4 mg/kg daily or every 2d IM for up to 15 doses[33]

* The letter d stands for day.

27. Unpublished data indicate triclabendazole may be effective in a dosage of 5 mg/kg once daily for 3 days or 10 mg/kg twice in one day.

28. Albendazole 400 mg daily x 5d has also been reported to be highly effective against giardiasis (A Hall and Q Nahar, Trans R Soc Trop Med Hyg, 87:84, 1993).

29. Not absorbed and not highly effective, but may be useful for treatment of giardiasis in pregnancy

30. Ivermectin has been reported to be effective in animals (MT Anantaphruti et al, Trop Med Parasitol, 43:65, 1992).

31. P Kraivichian et al, Trans R Soc Trop Med Hyg, 86:418, 1992

32. In sulfonamide-sensitive patients, such as some HIV-infected patients, pyrimethamine 50-75 mg daily has been effective (LM Weiss et al, Ann Intern Med, 109:474, 1988). In immunocompromised patients, it may be necessary to continue therapy indefinitely.

33. May be repeated or continued. A longer duration may be needed for some forms of visceral leishmaniasis.

34. Limited data indicate that ketoconazole, 400 to 600 mg daily for four to eight weeks, may be effective for treatment of cutaneous and mucosal leishmaniasis (RE Saenz et al, Am J Med, 89:147, 1990; V Ramesh et al, Arch Dermatol, 128:411, 1992). Some studies indicate that *L. donovani* resistant to sodium stibogluconate or meglumine antimonate may respond to recombinant human gamma interferon in addition to antimony (R Badaro and WD Johnson, J Infect Dis, 167 suppl 1:S13, 1993), pentamidine followed by a course of antimony (CP Thakur et al, Am J Trop Med Hyg, 45:435, 1991), or ketoconazole (JP Wali et al, J Infect Dis, 166:215, 1992). Liposomal encapsulated amphotericin B (*AmBisome,* Vestar, San Dimas, CA) has been used successfully to treat multiple-drug-resistant visceral leishmaniasis (RN Davidson et al, Lancet, 337:1061, 1991). Recently, aminosidine (parenteral paromomycin) plus sodium stibogluconate apparently decreased time to clinical and parasitological cure of visceral leishmaniasis (J Seaman et al, J Infect Dis, 168:715, 1993).

TABLE 5.7—Drugs for Treatment of Parasitic Infections *(continued)*

Infection		Drug	Adult Dosage*	Pediatric Dosage*
LICE infestation *(Pediculus humanus, capitis, Phthirus pubis)*[35]				
Drug of choice:		1% Permethrin[36]	Topically	Topically
	OR	0.5% Malathion	Topically	Topically
Alternatives:		Pyrethrins with piperonyl butoxide	Topically[37]	Topically[37]
		Lindane	Topically[37]	Topically[37]
Loa loa, see FILARIASIS				
MALARIA, Treatment of *(Plasmodium falciparum, P. ovale, P. vivax, and P. malariae)*				
Chloroquine-resistant *P. falciparum*[38]				
ORAL				
Drugs of choice:		Quinine sulfate	650 mg q8h x 3-7d[39]	25 mg/kg/d in 3 doses x 3-7d[39]
		plus pyrimethamine-sulfadoxine[40]	3 tablets at once on last day of quinine	<1 yr: ¼ tablet 1-3 yrs: ½ tablet 4-8 yrs: 1 tablet 9-14 yrs: 2 tablets
	OR	**plus** tetracycline[6]	250 mg qid x 7d	20 mg/kg/d in 4 doses x 7d[12]
	OR[41]	**plus** clindamycin[6]	900 mg tid x 3d	20-40 mg/kg/d in 3 doses x 3d
Alternatives:[42]		Mefloquine[43,44]	1250 mg once[45]	25 mg/kg once[46] (<45 kg)
		Halofantrine[47]	500 mg q6h x 3 doses; repeat in 1 week	8 mg/kg q6h x 3 doses (<40 kg); repeat in 1 week
PARENTERAL				
Drug of choice:[48,49]		Quinidine gluconate[50]	10 mg/kg loading dose (max. 600 mg) in normal saline slowly over 1 to 2 hrs, followed by continuous infusion of 0.02 mg/kg/min until oral therapy can be started	Same as adult dose
	OR	Quinine dihydrochloride[51]	20 mg salt/kg loading dose in 10 ml/kg 5% dextrose over 4 hrs, followed by 10 mg salt/kg over 2-4 hrs q8h (max. 1800 mg/d) until oral therapy can be started	Same as adult dose

35. For infestation of eyelashes with crab lice, use petrolatum.
36. FDA-approved only for head lice.

37. Some consultants recommend a second application one week later to kill hatching progeny. Seizures have been reported in association with the use of lindane. Do not use higher than recommended doses and avoid warm baths before application (M Tenenbein, J Am Geriatr Soc, 39:394, 1991). Prolonged use of lindane has been associated with aplastic anemia (AE Rauch et al, Arch Intern Med, 150:2393, 1990).

38. Chloroquine-resistant *P. falciparum* infections occur in all malarious areas except Central America west of the Panama Canal Zone, Mexico, Haiti, the Dominican Republic, and the Middle East (including Egypt).

39. In Southeast Asia and possibly in other areas, such as South America, relative resistance to quinine has increased and the treatment should be continued for seven days.

40. *Fansidar* tablets contain 25 mg of pyrimethamine and 500 mg of sulfadoxine. Resistance to pyrimethamine-sulfadoxine has been reported from Southeast Asia, the Amazon basin, East Africa, Bangladesh, and Oceania.

41. In pregnancy

42. For treatment of multidrug resistant *P. falciparum* in Southeast Asia, especially Thailand, where resistance to mefloquine and halofantrine frequently occur, a 7-day course of quinine and tetracycline is recommended (G Watt et al, Am J Trop Med Hyg, 47:108, 1992).

43. At this dosage, adverse effects including nausea, vomiting, diarrhea, dizziness, disturbed sense of balance, toxic psychosis, and seizures can occur. Mefloquine is teratogenic in animals and should not be used in pregnancy. It should not be given together with quinine or quinidine, and caution is required in using quinine or quinidine to treat patients with malaria who have taken mefloquine for prophylaxis. The pediatric dosage has not been approved by the FDA. Resistance to mefloquine has been reported in some areas, such as Thailand.

44. In the USA, a 250-mg tablet of mefloquine contains 228 mg of mefloquine base. Outside the USA, each 275-mg tablet contains 250 mg base.

45. Outside the USA, the manufacturer recommends dividing the 1250-mg dose into 750 mg followed 6-8 hours later by 500 mg (D Kingston, Med J Aust, 153:235, 1990).

46. NJ White, Eur J Clin Pharmacol, 34:1, 1988

47. May be effective in multiple-drug-resistant *P. falciparum* malaria, but treatment failures have been reported (GD Shanks et al, Am J Trop Med Hyg, 45:488, 1991), and the drug causes consistent dose-related lengthening of the PR and QTc intervals (A Castot et al, Lancet, 341:1541, 1993). Several patients have developed first degree block (F Nosten et al, Lancet 341:1054, 1993). It should not be taken one hour before to three hours after meals and probably should not be used for patients with cardiac conduction defects.

48. A recent study found artemether, a Chinese drug, effective for parenteral treatment of severe malaria in children (NJ White et al, Lancet, 339:317, 1992).

49. Exchange transfusion has been helpful for some patients with high-density (>10%) parasitemia, altered mental status, pulmonary edema, or renal complications (JR Zucker and CC Campbell, Infect Dis Clin North Am, 7:547, 1993).

50. EKG and blood pressure monitoring are recommended.

51. Not available in the USA. IV administration of quinine dihydrochloride can be hazardous; constant monitoring of the pulse and blood pressure is necessary to detect arrhythmia or hypotension. Use of parenteral quinine may also lead to severe hypoglycemia; blood glucose should be monitored.

TABLE 5.7—Drugs for Treatment of Parasitic Infections *(continued)*

Infection		Drug	Adult Dosage*	Pediatric Dosage*
MALARIA, Treatment of *(continued)*				
All *Plasmodium* except Chloroquine-resistant *P. falciparum*[38]				
ORAL				
Drug of choice:		Chloroquine phosphate[52,53]	600 mg base (1 gram), then 300 mg base (500 mg) 6 hrs later, then 300 mg base (500 mg) at 24 and 48 hrs	10 mg base/kg (max. 600 mg base), then 5 mg base/kg 6 hrs later, then 5 mg base/kg at 24 and 48 hrs
PARENTERAL				
Drug of choice:[49]		Quinidine gluconate[50]	same as above	same as above
	OR	Quinine dihydrochloride[51]	same as above	same as above
Prevention of relapses: *P. vivax* and *P. ovale* only				
Drug of choice:		Primaquine phosphate[54,55]	15 mg base (26.3 mg)/d x 14d or 45 mg base (79 mg)/wk x 8 wks	0.3 mg base/kg/d x 14d
MALARIA, Prevention of[56,57]				
Chloroquine-sensitive areas				
Drug of choice:		Chloroquine phosphate[58]	300 mg base (500 mg salt) orally, once/week[59]	5 mg/kg base (8.3 mg/kg salt) once/week, up to adult dose of 300 mg base
Chloroquine-resistant areas[38]				
Drug of choice:		Mefloquine[44,58,60]	250 mg oral once/week[59]	15-19 kg: ¼ tablet 20-30 kg: ½ tablet 31-45 kg: ¾ tablet >45 kg: 1 tablet
	OR	Doxycycline[58,61]	100 mg daily[61]	>8 years of age: 2 mg/kg/d orally, up to 100 mg/day
Alternatives:		Chloroquine phosphate[58] **plus** pyrimethamine-sulfadoxine[40] for presumptive treatment	same as above Carry a single dose (3 tablets) for self-treatment of febrile illness when medical care is not immediately available	same as above <1 yr: ¼ tablet 1-3 yrs: ½ tablet 4-8 yrs: 1 tablet 9-14 yrs: 2 tablets

or **plus** proguanil[62]   200 mg daily[62]
(in Africa south of
the Sahara)

<2 yrs: 50 mg daily
2-6 yrs: 100 mg daily
7-10 yrs: 150 mg daily
>10 yrs: 200 mg daily

52. If chloroquine phosphate is not available, hydroxychloroquine sulfate is as effective; 400 mg of hydroxychloroquine sulfate is equivalent to 500 mg of chloroquine phosphate.

53. In *P. falciparum* malaria, if the patient has not shown a response to conventional doses of chloroquine in 48-72 hours, parasitic resistance to this drug should be considered. *P. vivax* with decreased susceptibility to chloroquine has been reported from New Guinea (KH Rieckmann et al, Lancet, 2:1183, 1989) and from Indonesia (IK Schwartz et al, N Engl J Med, 324:927, 1991); a single dose of mefloquine, 15 mg/kg, has been recommended to treat these infections.

54. Some relapses have been reported with this regimen; relapses should be treated with chloroquine plus primaquine, 30 mg base/d x 14 days.

55. Primaquine phosphate can cause hemolytic anemia, especially in patients whose red cells are deficient in glucose-6-phosphate dehydrogenase. This deficiency is most common in African, Asian, and Mediterranean peoples. Patients should be screened for G-6-PD deficiency before treatment. Primaquine should not be used during pregnancy.

56. No drug regimen guarantees protection against malaria. If fever develops within a year (particularly within the first two months) after travel to malarious areas, travelers should be advised to seek medical attention. Insect repellents, insecticide-impregnated bed nets, and proper clothing are important adjuncts for malaria prophylaxis.

57. In pregnancy, chloroquine prophylaxis has been used extensively and safely, but the safety of other prophylactic antimalarial agents in pregnancy is unclear. Therefore, travel during pregnancy to chloroquine-resistant areas should be discouraged.

58. For prevention of attack after departure from areas where *P. vivax* and *P. ovale* are endemic, which includes almost all areas where malaria is found (except Haiti), some experts prescribe in addition primaquine phosphate 15 mg base (26.3 mg)/d or, for children, 0.3 mg base/kg/d during the last two weeks of prophylaxis. Others prefer to avoid the toxicity of primaquine and rely on surveillance to detect cases when they occur, particularly when exposure was limited or doubtful. See also footnotes 54 and 55.

59. Beginning one week before travel and continuing weekly for the duration of stay and for four weeks after leaving.

60. The pediatric dosage has not been approved by the FDA, and the drug has not been approved for use during pregnancy. Women should take contraceptive precautions while taking mefloquine and for two months after the last dose. Mefloquine is not recommended for children weighing less than 15 kg, or for patients with cardiac conduction abnormalities. Patients with a history of seizures or psychiatric disorders and those whose occupation requires fine coordination or spatial discrimination should probably avoid mefloquine (Medical Letter, 32:13, 1990). Resistance to mefloquine has been reported in some areas, such as Thailand; in these areas, doxycycline should be used for prophylaxis.

61. Beginning one day before travel and continuing for the duration of stay and for four weeks after leaving. Use of tetracyclines is contraindicated in pregnancy and in children less than eight years old. Doxycycline can cause gastrointestinal disturbances, vaginal moniliasis and photosensitivity reactions.

TABLE 5.7—Drugs for Treatment of Parasitic Infections *(continued)*

Infection	Drug	Adult Dosage*	Pediatric Dosage*
MICROSPORIDIOSIS			
Ocular (*Encephalitozoon hellem, Nosema corneum*)			
Drug of choice:	See footnote 63		
Intestinal (*Enterocytozoon bieneusi, Septata intestinalis*)			
Drug of choice:	See footnote 64		
Disseminated (*Encephalitozoon hellem, Encephalitozoon cuniculi Pleistophora sp.*)			
Drug of choice:	See footnote 65		
Mites, see SCABIES			
***MONILIFORMIS moniliformis* infection**			
Drug of choice:	Pyrantel pamoate[6]	11 mg/kg once, repeat twice, 2 wks apart	11 mg/kg once, repeat twice, 2 wks apart
***Naegleria* species,** see AMEBIC MENINGOENCEPHALITIS, PRIMARY			
Necator americanus, see HOOKWORM infection			
Oesophagostomum bifurcum			
Drug of choice:	See footnote 66		
Onchocerca volvulus, see FILARIASIS			
Opisthorchis viverrini, see FLUKE infection			
Paragonimus westermani, see FLUKE infection			
Pediculus capitis, humanus, Phthirus pubis, see LICE			
Pinworm, see ENTEROBIUS			
***PNEUMOCYSTIS carinii* pneumonia**[67]			
Drug of choice:	Trimethoprim-sulfamethoxazole	TMP 15-20 mg/kg/d, SMX 75-100 mg/kg/d, oral or IV in 3 or 4 doses x 14-21d	Same as adult dose
Alternatives:[68] OR	Pentamidine	3-4 mg/kg IV qd x 14-21 days	Same as adult dose
	Trimethoprim[8]	5 mg/kg PO q6h x 21 days	
	plus dapsone[6,69]	100 mg PO qd x 21 days	

Atovaquone[70]	750 mg tid PO x 21 d
Primaquine[6,55]	15 mg base PO qd x 21 days
plus clindamycin[6]	600 mg IV q6h x 21 days, or 300-450 mg PO q6h x 21 days
Trimetrexate	45 mg/m² IV qd x 21 days
plus folinic acid	20 mg/m² PO or IV q6h x 21 days

Primary and secondary prophylaxis

Drug of Choice:	Trimethoprim-sulfamethoxazole	1 DS tab PO qd or 3x/week
Alternatives:	Dapsone[6,69]	25-50 mg PO qd, or 100 mg PO 2x/week
	Aerosol pentamidine	300 mg inhaled monthly via *Respirgard II nebulizer or System 22 Mizer Jet Nebulizer*

62. Proguanil (*Paludrine* – ICI, England), which is not available in the USA but is widely available overseas, is recommended mainly for use in Africa south of the Sahara. Prophylaxis is recommended during exposure and for four weeks afterwards. Failures in prophylaxis with chloroquine and proguanil have been reported in travelers to Kenya (AJ Barnes, Lancet, 338:1338, 1991).

63. Ocular lesions due to *E. hellem* in HIV-infected patients have responded to fumagillin eyedrops prepared from *Fumidil-B*, a commercial product used to control a microsporidial disease of honey bees, available from Mid-Continent Agrimarketing, Inc., Lenexa, Kansas 66215 (MC Diesenhouse, Am J Ophthalmol, 115:293, 1993). In one report, a keratopathy due to *E. hellem* in an HIV-infected patient was treated successfully with surgical debridement, topical antibiotics, and itraconazole (RW Yee et al, Ophthalmology, 98:196, 1991). For lesions due to *N. corneum*, topical therapy is generally not effective and keratoplasty may be required (RM Davis et al, Ophthalmology, 97:953, 1990).

64. Octreotide (*Sandostatin*) has provided symptomatic relief of *E. bieneusi* infection (JP Cello et al, Ann Intern Med, 115:705, 1991). Albendazole, 400 mg b.i.d., may be helpful for *E. bieneusi* (DT Dieterich et al, J Infect Dis, 1994, in press) and can cure *S. intestinalis* (C Blanshard et al, AIDS, 6:311, 1992).

65. No established treatment

66. Albendazole or pyrantel pamoate may be effective (HP Krepel et al, Trans R Soc Trop Med Hyg, 87:87, 1993).

TABLE 5.7—Drugs for Treatment of Parasitic Infections *(continued)*

Infection	Drug	Adult Dosage*	Pediatric Dosage*
Roundworm, see ASCARIASIS			
SCABIES *(Sarcoptes scabiei)*			
Drug of choice:	5% Permethrin	Topically	Topically
Alternatives:	Lindane[37]	Topically	Topically
	10% Crotamiton	Topically	Topically
SCHISTOSOMIASIS *(Bilharziasis)*			
S. haematobium			
Drug of choice:	Praziquantel	40 mg/kg/d in 2 doses x 1d	40 mg/kg/d in 2 doses x 1d
S. japonicum			
Drug of choice:	Praziquantel	60 mg/kg/d in 3 doses x 1d	60 mg/kg/d in 3 doses x 1d
S. mansoni			
Drug of choice:	Praziquantel	40 mg/kg/d in 2 doses x 1d	40 mg/kg/d in 2 doses x 1d
Alternative:	Oxamniquine[71]	15 mg/kg once[72]	20 mg/kg/d in 2 doses x 1d[72]
S. mekongi			
Drug of choice:	Praziquantel	60 mg/kg/d in 3 doses x 1d	60 mg/kg/d in 3 doses x 1d
Sleeping sickness, see TRYPANOSOMIASIS			
STRONGYLOIDIASIS *(Strongyloides stercoralis)*[73]			
Drug of choice:	Thiabendazole	50 mg/kg/d in 2 doses (max. 3 grams /d) x 2d[10,74]	50 mg/kg/d in 2 doses (max. 3 grams/d) x 2d[10,74]
	OR Ivermectin[75]	200 µg/kg/d x 1-2d	
TAPEWORM infection — **Adult (intestinal stage)**			
Diphyllobothrium latum (fish), *Taenia saginata* (beef), *Taenia solium* (pork), *Dipylidium caninum* (dog)			
Drug of choice:	Praziquantel[6]	5-10 mg/kg once	5-10 mg/kg once
	OR Niclosamide	A single dose of 4 tablets (2 grams), chewed thoroughly	11-34 kg: a single dose of 2 tablets (1 gram); >34 kg: a single dose of 3 tablets (1.5 g)
Hymenolepis nana (**dwarf tapeworm**)			
Drug of choice:	Praziquantel[6]	25 mg/kg once	25 mg/kg once
Alternative:	Niclosamide	A single daily dose of 4 tablets (2 g), chewed thoroughly, then 2 tablets daily x 6d	11-34 kg: a single dose of 2 tablets (1 g) x 1d, then 1 tablet (0.5 grams) /d x 6d; >34 kg: a single dose of 3 tablets (1.5 g) x 1d, then 2 tablets (1 g)/d x6d

— Larval (tissue stage)

***Echinococcus granulosus* (hydatid cyst)**

Drug of choice: Albendazole[76,77]   400 mg bid x 28 days, repeated as necessary   15 mg/kg/d x 28 days, repeated as necessary

Echinococcus multilocularis

Treatment of choice: See footnote 78

***Cysticercus cellulosae* (cysticercosis)**

Drug of choice:[79]   Albendazole[80]   15 mg/kg/d in 3 doses x 28d, repeated as necessary   15 mg/kg/d in 3 doses x 28d, repeated as necessary

OR   Praziquantel[6]   50 mg/kg/d in 3 doses x 15d   50 mg/kg/d in 3 doses x 15d

Alternative: Surgery

---

67. HIV-infected patients should be treated for 21 days. In severe disease with room air $PO_2 \leq 70$ mmHg or Aa gradient ≥ 35 mmHg, prednisone should also be used (Medical Letter, 35:79, 1993).

68. For patients who have failed or are intolerant to standard therapy.

69. Assay for G-6-PD deficiency recommended before therapy.

70. Recommended in mild to moderate disease (room air $PO_2 > 60$ mmHg) (W Hughes, N Engl J Med, 328:1521, 1993).

71. Neuropsychiatric disturbances and seizures have been reported in some patients (H Stokvis et al, Am J Trop Med Hyg, 35:330, 1986).

72. In East Africa, the dose should be increased to 30 mg/kg, and in Egypt and South Africa, 30 mg/kg/d x 2d. Some experts recommend 40-60 mg/kg over 2-3 days in all of Africa (KC Shekhar, Drugs, 42:379, 1991).

73. In immunocompromised patients it may be necessary to continue therapy or use other agents.

74. In disseminated strongyloidiasis, thiabendazole therapy should be continued for at least five days.

75. C Naquira et al, Am J Trop Med Hyg, 40:304, 1989; M Lyagoubi et al, Trans R Soc Trop Med Hyg, 86:541, 1992

76. With a fatty meal to enhance absorption. Some patients may benefit from or require surgical resection of cysts (RK Tompkins, Mayo Clin Proc, 66:1281, 1991). Praziquantel may also be useful preoperatively or in case of spill during surgery.

77. Recently, percutaneous drainage with ultrasound guidance plus albendazole therapy has been effective for management of hepatic hydatid cyst disease (MS Khuroo et al, Gastroenterology, 104:1452, 1993).

78. Surgical excision is the only reliable means of treatment, although some reports have suggested use of albendazole or mebendazole (JF Wilson et al, Am J Trop Med Hyg, 37:162, 1987; A Davis et al, Bull WHO, 64:383, 1986).

79. Corticosteroids should be given for two to three days before and during drug therapy for neurocysticercosis. Any cysticercocidal drug may cause irreparable damage when used to treat ocular or spinal cysts, even when corticosteroids are used.

80. Albendazole should be taken with a fatty meal to enhance absorption.

81. In ocular toxoplasmosis, corticosteroids should also be used for an anti-inflammatory effect on the eyes.

TABLE 5.7—Drugs for Treatment of Parasitic Infections (continued)

Infection	Drug	Adult Dosage*	Pediatric Dosage*
Toxocariasis, see VISCERAL LARVA MIGRANS			
TOXOPLASMOSIS (*Toxoplasma gondii*)[81]			
Drugs of choice:[82]	Pyrimethamine	25-100 mg/d x 3-4 wks	2 mg/kg/d x 3d, then 1 mg/kg/d (max. 25 mg/d) x 4 wks[83]
	plus sulfadiazine[84]	1-2 grams qid x 3-4 wks	100-200 mg/kg/d x 3-4 wks
Alternative:	Spiramycin[85]	3-4 grams/d	50-100 mg/d x 3-4 wks
TRICHINOSIS (*Trichinella spiralis*)			
Drugs of choice:	Steroids for severe symptoms		
	plus mebendazole[6,86]	200-400 mg tid x 3d, then 400-500 mg tid x 10d	
TRICHOMONIASIS (*Trichomonas vaginalis*)			
Drug of choice:[87]	Metronidazole	2 grams once or 250 mg tid orally x 7d	15 mg/kg/d orally in 3 doses x 7d
OR	Tinidazole[4]	2 grams once	50 mg/kg once (max. 2 grams)
TRICHOSTRONGYLUS infection			
Drug of choice:	Pyrantel pamoate[6]	11 mg/kg once (max. 1 gram)	11 mg/kg once (max. 1 gram)
Alternative:	Mebendazole[6]	100 mg bid x 3d	100 mg bid x 3d
OR	Albendazole	400 mg once	400 mg once
TRICHURIASIS (*Trichuris trichiura*, whipworm)			
Drug of choice:	Mebendazole	100 mg bid x 3d	100 mg bid x 3d
OR	Albendazole	400 mg once[88]	400 mg once[88]
TRYPANOSOMIASIS			
***T. cruzi* (South American trypanosomiasis, Chagas' disease)**			
Drug of choice:	Nifurtimox[2,89]	8-10 mg/kg/d orally in 4 doses x 120d	1-10 yrs: 15-20 mg/kg/d in 4 doses x 90d; 11-16 yrs: 12.5-15 mg/kg/d in 4 doses x 90d
Alternative:	Benznidazole[90]	5-7 mg/kg/d x 30-120d	

T. brucei gambiense; T. b. rhodesiense (African trypanosomiasis, sleeping sickness)

hemolymphatic stage

Drug of choice:	Suramin²	100-200 mg (test dose) IV, then 1 gram IV on days 1,3,7,14, and 21	20 mg/kg on days 1,3,7,14, and 21
Alternative:	OR Eflornithine	See footnote 91	
	Pentamidine isethionate⁶	4 mg/kg/d IM x 10d	4 mg/kg/d IM x 10d

late disease with CNS involvement

Drug of choice:	Melarsoprol²·⁹²	2-3.6 mg/kg/d IV x 3 d; after 1 wk 3.6 mg/kg per day IV x 3d; repeat again after 10-21 days	18-25 mg/kg total over 1 month; initial dose of 0.36 mg/kg IV, increasing gradually to max. 3.6 mg/kg at intervals of 1-5d for total of 9-10 doses
Alternatives:	OR Eflornithine	See footnote 91	
	Tryparsamide	One injection of 30 mg/kg (max. 2g) IV every 5d to total of 12 injections; may be repeated after 1 month	
	plus suramin²	One injection of 10 mg/kg IV every 5d to total of 12 injections; may be repeated after 1 month	

82. Pyrimethamine is teratogenic in animals. To prevent hematological toxicity from pyrimethamine, it is advisable to give leucovorin (folinic acid), about 10 mg/day, either by injection or orally. To treat CNS toxoplasmosis in HIV-infected patients, some clinicians use pyrimethamine 50 to 100 mg daily after a loading dose of 200 mg with a sulfonamide and, when sulfonamide sensitivity developed, have given clindamycin 1.8 to 2.4 g/d in divided doses instead of the sulfonamide (JS Remington et al, Lancet, 338:1142, 1991; BJ Luft et al, N Engl J Med, 329:995, 1993). Atovaquone, 750 mg qid, appears to be an effective alternative in sulfa-intolerant patients (JA Kovacs et al, Lancet, 340:637, 1992). Dapsone-pyrimethamine can prevent first episodes of toxoplasmosis (P-M Girard et al, N Engl J Med, 328:1514, 1993). In HIV-infected patients, chronic suppressive treatment should continue indefinitely (Medical Letter, 35:79, 1993).

83. Congenitally infected newborns should be treated with pyrimethamine every two or three days and a sulfonamide daily for about one year (JS Remington and G Desmonts in JS Remington and JO Klein, eds, Infectious Disease of the Fetus and Newborn Infant, 3rd ed, Philadelphia:Saunders, 1990, page 89).

84. Available temporarily from the CDC, 404-488-4928.

85. For use during pregnancy, continue the drug until delivery.

86. Albendazole or flubendazole (not available in the USA) may also be effective.

TABLE 5.7—Drugs for Treatment of Parasitic Infections (continued)

Infection	Drug	Adult Dosage*	Pediatric Dosage*
VISCERAL LARVA MIGRANS[93]			
Drug of choice:	Diethylcarbamazine[6]	6 mg/kg/d in 3 doses x 7-10d	6 mg/kg/d in 3 doses x 7-10d
Alternatives:	Albendazole[94]	400 mg bid x 3-5d	
	Mebendazole[6,95]	100-200 mg bid x 5d	400 mg bid x 3-5d

Whipworm, see TRICHURIASIS

Wuchereria bancrofti, see FILARIASIS

87. Sexual partners should be treated simultaneously. Outside the USA, ornidazole has also been used for this condition. Metronidazole-resistant strains have been reported; higher doses of metronidazole for longer periods are sometimes effective against these strains (J Lossick, Rev Infect Dis, 12:S665, 1990).

88. In heavy infection it may be necessary to extend therapy for 3 days.

89. The addition of gamma interferon to nifurtimox for 20 days in a limited number of patients and in experimental animals appears to have shortened the acute phase of Chagas' disease (RE McCabe et al, J Infect Dis, 163:912, 1991).

90. Limited data

91. In *T. b. gambiense* infections, eflornithine is highly effective in both the hemolymphatic and CNS stages. Its effectiveness in *T. b. rhodesiense* infections has been variable. Some clinicians have given 400 mg/kg/d IV in 4 divided doses for 14 days, followed by oral treatment with 300 mg/kg/d for 3-4 wks (F Milord et al, Lancet, 340:652, 1992).

92. In frail patients, begin with as little as 18 mg and increase the dose progressively. Pretreatment with suramin has been advocated for debilitated patients. Corticosteroids have been used to prevent arsenical encephalopathy (J Pepin et al, Lancet, 1:1246, 1989).

93. For severe symptoms or eye involvement, corticosteroids can be used in addition.

94. D Stürchler et al, Ann Trop Med Parasitol, 83:473, 1989

95. One report of a cure using 1 gram tid for 21 days has been published (A Bekhti, Ann Intern Med, 100:463, 1984).

TABLE 5.8—Manufacturers of Antiparasitic Drugs

* albendazole — *Zentel* (SmithKline Beecham)
  atovaquone — *Mepron* (Burroughs-Wellcome)
** benznidazole — *Rochagan* (Roche, Brazil)
† bithionol — *Bitin* (Tanabe, Japan)
  chloroquine — *Aralen* (Sanofi Winthrop), others
  crotamiton — *Eurax* (Westwood-Squibb)
† dehydroemetine — (Hoffmann-LaRoche, Switzerland)
* diethylcarbamazine — *Hetrazan* (Lederle), others
† diloxanide furoate — *Furamide* (Boots, England)
* eflornithine (difluoromethylornithine, DFMO) — *Ornidyl* (Merrell Dow)
** flubendazole — (Janssen)
  furazolidone — *Furoxone* (Roberts)
** halofantrine — *Halfan* (SmithKline Beecham)
  hydroxychloroquine — *Plaquenil* (Sanofi Winthrop)
  iodoquinol (diiodohydroxyquin) — *Yodoxin* (Glenwood), others
† ivermectin — *Mectizan* (Merck)
  lindane (gamma benzene hexachloride) — *Kwell* (Reed & Carnrick), others
  malathion — *Ovide* (GenDerm)
  mebendazole — *Vermox* (Janssen)
  mefloquine — *Lariam* (Roche)
** meglumine antimonate — *Glucantime* (Rhône-Poulenc Rorer, France)
† melarsoprol — *Arsobal* (Rhône Poulenc Rorer, France)
  metronidazole — *Flagyl* (Searle), others
  niclosamide — *Niclocide* (Miles)
† nifurtimox — *Lampit* (Bayer, Germany)

** ornidazole — *Tiberal* (Hoffman-LaRoche, Switzerland)
  oxamniquine — *Vansil* (Pfizer)
  paromomycin — *Humatin* (Parke-Davis)
  pentamidine isethionate — *Pentam 300* (Fujisawa), *Nebu-Pent* (Fujisawa)
  permethrin — *Nix* (Burroughs Wellcome), *Elimite* (Herbert)
  praziquantel — *Biltricide* (Miles)
  primaquine phosphate — (Sanofi Winthrop)
** proguanil — *Paludrine* (Ayerst, Canada, ICI, England)
  pyrantel pamoate — *Antiminth* (Pfizer)
  pyrethrins and piperonyl butoxide — *RID* (Pfizer), others
  pyrimethamine — *Daraprim* (Burroughs Wellcome)
  pyrimethamine-sulfadoxine — *Fansidar* (Roche)
** quinacrine — *Atabrine* (Sanofi Winthrop)
  quinidine gluconate — (Lilly)
** quinine dihydrochloride
  quinine sulfate — many manufacturers
† sodium stibogluconate (antimony sodium gluconate) — *Pentostam* (Burroughs Wellcome, England)
‡ spiramycin — *Rovamycine* (Rhône-Poulenc Rorer)
† suramin — *Germanin* (Bayer, Germany)
  thiabendazole — *Mintezol* (Merck)
** tinidazole — *Fasigyn* (Pfizer)
** triclabendazole (Ciba-Geigy)
‡ trimetrexate — (US Bioscience)
** tryparsamide

---

* Available in the USA only from the manufacturer
** Not available in the USA
† Available from the CDC Drug Service, Centers for Disease Control and Prevention, Atlanta, Georgia 30333; 404-639-3670 (evenings, weekends, or holidays: 404-639-2888)
‡ Available from the National Institute of Allergy and Infectious Diseases, 1-800-537-9978

TABLE 5.9—Adverse Effects of Some Antiparasitic Drugs*

ALBENDAZOLE *(Zentel)*
Occasional: diarrhea; abdominal pain; migration of *ascaris* through mouth and nose
Rare: leukopenia; alopecia; increased serum transaminase activity

ATOVAQUONE *(Mepron)*
Frequent: rash, nausea
Occasional: diarrhea

BENZNIDAZOLE *(Rochagan)*
Frequent: allergic rash; dose-dependent polyneuropathy; gastrointestinal disturbances; psychic disturbances

BITHIONOL *(Bitin)*
Frequent: photosensitivity reactions; vomiting; diarrhea; abdominal pain; urticaria
Rare: leukopenia; toxic hepatitis

CHLOROQUINE HCI and CHLOROQUINE PHOSPHATE *(Aralen, and others)*
Occasional: pruritus; vomiting; headache; confusion; depigmentation of hair; skin eruptions; corneal opacity; weight loss; partial alopecia; extraocular muscle palsies; exacerbation of psoriasis, eczema, and other exfoliative dermatoses; myalgias; photophobia
Rare: irreversible retinal injury (especially when total dosage exceeds 100 grams); discoloration of nails and mucus membranes; nerve-type deafness; peripheral neuropathy and myopathy; heart block; blood dyscrasias; hematemesis

CROTAMITON *(Eurax)*
Occasional: rash; conjunctivitis

DEHYDROEMETINE
Frequent: cardiac arrhythmias; precordial pain; muscle weakness; cellulitis at site of injection
Occasional: diarrhea; vomiting; peripheral neuropathy; heart failure; headache; dyspnea

DIETHYLCARBAMAZINE CITRATE USP *(Hetrazan)*
Frequent: severe allergic or febrile reactions in patients with microfilariae in the blood or the skin; GI disturbances
Rare: encephalopathy

DILOXANIDE FUROATE *(Furamide)*
Frequent: flatulence
Occasional: nausea; vomiting; diarrhea
Rare: diplopia; dizziness; urticaria; pruritus

EFLORNITHINE (Difluoromethylornithine, DFMO, *Ornidyl*)
Frequent: anemia; leukopenia
Occasional: diarrhea; thrombocytopenia; seizures
Rare: hearing loss

FLUBENDAZOLE – similar to mebendazole

FURAZOLIDONE (*Furoxone*)
Frequent: nausea; vomiting
Occasional: allergic reactions, including pulmonary infiltration, hypotension, urticaria, fever, vesicular rash; hypoglycemia; headache
Rare: hemolytic anemia in G-6-PD deficiency and neonates; disulfiram-like reaction with alcohol; MAO-inhibitor interactions; polyneuritis

HALOFANTRINE (*Halfan*)
Occasional: diarrhea; abdominal pain; pruritus; prolongation of QTc and PR interval

IODOQUINOL (*Yodoxin*)
Occasional: rash; acne; slight enlargement of the thyroid gland; nausea; diarrhea; cramps; anal pruritus
Rare: optic neuritis; optic atrophy, loss of vision, peripheral neuropathy after prolonged use in high dosage (for months); iodine sensitivity

IVERMECTIN (*Mectizan*)
Occasional: Mazzotti-type reaction seen in onchocerciasis, including fever, pruritus, tender lymph nodes, headache, and joint and bone pain
Rare: hypotension

LINDANE (*Kwell*, and others)
Occasional: eczematous rash; conjunctivitis
Rare: convulsions; aplastic anemia

MALATHION (*Ovide*)
Occasional: local irritation

MEBENDAZOLE (*Vermox*)
Occasional: diarrhea; abdominal pain; migration of *ascaris* through mouth and nose
Rare: leukopenia; agranulocytosis; hypospermia

MEFLOQUINE (*Lariam*)
Frequent: vertigo; lightheadedness; nausea; other gastrointestinal disturbances; nightmares; visual disturbances; headache
Occasional: confusion
Rare: psychosis; hypotension; convulsions; coma; paresthesias

MEGLUMINE ANTIMONATE (*Glucantime*) Similar to sodium stibogluconate

MELARSOPROL (*Arsobal*)
Frequent: myocardial damage; albuminuria; hypertension; colic; Herxheimer-type reaction; encephalopathy; vomiting; peripheral neuropathy
Rare: shock

METRONIDAZOLE (*Flagyl*, and others)
Frequent: nausea; headache; dry mouth; metallic taste
Occasional: vomiting; diarrhea; insomnia; weakness; stomatitis; vertigo; paresthesias; rash; dark urine; urethral burning; disulfiram-like reaction with alcohol
Rare: seizures; encephalopathy; pseudomembranous colitis; ataxia; leukopenia; peripheral neuropathy; pancreatitis

NICLOSAMIDE (*Niclocide*)
Occasional: nausea; abdominal pain

TABLE 5.9—Adverse Effects of Some Antiparasitic Drugs* (continued)

NIFURTIMOX (Lampit)

Frequent: anorexia; vomiting; weight loss; loss of memory; sleep disorders; tremor; paresthesias; weakness; polyneuritis

Rare: convulsions; fever; pulmonary infiltrates and pleural effusion

ORNIDAZOLE (Tiberal)

Occasional: dizziness; headache; gastrointestinal disturbances

Rare: reversible peripheral neuropathy

OXAMNIQUINE (Vansil)

Occasional: headache; fever; dizziness; somnolence; nausea; diarrhea; rash; insomnia; hepatic enzyme changes; ECG changes; EEG changes; orange-red discoloration of urine

Rare: seizures; neuropsychiatric disturbances

PAROMOMYCIN (Aminosidine; Humatin)

Frequent: GI disturbances

Occasional: eighth-nerve damage (mainly auditory); renal damage

PENTAMIDINE ISETHIONATE (Pentam 300, NebuPent)

Frequent: hypotension; hypoglycemia often followed by diabetes mellitus; vomiting; blood dyscrasias; renal damage; pain at injection site; GI disturbances

Occasional: may aggravate diabetes; shock; hypocalcemia; liver damage; cardiotoxicity; delirium; rash

Rare: Herxheimer-type reaction; anaphylaxis; acute pancreatitis; hyperkalemia

PERMETHRIN (Nix, Elimite)

Occasional: burning; stinging; numbness; increased pruritus; pain; edema; erythema; rash

PRAZIQUANTEL (Biltricide)

Frequent: malaise; headache; dizziness

Occasional: sedation; abdominal discomfort; fever; sweating; nausea; eosinophilia; fatigue

Rare: pruritus; rash

PRIMAQUINE PHOSPHATE USP

Frequent: hemolytic anemia in G-6-PD deficiency

Occasional: neutropenia; GI disturbances; methemoglobinemia in G-6-PD deficiency

Rare: CNS symptoms; hypertension; arrhythmias

PROGUANIL (Paludrine)

Occasional: oral ulceration; hair loss; scaling of palms and soles; urticaria

Rare: hematuria (with large doses); vomiting; abdominal pain; diarrhea (with large doses); thrombocytopenia

PYRANTEL PAMOATE (Antiminth)

Occasional: GI disturbances; headache; dizziness; rash; fever

PYRETHRINS and PIPERONYL BUTOXIDE (RID, others)

Occasional: allergic reactions

PYRIMETHAMINE USP (Daraprim)

Occasional: blood dyscrasias; folic acid deficiency

Rare: rash; vomiting; convulsions; shock; possibly pulmonary eosinophilia; fatal cutaneous reactions with **pyrimethamine-sulfadoxine** (Fansidar)

QUINACRINE HCl USP *(Atabrine)*
Frequent: dizziness; headache; vomiting; diarrhea
Occasional: yellow staining of skin; toxic psychosis; insomnia; bizarre dreams; blood dyscrasias; urticaria; blue and black nail pigmentation; psoriasis-like rash
Rare: acute hepatic necrosis; convulsions; severe exfoliative dermatitis; ocular effects similar to those caused by chloroquine

QUININE DIHYDROCHLORIDE and SULFATE
Frequent: cinchonism (tinnitus, headache, nausea, abdominal pain, visual disturbance)
Occasional: deafness; hemolytic anemia; other blood dyscrasias; photosensitivity reactions; hypoglycemia; arrhythmias; hypotension; drug fever
Rare: blindness; sudden death if injected too rapidly

SODIUM STIBOGLUCONATE *(Pentostam)*
Frequent: muscle pain and joint stiffness; nausea; transaminase elevations; T-wave flattening or inversion
Occasional: weakness; colic; liver damage; bradycardia; leukopenia
Rare: diarrhea; rash; pruritus; myocardial damage; hemolytic anemia; renal damage; shock; sudden death

SPIRAMYCIN *(Rovamycine)*
Occasional: GI disturbances
Rare: allergic reactions

SURAMIN SODIUM *(Germanin)*
Frequent: vomiting; pruritus; urticaria; paresthesias; hyperesthesia of hands and feet; photophobia; peripheral neuropathy
Occasional: kidney damage; blood dyscrasias; shock; optic atrophy

THIABENDAZOLE *(Mintezol)*
Frequent: nausea; vomiting; vertigo
Occasional: leukopenia; crystalluria; rash; hallucinations; olfactory disturbance; erythema multiforme
Rare: shock; tinnitus; intrahepatic cholestasis; convulsions; angioneurotic edema; Stevens-Johnson syndrome

TINIDAZOLE *(Fasigyn)*
Occasional: metallic taste; nausea; vomiting; rash

TRIMETREXATE (with "leucovorin rescue")
Occasional: rash; peripheral neuropathy; bone marrow depression; increased serum aminotransferase concentrations

TRYPARSAMIDE
Frequent: nausea; vomiting
Occasional: impaired vision; optic atrophy; fever; exfoliative dermatitis; allergic reactions; tinnitus

* Drug interactions are generally not included here; see the current edition of *The Medical Letter Handbook of Adverse Drug Interactions.*

APPENDICES

Appendix I

Directory of Telephone Numbers

Organization or Source	Telephone Number
American Academy of Pediatrics	708/228-5005
Centers for Disease Control and Prevention (CDC)	
• Public Inquiries	404/639-3534
• National Immunization Program	404/639-8200
• Immunization, Infectious Diseases, and Other Health Information - Voice Information System	404/332-4553
• International Travelers Hotline	404/332-4559
• Vector-Borne Infectious Disease—Information on Japanese Encephalitis	303/221-6400
• FAX Information Service (including international travel)	404/332-4565
• Drug Service	404/639-3670
• Division of Parasitic Diseases	404/488-4050
• Division of Tuberculosis Control	404/639-8120
• National HIV and AIDS Hotline	800/342-AIDS
Food and Drug Administration:	
• Center for Biologics Evaluation and Research	301/594-2000
• Center for Drug Evaluation and Research	301/594-1012
Michigan Department of Public Health (Division of Biologic Products)	517/335-8120
National Vaccine Injury Compensation Program (For information on filing claims)	800/338-2382
National Vaccine Program Office	202/401-8141
Pediatric AIDS Drug Trials - Information:	
• Pediatric Branch, National Cancer Institute	301/402-0696
• Pediatric Clinical Trials Group (NIAID-sponsored)	800/TRIALS-A
Vaccine Adverse Events Reporting System (VAERS)	800/822-7967

Appendix II

Standards for Pediatric Immunization Practices*

Recommended by the
National Vaccine Advisory Committee
April 1992

Approved by the
United States Public Health Service
May 1992

Endorsed by the
American Academy of Pediatrics
May 1992

The Standards represent the consensus of the National Vaccine Advisory Committee (NVAC) and of a broad group of medical and public health experts about what constitute the most desirable immunization practices. It is recognized by the NVAC that not all of the current immunization practices of public and private providers are in compliance with the Standards. Nevertheless, the Standards are expected to be useful as a means of helping providers to identify needed changes, to obtain resources if necessary, and to actually implement the desirable immunization practices in the future.

STANDARDS FOR PEDIATRIC IMMUNIZATION PRACTICES

Preamble

Ideally, immunizations should be given as part of comprehensive child health care. This is the ultimate goal toward which the nation must strive if all of America's children are to benefit from the best primary disease prevention our health care system has to offer.

Overall improvement in our primary care delivery system requires intensive effort and will take time. However, we should not wait for changes in this system before providing immunizations more effectively to our children. Current health care policies and practices in all settings result in the failure to deliver vaccines on schedule to many of our vulnerable preschool-aged children. This failure is due primarily to barriers that impede vaccine delivery and to missed opportunities during clinic visits. Changes in policies and practices can immediately improve coverage. The present system should be geared to "user-friendly," family-centered, culturally sensitive, and comprehensive primary health care that can provide rapid, efficient, and consumer-oriented services to the users, ie, children and their parents. The failure to do so is evidenced by the recent resurgence of measles and measles-related childhood mortality, which may be an omen of other vaccine-preventable disease outbreaks.

Present childhood immunization practices must be changed if we wish to protect the nation's children and immunize 90% of two-year-olds by the year 2000.

The following standards for pediatric immunization practices address these issues. These standards are recommended for use by **all** health professionals in

---

*Reproduced from *Standards for Pediatric Immunization Practices*. Atlanta, GA: Centers for Disease Control and Prevention; 1993. US Dept of Health and Human Services.

the public and private sector who administer vaccines to or manage immunization services for infants and children. These **Standards** represent the most desirable immunization practices which health care providers should strive to achieve to the extent possible. By adopting these **Standards**, providers can begin to enhance and change their own policies and practices. It is recognized that not all providers will have the funds necessary to fully implement the **Standards** immediately. Nevertheless, those providers and programs lacking the resources to implement the **Standards** fully should find them a useful tool in better delineating immunization needs and in obtaining additional resources in the future in order to achieve the Healthy People 2000 immunization objective.

Standards

Standard 1. Immunization services are **readily available**.

Standard 2. There are **no barriers** or **unnecessary prerequisites** to the receipt of vaccines.

Standard 3. Immunization services are available **free** or for a minimal fee.

Standard 4. Providers utilize all clinical encounters to **screen** and, when indicated, **immunize** children.

Standard 5. Providers **educate** parents and guardians about immunization in general terms.

Standard 6. Providers **question** parents or guardians about **contraindications** and, before immunizing a child, **inform** them in specific terms about the risks and benefits of the immunizations their child is to receive.

Standard 7. Providers follow only true **contraindications**.

Standard 8. Providers administer **simultaneously** all vaccine doses for which a child is eligible at the time of each visit.

Standard 9. Providers use accurate and complete **recording procedures**.

Standard 10. Providers **co-schedule** immunization appointments in conjunction with appointments for other child health services.

Standard 11. Providers **report adverse events** following immunization promptly, accurately and completely.

Standard 12. Providers operate a **tracking system**.

Standard 13. Providers adhere to appropriate procedures for **vaccine management**.

Standard 14. Providers conduct semi-annual **audits** to assess immunization coverage levels and to review immunization records in the patient populations they serve.

Standard 15. Providers maintain up-to-date, easily retrievable **medical protocols** at all locations where vaccines are administered.

Standard 16. Providers operate with **patient-oriented** and **community-based** approaches.

Standard 17. Vaccines are administered by **properly trained** individuals.

Standard 18. Providers receive **ongoing education** and **training** on current immunization recommendations.

Discussion

1.

Immunization services are *readily available*.

Immunization services should be responsive to the needs of patients. For example, in large urban areas, public immunization clinic services should be available daily, 8 hours per day. In smaller cities and rural areas, clinics may operate less frequently. To be fully responsive, providers in many locations should consider offering immunization services each working day as well as during some off-hours (e.g., weekends, evenings, early mornings, or lunch-hours). Immunization services should be considered for all days and at all hours that other child health services in the same site are offered (e.g., Special Supplemental Food Program for Women, Infants, and Children, [WIC]). Private providers who offer primary care to infants and children should always include immunization services as a routine part of that care.

Ready availability of immunization services also requires that the supply of vaccines be adequate at all times.

2.

There are *no barriers* or *unnecessary prerequisites* to the receipt of vaccines.

Appointment-only systems often serve as barriers to immunization in both public and private settings. Thus, immunization services should also be available on a walk-in basis at all times for both routine and new enrollee visits. Waiting time should be minimized and generally not exceed 30 minutes. Furthermore, administration of needed vaccines should not be contingent on enrollment in a well-baby program unless enrollment is immediately available. Children presenting only for immunizations should be rapidly and efficiently screened without requiring other comprehensive health services. However, children receiving immunizations in such an "express lane" fashion and found not to have a primary care provider should be referred to one.

Physical examinations and temperature measurements prior to immunization should not be required if they delay or impede the timely receipt of immunizations (e.g., appointments for physical examination in some facilities may take weeks to months). A reliable decision to vaccinate can be based exclusively on the information elicited from a parent or guardian and on the provider's observations and judgment about the child's wellness at the time of vaccination. At a minimum, children should have pre-immunization assessments, including (a) observing the child's general state of health, (b) asking the parent or guardian if the child is well, and (c) questioning the parent or guardian about potential contraindications (see Table, page 611).

In public clinic settings, the administration of vaccines should not be dependent on individual written orders or on a referral from a primary care provider. Rather, standing orders should be developed and implemented.

3. **Immunization services are available *free* or for a minimal fee.**

In the public sector, immunizations should be free of charge. If fees must be collected, they should be kept to a minimum. In the private sector, charges should include the cost of the vaccine, and a reasonable administration fee. Affordable vaccinations will limit the fragmentation of care and help assure the immunization of the greatest number of children. Public and private providers charging a fee to administer vaccines obtained through a consolidated federal contract should prominently display a state approved sign indicating that no one will be denied immunization services because of inability to pay the fee.

4. **Providers utilize all clinical encounters to *screen* for needed vaccines and, when indicated, *immunize* children.**

Each encounter with a health care provider, including an emergency room visit or hospitalization, is an opportunity to screen the immunization status and, if indicated, administer needed vaccines. Before discharge from the hospital, children should receive immunizations for which they are eligible by age and/or health status. The child's regular health care provider should be informed about the immunizations administered. Implementation of this standard minimizes the number of missed opportunities to vaccinate.

In addition, children accompanying parents or siblings who are seeking any service should also be screened and, when indicated, given needed vaccines.

Providers in subspecialty clinics (eg, oncology) who care for children should pay particular attention to the immunization status of their patients and vaccinate or refer them to immunization services or primary health care providers as appropriate.

Providers in other specialties should also note the immunization status of children and refer or immunize as appropriate.

5. **Providers *educate* parents and guardians about immunization in general terms.**

Providers should educate parents and guardians in a culturally sensitive way, preferably in their own language, about the importance of immunizations, the diseases they prevent, the recommended immunization schedules, the need to receive immunizations at recommended ages and the importance of bringing their child's immunization record to each visit. Parents should be encouraged to take responsibility for ensuring that their child completes the full series. Providers should answer all questions parents and guardians may have and provide appropriate educational materials at suitable reading levels in pertinent languages.

6. Providers *question* parents or guardians about *contraindications* and, before immunizing a child, *inform* them in specific terms about the risks and benefits of the immunizations their child is to receive.

Minimal acceptable screening procedures for precautions and contraindications include asking questions to elicit a possible history of adverse events following prior immunizations and determining any existing precautions or contraindications (see Table, page 611).

The Vaccine Information Pamphlets (required by regulation* to be used universally beginning April 15, 1992, for Measles, Mumps, Rubella, Diphtheria, Tetanus, Pertussis, and Polio by all providers administering vaccine purchased from the federal contract) should be provided and reviewed with parents or guardians. Private physicians who purchase their own vaccines must use these pamphlets or must develop and use alternative vaccine information materials that meet all the requirements of the law. Similar information contained in the Important Information Statements for other vaccines (e.g., hepatitis B and *Haemophilus influenzae* type b) should be provided to all parents or guardians in public clinics and use of these statements should be considered by private providers. Providers should ensure that information materials are current and available in appropriate languages. Providers should ask parents or guardians if they have questions about what they have read and should ensure that they receive satisfactory answers to their questions.

Providers should explain where and how to obtain medical care during day- and night-time hours in case of an adverse event following vaccination.

7. Providers follow only true *contraindications*.

Accepting conditions which are not true contraindications as being true contraindications (see Table, page 611) often results in the needless deferment of indicated immunizations. The table of true contraindications is based on the recommendations of the Advisory Committee on Immunization Practices (ACIP) and the recommendations of the Committee on Infectious Diseases (*Red Book* Committee) of the American Academy of Pediatrics (AAP). Sometimes these recommendations may vary from those contained in the manufacturer's package inserts. For more detailed information, providers should consult the published recommendations of the ACIP, the AAP, the American Academy of Family Physicians (AAFP), and the manufactur's package inserts.

---

*Federal Register 1991;56(199):51798-51818, Codified at 42 Code of Federal Regulations Part 110

8. **Providers administer *simultaneously* all vaccine doses for which a child is eligible at the time of each visit.**

Available evidence suggests that the simultaneous administration of childhood immunizations is safe and effective. In addition, evidence suggests that the simultaneous administration of multiple needed vaccines can potentially raise immunization coverage by 9%-17%. If providers elect not to administer a needed vaccine simultaneously with others (based either on their judgment that this action will not compromise the timely immunization of the child or on a request by the parent or guardian), they should document such actions and the reasons why the vaccine was not administered. The record should be flagged with an automatic recall for an appointment to receive the needed vaccine(s). This next appointment should be discussed with the parent or guardian of the child.

Measles, Mumps, Rubella (MMR) vaccine should always be used in combined form when providing routine childhood immunizations.

9. **Providers use accurate and complete *recording procedures*.**

Providers are required by statute to record what vaccine was given, the date the vaccine was given (month, day, year), the name of the manufacturer of the vaccine, the lot number, the signature and title of the person who gave the vaccine, and the address where the vaccine was given.* In addition, providers should record on the child's personal immunization record card (preferably the official state version) what vaccine was given, the date the vaccine was given and the name of the provider. Providers should encourage parents or guardians to maintain a copy of their child's personal immunization record card. This card should be updated at each visit for immunizations. If a parent fails to bring their child's card, a new one should be issued containing all previous immunizations and designated as a replacement record card. When accepting immunization record data from parents, providers should confirm that prior doses of vaccines have actually been administered, either by reviewing immunization record cards or by contacting former providers and entering this verified information onto their records. When a provider who does not routinely vaccinate or care for a child administers a vaccine to that child, the regular provider should be informed.

Providers with manual record-keeping systems should maintain separate or easily retrievable files of the immunization records of preschoolers to facilitate assessment of coverage as well as the identification and recall of children who miss appointments. In addition, preschooler immunization files should be sorted periodically, with inactive records placed into a separate file. Providers should indicate in their records, or in an appropriately identified place, all primary care services that each child receives in order to facilitate co-scheduling with other services.

---

*42 US Code 300aa-25

10. Providers *co-schedule* immunization appointments in conjunction with appointments for other child health services.

Providers of immunization-only services which require an appointment should co-schedule immunization appointments with other needed health care services such as WIC, dental exams or developmental screening **provided such scheduling does not create a barrier** by delaying needed immunizations.

11. Providers *report adverse events* following immunization promptly, accurately, and completely.

Providers should encourage parents or legal guardians to inform them of adverse events following immunization. Providers should report all such clinically significant events, including those required by law, to the Vaccine Adverse Event Reporting System (VAERS), regardless of whether or not they believe the events are caused by the vaccines. Report forms and assistance are available by calling 1-800/822-7967. Providers should document fully the adverse event in the medical record at the time of the event or as soon as possible thereafter.

12. Providers operate a *tracking system*.

A tracking system should produce reminders of upcoming immunizations as well as recalls for children who are overdue. A system may be automated or manual and may include mailed or telephone messages. In the public sector, health department staff may also make home visits. All providers should identify, for additional intensive tracking efforts, children considered at high risk of failing to complete the immunization series on schedule (e.g., children who start their series late).

13. Providers adhere to appropriate procedures for *vaccine management*.

Vaccines should be handled and stored as recommended in the manufacturer's package inserts. The temperatures at which vaccines are stored and transported should be monitored daily and the expiration date for each vaccine should be noted.

Providers using publicly purchased vaccine should periodically report usage, wastage, loss and inventory as required by state or local public health authorities.

14. **Providers conduct semi-annual *audits* to assess immunization coverage levels and to review immunization records in the patient populations they serve.**

In both the public and private sector, the assessment of immunization services for pre-school-aged patients should include audits of immunization records or inspection of a random sample of records (1) to determine the immunization coverage level (i.e., the percentage of children that are up-to-date by their second birthday), (2) to identify how frequently opportunities for simultaneous immunization are missed and (3) to assess the quality of documentation. The results of such assessments should be discussed by providers as part of their ongoing quality assurance reviews and used to develop solutions to the problems identified.

15. **Providers maintain up-to-date, easily retrievable *medical protocols* at all locations where vaccines are administered.**

Providers administering vaccines should maintain a protocol which, at a minimum, discusses the appropriate vaccine dosage, vaccine contraindications, the recommended sites and techniques for vaccine administration as well as possible adverse events and their emergency management. Such protocols should specify the necessary emergency medical equipment, drugs (including dosage) and personnel to safely and competently deal with any medical emergency which may arise after the administration of a vaccine. All providers should be familiar with the content of these protocols, their location and how to follow them. Vaccines can be administered in any setting (e.g., schools, churches) where providers can adhere to these protocols.

16. **Providers practice *patient-oriented* and *community-based* approaches.**

Public providers should routinely seek the input of their patients on specific approaches to better serve their immunization needs and implement the changes necessary to provide more user-friendly services.

Public providers should adopt a community-based approach to the provision of immunization services which calls for reaching high coverage levels in their catchment area populations and not only in the active patient populations they serve. Such a community-based approach requires all public providers to publicize the availability of their immunization services and to conduct community outreach activities to increase demand for immunization services. Private providers should cooperate with local health officials in their efforts to assure high coverage levels throughout the community. Without high immunization coverage levels, no community is completely protected against vaccine-preventable diseases. All providers share in the responsibility to achieve the highest possible degree of community protection.

17. **Vaccines are administered by *properly trained* individuals.**

Only properly trained individuals should administer vaccines. However, the task of administering vaccines need not be assigned exclusively to physicians and nurses. With appropriate training, including the management of emergency situations, and under professional supervision, other personnel can skillfully and safely administer vaccines. In some jurisdictions, statutory requirements may limit the administration of vaccines to licensed physicians and/or nurses which could therefore create barriers to immunization. If so, legal opinion should be sought locally to determine the necessary steps to overcome this barrier.

18. **Providers receive *ongoing education* and *training* on current immunization recommendations.**

Providers include all individuals who are involved in the administration of vaccines, the management of immunization clinics, or the support of these functions. Training and education should cover current guidelines and recommendations of the ACIP, AAP and the AAFP, as well as the Standards for Pediatric Immunization Practices and other immunization information sources such as the manufacturer's package inserts. Providers should also receive information about ongoing national efforts to reach the year 2000 goal of 90% series complete immunization by the second birthday.

Contraindications

Guide to Contraindications and Precautions to Immunizations, May 1992

Vaccine	True Contraindications and Precautions	Not True (Vaccines may be given)
GENERAL FOR ALL VACCINES	Anaphylactic reaction to a vaccine contraindicates further doses of that vaccine	Mild to moderate local reaction (soreness, redness, swelling) following a dose of an injectable antigen
	Anaphylactic reaction to a vaccine constituent contraindicates the use of vaccines containing that substance	
	Moderate or severe illnesses with or without a fever	Mild acute illness with or without low-grade fever
[DTP/DTaP, OPV, IPV, MMR, Hib, HBV]		Current antimicrobial therapy
		Convalescent phase of illnesses
		Prematurity (same dosage and indications as for normal, full-term infants)
		Recent exposure to an infectious disease
		History of penicillin or other nonspecific allergies or fact that relatives have such allergies

This information is based on the recommendations of the Advisory Committee on Immunization Practices (ACIP) and those of the Committee on Infectious Diseases (Red Book Committee) of the American Academy of Pediatrics (AAP). Sometimes these recommendations vary from those contained in the manufacturers' package inserts. For more detailed information, providers should consult the published recommendations of the ACIP, the AAP, the AAFP, and the manufacturers' package inserts.

Guide to Contraindications and Precautions to Immunizations, May 1992 (continued)

Vaccine	True Contraindications and Precautions		Not True (Vaccines may be given)
DTP/DTaP	Encephalopathy within 7 days of administration of previous dose of DTP		Temperature of <40.5°C (105°F) following a previous dose of DTP
	Fever of ≥40.5°C (105°F) within 48 hrs after vaccination with a prior dose of DTP		Family history of convulsions*
	Collapse or shocklike state (hypotonic-hyporesponsive episode) within 48 hrs of receiving a prior dose of DTP		Family history of sudden infant death syndrome
	Precautions*	Seizures within 3 days of receiving a prior dose of DTP (see footnote** regarding management of children with a personal history of seizures at any time)	Family history of an adverse event following DTP administration
		Persistent, inconsolable crying lasting ≥3 hrs, within 48 hrs of receiving a prior dose of DTP	

*The events or conditions listed as precautions, although not contraindications, should be carefully reviewed. The benefits and risks of administering a specific vaccine to an individual under the circumstances should be considered. If the risks are believed to outweigh the benefits, the immunization should be withheld; if the benefits are believed to outweigh the risks (for example, during an outbreak or foreign travel), the immunization should be given. Whether and when to administer DTP to children with proven or suspected underlying neurologic disorders should be decided on an individual basis. It is prudent on theoretical grounds to avoid vaccinating pregnant women. However, if immediate protection against poliomyelitis is needed, OPV, not IPV, is recommended.

**Acetaminophen given prior to administering DTP and thereafter every 4 hours for 24 hours should be considered for children with a personal or with a family history of convulsions in siblings or parents.

Vaccine	True Contraindications and Precautions		Not True (Vaccines may be given)
OPV***	Infection with HIV or a household contact with HIV		Breast feeding
	Known altered immunodeficiency (hematologic and solid tumors; congenital immunodeficiency; and long term immunosuppressive therapy)		Current antimicrobial therapy
	Immunodeficient household contact		Diarrhea
	Precaution*	Pregnancy	
IPV	Anaphylactic reaction to neomycin or streptomycin		
	Precaution*	Pregnancy	

*The events or conditions listed as precautions, although not contraindications, should be carefully reviewed. The benefits and risks of administering a specific vaccine to an individual under the circumstances should be considered. If the risks are believed to outweigh the benefits, the immunization should be withheld; if the benefits are believed to outweigh the risks (for example, during an outbreak or foreign travel), the immunization should be given. Whether and when to administer DTP to children with proven or suspected underlying neurologic disorders should be decided on an individual basis. It is prudent on theoretical grounds to avoid vaccinating pregnant women. However, if immediate protection against poliomyelitis is needed, OPV, not IPV, is recommended.

***There is a theoretical risk that the administration of multiple live virus vaccines (OPV & MMR) within 30 days of one another if not given on the same day will result in a suboptimal immune response. There are no data to substantiate this.

Guide to Contraindications and Precautions to Immunizations, May 1992 (continued)

Vaccine	True Contraindications and Precautions		Not True (Vaccines may be given)
MMR***	Anaphylactic reactions to egg ingestion and to neomycin****		Tuberculosis or positive PPD
			Simultaneous TB skin testing*****
	Pregnancy		Breast feeding
	Known altered immunodeficiency (hematologic and solid tumors; congenital immunodeficiency; and long term immunosuppressive therapy		Pregnancy of mother of recipient
			Immunodeficient family member or household contact
	Precaution*	Recent (within 3 months) IG administration	Infection with HIV
			Nonanaphylatic reactions to eggs or neomycin
Hib			
HBV			Pregnancy

*The events or conditions listed as precautions, although not contraindications, should be carefully reviewed. The benefits and risks of administering a specific vaccine to an individual under the circumstances should be considered. If the risks are believed to outweigh the benefits, the immunization should be withheld; if the benefits are believed to outweigh the risks (for example, during an outbreak or foreign travel), the immunization should be given. Whether and when to administer DTP to children with proven or suspected underlying neurologic disorders should be decided on an individual basis. It is prudent on theoretical grounds to avoid vaccinating pregnant women. However, if immediate protection against poliomyelitis is needed, OPV, not IPV, is recommended.

***There is a theoretical risk that the administration of multiple live virus vaccines (OPV & MMR) within 30 days of one another if not given on the same day will result in a suboptimal immune response. There are no data to substantiate this.

****Persons with a history of anaphylactic reactions following egg ingestion should be vaccinated only with extreme caution. Protocols have been developed for vaccinating such persons and should be consulted (*J Pediatr* 1983;102:196-9, *J Pediatr* 1988;113:504-506).

*****Measles vaccination may temporarily suppress tuberculin reactivity. If testing can not be done on the day of MMR vaccination, the test should be postponed for 4-6 weeks.

Appendix III

National Vaccine Injury Compensation Table (as of December 1993)[1,2]

The following excerpt from the National Childhood Vaccine Injury Act of 1986 lists the vaccination-associated events and time period in which the first symptom, manifestation, or significant aggravation occurred for which compensation will be provided.

Sec 2114. (a)

Vaccine Injury Table

I. DTP; P; DTP/Polio Combination; or Any Other Vaccine Containing Whole Cell Pertussis Bacteria, Extracted or Partial Cell Bacteria, or Specific Pertussis Antigen(s).

Illness, disability, injury, or condition covered:	Time period for first symptom or manifestation of onset or of significant aggravation after vaccine administration:
A. Anaphylaxis or anaphylactic shock	24 hours
B. Encephalopathy (or encephalitis)	3 days
C. Shock-collapse or hypotonic-hyporesponsive collapse	3 days
D. Residual seizure disorder in accordance with subsection (b)(2)	3 days
E. Any acute complication or sequela (including death) of an illness, disability, injury, or condition referred to above which illness, disability, injury, or condition arose within the period prescribed	Not applicable

II. Measles, mumps, rubella, or any vaccine containing any of the foregoing as a component; DT; Td; or Tetanus Toxoid.

A. Anaphylaxis or anaphylactic shock	24 hours
B. Encephalopathy (or encephalitis)	15 days (for mumps, rubella, measles, or any vaccine containing any of the foregoing as a component). 3 days (for DT, Td, or tetanus toxoid).
C. Residual seizure disorder in accordance with sub-section (c)(2)	15 days (for mumps, rubella, measles, or any vaccine containing any of the foregoing as a component). 3 days (for DT, Td, or tetanus toxoid).
D. Any acute complication or sequela (including death) of an illness, disability, injury, or condition referred to above which illness, disability, injury or condition arose within the time period prescribed	Not applicable

---

[1]Public Law 99-660; amended by Public Law 101-239 (1987), effective January 1, 1988.

[2]This table may be revised in the near future for prospective cases, since modifications recommended by the Advisory Commission on Childhood Vaccines to the Secretary of Health and Human Services currently are under review.

Vaccine Injury Table *(continued)*

III. Polio Vaccines (other than Inactivated Polio
    Vaccine).
    A. Paralytic polio
        - in a nonimmunodeficient recipient .... 30 days
        - in an immunodeficient recipient .... 6 months
        - in a vaccine-associated community case .... Not applicable
    B. Any acute complication or sequela (including
        death) of an illness, disability, injury, or
        condition referred to above which illness,
        disability, injury, or condition arose within
        the time period prescribed.. Not applicable
IV. Inactivated Polio Vaccine.
    A. Anaphylaxis or anaphylactic shock .... 24 hours
    B. Any acute complication or sequela (including
        death) of an illness, disability, injury, or
        condition referred to above which illness,
        disability, injury, or condition arose within
        the time period prescribed.. Not applicable

"(b) Qualifications and Aids to Interpretation.—The following qualifications and aids to interpretation shall apply to the Vaccine Injury Table in subsection (a):

"(1) A shock-collapse or a hypotonic-hyporesponsive collapse may be evidenced by indicia or symptoms such as decrease or loss of muscle tone, paralysis (partial or complete), hemiplegia or hemiparesis, loss of color or turning pale white or blue, unresponsiveness to environmental stimuli, depression of consciousness, loss of consciousness, prolonged sleeping with difficulty arousing, or cardiovascular or respiratory arrest.

"(2) A petitioner may be considered to have suffered a residual seizure disorder if the petitioner did not suffer a seizure or convulsion unaccompanied by fever or accompanied by a fever of less than 102 degrees Fahrenheit before the first seizure or convulsion after the administration of the vaccine involved and if—

"(A) in the case of measles, mumps, or rubella vaccine or any combination of such vaccines, the first seizure or convulsion occurred within 15 days after administration of the vaccine and 2 or more seizures or convulsions occurred within 1 year after the administration of the vaccine which were unaccompanied by fever or accompanied by a fever of less than 102 degrees Fahrenheit, and

"(B) in the case of any other vaccine, the first seizure or convulsion occurred within 3 days after administration of the vaccine and 2 or more seizures or convulsions occurred within 1 year after the administration of the vaccine which were unaccompanied by fever or accompanied by a fever of less than 102 degrees Fahrenheit.

"(3)(A) The term encephalopathy means any significant acquired abnormality of, or injury to, or impairment of function of the brain. Among the frequent manifestations of encephalopathy are focal and diffuse neurologic signs, increased intracranial pressure, or changes lasting at least 6 hours in level of consciousness, with or without convulsions. The neurological signs and symptoms of encephalopathy may be temporary, with complete recovery, or may result in various degrees of permanent impairment. Signs and symptoms such as high pitched and unusual screaming, persistent unconsolable crying, and bulging fontanel are compatible with an encephalopathy, but in and of themselves are not conclusive evidence of encephalopathy. Encephalopathy usually can be documented by slow wave activity on an electroencephalogram.

"(B) If in a proceeding on a petition it is shown by a preponderance of the evidence that an encephalopathy was caused by infection, toxins, trauma, or metabolic disturbances the encephalopathy shall not be considered to be a condition set forth in the table. If at the time a judgment is entered on a petition filed under section 2111(b) for a vaccine-related injury or death it is not possible to determine the cause, by a preponderance of the evidence, or an encephalopathy, the encephalopathy shall be considered to be a condition set forth in the table. In determining whether or not an encephalopathy is a condition set forth in the table, the court shall consider the entire-medical record.

"(4) For purposes of paragraphs (2) and (3), the terms "seizure" and "convulsion" include grand mal, petit mal, absence, myoclonic, tonic-clonic, and focal motor seizures and signs. If a provision of the table to which paragraph (1), (2), (3), or (4) applies is revised under subsection (c) or (d), such paragraph shall not apply to such provision after the effective date of the revision unless the revision specifies that such paragraph is to continue to apply."

Appendix IV

Diseases Transmitted by Animals

The transmission of diseases of animals to humans is of special interest in the care of children who may share a household with pets or unwanted rodents, or who are otherwise in contact with animals. Important zoonoses that may be encountered in North America and that are reviewed in the *Red Book* (see chapters on specific diseases in Section 3 for further information) are given in the table below. The emphasis in this table is given to primary modes of transmission involving animals. However, other modes of spread, including human-to-human, may occur. For a more complete listing of these diseases, see *The Zoonoses* (prepared jointly by the US Department of Health and Human Services, the US Public Health Service, the Centers for Disease Control and Prevention, the Centers for Infectious Diseases, and the Office of Biosafety, Atlanta, GA 30333; and the University of Texas, School of Public Health, Science Center, Houston, TX 77025). Additional resources are the following: Acha PM, Szyfres B. *Zoonoses and Communicable Diseases Common to Man and Animals*, Scientific Publication No 354, 1980, Pan American Health Organization, Pan American Sanitary Bureau, Regional Offices of the World Health Organization, 525 23rd Street, NW, Washington, DC 20037; and Chomel BB, Zoonose of house pets other than dogs, cats, and birds. *Pediatr Infect Dis.* 1992;11:479-487. Morbidity resulting from zoonotic diseases in the United States is reported annually by the Centers for Disease Control and Prevention (*Summary of Notifiable Diseases*).

Diseases Transmitted by Animals

Disease or Organism	Common Animal Sources	Vector or Means of Spread
Bacterial Diseases		
Borreliosis Lyme disease	Deer, rodents	Tick Bite
Relapsing fever	Wild rodents	Tick Bite
Brucellosis	Cattle, goats, sheep, swine, rarely dogs	Direct contact with birth products, ingestion of contaminated milk, inhalation of aerosols
Campylobacteriosis (*Campylobacter jejuni*)	Dogs, cats, ferrets, poultry	Direct contact, particularly with diarrheic animals, ingestion of contaminated food
*Capnocytophaga canimorsus**	Dogs, rarely cats	Bites, contact

*Formerly dysgonic fermenter-2 (DF-2).

Disease or Organism	Common Animal Sources	Vector or Means of Spread
Leptospirosis	Dogs, rats, livestock	Contact with urine, particularly in contaminated water
Mycobacteriosis (*Mycobacteria marinum*, others)	Fish, aquaria	Wound infection
Pasteurella multocida	Cats, infrequently dogs	Bites, scratches
Plague (*Yersinia pestis*)	Wild rabbits, rodents, fleas, rabbits, cats, dogs	Bite of rodent fleas, direct contact
Rat-bite fever (*Streptobacillus moniliformis*, *Spirillum minus*)	Rodents (particularly rats)	Bites
Salmonellosis	Poultry, dogs, cats, rodents, ferrets, turtles, reptiles, and other wild and domestic animals	Ingestion of contaminated food; direct contact
Tetanus	Any animal, usually indirect via soil	Wound infection, contaminated bites
Tularemia	Rabbits, squirrels	Direct contact, ingestion of contaminated water, bite of infected insect vector (eg, tick, deerfly), inhalation of aerosols
Yersiniosis	Rodents, swine; rarely dogs, cats	Direct contact, ingestion of contaminated food or water

Fungal Diseases

Disease or Organism	Common Animal Sources	Vector or Means of Spread
Cryptococcosis	Birds, particularly pigeons	Inhalation of aerosols from accumulations of pigeon feces
Histoplasmosis	Bats, birds, particularly starlings	Inhalation of aerosols from accumulations of bat and bird feces
Ringworm (*Microsporum* and *Trichophyton* species)	Cats, dogs, rabbits, rodents	Direct contact

Diseases Transmitted by Animals *(continued)*

Disease or Organism	Common Animal Sources	Vector or Means of Spread
Parasitic Diseases		
Anisakiasis	Saltwater and anadromous fish	Ingestion of raw or insufficiently cooked fish
Babesiosis	Wild rodents	Bite of tick
Cestoidiasis (*Hymenodepsis nana*)	Hamsters, rodents	Ingestion of eggs from feces (contaminated food, water)
Cryptosporidiosis	Domestic animals, particularly cattle	Ingestion of oocysts shed in feces
Cutaneous larva migrans (*Ancyclostoma brazilense*)	Dogs, cats	Contact with larvae, which develop in soil contaminated with eggs shed in feces and penetrate skin
Cysticercosis (*Taenia solium*)	Swine (intermediate host)	Ingestion of ova (fecal-oral contact or contaminated food, water)
Echinococcosis (Hydatid disease)	Dogs, foxes, possibly other carnivores	Ingestion of eggs shed in feces
Fish tapeworm (Diphyllobothriasis)	Saltwater and freshwater fish	Ingestion of raw or insufficiently cooked fish
Giardiasis	Wild animals, particularly beavers	Ingestion of cysts (fecal-oral contact or in contaminated food, water)
Toxoplasmosis	Cats, livestock	Ingestion of oocysts from infected cat feces, consumption of insufficiently cooked meat, contact with birth products of sheep, goats
Trichinosis	Swine, bears, possibly other wild carnivores	Ingestion of raw or insufficiently cooked meat
Visceral larva migrans (toxocariasis)	Dogs, cats	Ingestion of eggs, usually from soil contaminated by feces
Chlamydial and Rickettsial Diseases		
Cat scratch disease (*Rochalimea henselae*)	Cats, rarely dogs (<10%)	Scratches, bites

Disease or Organism	Common Animal Sources	Vector or Means of Spread
Ehrlichiosis (*Ehrlichea chaffeensis*)	Unknown	Tick bite
Psittacosis (*Chlamydia psittaci*)	Psittacine and domestic birds	Inhalation of aerosols from feces
Q fever (*Coxiella burnetii*)	Sheep, other livestock, wild rodents, rabbits	Direct contact and aerosols from birth products, ingestion of contaminated milk, occasionally tick bite
Rickettsialpox (*Rickettsia akari*)	House mouse	Mite bite
Rocky Mountain spotted fever	Dogs, wild rodents, rabbits	Tick bite
Typhus Endemic (*Rickettsia typhi*)	Rats, opossums	Flea bite
Epidemic (zoonotic) (*Rickettsia prowazekii*)	Flying squirrels	Contact with squirrels, their nests, or ectoparasites

Viral Diseases

Colorado tick fever	Wild rodents, particularly squirrels	Tick bite
Encephalitis		
California	Wild rodents	Mosquito bite
Eastern equine	Wild birds, poultry, horses	Mosquito bite
Western equine	Wild birds, poultry, horses	Mosquito bite
St Louis	Wild birds, poultry	Mosquito bite
Lymphocytic choriomeningitis	Rodents, particularly hamsters	Direct contact, inhalation of aerosols, ingestion of contaminated food
Rabies	Dogs, skunks, cats, raccoons, bats, foxes	Bites

Appendix V

Raw Milk*

Serious systemic infections due to *Salmonella* and *Campylobacter* have been attributed to the consumption of raw milk, including certified raw milk. The American Academy of Pediatrics strongly recommends that parents and public health officials be fully informed of the important risks inherent in the consumption of all raw milk, and endorses pasteurized milk.

---

*Interstate sale of raw milk is banned by the Food and Drug Administration.

Appendix VI

State Immunization Requirements for School Attendance

All states require immunization of children at the time of entry into licensed child care and entry into school. In addition, many states have regulations requiring immunization of older children in upper grades as well as those entering college. The best and most up-to-date information about which vaccines are required in a specific state and groups affected by regulation can be obtained from the immunization program manager of each state health department as well as from a number of local health departments.

The Centers for Disease Control and Prevention collects and publishes data on the current school entry laws, child care and Head Start immunization regulations, and college immunization requirements in effect in the various states. This survey of school laws is published yearly. Copies of the latest survey, "State Immunization Requirements for School Attendance," may be obtained by sending a request for single copies to the following: Centers for Disease Control and Prevention, National Immunization Program, Mailstop E-52, Atlanta, GA 30333.

Appendix VII

Nationally Notifiable Infectious Diseases in the United States

Reporting of specific diseases, which are listed below, is required in all states and territories. Additional and specific requirements should be obtained from the responsible state health department. A more complete listing of infectious diseases that are reportable to state health departments can be found in the following publication: Centers for Disease Control. Mandatory reporting of infectious diseases by clinicians. *MMWR*. 1990;39(RR-9):1-17.

Acquired immunodeficiency syndrome	Lymphogranuloma venereum
Amebiasis	Malaria
Anthrax	Measles (rubeola)
Botulism	Meningitis, aseptic
Brucellosis	Meningococcal infections
Chancroid	Mumps
Chickenpox	Pertussis
Cholera	Plague
Congenital rubella	Poliomyelitis
Congenital syphilis	Psittacosis
Diphtheria	Rabies, animal and human
Encephalitis	Rheumatic fever
Gonorrhea	Rocky Mountain spotted fever
Granuloma inguinale	Rubella
Haemophilus influenzae, type b infections (invasive)	*Salmonella* infections
	Shigella infections
Hepatitis A	Syphilis
Hepatitis B	Tetanus
Hepatitis non-A, non-B	Toxic shock syndrome
Hepatitis, unspecified	Trichinosis
Herpes zoster	Tuberculosis
Legionellosis	Tularemia
Leprosy	Typhoid fever
Leptospirosis	Typhus
Lyme disease	Yellow fever

In partnership with the Council of State and Territorial Epidemiologists (CSTE), the Centers for Disease Control and Prevention (CDC) operates the National Notifiable Diseases Surveillance System. The system provides weekly provisional information for reportable diseases. Cases of diseases reported by physicians to state epidemiologists are forwarded to CDC for publication in the *Morbidity and Mortality Weekly Report* (*MMWR*) and in the *Summary of Notifiable Diseases, United States*. Notifiable disease surveillance data are used by public health officials at the local, state, and federal levels as part of disease prevention and control activities.

Appendix VIII

Services of the Centers for Disease Control and Prevention (CDC)

The Centers for Disease Control and Prevention (US Public Health Service, Department of Health and Human Services, Atlanta, Georgia) is the federal agency charged with protecting the public health of the nation by preventing disease and other disabling conditions. The CDC administers national programs for the prevention and control of (1) infectious diseases, (2) occupational diseases and injury, (3) chronic diseases, and (4) environment-related injury and illness. The CDC also provides consultation to other nations and participates with international agencies in the control of preventable diseases. In addition, the CDC directs and enforces foreign quarantine activities and regulations, and it provides consultation and assistance in upgrading the performance of clinical laboratories.

The CDC provides a number of services related to infectious disease management and control. Although the CDC is principally a resource for state and local health departments, it also offers direct and indirect services to hospitals and practicing physicians. The range of services includes reference laboratory diagnosis and epidemiologic consultation, both usually arranged through the state health department. In addition, the CDC Drug Service supplies some specific prophylactic or therapeutic drugs and biologic agents.

Specific immunobiologic products available include botulinal equine (trivalent, ABE) antitoxin, diphtheria equine antitoxin, vaccinia immune globulin (VIG), botulinus pentavalent toxoid, and western equine encephalomyelitis (WEE) immune globulin.

Additionally, several drugs for the treatment of parasitic disease, which are not currently licensed for use in the United States, are handled under the Investigational New Drug (IND) permit. These antiparasitic drugs include suramin, nifurtimox, bithionol, dehydroemetine, diloxanide furoate (furamide), ivermectin, melarsoprol, quinine (for parenteral use), and stibogluconate sodium.

Requests for biologic products, antiparasitic drugs, and related information should be directed to the CDC Drug Service (see Directory of Telephone Numbers, p 601).

INDEX

Page numbers in boldface indicate a main discussion.
Page numbers followed by a "*t*" indicate a table.

in American trypanosomiasis, 479
in arboviruses, 123
in babesiosis, 133
in cytomegalovirus infection, 177
in hepatitis A, 222
in hepatitis B, 225, 233, 237
in hepatitis C, 239
in hepatitis delta virus, 240
in HIV infection, 257, 268, 269
in infectious mononucleosis, 274
in Lyme disease, 300
in malaria, 302
in parvovirus B19 infections, 346
in rat-bite fever, 395-396
in Rocky Mountain spotted
  fever, 402
in *Toxoplasma gondii* infections, 471
Blood donation as contraindicated
in African trypanosomiasis, 478
in American trypanosomiasis, 480
in infectious mononucleosis, 275
in Lyme disease, 300
Blurred vision, in *Clostridium botulinum,*
160
Body fluids. *See also* Blood and blood
products
and hepatitis B, 225
and HIV infection, 268
Bolivian hemorrhagic fever, 217-218
Bone marrow transplantation, 44
Bordetella parapertussis, 355
Bordetella pertussis, 355
antimicrobial prophylaxis for, 522*t*
transmission of, in out-of-home child
  care, 84
Borrelia burgdorferi, 142, 297, 298
Borrelia hermsii, 141
Borrelia parkeri, 141
Borrelia recurrentis, 141
Borrelia (relapsing fever), **141-142**
clinical manifestations, 141
control measures, 142
diagnostic tests, 142
epidemiology, 141, 618*t*
etiology, 141
isolation of hospitalized patient, 142
treatment, 142
Borrelia turicatae, 141
Borreliosis. *See* Lyme disease
Botulism (*Clostridium botulinum*),
160-162
clinical manifestations, 160
control measures, 162, 624*t*
diagnostic tests, 161
epidemiology, 160
food-borne, 161
infant, 160
isolation of hospitalized patient, 161

treatment, 161
wound, 160, 161
Boutonneuse fever, *Rickettsia conorii* as
etiologic agent of, 400
Bradycardia
in bunyavirus infections, 219
in *Malassezia furfur* invasive
  infections, 307
Brain damage
in cytomegalovirus infection, 173
from pertussis vaccination, 363-364,
  365-366
Branhamella catarrhalis, 328
Breast-feeding
benefits of, 73
and hepatitis B, 236
and herpes simplex virus infection,
  248
and HIV infection, 269
and poliovirus infection vaccine, 19,
  382
and rotavirus infections, 405
and tuberculosis, 491
Brill-Zinsser disease (relapsing epidemic
typhus), 508
Bronchiectasis, in paragonimiasis, 340
Bronchiolitis
in adenovirus infections, 116
in parainfluenza virus infections, 341
in respiratory syncytial virus
  infections, 396
Bronchitis
in influenza, 276
in *Pasteurella multocida* infections,
  348
in rhinovirus infections, 398
in respiratory syncytial virus
  infections, 396
Bronchopneumonia, in measles, 308
Bronchopulmonary dysplasia, and
influenza, 276
Bronchoscopy, and alpha-hemolytic
(viridans) streptococci following dental
procedures, 528
Bronchospasm, in *Chlamydia
pneumoniae,* 152
Brucella abortus, 143
Brucella canis, 143
Brucella melitensis, 143
Brucella suis, 143
Brucellosis, **143-144**
clinical manifestations, 143
control measures, 144, 624*t*
diagnostic tests, 143-144
epidemiology, 143, 618*t*
etiology, 143
isolation of hospitalized patient, 144
treatment, 144

Human bites
in *Bacteroides* infections, 137
chemoprophylaxis of, 523
and hepatitis B transmission, 88
Human diploid cell vaccine (HDCV)
for rabies, 25, 392
adverse reactions and precautions
with, 392-393
Human herpesvirus 6 infections,
272-273
clinical manifestations, 272
control measures, 273
diagnostic tests, 273
epidemiology, 272-273
isolation of hospitalized
patient, 273
treatment, 273
Human immunodeficiency virus DNA,
258
Human immunodeficiency virus (HIV).
See HIV infection and AIDS
Human immunodeficiency virus
type 1, 257
Human milk, **73-79**
antimicrobial agents in, 76-79,
77*t*, 78*t*
and immunization of mothers
and infants, 73-74
transmission of
cytomegalovirus infection in, 177
infectious agents, 74-76
Human papillomavirus (HPV) infections,
338. *See also* Papillomaviruses
and sexual abuse, 110
Human plasma, 46
Human T-cell leukemia virus type 1
(HTLV-1) transmission of, via human
milk, 75
Hydatid disease, 457, 458, 620*t*
Hydrocephalus
in coccidioidomycosis, 167
in lymphocytic choriomeningitis, 300
in *Toxoplasma gondii* infections, 471
Hydroxocobalamin, for tapeworm
infections, 457
Hymenolepis nana, **457**
Hyperbaric oxygen, for clostridial
myonecrosis, 165
Hypereosinophilia, in toxocariasis,
470
Hypergammaglobulinemia, in
toxocariasis, 469, 470
Hyperglycemia, in *Pneumocystis carinii*
infections, 377
Hypersensitivity reactions to vaccine
constituents, 36-38
Hypogammaglobulinemia, in chronic
lymphocytic leukemia, 44

Hypoglycemia
in cholera, 157
in *Pneumocystis carinii*
infections, 377
Hypokalemia, in cholera, 157
Hyponatremia, in ehrlichiosis, 182
Hypoproteinemia, in hookworm
infections, 270
Hypotension
in bunyaviruses, 219
in clostridial myonecrosis, 164
in *Pneumocystis carinii* infections,
377
in staphylococcal toxic shock
syndrome, 428
Hypotonia, in botulism, 160
Hypovolemic shock, in cholera, 157

I

Idiopathic thrombocytopenia purpura,
and administration of immune
globulin, 40
IG. *See* Immune globulin
IGIV. *See* Intravenous immune globulin
(IGIV)
Ileitis, in *Yersinia* infections, 519
Illness, management and prevention
of, in out-of-home child care, 80-81,
82*t*
Imipenem-cilastatin, dose of, for pediatric
patients, 550*t*
for *Bacillus cereus* infections, 135
for *Bacteroides* infections, 138
Immigrants and refugees
American trypanosomiasis in, 479
hepatitis B in, 225
hepatitis delta virus in, 240
immunizations for, 66-67
leprosy in, 292
parasitic diseases in, 342
tuberculosis in, 481
Immune globulin (IG), **40-51**
active immunization of persons
who recently received, 28
adverse reactions to, 42-43
and exposure to measles, 60-61
for exposure to rubella, 408
for hepatitis A, 223
for hepatitis B, 228
indications for use of, 41, 43-45
indications for use of intravenous,
43-45
for measles, 311
and measles vaccine, 318, 320
and mumps, 332
nonproven uses of, 41-42
precautions in use of, 42